AAOS

AMERICAN ACADEMY OF ORTHOPAEDIC SURGEONS

Nancy Caroline's

Emergency Care in the Streets

Author: Bob Elling, MPA, EMT-P

Student Workbook

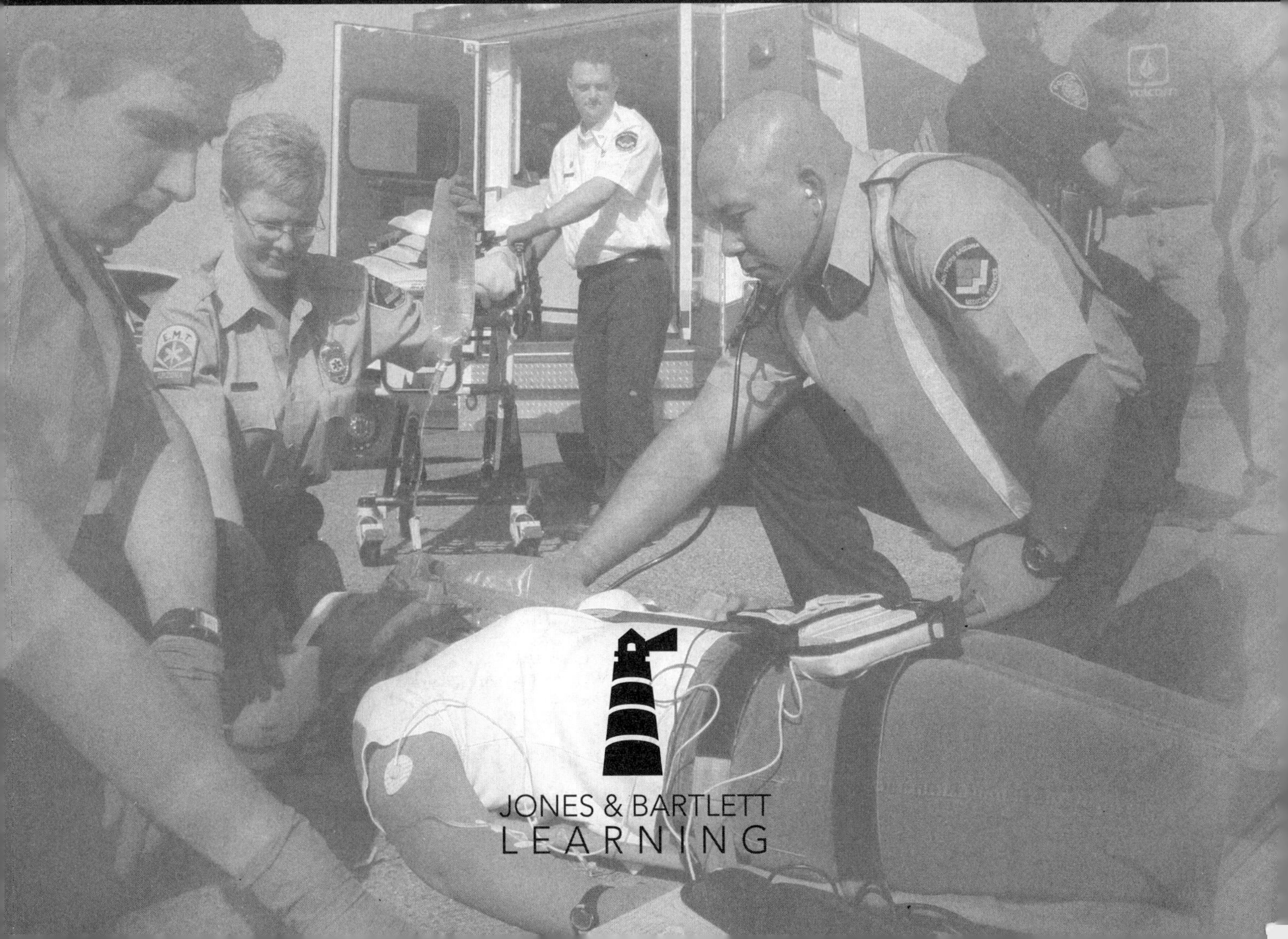

JONES & BARTLETT LEARNING

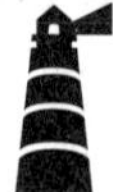

World Headquarters
Jones & Bartlett Learning
5 Wall Street
Burlington, MA 01803
978-443-5000
info@jblearning.com
www.jblearning.com

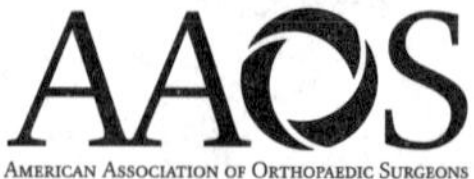

Substantial discounts on bulk quantities of Jones & Bartlett Learning publications are available to corporations, professional associations, and other qualified organizations. For details and specific discount information, contact the special sales department at Jones & Bartlett Learning via the above contact information or send an email to specialsales@jblearning.com.

Jones & Bartlett Learning books and products are available through most bookstores and online booksellers. To contact Jones & Bartlett Learning directly, call 800-832-0034, fax 978-443-8000, or visit our website, www.jblearning.com.

14225-9

Production Credits
General Manager and Executive Publisher: Kimberly Brophy
VP, Product Development: Christine Emerton
Senior Acquisitions Editor: Tiffany Sliter
Senior Editor: Carol B. Guerrero
Editorial Assistant: Jessica Sturtevant
Editorial Assistant: Ashley Procum
Vendor Manager: Nora Menzi
VP, Sales, Public Safety Group: Matthew Maniscalco
Director of Sales, Public Safety Group: Patricia Einstein
Director of Marketing Operations: Brian Rooney
VP, Manufacturing and Inventory Control: Therese Connell
Composition and Project Management: S4Carlisle Publishing Services
Cover Design: Kristin E. Parker
Rights & Media Specialist: Robert Boder
Media Development Editor: Troy Liston
(Title Page, Part Opener, Chapter Opener): © Jones & Bartlett Learning. Courtesy of MIEMSS. Background: © Photos.com/Getty
Printing and Binding: Edwards Brothers Malloy
Cover Printing: Edwards Brothers Malloy

6048

Printed in the United States of America
21 20 19 18 17 10 9 8 7 6 5 4 3 2 1

Contents

CHAPTER 1

EMS Systems

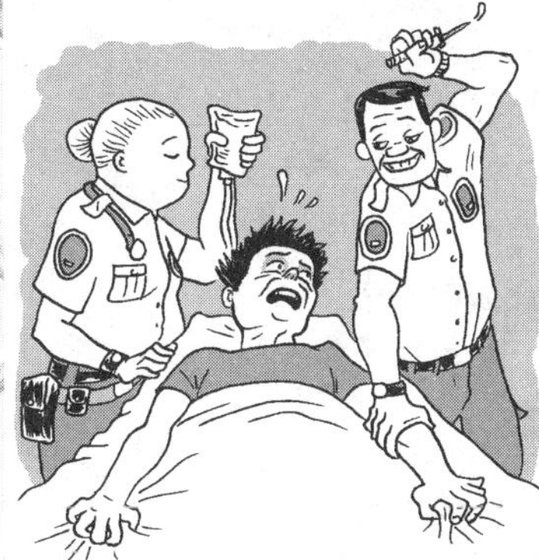

Try seeing it from the patient's point of view.

Matching

Match each of the definitions in the left column to the appropriate term in the right column.

______	**1.** Outlined measures that may be difficult to obtain in a research project.	**A.** Systematic sampling
______	**2.** A research format that uses a hypothesis to prove one finding from another.	**B.** Reciprocity
______	**3.** A computer-generated list of subjects or groups for research.	**C.** Parameters
______	**4.** A type of study in which the subjects are advised of all aspects of the study.	**D.** Inferential
______	**5.** A process in which a person, an institution, or a program is evaluated and recognized as meeting certain predetermined standards to provide safe and ethical care.	**E.** Evidence-based practice
______	**6.** The process of granting licensure or certification to a provider from another state or agency.	**F.** Unblinded study
______	**7.** Time parameters set during a research project.	**G.** Certification
______	**8.** The process used by medical magazines, journals, and other publications to ensure the quality and validity of an article before publishing it; it involves sending the article to subject matter experts for review of the content and research methods.	**H.** Peer review
______	**9.** The use of practices that have been proven to be effective in improving patient outcomes.	**I.** Online (direct) medical control
______	**10.** Medical direction given in real time to an EMS service or provider.	**J.** Alternative time sampling

Multiple Choice

Read each item carefully, and then select the best response.

______ **1.** In which year did the National Academy of Science and the National Research Council release the white paper entitled "Accidental Death and Disability: The Neglected Disease of Modern Society"?

- **A.** 1965
- **B.** 1967
- **C.** 1968
- **D.** 1969

______ **2.** Which of the following was NOT an emergency medical services (EMS) system element during the 1980s and 1990s?

- **A.** Resource management
- **B.** Public information and education
- **C.** Decrease in number of providers
- **D.** Medical direction

______ **3.** What does EMR stand for?
- **A.** Emergency medical reaction
- **B.** Emergency medical receiver
- **C.** Emergency management response
- **D.** Emergency medical responder

______ **4.** Which of the following may involve radio or electronic communications during patient care?
- **A.** Off-line medical control
- **B.** Online medical control
- **C.** Protocols
- **D.** Standing orders

______ **5.** Which type of research is considered a basic observation only, may involve interviews with subjects, and specifies that no alterations occur?
- **A.** Experimental
- **B.** Descriptive
- **C.** Cross-sectional
- **D.** Qualitative

______ **6.** Attributes of professionalism, as a paramedic, include all of the following, EXCEPT:
- **A.** communication.
- **B.** patient advocacy.
- **C.** empathy.
- **D.** reciprocity.

______ **7.** Which of the following is considered a high-risk activity from a continuous quality improvement point of view?
- **A.** Taking vital signs
- **B.** Intravenous therapy
- **C.** Handing off patients
- **D.** Basic airway management

______ **8.** Who is considered the father of paramedicine?
- **A.** Dr. David Boyd
- **B.** Dr. Eugene Nagel
- **C.** Dr. Jean Larrey
- **D.** Dr. Peter Safar

______ **9.** Who is usually the first EMS professional with whom the public deals?
- **A.** EMT
- **B.** Law enforcement officer
- **C.** Dispatcher
- **D.** Paramedic

______ **10.** Which level of EMS was changed to Advanced EMT in the most recent National EMS Education Standards?
- **A.** EMR
- **B.** EMT
- **C.** EMT-Intermediate
- **D.** Paramedic

______ **11.** Which of the following is NOT considered a traditional EMS employment career for paramedics?
- **A.** Fire-based EMS
- **B.** Third-service EMS
- **C.** Emergency department technicians
- **D.** Private EMS agency

_____ **12.** In a community where the municipality operates the EMS agency, and it is not part of a public safety entity, this is referred to as:
- **A.** hospital-based EMS.
- **B.** a hybrid system.
- **C.** fire-based EMS.
- **D.** third-service EMS.

_____ **13.** When a paramedic is employed to work with a physician or other primary care provider to provide specific services to the physician's patients, this is referred to as:
- **A.** a municipal EMS system.
- **B.** a hybrid system.
- **C.** hospital-based EMS.
- **D.** a private EMS agency.

Fill in the Blank

Read each item carefully, and then complete the statement by filling in the missing word(s).

1. In the late 1950s and early 1960s, the __________ __________ __________ __________ were staffed by specially trained physicians.
2. The __________ receives and enters all information on the call, interprets the information, and relays it to the appropriate resources.
3. When a state grants certification (or licensure) to a provider from another state, it is known as __________.
4. The paramedic who can demonstrate to the patient, the patient's family members, and other health care providers the ability to identify and understand their feelings is showing __________.
5. During scene management, ensuring your own safety and the safety of your crew is your __________ __________.
6. The tool often used to continually evaluate your care is called __________ __________ __________.
7. __________ research is based on a clearly defined problem or question and gathers information as events occur in real time.

Ambulance Calls

The following case scenarios provide an opportunity to explore the concerns associated with patient management and paramedic care. Read each scenario, and then answer each question.

1. You are exiting a theater after watching a movie, when suddenly the woman in front of you falls down on the carpeted floor, landing on her knees and hands. She apparently has tripped in the dark on the steps. As you try to help her to a seated position, you find that she is not responding to you as she should. She says she feels very faint, so you lower her back to the ground. She then loses consciousness, and you lower her all the way to a supine position and make sure that her airway is open and that she is breathing. You ask your spouse to call 9-1-1 on her cell phone and to find management to bring up the theater lights and get the nearest automated external defibrillator (AED). Your patient is a 60-year-old woman who wakes up and says she is fine and doesn't want anyone making a fuss over her. She just wants to go home.
   a. Which information should you give your spouse to tell the dispatcher?

   ____

   ____

   ____

b. What are some reasons this patient should go to the hospital to get checked out?

____

____

____

2. Wow, what an evening at the theater! After your patient has left in an ambulance, you head out the door to go home. Just as you are getting into your vehicle, you hear a woman scream. It seems she has been hit by a small pickup truck that was backing up to get a good parking spot. You hurry over to find a 40-year-old woman who is conscious and alert. She is sprawled out on the ground. She is screaming about her left leg, which is where the bumper of the pickup impacted her. She was knocked to the pavement. The driver of the pickup stopped when he heard the impact and then pulled forward, which caused no more injury to the woman. She has an obvious deformity at midthigh on the left leg. An emergency medical technician (EMT) comes running to help because several people have already called 9-1-1. Because you are first on scene and the more highly trained responder, you take charge of this patient.

a. What is the first thing you should do on this scene?

____

____

____

b. Which steps should you take in treating this patient before the ambulance arrives?

____

____

____

True/False

If you believe the statement to be more true than false, write the letter "T" in the space provided. If you believe the statement to be more false than true, write the letter "F."

_____ **1.** The *first* documented ambulance service was started in 1869 in New York City out of Bellevue Hospital.

_____ **2.** "The White Paper" provided authority and financial support for the development of basic and advanced life support services.

_____ **3.** An emergency medical dispatcher can give simple medical instructions to the caller.

_____ **4.** The primary and backbone level of employment in the traditional EMS system is the EMR.

_____ **5.** In EMS, paramedics constitute the greatest number of trained and certified individuals in the field.

_____ **6.** The first priority at the scene is assessment of the patient.

_____ **7.** Peer review is used as a means of continuous quality improvement.

_____ **8.** Retrospective research uses available data from medical records or patient care reports (PCRs).

_____ **9.** Only the emergency vehicle operator is responsible for restocking the unit after a call.

_____ **10.** Injury prevention in the home is a topic the paramedic should be comfortable discussing with patients and bystanders.

Short Answer

Complete this section with short written answers using the space provided.

1. Pretend you are a fly on the wall during this scene: A team of paramedics arrives on scene for a routine geriatric call. The woman fell and has a broken hip. Her daughter found her and called 9-1-1. List the professional attributes the paramedics should demonstrate on this and every call.

   a. ______________________________

   b. ______________________________

   c. ______________________________

   d. ______________________________

   e. ______________________________

   f. ______________________________

   g. ______________________________

   h. ______________________________

   i. ______________________________

   j. ______________________________

   k. ______________________________

2. Paramedics follow an important sequence of procedures for every emergency call. List the eight procedures.

   a. ______________________________

   b. ______________________________

   c. ______________________________

   d. ______________________________

   e. ______________________________

   f. ______________________________

   g. ______________________________

   h. ______________________________

3. No paramedic service in the United States can perform advanced life support procedures without medical direction. What is medical direction, and why is it necessary?

   ____

   ____

   ____

4. Medical control consists of several different parts. Give an example of each of the following:

a. Online medical control: ______________________________

b. Protocols: ______________________________

c. Standing orders: ______________________________

CHAPTER 2

Workforce Safety and Wellness

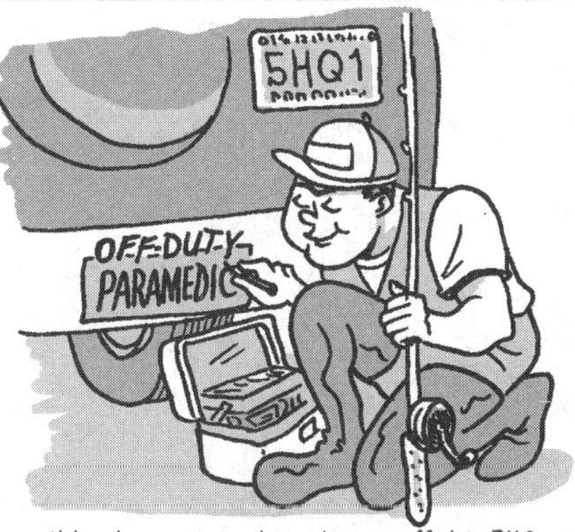

© Jones & Bartlett Learning.

Although some states do require even off-duty EMS providers to stop at the scene of an accident, this law can vary from state to state. Make sure you know the laws in your area.

Matching

Part I

Stress is a major part of a paramedic's job. Indicate which of the following two types of stress you are more likely to experience in the following scenarios.

A. Eustress B. Distress

______ **1.** You are running a 10-km road race with your best friend. You have been training to beat her, and she is about 15 steps in front of you.

______ **2.** You respond to a rollover collision and find out that the unrestrained driver of the vehicle is your 17-year-old daughter.

______ **3.** You are assigned to work with Billy Bob for the next month. Billy Bob is not your favorite person and is always criticizing every move you make.

______ **4.** You are taking your National Registry Paramedic exam next week, and you are studying in hopes of passing the test with an excellent grade the first time you take it.

______ **5.** You find out the ambulance service that you work for is merging with a larger service. There is talk that your position will be eliminated.

______ **6.** You are climbing Pikes Peak, and you are about to make the summit (your lifelong dream), but you don't feel that you have enough energy left to climb the last 500 feet.

______ **7.** Your spouse has just left a letter explaining to you that he/she is divorcing you and that he/she has already cleaned out the bank accounts.

Part II

Match each psychological defense mechanism with the situation in which it is most likely to be used.

A. Projection **B.** Denial **C.** Regression

______ **1.** Your patient is ignoring the symptoms he has been having over the past few days.

______ **2.** Your school-aged patient is upset by her injuries and seems to be acting like a toddler.

______ **3.** Your patient seems to be blaming his symptoms on the bad behaviors of his family members.

Part III

Match each of the definitions in the left column to the appropriate term in the right column.

	Definition	Term
______	**1.** A fear reaction in which a person's judgment seems to disappear entirely; it is particularly dangerous because it may precipitate mass panic among others.	**A.** Defense mechanism
______	**2.** Pathogenic microorganisms that are present in human blood and can cause disease in humans; they include, but are not limited to, hepatitis B virus and human immunodeficiency virus.	**B.** Transmission
______	**3.** Any disease that can be spread from person to person or from animal to person.	**C.** Denial
______	**4.** An event that overwhelms a person's ability to cope with the experience, either at the scene or later.	**D.** Blind panic
______	**5.** Psychological ways to relieve stress; they are usually automatic or subconscious (eg, denial, regression, projection, and displacement).	**E.** Standard precautions
______	**6.** An early response to a serious medical emergency in which the severity of the emergency is diminished or minimized.	**F.** Bloodborne pathogens
______	**7.** Exposure to, or transmission of, a communicable disease from one person to another by physical contact.	**G.** Direct contact
______	**8.** A disease that is caused by the growth and spread of small harmful organisms within the body or one that is capable of being transmitted with or without direct contact.	**H.** Communicable disease
______	**9.** Protective measures that have traditionally been developed by the Centers for Disease Control and Prevention for use in dealing with objects, blood, body fluids, or other potential exposure risks of communicable disease.	**I.** Infectious disease
______	**10.** The way in which an infectious agent is spread: contact, airborne, foodborne, or by vectors.	**J.** Critical incident

Multiple Choice

Read each item carefully, and then select the best response.

______ **1.** You respond to a 12-year-old boy who has been hit by a car. He is alert but has a deformity of his lower left leg. The boy "baby talks" as he is answering your questions. This is a form of:

- **A.** denial.
- **B.** projection.
- **C.** regression.
- **D.** displacement.

______ **2.** You respond to a multiple-casualty incident (MCI) involving a collision of a charter bus of senior citizens and a car with four teenagers. At the scene, you find one teen with no obvious injuries. You have to tell him numerous times to sit on the side of the road and stay away from the moving traffic. His judgment seems impaired, and he may be experiencing:

- **A.** conversion hysteria.
- **B.** projection.
- **C.** depression.
- **D.** blind panic.

______ **3.** Which of the following would NOT be a symptom of impending paramedic burnout?

- **A.** Increased interest in hobbies
- **B.** Chronic fatigue and irritability
- **C.** Cynical, negative attitude
- **D.** Decreasing ability to concentrate

_____ **4.** As a result of your partner's careless behavior, you have been stuck by a needle that was used to start an IV on your patient. Which of the following should be done immediately?

A. Get a medical evaluation from the emergency department physician.
B. Document the negligence of your partner.
C. Wash the area of the exposure with soap and water.
D. Get a booster shot for all of your immunizations.

_____ **5.** According to the Centers for Disease Control and Prevention, when should you wear an N95 or N100 respirator?

A. Between patient contacts
B. When working with a patient who has tuberculosis
C. When touching mucous membranes
D. When dealing with blood or body fluids

_____ **6.** You are on your first "code." As you arrive on scene, you feel stressed. Which of the following management techniques would NOT help you during this call?

A. Focusing on the immediate situation
B. Controlled deep breathing
C. Progressive relaxation
D. Regression

_____ **7.** You are on the scene of a major car crash. Your patient is an elderly man who has now accepted the fact that he is really hurt and could be in the hospital for a long time. Which of the following reactions might the patient experience?

A. Depression
B. Fear
C. Anger
D. All of the above

_____ **8.** At a vehicle collision, you believe that you have everyone accounted for and managed. Suddenly you hear a baby crying and realize there is a child whom you have not found yet. Your heart begins to race; this is an example of a(n):

A. delayed reaction.
B. alert response.
C. defense mechanism.
D. fight-or-flight response.

_____ **9.** After being told she might be having a heart attack, a 66-year-old female patient hits the paramedic in anger and tells him that he doesn't know what he is talking about. Which defense mechanism is associated with this kind of reaction?

A. Displacement
B. Projection
C. Alarm reaction
D. Denial

_____ **10.** A paramedic who has been on duty for 6 months of double shifts (without a personal day) begins to show signs of physical and emotional breakdown. He is cynical and doesn't seem to be able to sleep. These are signs of:

A. eustress.
B. burnout.
C. anxiety.
D. alert response.

Fill in the Blank

Read each item carefully, and then complete the statement by filling in the missing word(s).

1. The following paragraphs describe behaviors of different individuals under stress. For each description, fill in the defense mechanism that the individual is apparently using.
   - **a.** Your partner has been irritable and ill-tempered ever since he arrived at work today. You are doing your best to keep a low profile and not annoy him further, but nonetheless he snaps at you, "You sure are in a lousy mood today." Your partner is showing the mechanism of defense known as __________.
   - **b.** You are called by a very distraught woman to treat her husband, who has been having chest pain. When you reach the patient's house, he says, "I can't understand why my wife called for an ambulance; I'm just having a little indigestion, that's all." His face is gray, and he is sweating profusely. He is using the psychological defense mechanism known as __________.
   - **c.** A 22-year-old woman is extricated from a wrecked automobile in which her boyfriend remains trapped. She says she has lost all sensation in her hands and feet. She does not appear terribly upset about that fact, and you cannot find any signs of injury on her body. She is using the psychological defense mechanism known as __________.
   - **d.** At the scene of a car crash, you are trying to extricate an entrapped front-seat passenger who is seriously injured. The driver, who has not suffered any apparent injury, is giving you a hard time. "Be careful, will you! Don't drop her! Watch what you're doing, you damn idiot!" He is very aggressive toward you, but you realize that his behavior is simply a(n) __________ of the anger he feels toward himself for having caused the injury to his passenger.

2. Being a paramedic is a stressful job. For some, the stresses are too much, and burnout can occur. The time to start thinking about burnout—and how to prevent it—is now, during your training. Develop strategies that will keep burnout from happening to you by listing some of the steps you plan to take to keep from burning out as a paramedic.
   - **a.** ______________________________
   - **b.** ______________________________
   - **c.** ______________________________
   - **d.** ______________________________
   - **e.** ______________________________
   - **f.** ______________________________
   - **g.** ______________________________
   - **h.** ______________________________

Identify

In the following case study, list the six pertinent negatives with regard to the well-being of your partner, Tommy Jones. Also, identify two stress reactions of the patient.

It is midnight, and Tommy Jones is still awake, watching a horror movie on TV and drinking his last soda out of the six-pack that he brought to work today. You are both on a 24-hour shift, and he has just been lying around the TV room when he was not out on calls. He skipped his workout today so that he could watch his favorite soap opera. He is bummed out that he is out of cigarettes and is searching the kitchen for yet another bag of popcorn when the tones go off, indicating another call.

As you head from the bunk room to the ambulance, Tommy is yelling that it is all your fault there is another call. "If you hadn't gone to bed, we wouldn't have had another call tonight," he grumbles.

You arrive at the scene to find a 72-year-old woman who has fallen and fractured her hip. As you begin your treatment, the patient begins to blame you for all of her problems. As you load her into the ambulance, the patient reaches out and pinches your arm as hard as she can.

After you deliver your patient to the hospital, Tommy stops to grab another pack of smokes and a bean burrito. As you pull into the bay, Tommy tells you to restock because he wants to watch the end of the movie. As he heads into the TV room, he tells you that his stomach is killing him and that he might be your next patient.

1. Pertinent negatives

   a. ______________________________

   b. ______________________________

   c. ______________________________

   d. ______________________________

   e. ______________________________

   f. ______________________________

2. Stress reactions

   a. ______________________________

   b. ______________________________

Ambulance Calls

The following case scenarios provide an opportunity to explore the concerns associated with patient management and paramedic care. Read each scenario, and then answer each question.

1. Your unit responds to a call for a 3-month-old boy who is not breathing. When you enter the house, you find a mother holding the boy, who is not breathing and is very pale. You and your partner, John, begin working the code. You start the steps of cardiopulmonary resuscitation (CPR), with compressions, while gathering as much information as possible about what has happened. As you arrive at the hospital with the infant, you know in your heart that the child is dead. The code team works further on the child, and finally, the doctor calls for the time of death. John storms out of the room and out to the ambulance to begin cleanup. John begins to yell about the fact that the child died and how if he hadn't missed the first IV on the child, he might still be alive. You finish your patient care report (PCR) and then head back to the station. At the station, John refuses to talk about the call and says he wants to be alone. He ends up sitting at the table just staring off into space for the rest of the afternoon. At the next shift, John is very negative and flies off the handle at everyone that day. After the shift is over, John heads for the local bar instead of going home to his wife and his 2-month-old son. Two weeks later, John is put on mandatory leave for his mental well-being.

   a. Explain how this one incident could have triggered John's decline.

   ____

   ____

   ____

   b. What are some steps that every paramedic can take to reduce stress on the job?

   ____

   ____

   ____

2. A call comes in for a motor vehicle crash involving a small car and a pickup truck. It was a head-on collision, with both vehicles going 60 mi/h. Your patient is a 56-year-old man. He was not wearing his seat belt when the crash occurred. He has multiple breaks of both arms and legs. He has a large cut on his forehead that is bleeding profusely. You begin your trauma assessment on him after doing a rapid extrication with a long backboard. In the back of the ambulance, you begin treatment by applying oxygen and starting two large-bore IVs en route to the hospital. The patient is alert and is able to respond to you correctly. His blood pressure is 78/40 mm Hg, and respirations are 32 breaths/min and

shallow. His skin is cool and clammy, and you have no pulses in the wrists or the feet. The cardiac monitor is showing sinus tachycardia with multifocal premature ventricular complexes (PVCs) that are becoming very frequent. You don't hear good lung sounds, and you prepare for needle decompression of the right chest. You know that this patient is approaching death and will more than likely turn into a trauma code.

a. Your patient looks up at you and asks, "Am I going to die?" How do you respond to him?

____

____

____

b. What are the five stages that you might witness in this patient, and how will the patient act during these stages?

(1)____

(2)____

(3)____

(4)____

(5)____

True/False

If you believe the statement to be more true than false, write the letter "T" in the space provided. If you believe the statement to be more false than true, write the letter "F."

_____ **1.** The USDA 2015 dietary guidelines contain five different food groups.

_____ **2.** You should avoid caffeine and keep a regular sleep schedule.

_____ **3.** When lifting, you should use your back, so you don't injure your knees.

_____ **4.** Indirect contact involves the spread of infection between the patient with an infection to another person through a contaminated inanimate object.

_____ **5.** You should sanitize your stethoscope with alcohol or disinfectant wipes.

_____ **6.** Anger is a defense mechanism.

_____ **7.** Blind panic is present when a patient converts anxiety to a bodily dysfunction, such as a paralyzed extremity.

_____ **8.** Burnout is a consequence of chronic, unrelieved stress.

_____ **9.** The stages of the grieving process, in order, are denial, anger, bargaining, depression, and acceptance.

_____ **10.** Gloves are absolutely essential on every emergency medical services (EMS) call.

_____ **11.** Gloves are the only personal protective equipment (PPE) needed when suctioning a patient.

_____ **12.** A mask worn by you can protect the patient from your germs.

_____ **13.** Your maximum heart rate during exercise should be 320 minus your age.

_____ **14.** The redirecting of one's emotions from the original source to the paramedic is known as displacement.

Short Answer

Complete this section with short written answers using the space provided.

1. When faced with a perceived threat, the body reacts with a fight-or-flight response. From your own experience, list four signs or symptoms of the fight-or-flight response.

   a. ______________________________

   b. ______________________________

   c. ______________________________

   d. ______________________________

2. At times, you are the person who will be dealing with a grieving family. List the six guidelines for helping the family begin the process of coping with their loss.

   a. ______________________________

   b. ______________________________

   c. ______________________________

   d. ______________________________

   e. ______________________________

   f. ______________________________

3. In general, people who have any of five types of reactions to mass casualties should be removed from the scene. These five types of reactions are:

   a. ______________________________

   b. ______________________________

   c. ______________________________

   d. ______________________________

   e. ______________________________

Problem Solving

Calculate the maximum heart rate and target heart rate for a person with a resting heart rate of 76 beats/min and an age of 46 years.

1. a. Resting heart rate __________

   b. 220 – __________ (age in years) = __________ (Maximum heart rate)

   c. __________ (Maximum heart rate) – __________ (Resting heart rate) = __________ × 0.7 = __________ (round up)

   d. __________ (Total) + __________ (Resting heart rate) = __________ (Target heart rate)

Public Health

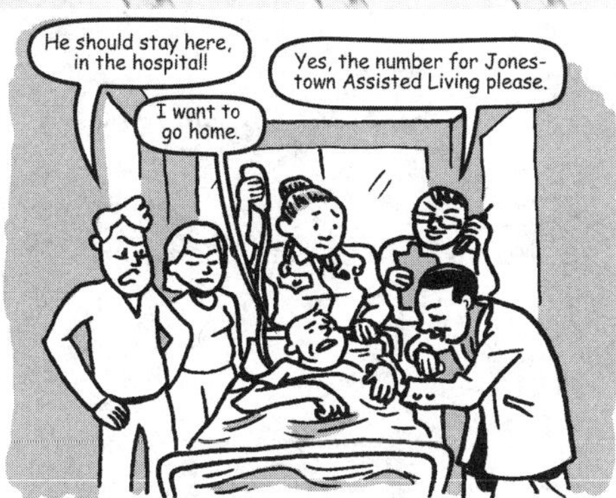

As a paramedic, you will encounter ethical dilemmas on an almost daily basis. It is best to work through these issues as they arise by communicating calmly and directly with everyone involved.

Matching

Part I

Match each of the definitions in the left column to the appropriate term in the right column.

	Definition	Term
______	**1.** A way of measuring and comparing the overall impact of deaths resulting from different causes; calculated based on a fixed age minus the age at death.	**A.** Epidemiology
______	**2.** Injuries that occur without intent to harm (commonly called accidents); examples are motor vehicle crashes, poisonings, drownings, falls, and most burns.	**B.** Evaluation
______	**3.** Monitoring and comparing the current number and nature of medical cases against the expected volume of these cases at a given time and place in the community.	**C.** Intentional injuries
______	**4.** The ongoing systematic collection, analysis, and interpretation of injury data essential to the planning, implementation, and evaluation of public health practice.	**D.** Interventions
______	**5.** Reducing the effects of an injury or illness that has already happened.	**E.** Morbidity
______	**6.** Deaths caused by injury and disease usually expressed as a rate; the number of deaths in a certain population in a given time period divided by the size of the population.	**F.** Mortality
______	**7.** Number of nonfatally injured or disabled people, usually expressed as a rate; the number of nonfatal injuries in a certain population in a given time period divided by the size of the population.	**G.** Passive interventions
______	**8.** In the context of prevention, specific measures or activities designed to meet a program objective; categories include education/behavior change, enforcement/legislation, engineering/technology, and economic incentives.	**H.** Primary prevention
______	**9.** Injuries that are purposefully inflicted by a person on himself or herself or on another person; examples include suicide or attempted suicide, homicide, rape, assault, domestic abuse, elder abuse, and child abuse.	**I.** Process objectives
______	**10.** Collection of the methods, skills, and activities necessary to determine whether a service or program is needed, is likely to be used, is conducted as planned, and actually helps people.	**J.** Public health
______	**11.** The study of the causes, patterns, prevalence, and control of disease in groups of people.	**K.** Risk
______	**12.** A potentially hazardous situation that puts people in a position in which they could be harmed.	**L.** Secondary prevention

______	**13.** An industry whose mission is to prevent disease and promote good health within groups of people.	**M.** Surveillance
______	**14.** Statements of how a program will be implemented, describing the service to be provided, the nature of the service, and to whom it will be directed.	**N.** Syndromic surveillance
______	**15.** Keeping an injury or illness from occurring.	**O.** Unintentional injuries
______	**16.** Something that offers automatic protection from injury or illness, often without requiring any conscious change of behavior by the person; child-resistant bottles and airbags are examples.	**P.** Years of potential life lost

Part II

Match the following prevention methods with the correct situation.

______	**1.** New guardrails are installed on a road in the area because a lot of crashes have occurred there.	**A.** Education
______	**2.** The emergency medical services (EMS) agency holds a free "Learn CPR Week" for residents of the town.	**B.** Enforcement
______	**3.** A vehicle insurance company offers a discounted rate to 16-year-olds for taking driver's education.	**C.** Engineering/ environment
______	**4.** The police stop students on the way to school and hand out coupons for a free iTunes music download to students who are wearing their seat belts.	**D.** Economic incentives
______	**5.** A car dealership offers a free child car seat check this weekend.	
______	**6.** An adolescent is stopped for speeding in a work zone and is given a ticket that costs him $250.	
______	**7.** The new car seats available have a five-point harness system instead of a bar that holds the child in the seat.	
______	**8.** The ambulance crew offers to do an inspection of any elderly person's home to determine potential risk areas. This service is provided free of charge.	
______	**9.** Because of the law, all poisons must be listed on the front of every container that contains products that can cause poisoning.	
______	**10.** Homeowners receive a discount on their home insurance because they have a smoke alarm and carbon monoxide (CO) monitor on every floor of the house.	

Multiple Choice

Read each item carefully, and then select the best response.

______ **1.** Fred is on the roof, trying to reposition the "dish" during the big game. He falls off and hurts his back. This is considered a(n) __________ injury.

- **A.** intentional
- **B.** unintentional
- **C.** secondary
- **D.** environmental

______ **2.** Which of the following is NOT an intentional injury?

- **A.** Rape
- **B.** Motor vehicle crash
- **C.** Suicide
- **D.** Elder abuse

______ **3.** When choosing objectives as you build an implementation plan, the *S* in SMART stands for:

- **A.** signs.
- **B.** swelling.
- **C.** simple.
- **D.** success.

_____ **4.** Which of the following patients could benefit from a "teachable moment"?
- **A.** An 18-year-old not wearing his seat belt who received cuts and bruises as a result of a motor vehicle crash
- **B.** A 3-year-old drowning patient
- **C.** An elderly person suffering from dementia
- **D.** A 45-year-old woman with a dog bite

_____ **5.** Which of the following is NOT a primary injury prevention measure?
- **A.** Wearing your seat belt
- **B.** Using safe lifting techniques
- **C.** Smoking only a pack a day
- **D.** Wearing gloves at the scene of a crash

_____ **6.** When developing a prevention program, what is the second step of the five steps discussed in the text?
- **A.** Plan and test interventions.
- **B.** Conduct a community assessment.
- **C.** Set goals and objectives.
- **D.** Define the problem.

_____ **7.** According to the Centers for Disease Control and Prevention (CDC), more than __________ children and teenagers are evaluated in the emergency department (ED) for _____________.
- **A.** 0.5 million; home injuries
- **B.** 1.5 million; motor vehicle injuries
- **C.** 2.6 million; sports-related injuries
- **D.** 5 million; abuse-related injuries

_____ **8.** What is the primary focus for an EMS provider when dealing with prevention?
- **A.** Primary injury prevention
- **B.** Secondary injury prevention
- **C.** Illness prevention
- **D.** Intervention research

_____ **9.** Which of the following is NOT a reason EMS should be involved in the prevention field?
- **A.** EMS providers reflect the composition of the community.
- **B.** EMS providers are high-profile role models.
- **C.** EMS personnel are contacted by auto makers for safety recommendations.
- **D.** EMS providers are welcomed by school systems.

_____ **10.** What is the leading killer among those aged 1 to 19 in the United States?
- **A.** Heart disease and congenital defects of the heart
- **B.** Diabetes
- **C.** Influenza and pneumonia
- **D.** Injury

Fill in the Blank

Read each item carefully, and then complete the statement by filling in the missing word(s).

1. A(n) __________ is a specific prevention measure that increases safety and positive health outcomes.

2. Assault, suicide, and intentional overdose are defined as __________ injuries.

3. The four Es of prevention are __________, __________, __________/__________, and __________ __________.

4. A toy manufacturer no longer sews buttons on the teddy bears for eyes; instead, it paints on the eyes with nontoxic paint. An automatic protection for our children such as this is known as __________ __________.

5. The top five causes of death in 2014 were ______, _______, ________, ________, and ___________.

6. When developing a prevention program, the type of objective that declares that all mobile homes will be provided with a smoke alarm and CO monitor is known as a(n) __________ __________.

7. Specific, nonjudgmental advice given on a scene to a patient who is receptive to the message is called a(n) __________ __________.

Identify

In the following case study, list the pertinent negatives that can lead to injury.

Mrs. M is so tired. She is 6 months pregnant with Katie's new brother. She works a night shift and takes care of curious 3-year-old Katie during the day. Their day starts with a bath for Katie. Mrs. M takes her out, dries her off, and gets her dressed but forgets to pull the plug in the tub because the phone is ringing. Katie runs off to get some breakfast in the kitchen, where she finds a pot of hot water for oatmeal boiling on the stove. Meanwhile, Mrs. M is still on the phone with her overbearing mother. Because Katie can't find anything to eat, she decides to go outside and play on the trampoline. Mr. M didn't get the safety net up last night when he put it together. Mrs. M finally gets off the phone with her mother and has a hard time finding Katie. Later on in the day, Mrs. M sneaks a nap while Katie is playing on the floor. Katie decides she wants to play that she is sewing like her mommy and finds the knitting needles and scissors in mommy's bag beside the chair. Luckily, Katie decides to play barber shop instead of doctor on her mommy. When Mrs. M wakes up, she is horrified to find lots of her own hair on the chair. Mrs. M. decides it would be better to take Katie to day care in the mornings while she catches up on her sleep!

1. Pertinent negatives
   a. ______________________________
   b. ______________________________
   c. ______________________________
   d. ______________________________

Ambulance Calls

The following case scenarios provide an opportunity to explore the concerns associated with patient management and paramedic care. Read each scenario, and then answer each question.

2. Mary and Jake are on duty when the tones go off for a man down. As they respond to the call, they radio dispatch for more information. Dispatch tells them that this is a lifeline call, and they are unable to get any response when they call the residence. Not knowing what they will encounter, Mary and Jake radio for law enforcement backup. When they arrive at the residence and first knock on the door, they can hear shouts for help from inside the house. A police officer shows up to help, and they determine that all doors and windows are locked, and there is no way into the house. The officer determines the basement window is the best one to break. Because Mary is the smallest person there, she is chosen to crawl through the basement window. She enters the house and finds an elderly man on the bathroom floor. After checking on the patient, she goes to unlock the front door. Mary and Jake determine that the man fell when trying to get from the toilet back to his wheelchair. He has no injuries and doesn't want to go to the hospital. He just needs a hand getting up. After calling a neighbor to come stay with the gentleman until his caregiver gets home, they load up and head back.

   a. Why is it a good idea that Mary and Jake call for an officer before they get to the scene?

   ____

   ____

   b. Which equipment should Mary have taken with her when she entered the home through the basement window?

   ____

   ____

c. During this call, Mary and Jake can apply the teachable moment. What are some things they can teach their patient?

____

____

3. Courtney and Larry have been called by the local elementary school to do a program for the third and fourth grades. They decide to educate the children on how and why to call 9-1-1. They arrive with a video of a dispatcher taking a "call" from a child. They show all the steps of how and when to call, what the dispatcher will say, and how the ambulance will respond to them. The video shows a child calling 9-1-1 after she finds her grandpa "asleep" on the floor and is unable to wake him up. Three days later during their shift, Courtney and Larry get a call for a woman who won't wake up. The dispatcher has the woman's 8-year-old son on the phone. When they arrive, they find a woman who won't wake up on the couch and a very upset little boy. With a few good questions, they determine the mother has diabetes. After getting a reading of 66 on the glucometer, they start an IV and give her D_{50}. The woman wakes up, and after eating a peanut butter and jelly sandwich, her glucose level stabilizes. Courtney and Larry stay a little longer to make sure everything is going well and wait for her neighbor to arrive. After receiving approval from medical control, they allow the patient to sign off and not be transported. During this time, they find out the boy, Ryan, was at their demonstration a few days ago.

a. When Larry and Courtney created an implementation plan for their program, they developed their objective with the SMART plan. What does the SMART plan stand for?

S ____

M ____

A ____

R ____

T ____

b. How did their program help Ryan decide to get help for his mother?

____

____

True/False

If you believe the statement to be more true than false, write the letter "T" in the space provided. If you believe the statement to be more false than true, write the letter "F."

_____ **1.** Primary prevention is defined as reducing the effects of an injury that has already happened.

_____ **2.** Unintentional injuries are the leading cause of death for people between 1 and 19 years of age.

_____ **3.** The three factors used in making a Haddon injury matrix are the host, the event, and the post-event.

_____ **4.** The process of collecting, analyzing, and interpreting injury data is called injury surveillance.

_____ **5.** A risk factor for an intentional injury would be not wearing your seat belt.

_____ **6.** In creating an implementation plan, you need a realistic time line to complete your project.

_____ **7.** Two of the five steps in developing a prevention plan are conducting a community assessment and setting goals and objectives.

_____ **8.** When using SMART to meet your objectives, the *R* in this acronym stands for risk.

_____ **9.** Funding for a prevention program can include donations from local media, grants, and sponsorships from different organizations.

_____ **10.** Every EMS call includes a teachable moment.

Short Answer

Complete this section with short written answers using the space provided.

1. Define primary injury prevention and secondary injury prevention, and give an example of each.

Primary injury prevention: ______

Secondary injury prevention: ______

2. Give three examples of why EMS providers should be active in the prevention field.

a. ______

b. ______

c. ______

3. List the four Es of prevention, and explain each one.

a. ______

b. ______

c. ______

d. ______

4. A public health model will help to identify a problem and how to approach the problem. Use this approach to list the three key factors involved in the problem of children and swimming-pool drowning deaths.

a. ______

b. ______

c. ______

Fill in the Table

Fill in the missing parts of the table.

The Five Steps to Developing a Prevention Program
1. ______
2. ______
3. Set goals and objectives.
4. ______
5. ______

CHAPTER 4

Medical, Legal, and Ethical Issues

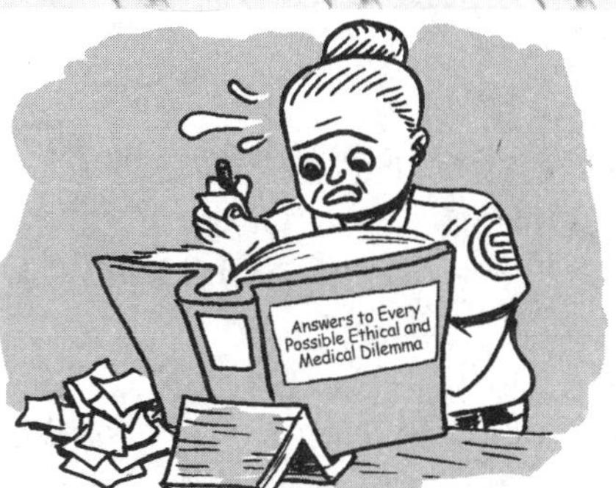

As a paramedic you will frequently encounter situations for which there is no right or wrong answer—and for which no amount of studying can prepare you. Use your best judgment, consult with supervisors if possible, and ask yourself, "What is best for the patient?"

Matching

Part I

Match the following sentences with the correct situation. For questions 1 to 6, indicate whether:

A. You may treat the patient without obtaining the patient's expressed consent.

B. You may NOT treat the patient without obtaining the patient's expressed consent.

_____ **1.** A 10-year-old child is struck by a car. He is bleeding profusely. His parents cannot be located.

_____ **2.** A 48-year-old man is injured in a motor vehicle crash in which his car was demolished. He has bruises on his forehead. He seems confused. He says, "I'm all right. Let me alone. I just called for an Uber car."

_____ **3.** A 56-year-old woman has chest pain. Her husband phoned for an ambulance. The patient says, "It's nothing, just my gastroesophageal reflux disease." She refuses to be examined or treated.

_____ **4.** A 26-year-old woman is pulled from the beach surf in cardiac arrest.

_____ **5.** A 23-year-old man is injured in a barroom altercation. He is bleeding profusely from his nose and mouth. He smells strongly of alcohol. He is very belligerent and shouts at you, "Leave me alone, you creeps. If you come any closer, I'll knock your teeth in."

_____ **6.** An 82-year-old woman has fainted at home. Her son found her on the floor and called for an ambulance. She is conscious when you arrive. She says to you, "You are all very sweet, but one can't live forever, you know, and I don't fancy hospitals."

For questions 7 to 10, match the following words to the correct situation.

A. Slander

B. Defamation

C. Battery

D. Assault

_____ **7.** The reporting paramedic wrote on his patient care report (PCR) that Mr. Paul was obviously drunk. The paramedic made that statement because he has a long-running feud with Mr. Paul and thought this was a great way to pay him back.

_____ **8.** Mrs. O'Malley told the emergency medical technician (EMT) not to touch her. She did not want any help. The EMT went ahead and tried to grab Mrs. O'Malley and put her on the cot.

_____ **9.** Mitch is taking a patient into the hospital. The patient asks about the doctor on staff. Mitch tells the patient, "Sorry, buddy, but I wouldn't want that witch doctor treating me. Good luck, partner."

_____ **10.** Ryan is in the back of the ambulance with his patient, Jake, who is 16 years old and has just rolled his car. Jake is really wound up and wants out of the ambulance. Ryan tells Jake that if he doesn't calm down, he is going to strap him down and give him a shot.

Match each of the following items to the appropriate situation.

E = Ethical **M** = Moral **UE** = Unethical practice

_____ **11.** The patient's religion determines that no matter how sick the person is, the person will not seek medical attention.

_____ **12.** The physician believes that Mother is terminal, but he wants to try at least one more medication to see if it can help her.

_____ **13.** My patient has overdosed on crack cocaine, so he is not worth working on.

_____ **14.** Even though my patient, who was drinking and driving, has just killed a family of four in a car crash, I will do my best to provide medical attention to him.

_____ **15.** A 40-year-old woman has tried to commit suicide by overdosing; if she wants to die, let's give her that wish by working this as a "slow code."

_____ **16.** The patient does not want any pain medication because he feels that those medications are considered "drugs."

_____ **17.** This patient obviously doesn't have the money for this emergency department (ED) visit; let's wait until all of the other patients have been taken care of before we work on this welfare case.

_____ **18.** Mark intentionally left out the fact that he gave five times the normal epinephrine dose on the PCR.

_____ **19.** After helping the mother give birth to a premature stillborn child, the paramedic blessed the infant because the mother requested that the child be blessed.

_____ **20.** The paramedic gave the apparently "drunk" 18-year-old patient Lasix on the long transport to the hospital. He wanted to teach the patient a lesson. He thought that if the patient wet himself, it would be funny.

Part II

Match each of the definitions in the left column to the appropriate term in the right column.

_____	**1.** Unauthorized act committed outside the scope of medical practice defined by law.	**A.** Abandonment
_____	**2.** A person who is younger than the legal age (generally 18 years) in a given state but is legally considered an adult because of other circumstances.	**B.** Advance directive
_____	**3.** Legal protection from penalties that could normally be incurred under the law.	**C.** Borrowed servant doctrine
_____	**4.** A right to a fair procedure for a legal action against a person or agency; has two components: notice and opportunity to be heard.	**D.** Common law
_____	**5.** Act(s) committed by a plaintiff that contribute(s) to adverse outcomes.	**E.** Contributory negligence
_____	**6.** A principle that absolves an institution of liability when one of its members acts beyond his or her scope of certification or training by following someone else's orders.	**F.** Defamation
_____	**7.** Termination of medical care for the patient without giving the patient sufficient opportunity to find another suitable health care professional to take over his or her medical treatment.	**G.** Due process
_____	**8.** A decision that has been made by a judge through a court case based on his or her interpretation of the statutes and constitutions; it can be overturned either by another court with a higher authority or the issuing court at a later time; also called case law.	**H.** Emancipated minor
_____	**9.** A written document or oral statement that expresses the wants, needs, and desires of a patient in reference to future medical care; examples include living wills, do not resuscitate (DNR) orders, and organ donation orders.	**I.** Immunity
_____	**10.** Intentionally making a false statement, through written or verbal communication that injures a person's good name or reputation.	**J.** Malfeasance

Multiple Choice

Read each item carefully, and then select the best response.

_____ **1.** You have responded to a fender bender, where your patient is conscious and alert. The patient is able to answer all questions correctly and declines treatment. Your overzealous partner starts to put a cervical collar on the patient. What could he be charged with?

- **A.** Assault
- **B.** Battery
- **C.** False imprisonment
- **D.** Libel

_____ **2.** You are on a volunteer squad in a small town. At the grocery store, your neighbor starts asking you what happened the night before. You proceed to tell her that the local dentist was hitting his wife, and you had to take her up to the hospital for a broken jaw. Along the way, you let slide a few of your own opinions about the dentist. Soon the story is all over town. The dentist is upset and contacts a lawyer to initiate a lawsuit against you. What will you be charged with?

- **A.** Defamation
- **B.** Libel
- **C.** Slander
- **D.** Assault

_____ **3.** What does the Health Insurance Portability and Accountability Act (HIPAA) guarantee the patient?

- **A.** The hospital cannot transfer a mother in labor.
- **B.** The paramedic can treat the patient without consent if she or he believes the patient has a life-threatening problem.
- **C.** The paramedic meets minimum qualifications.
- **D.** The patient's medical information will remain confidential at all times.

_____ **4.** Which of the following is NOT needed to prove the negligence of the paramedic?

- **A.** The paramedic treated an unconscious patient.
- **B.** The paramedic had a legal duty to act.
- **C.** The paramedic breached his or her duty to act.
- **D.** The patient was harmed by the paramedic.

_____ **5.** You arrive at the ED with a patient complaining of "chest pain" as your pager goes off for the next call of the night. In your hurry to get out of the hospital, you hand off your patient to the ward clerk, knowing that a registered nurse (RN) will be coming soon to take over. You are guilty of:

- **A.** proximate cause.
- **B.** ordinary negligence.
- **C.** gross negligence.
- **D.** abandonment.

_____ **6.** You are called to the local elementary school for a child who has fallen from the top of the slide. The child is not making any sense and is vomiting. The school is unable to reach her parents. Under which type of consent can you treat and transport this child?

- **A.** Informed
- **B.** Implied
- **C.** Expressed
- **D.** Involuntary

_____ **7.** You respond to a man down. You find a homeless person in an alley. Which of the following findings would allow you to take the man to the hospital under implied consent?

- **A.** He has not eaten for at least 6 hours.
- **B.** He does not appear clean.
- **C.** His oxygen level is 82%.
- **D.** His blood glucose level is normal.

______ **8.** After transferring care of the homeless man in the preceding question to the nurse, which of the following does NOT belong in your PCR?

A. The patient was unkempt and stunk badly.
B. The patient had an oxygen level of 92%.
C. The patient has not had anything to eat.
D. The patient's blood glucose was 100 mg/dL.

______ **9.** Which of the following patients must be reported?

A. A 16-year-old girl who refuses to eat
B. A new mother who is feeling very depressed
C. A 10-year-old boy who was bitten by a dog
D. A 25-year-old man who was binge drinking

______ **10.** How are most civil cases resolved?

A. A settlement process
B. A trial by a judge
C. A trial by jury
D. None of the above

______ **11.** What is the paramedic's best protection in court?

A. A voice recording of every call
B. A complete and accurate PCR
C. Rewriting the PCR at a later date or time
D. Video cameras in the back of the units

______ **12.** In which of the following situations would you work "the code"?

A. A woman who was found in rigor mortis in her bathroom
B. A patient who was decapitated in a car wreck
C. A 6-year-old child who was trapped under ice for 20 minutes
D. A 56-year-old man who had a tractor crush his chest area and has been trapped for 40 minutes

______ **13.** What is the person (or procedure) called when one adult has the legal authority to make the health care decisions for another?

A. Power of attorney
B. Parents
C. Surrogate decision maker
D. None of the above

______ **14.** Which of the following is NOT an advance directive?

A. The doctor's recommendations
B. A DNR order
C. A living will
D. A health care power of attorney

______ **15.** In the National Association of Emergency Medical Technicians (NAEMT) *Code of Ethics for Emergency Medical Technicians*, which of the following is NOT a fundamental responsibility?

A. Alleviating suffering
B. Promoting health
C. Conserving life
D. Providing moral support

Fill in the Blank

Read each item carefully, and then complete the statement by filling in the missing word(s).

1. Failure to obtain consent before providing medical treatment might give rise to charges of technical assault and battery. What are the requirements for obtaining consent to treat in the following scenarios?

   a. From a conscious, mentally competent adult, consent must be __________.

   b. To treat a child, consent must be obtained from the __________ __________ or __________ __________.

2. The patient is claiming that he was harmed by the paramedic's actions. In a lawsuit, the patient will be the __________, and the paramedic will be the __________.

3. The paramedic is permitted by the medical director to carry out certain treatments. This is known as the paramedic's __________ __________ __________.

4. A document that expresses the patient's wants, needs, and desires in relation to the patient's future medical care is known as a(n) __________ __________.

5. A minor who has been __________ is a minor younger than legal age but is treated as an adult because of marriage, pregnancy, or active military service.

6. Another significant __________ and __________ problem that has occurred in emergency medical services (EMS) is the __________ of training and certification records.

Identify

In the following case study, list the chief complaint, vital signs, and pertinent negatives.

You are called to the local sports bar for a man not feeling well. When you arrive, you are confronted by a 30-year-old man who is acting very strangely. He is yelling that he doesn't need anyone's help and just to leave him alone. All he wants is a sandwich and a beer. The patient refuses any type of help and correctly answers all of your questions. Once again, he says he wants to be left alone. Without consent and with a cranky patient, you don't feel that you can treat this patient. As you are ready to leave, the man falls off the barstool and is unconscious. You begin treatment by opening his airway and checking for breathing. He is breathing 20 breaths/min with an oxygen saturation level of 97%. The patient moans but makes no other noises. Your partner notices a medical ID bracelet stating the man has diabetes. You take a blood glucose reading and find it to be 42 mg/dL. Your partner applies oxygen by a non-rebreathing mask and starts an IV on the patient. Vital signs for this patient are as follows: blood pressure is 132/70 mm Hg, pulse is 96 beats/min, lung sounds are clear bilaterally, skin is cool, and pupils are a bit sluggish. You give 25 g of D_{50} by IV. The patient begins to wake up very quickly and asks what is going on. He tells you he had taken his sugar reading earlier and realized he needed to eat, so he stopped for food. He is now competent and does not want to be transported to the ED. After making sure that his vital signs are within normal ranges and that his blood glucose level has come up to a reading of 118 mg/dL, you discontinue the IV. Your partner writes up a report, and once again you check all of the patient's vital signs, finding them normal. The patient again refuses transport after you have determined that he is competent. With approval from medical control, you have the patient sign off, and you return to your unit, back in service for the next call.

1. Chief complaint: ______________________________

   ____

   ____

2. Vital signs: ______________________________

   ____

   ____

3. Pertinent negatives: ______________________________

____

____

Ambulance Calls

The following case scenarios provide an opportunity to explore the concerns associated with patient management and paramedic care. Read each scenario, and then answer each question.

1. Six emergency calls are described in the following list. Circle the letter beside those calls in which it is permissible for a paramedic to give treatment without obtaining expressed consent from the patient. In those cases in which you may *not* treat the patient without expressed consent, describe which action you would take.
   a. A 10-year-old boy has fallen at school and sprained his right ankle. The school authorities have so far been unable to reach the boy's parents.

   ____

   ____

   b. A 45-year-old woman is found in cardiac arrest.

   ____

   ____

   c. A 21-year-old man called for an ambulance after his 19-year-old girlfriend swallowed a large number of sleeping pills. She is awake and refuses treatment. She says, "Go away and let me die."

   ____

   ____

   d. A 20-year-old man has taken PCP (a psychedelic drug that often induces violent behavior) and has tried to gouge out his eyes. He is bleeding profusely from the face and screaming, "Don't come near me."

   ____

   ____

   e. A 14-year-old boy was knocked from his bicycle and hit by a truck. He is unconscious and bleeding. Both legs appear fractured. Bystanders do not know the boy or his parents.

   ____

   ____

   f. A 48-year-old man has crushing chest pain. His wife called for the ambulance. The man says he doesn't need an ambulance; he just has indigestion. His face is gray, and he is sweating profusely.

   ____

   ____

2. You are called to the scene of a crash in which a pedestrian has been struck by a car. The driver of the car says the pedestrian staggered out into the street in front of him. The pedestrian is now sitting on the curb. He has an obvious bruise on his head. He is unkempt and smells strongly of alcohol. He tells you that he doesn't want to go to the hospital. You suspect that the patient might not be competent to make that decision. List three things you can check to assess his mental competence.

   a. ______________________________

   b. ______________________________

   c. ______________________________

True/False

If you believe the statement to be more true than false, write the letter "T" in the space provided. If you believe the statement to be more false than true, write the letter "F."

_____ 1. You can be sued for slander when you write a false statement on your PCR.

_____ 2. The discovery period during a lawsuit can take anywhere from a few months to more than 2 years.

_____ 3. You should contact medical control in the case of a physician's orders on a scene if the orders do not fit the emergency situation.

_____ 4. HIPAA protects the patient's right to confidentiality.

_____ 5. Good Samaritan laws are designed to protect all paramedics from lawsuits.

_____ 6. To prove negligence on the part of the paramedic, the plaintiff must prove legal duty, breach of duty, failure to act, and harm.

_____ 7. A DNR order is not considered an advance directive.

_____ 8. You must gain informed consent from every competent adult before beginning treatment.

_____ 9. You must have parental consent even for an emancipated minor.

_____ 10. The paramedic's best defense in a lawsuit is his or her written report on the patient.

_____ 11. Ethics is a code of conduct that is defined by society and religion along with a person's conscience.

_____ 12. The *Code of Ethics for Emergency Medical Technicians* states that EMTs should adhere to standards of personal ethics that reflect credit upon the profession.

_____ 13. You should always place the welfare of your patient ahead of any personal considerations, except for your own safety.

_____ 14. Patient autonomy is the power of attorney making medical decisions for the patient.

_____ 15. A DNR order can be printed on a medical ID bracelet.

_____ 16. Advance directives are usually created once the patient can no longer make the decisions for his or her own health care.

_____ 17. A person who makes health care decisions for another or carries the power of attorney is called a surrogate decision maker.

_____ 18. Your general focus during resuscitation should be to provide at least 30 minutes of your best efforts.

_____ 19. If you witness misconduct by another EMS provider, you should report that person immediately to the chain of command.

_____ 20. You should always work on a baby with sudden infant death syndrome (SIDS), even if the baby is in rigor mortis.

Short Answer

Complete this section with short written answers using the space provided.

1. Every state in the United States defines certain cases as "coroner's cases"—that is, cases of death that you are obliged to report to law enforcement authorities. Although regulations vary somewhat from state to state, certain categories of cases are nearly universally regarded as coroner's cases. List three such categories.

a. ______________________________

b. ______________________________

c. ______________________________

2. Good Samaritan legislation was written to prevent lawsuits from being brought against people who try to assist at an emergency scene. Explain why the Good Samaritan laws would not be a good defense for a paramedic who has a lawsuit brought against him or her.

____

____

____

3. If legal action is taken against a paramedic, the charge most likely to be brought is that of professional negligence (malpractice). To prove that the paramedic was negligent, the plaintiff must demonstrate four things. List the four elements required to prove negligence.

a. _______________

b. _______________

c. _______________

d. _______________

4. List four types of cases that paramedics or other health care professionals in your state are required to report to the appropriate authorities.

a. _______________

b. _______________

c. _______________

d. _______________

5. **(a)** What is MOLST?
(b) Is it used in your state?

a. _______________

b. _______________

6. Ethics refers to the rules of right and wrong that we live by. Medical ethics refers to rules of right and wrong that guide the behavior of health care professionals. State in one or two sentences what you regard as the guiding principle of your work as a paramedic.

____

____

____

7. How would you handle a paramedic who continually makes racist remarks about your patients?

____

____

____

8. Explain the things you would look for in a DNR order when you arrive on scene and find the patient in cardiac arrest.

____

____

____

CHAPTER 5

Communications

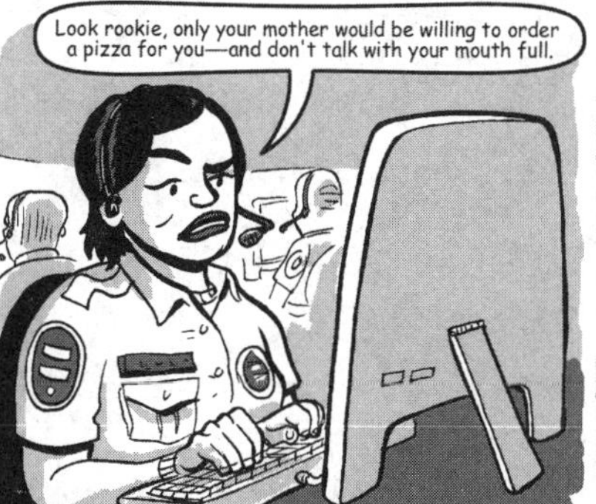

Matching

Part I

Indicate whether each of the following questions from a patient interview is an open-ended question or a closed-ended question.

O = open-ended question

C = closed-ended question

_____ **1.** What happened today?

_____ **2.** Do you remember the collision?

_____ **3.** What does your blood pressure usually run?

_____ **4.** Are you pregnant?

_____ **5.** Have you been sick in the last few weeks?

_____ **6.** Do you have asthma?

_____ **7.** Which medications do you take daily?

_____ **8.** What does the pain feel like to you?

_____ **9.** Do you wear contact lenses?

_____ **10.** How much do you weigh?

Part II

Match each of the definitions in the left column to the appropriate term in the right column.

_____ **1.** The number of cycles (oscillations) per second of a radio signal.

_____ **2.** Radio system using paired frequencies to permit the use of remote repeaters or simultaneous transmission and reception.

_____ **3.** The location to which 9-1-1 calls are routed, which may or may not serve as the dispatch center.

_____ **4.** Remote radio transceiver that receives radio signals and rebroadcasts them at a higher power, extending the range of a radio communications system.

_____ **5.** Public safety communications systems that are compatible across all local, tribal, state, and federal agencies.

_____ **6.** Computer-based system permitting real-time two-way audio, video, and data communication between the paramedic and the medical control physician.

_____ **7.** Simultaneous transmission of multiple data streams, most often voice and electrocardiogram signals.

A. Base station

B. Biotelemetry

C. Computer-assisted dispatch (CAD)

D. Crew resource management (CRM)

E. Cultural competence

F. Digital radio

G. Duplex

______	**8.** Computerized sharing of radio frequencies by multiple units, agencies, or systems.	**H.** Frequency
______	**9.** A radio at a fixed location consisting of a transmitter, receiver, and antenna.	**I.** Interoperability
______	**10.** Linked dispatch center computer consoles and vehicle-mounted mobile data terminals.	**J.** Multiplex
______	**11.** The transmission of information via radio waves using native digital data or analog (voice) signals that have been converted to a digital signal and compressed.	**K.** Public safety answering point (PSAP)
______	**12.** An understanding of the predominant cultures that exist in the geographic area in which the paramedic provides patient care.	**L.** Repeater
______	**13.** Transmission of physiologic data, such as electrocardiogram, from the patient to a distant point of reception (commonly referred to in emergency medical services as telemetry).	**M.** Telemedicine
______	**14.** An operational practice designed to enhance communication and teamwork, thereby reducing preventable errors.	**N.** Trunked radio system

Part III

The following statements come from a patient's case history. Arrange them in the correct order for a paramedic radio transmission to medical command.

1. **A.** Pulse is 50 beats/min and regular, respirations are 36 breaths/min and deep, blood pressure (BP) is 180/126 mm Hg, and Spo_2 is 94%.
   B. The patient has a history of hypertension.
   C. The deep tendon reflexes are hyperactive.
   D. Her daughter says the patient complained of a severe headache before she collapsed.
   E. The patient was still responsive on our arrival, but she rapidly became unresponsive.
   F. The patient is a 60-year-old woman who collapsed in the bathroom while sitting on the toilet.
   G. We are administering supplemental oxygen at 4 L/min by nasal cannula.
   H. The patient's medications include nitroglycerin and Aldomet (methyldopa).
   I. Her left pupil is larger than the right and does not react to light.
   J. Her daughter states, "She was well until 9:00 a.m. this morning."
   K. Her neck is somewhat stiff.
   L. She was hospitalized 6 years ago for an acute myocardial infarction (AMI).

(1)________	(5)________	(9)________
(2)________	(6)________	(10)________
(3)________	(7)________	(11)________
(4)________	(8)________	(12)________

Multiple Choice

Read each item carefully, and then select the best response.

______ **1.** Which of the following best describes the use of slang terms?
- **A.** Helpful when communicating with the hospital because of patient confidentiality
- **B.** Breaks up the stress of the job by interjecting "dark humor"
- **C.** Unprofessional and disrespectful
- **D.** Helpful when communicating with other paramedics

______ **2.** Emergency medical services (EMS) systems require a large number of personnel to work and communicate together. All of the following are part of this communication EXCEPT:
- **A.** an emergency medical dispatcher (EMD).
- **B.** a citizen notifier.
- **C.** computer-aided dispatch (CAD).
- **D.** online medical control with base station physician.

_____ **3.** Federal oversight of emergency medical communication is accomplished by the:
A. State Emergency Management Organization.
B. Department of Homeland Security.
C. Federal Emergency Management Agency (FEMA).
D. Federal Communications Commission (FCC).

_____ **4.** What is the mode of two-way radio transmission that allows users to talk and listen simultaneously by using two separate radio frequencies at once?
A. Multiplex
B. Stereo
C. Duplex
D. Simplex

_____ **5.** Which of the following is a method of transmitting information to communicate with a patient?
A. Verbal
B. Nonverbal
C. Electronic
D. All of the above

_____ **6.** What is the best way to develop rapport with a patient?
A. Have genuine concern for the patient.
B. Always call the patient by a pet name.
C. Hug the patient.
D. Always use medical terminology.

_____ **7.** Which of the following would suggest a mental impairment when first addressing the patient?
A. The patient responds with a coherent speech pattern.
B. The patient does not turn and look at you when you speak.
C. The patient waits a second before answering your question.
D. The patient has a meaningful response to your greeting.

_____ **8.** When dealing with a fearful patient, which of the following will NOT be useful?
A. Showing concern for the patient
B. Standing with your arms crossed
C. Acting like a professional
D. Telling the patient about his electrocardiogram (ECG) rhythm

_____ **9.** Which of the following strategies will help you get a useful response from the patient?
A. Asking questions with specific medical terms
B. Talking constantly with the patient
C. Being quiet and letting the patient talk
D. Speaking calmly and clearly

_____ **10.** If you do not understand what the patient is trying to say to you, you should:
A. just nod and say, "I understand."
B. let the patient continue until you do catch something you understand.
C. ask the patient to explain in more detail.
D. ask the patient a closed-ended question.

_____ **11.** What is the best way to demonstrate to the patient that you are honest?
A. Using frequent and direct eye contact
B. Patting the patient on the arm
C. Kneeling on the floor in front of the patient
D. Always having a smile on your face

_____ 12. When assessing a patient's memory, which of the following is NOT a useful tool?
- A. Asking the patient his or her name
- B. Asking the patient what he or she had for breakfast the day before
- C. Asking the patient where she or he is
- D. Asking the patient what happened to her or him

_____ 13. Which of the following cultures considers direct eye contact to be rude?
- A. Islamic
- B. French
- C. Brazilian
- D. Asian

_____ 14. When treating a patient from another culture, what is a good rule of thumb?
- A. Always use hand gestures to make your points.
- B. Never use hand gestures when communicating.
- C. Always use medical terms in your conversation with the patient.
- D. Use pet names for the patient because it makes the patient feel that you like him or her.

Fill in the Blank

You have just been appointed the communications director for your regional EMS system, and you have been asked to draw up plans for an EMS communications system. To do so, you have to figure out who needs to communicate with whom in such a system and what is the best technical means (pager, radio, landline, or cellular phone) to achieve each link in the communications chain. Complete the following statements.

1. The __________ needs to be able to talk with __________. The best technical means of establishing that link is __________.

2. The __________ needs to be able to talk with __________. The best technical means of establishing that link is __________.

3. The __________ needs to be able to talk with __________. The best technical means of establishing that link is __________.

4. The __________ needs to be able to talk with __________. The best technical means of establishing that link is __________.

5. The __________ needs to be able to talk with __________. The best technical means of establishing that link is __________.

6. The act of transmitting information to another person is called __________.

7. When dealing with a crisis, your challenge is to remain __________.

8. A(n) __________ __________ __________ is a question that does not have a yes or no answer.

9. When using touch to assure a patient, you should touch a(n) __________ part of the patient's body.

10. If the patient is hostile and you are unable to diffuse the patient's anger, you should call the __________.

11. When treating a child, __________ are useful tools for bridging the emotional gap with the child.

12. The best way for you to recognize cross-cultural differences and understand how they may affect interactions with the diverse population you serve is to learn more about __________ __________.

Identify

After reading the following case history, provide the indicated assessment information.

The patient is a 52-year-old man who called for an ambulance because of chest pain. The pain was "squeezing" in character, was a 6 out of 10 in severity, radiated to the left shoulder and jaw, and had been present for 2 hours. The pain was accompanied by increasing difficulty in breathing, relieved somewhat by sitting upright. The patient denied nausea, vomiting, sweating, or palpitations. He is known to be a cardiac patient and takes nitroglycerin at home; he took two nitroglycerin doses today, without relief. He denies any history of hypertension or diabetes. He has been treated for a peptic ulcer in the past.

On physical examination, the patient was sitting bolt upright; he appeared alert and apprehensive and was in moderate respiratory distress, breathing shallowly at 30 breaths/min. Pulse was 130 beats/min, weak and regular; BP was 200/90 mm Hg; and Spo_2 was 94%. His neck veins were distended to the angle of the jaw at 45°. Wet crackles were heard at both lung bases, and auscultation of the heart revealed a gallop rhythm. The abdomen was not distended. There was 1+ presacral and ankle edema.

The patient was given supplemental oxygen by non-rebreathing mask at 12 L/min, a 12-lead ECG, and an IV of normal saline, then transported to the regional cardiac center in semi-Fowler position. His vital signs remained stable throughout transport.

1. Chief complaint:

____

____

2. History of the present illness:

____

____

3. Other medical history:

____

____

4. General appearance:

____

____

5. Vital signs:

____

____

6. Physical exam:

____

____

7. Treatment given:

____

____

8. Pertinent negatives:

____

____

Ambulance Calls

Part I

The following case scenarios provide an opportunity to explore the concerns associated with patient management and paramedic care. Read each scenario, and then answer each question.

1. Following is a transcript of a transmission between a paramedic unit in the field and a local hospital. **The transmission does *not* follow the guidelines for good radio communications.** Read through the transmission, and then list all the errors in it that you can find.
Ambulance: Medic 12 to County Hospital.
Hospital: Who's calling County Hospital?
Ambulance: This is Medic 12.
Hospital: Go ahead, Medic 12.
Ambulance: Be advised that we are en route to your location with Maggie Jones, a lady well endowed with adipose tissue who's complaining of SOB.
Hospital: Could you please 10-9 that chief complaint?
Ambulance: What's the matter, are you deaf or something? S. O. B. S as in silly, O as in old, B as in bag. Stand by for the ECG.
[Pause.]
Ambulance: Medic 12 to County Hospital. Did you get the strip?
Hospital: Yes.
Ambulance: Say again.
Hospital: Yes, we received the strip. The doctor wants to know how old the patient is.
Ambulance: She's 58.
Hospital: And does she have any medical history?
Ambulance: Yeah, she's a cardiac patient and takes digitalis, atenolol, potassium chloride, chlorothiazide, and a whole bunch of other stuff.
Hospital: Did you get any vitals?
Ambulance: That's affirmative. The blood pressure is 180/120 mm Hg, the pulse is 44 beats/min, and the respirations are. . .let's see. . .here it is. . .the respirations are 30 breaths/min.
Hospital: Doctor's orders are to give 1 mg of atropine IV.
Ambulance: That's a 10-4. Will do.
Hospital: What's your ETA?
Ambulance: About 10 minutes.
Hospital: We'll see you then.
Ambulance: Roger. Pop a few doughnuts into the microwave for us, will you?
What's wrong with this transmission?

a. ______________________________

b. ______________________________

c. ______________________________

d. ______________________________

e. ______________________________

f. ______________________________

g. ______________________________

h. ______________________________

2. You are covering for the dispatcher during his lunch break. ("Don't worry about a thing," you tell him as he heads out the door. "This job's a piece of cake.") The dispatcher has no sooner departed than the telephone rings. You answer on the first ring, and a caller blurts out, "There's been a terrible crash. Oh my God, it's terrible, it's terrible," and he starts sobbing. List the questions you will ask this caller, and indicate at which point you will dispatch an ambulance.

____

____

____

Part II

The following case scenarios provide an opportunity to explore the concerns associated with patient management and paramedic care. Read each scenario, and then answer each question.

1. You are called to the scene of a bad motor vehicle crash in which a semitrailer plowed head-on into a passenger car. The driver of the car is pinned inside his vehicle, very seriously injured. You manage to gain access to the patient and start tending to him while you await help in what will be a lengthy extrication procedure. The patient is still conscious, and he asks you, "Am I going to die?" There is, in fact, a high probability that he will die. Describe how you would reply to this patient's question.

____

____

____

2. You are called to a suburban neighborhood where a 32-year-old female patient with diabetes is having some problems with her glucose levels. Your assessment determines that you need to start an IV and give the patient D_{50}. How would you explain to your patient what you are about to do?

____

____

____

3. You are dispatched to a call for chest pain. The scene is a large farm in the rural Midwest. Upon your arrival, a man in a pickup truck meets you at the front gate. He waves for you to follow him. He leads you to a large area on the farm where many camper-trailers are parked. As you get out of your ambulance, the driver of the truck approaches you. He introduces himself as the owner of the farm and tells you that the grandmother of his harvest foreman is experiencing chest pain. He also explains that the foreman and his family are migrant farm workers who speak mostly Spanish.

As you enter a camper, a worried Hispanic gentleman meets you, and the farmer introduces you as "el paramedico." The man extends his hand to you to shake it and says, "Gracias, gracias, señor," and gestures for you follow him. You are led to a cramped bedroom, where an elderly Hispanic woman is lying on a bed, propped up with several blankets. There are several Catholic icons on the wall, as well as a statue of the Virgin Mary at the bedside. The woman has a string of beads in her hand. You notice several small candles burning on a dresser next to the bed. The man gestures toward her and says, "Mi abuela." The woman presents with pale complexion, diaphoresis, obvious dyspnea, and a facial grimace that you associate with severe pain. You have an emergency medical technician (EMT) partner and an EMT student intern riding with you, so you direct your partner to start setting up the ECG monitor and the student to take vital signs. The excited student says, "Yo," and starts to work. Knowing the patient needs oxygen, you bend over and blow out the candles, not wanting the hazard of open flame around the oxygen. This action really seems to upset the woman, who lets out a little cry. You don't speak any Spanish, so you kneel beside the bed and very slowly ask, "What... is... your... name?" The woman looks in confusion to her grandson, who says "nombre." The woman tells you, very proudly, "Mi nombre es Señora Talia Elizabet Cordoba de Castille." You feel around your uniform for your pen to write it down and realize you left it in the ambulance. You find the red pen you have been using to correct the students' reports and begin to write down her name. The woman lets out a hysterical shriek and tries to back away from you on the bed. There is suddenly much excited confusion in the room, and the grandson is trying desperately to calm his grandmother.

The woman is very agitated, and the ECG monitor shows you a sinus tachycardia with several premature ventricular complexes (PVCs). You tell the EMT student to run and get the cot. He responds with another "yo" and makes the "rock on" sign with his left hand. The woman's eyes get wide, and she shrieks again, and this time she faints. The grandson cries out, "Abuela!" and then tearfully asks you to perform last rites. You inform the grandson that his grandmother is not dead but needs to be transported immediately. You really don't like the way this call is progressing and just want to get back in the ambulance.

In the preceding scenario, you not only have a language barrier but a religious one as well. Hispanic families are very close-knit, and older Hispanics are generally very religious, especially those who have come from the "old country." The majority practice Roman Catholicism and may also be very superstitious. Old World beliefs in the forces of good and evil may be very prevalent, and traditional religious practices may also be interspersed with additional spiritual beliefs. Some of these may include Candomble, which is a mixture of Roman Catholicism and African Voodoo, practiced predominately in the Pan-Caribbean regions and South America; Santeria, which is popular in Cuba, the Caribbean, and South America; espiritismo, which is practiced predominately in Puerto Rico and Central America; and curanderismo, which is found in Mexico and the American Southwest and still exists in "Old Spain."

In some of these traditions, the color yellow is associated with death, the color red with witchcraft, and white with resisting evil spells. Thus, writing a person's name in red ink may be perceived as an attempt to "cast a spell" and gain power over the individual.

Hispanic people generally use two surnames. The first surname listed is from the father, and the second surname listed is from the mother. When speaking to someone, use his or her father's surname. A married woman may attach her husband's surname to the end of hers with a *de*. A widow may indicate her widowed status by including *-vda* ("widow of") in her name as well. Hispanics are very proud of their family names, and a good name is often more important than wealth or status. They also expect to be treated with dignity and respect (familiar theme, no?) and will reciprocate the same. It is very important in the paramedic–patient relationship to treat the Hispanic patient with polite formality and address him or her by title (Mr., Mrs., Señor, Señora). Once rapport is established, the paramedic can gain valuable inroads in the trust factor by politely asking about family members or loved ones. Hispanics, especially older Hispanics, base clinical trust on *individual* perception, not an institutional one.

a. What should you have asked the farmer before you entered the residence?

____

____

____

b. Upon seeing all the religious symbols in the room, what should you have done before blowing out the candles?

____

____

____

c. Why did the student intern upset the woman?

____

____

____

d. Why is a translator so important at this scene?

____

____

____

True/False

If you believe the statement to be more true than false, write the letter "T" in the space provided. If you believe the statement to be more false than true, write the letter "F."

_____ **1.** EMS may use very high frequency (VHF), ultra high frequency (UHF), and "trunking systems."

_____ **2.** aramedics skilled in dysrhythmia recognition do not rely heavily on ECG telemetry.

_____ **3.** An EMS base station consisting of a transmitter, receiver, and antenna is usually mounted in the front console of an ambulance for emergency communications.

_____ **4.** To have clarity of transmission, there must be a sender, a clear message, a receiver, and a feedback loop.

_____ **5.** Most EMS agencies use radio codes to comply with Health Insurance Portability and Accountability Act (HIPAA) requirements for transmitting patient information over the radio.

_____ **6.** Sometimes it might be more practical to step out of the patient exam room or to speak in a softer tone to provide the history and transfer information to the receiving medical practitioner.

_____ **7.** An EMD is nothing more than a "call taker" who relays the initial dispatch information.

_____ **8.** The description of "feeling what the patient is feeling" is used to describe empathy.

_____ **9.** Saying to the patient, "Please feel welcome to tell me about that" is referred to as facilitation.

_____ **10.** People in a crisis could not care less about your nonverbal communications.

_____ **11.** It is okay to use pet names like "dolly" or "chief" with your patients.

_____ **12.** One of the most important treatments you can provide is reassurance.

_____ **13.** When caring for patients with alcoholism or behavioral problems, you will need to use patience and persistence.

_____ **14.** A paramedic who frowns or smirks during a patient interview is demonstrating empathy.

_____ **15.** You show respect to other cultures when you make an effort to learn their language.

Short Answer

Complete this section with short written answers using the space provided.

1. You are planning a radio system for your ambulance service, which consists of six vehicles serving an area of 150 square miles. List the components you will need, and state the function of each component.

Component	Function

2. To the paramedic who is knee-deep in mud while trying to extricate a patient involved in a motor vehicle crash, the dispatcher's job looks pretty easy. In fact, the job is not easy at all. List four tasks the dispatcher has to perform to ensure that the EMS system operates as it should.

a. ____

b. ____

c. ______________________________

d. ______________________________

3. According to the dictionary, communication is a process by which information is exchanged. In EMS, information must go back and forth in several different channels. Suppose you had to design the communications network for *your* EMS system. Who needs to be connected to whom? Draw a diagram to show those connections, or describe which parties should be in contact with one another.

4. Create a radio report from the ambulance to the emergency department (ED) for the following patient scenario. Be sure to include all findings, the care provided, and the status of improvement of the patient.

   You are en route to the hospital with a conscious, alert 58-year-old man who appears to be having an AMI. The estimated time of arrival (ETA) is about 20 minutes. With the patient's consent, you have mutually decided that the most appropriate facility to treat him is one that has a 24-hour interventional cardiac catheter lab.

   The patient's chief complaint is substernal chest pressure that was radiating down his left arm. It began after he started shoveling snow. He describes the pain initially to be 10 on a 10-point scale, with 10 being the worst pain he ever felt. He also states feeling nauseated and appears to be anxious and sweaty.

   His previous medical history includes hypertension and hypercholesterolemia. The patient states that he believes that his father had a heart attack when he was in his 40s. The patient is allergic to Novocain (procaine; causes nausea). He takes 81 mg of aspirin daily PO. He also takes atorvastatin (Lipitor). The patient ate lunch 3 hours ago and was directed to self-administer 162 mg of aspirin by the EMD.

   The patient's exam includes bilateral crackles in the bases, pulse of 110 beats/min, BP of 146/82 mm Hg, and Spo_2 of 94%. He is on high-flow supplemental oxygen via non-rebreathing mask. The 12-lead ECG indicates a sinus tachycardia and elevations in V_3 and V_4.

   The patient has been treated with morphine, oxygen, nitroglycerin, and self-administered aspirin.

____

____

____

____

____

____

____

____

____

____

____

____

____

____

____

Fill in the Table

Fill in the table with the International Radiotelephony Phonetic Alphabet.

A		J		S	
B		K		T	
C		L		U	
D		M		V	
E		N		W	
F		O		X	
G		P		Y	
H		Q		Z	
I		R			

CHAPTER 6

Documentation

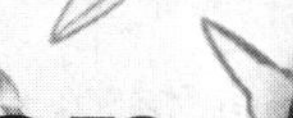

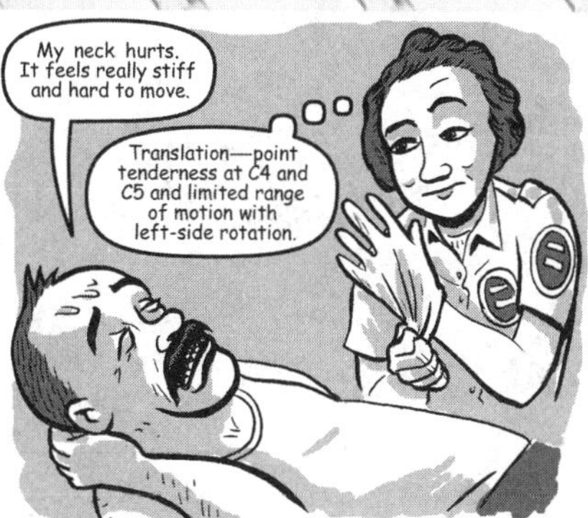

Matching

Part I

It does little good to take a careful history and conduct a thorough physical examination if you cannot communicate your findings to others. To do so, you need to know how to organize those findings in such a way that other medical professionals will be able to read your patient care report (PCR) and get a good understanding of your assessment findings and management of the patient.

Label each of the following statements to indicate which part of the PCR pertains to each item.

______ **1.** There was no pedal edema (edema of the ankles).
______ **2.** The patient is allergic to penicillin.
______ **3.** The pain came on while he was watching television.
______ **4.** The blood pressure was 190/110 mm Hg.
______ **5.** He was administered supplemental oxygen by non-rebreathing mask at 12 L/min.
______ **6.** The patient is a 51-year-old man with chest pain.
______ **7.** The chest was clear.
______ **8.** His skin was pale, cold, and sweaty (diaphoretic).
______ **9.** The patient was transported in semi-Fowler position.
______ **10.** Nothing seemed to make the pain better or worse.
______ **11.** The pulse was 52 beats/min and full, with an occasional premature beat.
______ **12.** The neck veins were not distended.
______ **13.** There was no cyanosis of the lips.
______ **14.** The patient takes alumina/magnesia (Maalox) and cimetidine (Tagamet) regularly.
______ **15.** He also felt nauseated.
______ **16.** His abdomen was soft and nontender.
______ **17.** His respirations were 20 breaths/min and unlabored.
______ **18.** He was sitting in a chair and appeared to be frightened.
______ **19.** He is under the care of Dr. Tums for an ulcer.
______ **20.** He was alert and oriented to person, place, and day.
______ **21.** He denies any shortness of breath.
______ **22.** An 18-gauge IV was started with normal saline at TKO rate.
______ **23.** The pain radiates down his left arm.
______ **24.** The blood pressure came down to 170/90 mm Hg during transport.

A. Chief complaint
B. Part of the history of the present illness
C. Part of the patient's other medical history
D. Part of the description of the patient's general appearance
E. Part of the vital signs
F. Part of the physical examination
G. Part of the management
H. Part of the patient's condition during transport

_____ **25.** He describes the pain as squeezing.
_____ **26.** Breath sounds were clear bilaterally.
27. Rearrange the preceding 26 statements into the order in which they should be presented.

(1)_________	(10)_________	(19)_________
(2)_________	(11)_________	(20)_________
(3)_________	(12)_________	(21)_________
(4)_________	(13)_________	(22)_________
(5)_________	(14)_________	(23)_________
(6)_________	(15)_________	(24)_________
(7)_________	(16)_________	(25)_________
(8)_________	(17)_________	(26)_________
(9)_________	(18)_________	

Part II

Now try the same exercise with a patient who has been injured. Keeping in mind what you will need to document on your PCR, label each of the following statements to indicate which part of the PCR pertains to each item.

_____ **1.** The right leg was severely angulated at the midfemur.
_____ **2.** The pulse was 92 beats/min, weak, and regular.
_____ **3.** Bystanders state, "The car that hit him was traveling very fast."
_____ **4.** His medical ID bracelet says he is a diabetic.
_____ **5.** There is a bruise on the left forehead.
_____ **6.** His skin is pale, cool, and moist.
_____ **7.** He was secured to a scoop stretcher.
_____ **8.** The patient is a middle-aged man who was struck by a car while crossing the street.
_____ **9.** Respirations were 30 breaths/min, deep, and noisy; blood pressure was 160/100 mm Hg.
_____ **10.** The patient was unresponsive and did not withdraw from painful stimuli.
_____ **11.** An OPA was inserted, and supplementary oxygen was given by non-rebreathing mask at 12 L/min.
_____ **12.** He apparently staggered into the street without looking, as if he were drunk.
_____ **13.** Chest wall was stable, and breath sounds were equal bilaterally.
_____ **14.** We put the right leg in a traction splint.
_____ **15.** The pupils were equal, midposition, and reactive to light.
_____ **16.** There was no change in his condition during transport.
_____ **17.** There was no blood or fluid draining from his nose or ears.
_____ **18.** His abdomen was soft.
_____ **19.** The dorsalis pedis pulses were equal.

A. Chief complaint
B. Part of the history of the present illness
C. Part of the patient's other medical history
D. Part of the description of the patient's general appearance
E. Part of the vital signs
F. Part of the physical examination
G. Part of the management condition during transport
H. Part of the patient's condition during transport

20. Rearrange the preceding 19 statements in the correct order for presentation.

(1)________ (8)________ (14)________

(2)________ (9)________ (15)________

(3)________ (10)________ (16)________

(4)________ (11)________ (17)________

(5)________ (12)________ (18)________

(6)________ (13)________ (19)________

(7)________

Part III

Sometimes you will be given information or obtain it in a sequence that needs to be rearranged into the standardized flow of information in which all health care professionals process a case. The following statements come from a patient's case history. Arrange them in the correct order for documentation on the PCR.

1. **A.** Pulse is 50 beats/min and regular, respirations are 36 breaths/min and deep, blood pressure is 180/126 mm Hg, and Spo_2 is 94%.
B. The patient has a history of hypertension.
C. The deep tendon reflexes are hyperactive.
D. Her daughter says the patient complained of a severe headache before she collapsed.
E. The patient was still conscious when we arrived, but she rapidly lost consciousness.
F. The patient is a 60-year-old woman who collapsed in the bathroom while sitting on the toilet.
G. We are administering supplemental oxygen at 12 L/min by non-rebreathing mask.
H. The patient's medications include nitroglycerin and methyldopa (Aldomet).
I. Her left pupil is larger than the right and does not react to light.
J. Daughter states, "She was well until this morning."
K. Her neck is somewhat stiff.
L. She was hospitalized 6 years ago for an AMI.

(1)________ (5)________ (9)________

(2)________ (6)________ (10)________

(3)________ (7)________ (11)________

(4)________ (8)________ (12)________

Multiple Choice

Read each item carefully, and then select the best response.

______ **1.** Which of the following would NOT be an example of a significant finding that indicates medical necessity for ambulance transport?

A. Patient is transported in an emergency mode per standard operating procedure (SOP).
B. Patient needs to be chemically and physically restrained.
C. Patient has no other means of transport for his doctor's appointment.
D. Patient has uncontrollable hemorrhage.

______ **2.** Patient data include the basic patient information collected on a PCR, which documents such information as the chief complaint and the:

A. call location.

B. assessment findings.

C. arrival time at the hospital.

D. disposition hospital.

______ **3.** A thorough patient refusal should involve documentation on the PCR of each of the following, EXCEPT:

A. your opinion that the patient is a system abuser.

B. the willingness of EMS to return.

C. evidence that the patient is able to make rational, informed decisions.

D. discussion with medical control according to protocols.

______ **4.** In most states, the paramedic is required to provide a supplemental report, aside from the PCR, in the case of a:

A. patient injured in a car crash.

B. cardiac arrest patient.

C. child who was abused.

D. burn patient.

______ **5.** Each of the following is a method used to organize the narrative section of the PCR, EXCEPT:

A. body systems/parts approach.

B. AVPU.

C. CHARTE method.

D. SOAP method.

______ **6.** Proper documentation is an essential job function of a paramedic. Today, in the majority of the jurisdictions in the United States, this formal *written* report is referred to as a:

A. trip sheet.

B. patient care report.

C. call sheet.

D. contact file.

______ **7.** PCRs may be used as all of the following, EXCEPT:

A. a patient description for the media.

B. legal documents.

C. quality assurance reviews.

D. billing documents.

______ **8.** Different EMS systems might use a variety of report-writing formats. Which of the following is an example of a report-writing format?

A. HEARSAY

B. TALK

C. SOAP

D. SAMPLE

______ **9.** Patients may have the ability and right to refuse medical care. Which of the following patients would have an appropriate case for refusing care?

A. A 10-year-old boy who was injured in a skateboard crash

B. A 28-year-old woman who fell off a barstool and struck her head

C. A 19-year-old woman who is conscious and alert

D. A 70-year-old man who called for assistance and was found shivering in an unheated house

______ **10.** When a paramedic discovers that he or she has made a documentation error on a paper PCR, it is okay for the paramedic to take which of the following actions?

A. Erase or "white out" the mistake.

B. Destroy the original report, and rewrite the report without the error.

C. Draw a single line through the error, initial it, and insert the correct information next to it.

D. Have the paramedic's partner write an addendum.

Fill in the Blank

How to Write a Narrative

Paramedics write a narrative on almost every call. Next to each topic in the following list, fill in the items you should include for each.

1. Standard precautions: ______________________________

2. Scene safety: ______________________________

3. MOI/NOI: ______________________________

4. Number of patients: ______________________________

5. Additional resources: ______________________________

6. Cervical spine: ______________________________

7. Initial general impression: ______________________________

8. LOC: ______________________________

9. Chief complaint: ______________________________

10. Life threats: ______________________________ ______________

11. ABCDE: ______________________________ ______________

12. Oxygen: ______________________________ ______________

13. Primary survey, patient history, secondary assessment, or reassessment: ________ ______________

____

14. SAMPLE/OPQRST: ______________________________ ______________

15. Vital signs: ______________________________ ______________

16. Medical direction: ______________________________ ______________

17. Management of secondary injuries/treat for shock: ______________ ______________

Identify

After reading the following case history, provide the indicated information for a PCR.

The patient is a 53-year-old woman who called 9-1-1 because she was having chest pain. She described the pain as a pressure in the center of the chest, with numbness of her left arm, which was present for 30 minutes. The pain was accompanied by difficulty in breathing with no relief. The patient denied vomiting but has some nausea and has been sweating profusely. She is known to have angina and takes nitroglycerin at home; she took one nitroglycerin dose today, without relief. She denies any history of hypertension or diabetes. She has been treated for asthma in the past.

On physical examination, the patient was sitting bolt upright; she appeared alert and apprehensive and was in moderate respiratory distress, breathing shallowly at 26 breaths/min. Pulse was 136 beats/min, weak and regular; blood pressure was 180/82 mm Hg; and Spo_2 was 95%. Her neck veins were distended to the angle of the jaw at 45°. Rales were heard at both lung bases, and auscultation of the heart revealed a gallop rhythm. The abdomen was not distended. There was no pedal edema.

The patient was given supplemental oxygen by non-rebreathing mask at 12 L/min, and a 12-lead ECG was acquired and transmitted because there was evidence of an ST segment elevation myocardial infarction (STEMI). She was transported to St.

Joseph's Hospital cath lab in semi-Fowler position. An IV of normal saline at to keep open (TKO) was started, and she was given 5 mg morphine, 324 mg acetylsalicylic acid (ASA), and nitroglycerin. Her vital signs remained stable throughout transport.

1. Chief complaint:

____

____

2. History of the present illness:

____

____

3. Other medical history:

____

____

4. General appearance:

____

____

5. Vital signs:

____

____

6. Physical exam:

____

____

7. Management:

____

____

8. Pertinent negatives:

____

____

True/False

If you believe the statement to be more true than false, write the letter "T" in the space provided. If you believe the statement to be more false than true, write the letter "F."

_____ 1. Times used to document actions on a PCR generally use Greenwich Mean Time (GMT).

_____ 2. To document time accurately, paramedics should "synchronize" their watches with the public safety access point (PSAP).

_____ 3. Accurate documentation depends on all information being provided, including times, narrative, and check boxes.

_____ 4. A false statement written about a patient could be considered libel.

_____ 5. It is not acceptable practice to "document findings to meet medical necessity standards" to help bring in revenue.

______ 6. To ensure that data can be shared on a national level, electronic documentation systems need not be National Emergency Medical Services Information System (NEMSIS) compliant.

______ 7. The military time for 1 hour after noon is 1300 hours.

______ 8. In a suspected child abuse case, it is best to document your objective findings and allow the legal system to investigate and make the ultimate determination of abuse or neglect.

______ 9. Your PCR may be used in legal proceedings against you or someone else and is the only record of the care you provided and why.

______ 10. Falsifying information on the PCR may result in suspension and/or revocation of your certification/license.

Short Answer

Complete this section with short written answers using the space provided.

1. A PCR must also contain other information besides that found in a traditional medical history. List at least one other item of information that needs to be recorded on a PCR, and explain why that information is important.

   a. Information that should be recorded:

   ____

   ____

   ____

   b. Why that information is important:

   ____

   ____

   ____

2. Give two reasons why you should make certain that your PCR is as accurate and complete as possible.

   a.

   ____

   ____

   ____

   b.

   ____

   ____

   ____

3. Give specifics to document for each of the following topics:

   a. Number of patients:

   ____

   ____

   ____

b. Standard precautions:

____

____

____

c. MOI/NOI:

____

____

____

d. Oxygen:

____

____

____

Complete the Patient Care Report

This feature will be found in a number of the chapters of this workbook. Read the incident scenario, and then complete the following PCR.

You and your partner are posted at the corner of 2nd Avenue and 14th Street, completing the paperwork for a recent diabetic call, when the dispatcher calls your unit. "Medic 185," the dispatcher says immediately.

"Medcom 185," you respond.

"Medic 185, Charlie response to 3-5-5 East 16th Street for a male with severe bleeding. Show your time of dispatch at sixteen fifty-three."

You copy the assignment and slowly roll out into traffic after activating the lights and siren, proceeding to the address, which is about six blocks away.

Five minutes later, you pull up outside a well-kept apartment house with a parking spot right in front of the building and are met by a woman frantically waving her arms.

"Please hurry!" She shouts as you open your door. "My husband was working with an electric saw in the basement and has a really deep cut on his leg. He's bleeding really bad!"

You and your partner grab your bags and walk down a flight of stairs into the basement area, where there is a woodshop. The man, whom you estimate to weigh about 170 pounds, is sitting on a pile of wood, pale and shaking, holding an old, bloody T-shirt against his lower left leg. A huge circle of blood is soaking into the wood pile under him.

"Sir, we're from the ambulance service, and we're here to help you," you say, kneeling next to the man. "Can you tell me what happened?"

As the 42-year-old man describes how the saw glanced off of a knot in the shelving he was cutting, sending it deep into the flesh of his leg, you remove the T-shirt from the wound—observing a jagged laceration approximately 9 cm long—and replace it with a wide trauma dressing. Your partner then places a non-rebreathing mask on the patient with the supplemental oxygen set to 15 L/min and begins assessing vital signs.

At 1704 hours, your partner reports the patient's vital signs as follows: systolic blood pressure (BP), 136; diastolic BP, 86; pulse, 128, strong and regular; respirations, 16, with good tidal volume; pale, cool, and diaphoretic skin; and pulse oximetry, 94%.

About 5 minutes after obtaining vital signs, you have stopped the bleeding using a pressure bandage and are loading the patient into the ambulance, keeping him covered with a blanket and in the supine position.

His wife tells you that he is allergic to amoxicillin and that he has been taking a cholesterol medication called Crestor ever since he suffered a transient ischemic attack in the spring of last year. You thank her for the information and climb into the patient compartment while your partner jumps into the driver's seat. Within a minute, you are en route to the emergency department (ED) and taking the patient's vital signs again.

This time they are as follows: systolic BP, 122; diastolic BP, 76; pulse, 136, weak and regular; respirations, 20 and shallow but with adequate tidal volume; skin still pale, cool, and diaphoretic; and pulse oximetry, 94%.

At 1715, you arrive at the ambulance bay of the Beth Israel Medical Center, quickly move the patient inside, and transfer his care to the ED staff. After giving a full report to the receiving nurse and properly cleaning and preparing the ambulance, you and your partner go back available at 1735.

EMS Patient Care Report (PCR)

Date:	Incident No.:	Nature of Call:	Location:

Dispatched:	En Route:	At Scene:	Transport:	At Hospital:	In Service:

Patient Information

Age:	Allergies:
Sex:	Medications:
Weight (in kg [lb]):	Past Medical History:
	Chief Complaint:

Vital Signs

Time:	BP:	Pulse:	Respirations:	SpO_2:
Time:	BP:	Pulse:	Respirations:	SpO_2:
Time:	BP:	Pulse:	Respirations:	SpO_2:

EMS Treatment
(circle all that apply)

Oxygen @ ______ L/min via (circle one): NC NRM Bag-mask device		Assisted Ventilation	Airway Adjunct	CPR
Defibrillation	Bleeding Control	Bandaging	Splinting	Other:

Narrative

CHAPTER 7

Medical Terminology

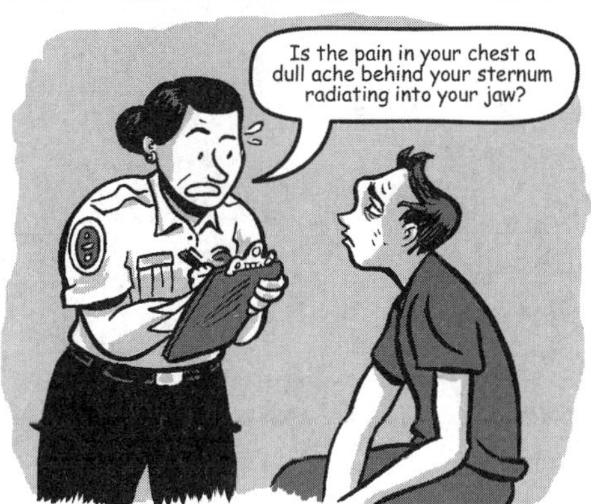

Beware the leading question!

Matching

Part I

Match each of the definitions in the left column to the appropriate term in the right column.

	Definition	Term
_____	**1.** The straightening of a joint.	**A.** Abduction
_____	**2.** The posterior surface of the body, including the back of the hand.	**B.** Adduction
_____	**3.** Farther inside the body and away from the skin.	**C.** Anatomic position
_____	**4.** An imaginary plane in which the body is cut into front and back portions.	**D.** Anterior
_____	**5.** A word containing more than one word root.	**E.** Anteroposterior axis
_____	**6.** A word root followed by a vowel.	**F.** Antonyms
_____	**7.** Rotating an extremity at its joint away from the midline.	**G.** Apex
_____	**8.** The name of a disease, device, procedure, or drug that is based on the person who invented, discovered, or first described it.	**H.** Bilateral
_____	**9.** Farther from the trunk and nearer to the free end of the extremity.	**I.** Combining form
_____	**10.** The product of slicing an object cross-wise, perpendicular to its long axis.	**J.** Combining vowel
_____	**11.** On the opposite side of the body.	**K.** Compound word
_____	**12.** The vowel used to combine two word roots or a word root and a prefix or suffix.	**L.** Contralateral
_____	**13.** In anatomy, a body part or condition that appears on both sides of the midline.	**M.** Coronal plane
_____	**14.** Pairs of word roots, prefixes, or suffixes that have opposite meanings.	**N.** Cross section
_____	**15.** The front surface of the body; the side facing you in the anatomic position.	**O.** Deep
_____	**16.** Movement of a limb toward the midline.	**P.** Distal
_____	**17.** The pointed extremity of a conical structure.	**Q.** Dorsal
_____	**18.** The axis that runs perpendicular to the coronal plane.	**R.** Eponym
_____	**19.** The position of reference, in which the patient stands facing you, arms at the side, with the palms of the hands facing forward.	**S.** Extension
_____	**20.** Movement of a limb away from the midline.	**T.** External rotation

Part II

Match each of the definitions in the left column to the appropriate term in the right column.

	Definition	Term
_____	**1.** Turning the palms downward.	**A.** Flexion
_____	**2.** In anatomy, the back surface of the body; the side away from you in the standard anatomic position.	**B.** Fowler position
_____	**3.** The forward-facing part of the hand in the anatomic position.	**C.** Homonyms
_____	**4.** Lying flat, face down.	**D.** Horizontal axis

______	5. Part of a term that appears before a word root, changing the meaning of the term.	E. Hyperextension
______	6. The sole or bottom surface of the foot.	F. Hyperflexion
______	7. An imaginary vertical line drawn from the middle of the forehead through the nose and the umbilicus to the floor.	G. Inferior
______	8. The view of an object cut along its long axis.	H. Internal rotation
______	9. In anatomy, parts of the body that lie farther from the midline.	I. Ipsilateral
______	10. Rotating the anterior surface of an extremity toward the midline.	J. Lateral
______	11. Maximum flexion or flexion beyond the normal range of motion.	K. Longitudinal axis
______	12. The axis that runs perpendicular to the sagittal plane; also called the mediolateral axis.	L. Longitudinal section
______	13. A sitting position, with the head elevated at a 90° angle.	M. Medial
______	14. The bending of a joint.	N. Midsagittal plane
______	15. Words that sound alike but are spelled differently and have different meanings.	O. Palmar
______	16. Maximum extension or extension beyond the normal range of motion.	P. Plantar
______	17. Below or closer to the feet.	Q. Posterior
______	18. On the same side of the body.	R. Prefix
______	19. The axis that runs perpendicular to the transverse plane.	S. Pronation
______	20. Closer to the midline.	T. Prone

Multiple Choice

Read each item carefully, and then select the best response.

______ **1.** Most medical terms have origins in the _______ or ________ language.

A. French; Italian
B. English; Roman
C. Greek; Latin
D. German; Russian

______ **2.** The language of medicine includes many eponyms and terms that have resulted from advances and discoveries. Which of the following is NOT considered an eponym?

A. McBurney point
B. Dysphagia
C. Apgar score
D. Levine sign

______ **3.** The portion of a medical term that appears before the root word is called the:

A. combining vowel.
B. suffix.
C. prefix.
D. antonym.

______ **4.** When comparing the terms or parts of terms listed here, which are NOT synonyms?

A. pulmon/o and pneum/o
B. dextro and sinister/o
C. nephr/o and ren/o
D. angi/o and vas/o

______ **5.** Each of the following is considered a common numerical prefix, EXCEPT:

A. deca-.
B. octo-.
C. quad-.
D. cardio-.

_____ **6.** Which common numerical prefix would be found in the word used to describe a congenital anomaly involving four anatomic abnormalities of the heart?
A. bi-
B. tetra-
C. quint-
D. multi-

_____ **7.** The root words used in medicine often describe a color. Which root is used for the color green?
A. alb-
B. polio/o
C. chlor/o
D. cirrh/o

_____ **8.** The imaginary plane that would divide the body into right and left sides is called the:
A. coronal plane.
B. sagittal plane.
C. transverse plane.
D. frontal plane.

_____ **9.** Terminology associated with the body region of the stomach would use the term:
A. buccal.
B. axillary.
C. cutaneous.
D. gastric.

_____ **10.** Which of the following terms means "pertaining to the skin"?
A. Gluteal
B. Inguinal
C. Cutaneous
D. Lumbar

_____ **11.** Which of the following terms means "pertaining to the armpit"?
A. Brachial
B. Axillary
C. Hepatic
D. Cranial

_____ **12.** Which of the following terms means "pertaining to the sole of the foot or the palm of the hand"?
A. Volar
B. Sacral
C. Perineal
D. Renal

_____ **13.** The common directional term used to describe the area closest to the point of attachment is:
A. posterior.
B. distal.
C. lateral.
D. proximal.

_____ **14.** The common directional term used to describe the area closest to the head is:
A. superficial.
B. superior.
C. inferior.
D. ventral.

_____ 15. To avoid potentially dangerous mistakes, the paramedic should always write down medication doses:
- **A.** by spelling out the full trade name.
- **B.** without trailing zeros and naked decimals.
- **C.** twice for clarity.
- **D.** All of the above

Fill in the Blank

Read each item carefully, and then complete the statement by filling in the missing word(s).

1. The __________ around the heart is called the _________.
2. The term __________ refers to ______ or through the vagina.
3. The term __________ refers to below or at the _______ of the thorax.
4. During pregnancy, when the embryo develops outside the _______, it is called a(n) _________ pregnancy.
5. A(n) __________ who is pregnant for the ________ time is called a primigravida.
6. A woman who has had __________ pregnancies resulting in ______ live births is called a quintipara.
7. The inflammation of an organ, such as __________ of the liver, causes yellow-orange pigmentation of the ________.
8. The __________ blood cell that contains hemoglobin to carry ______ is called a(n) __________.
9. The ___________ passing horizontally through the body at the waist, creating top and bottom portions, is referred to as the ________ plane.
10. The __________ in the __________ is referred to as the deltoid.

True/False

If you believe the statement to be more true than false, write the letter "T" in the space provided. If you believe the statement to be more false than true, write the letter "F."

_____ 1. *Abdominal* means "pertaining to the abdomen."

_____ 2. *Brachial* means "pertaining to the upper arm."

_____ 3. *Cranial* means "pertaining to the superior segment."

_____ 4. The term meaning "pertaining to the buttocks" is *buccal*.

_____ 5. *Inguinal* means "pertaining to the depressions in the abdominal wall near the thighs."

_____ 6. *Lumbar* means "pertaining to the loin."

_____ 7. *Plantar* means "relating to the palm of the hand."

_____ 8. The inferior, posterior region of the head is called the occipital.

_____ 9. Males do not have an umbilical region.

_____ 10. The vessel in the posterior knee is the popliteal.

_____ 11. The range of motion is the full range over which a joint can move.

_____ 12. In the anatomic position, all extremities are in extension.

_____ 13. The abduction of an extremity moves it toward the midline.

_____ 14. *Internal rotation* means turning the anterior portion of an extremity away from the midline.

_____ 15. The term *ipsilateral* refers to the same side of the body.

CHAPTER 8

Anatomy and Physiology

You have to consume something besides caffeine, fat, and sugar. How else can you pass the recertification exam?

Nutritional deficiencies have been shown to result in depression of bone marrow function and reduction in white blood cell development.

Matching

Part I

Match each of the definitions in the left column to the appropriate term in the right column.

_____ **1.** A pathologic condition resulting from the accumulation of acids in the body (blood pH less than 7.35).

_____ **2.** Any molecule that can give up a hydrogen ion, thereby increasing the concentration of hydrogen ions in a water solution.

_____ **3.** The socket formed by the coxal (hip) bone into which the ball-shaped femoral head fits snugly.

_____ **4.** A neurotransmitter released at synapses within the autonomic nervous system and by motor neurons to stimulate skeletal muscle contraction.

_____ **5.** The commonly used blood classification system, based on the antigens present or absent in the blood.

_____ **6.** The muscles not normally used during quiet breathing; examples include the sternocleidomastoid muscles of the neck, the chest pectoralis major muscles, and the abdominal muscles.

_____ **7.** The ability of the lens of the eye to change its shape to focus on a close object.

_____ **8.** The building of larger substances from smaller substances, such as the building of proteins from amino acids.

_____ **9.** The air sacs of the lungs in which the exchange of oxygen and carbon dioxide takes place; also, the bony sockets for the teeth that reside in the mandible and maxilla.

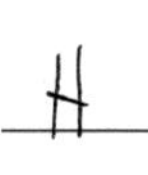 **10.** The tip of the shoulder and the site of attachment for the clavicle and various shoulder muscles.

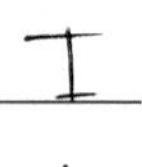 **11.** The sequence of changes in the membrane potential that occurs when an excitable cell (neuron or muscle) is stimulated.

_____ **12.** The outer layer of the adrenal gland; it produces hormones that are important in regulating the water and salt balance of the body.

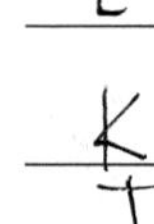 **13.** The temporary or permanent reduction of sensitivity to a particular stimulus.

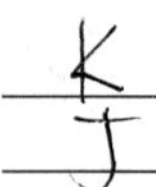 **14.** A method used to move compounds across a cell membrane to create or maintain an imbalance of charges, usually against a concentration gradient and requiring the expenditure of energy.

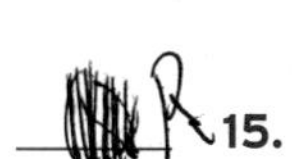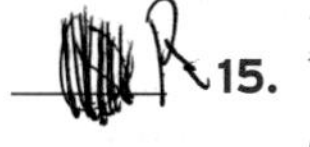 **15.** Variant forms of a gene, which can be identical or slightly different in a sequence of deoxyribonucleic acid.

A. ABO system
B. Accessory muscles
C. Accommodation
D. Acetabulum
E. Acetylcholine
F. Acid
G. Acidosis
H. Acromion process
I. Action potential
J. Active transport
K. Adaptation
L. Adrenal cortex
M. Adrenergic
N. Aerobic metabolism
O. Afterload

	Definition	Term
______	**16.** A pathologic condition resulting from the accumulation of bases in the body (blood pH greater than 7.45).	**P.** Aldosterone
______	**17.** The pressure in the aorta against which the left ventricle must pump blood.	**Q.** Alkalosis
______	**18.** A hormone responsible for the reabsorption of sodium and water from the kidney tubules.	**R.** Alleles
______	**19.** Metabolism that can proceed only in the presence of oxygen.	**S.** Alveoli
______	**20.** Having the characteristics of the sympathetic division of the autonomic nervous system.	**T.** Anabolism

Part II

Match each of the definitions in the left column to the appropriate term in the right column.

	Definition	Term
______	**1.** Nerve endings that are stimulated by pressure changes, including increased arterial blood pressure; they are located in the aortic arch and carotid sinuses.	**A.** Angle of Louis
______	**2.** White blood cells that contain histamine granules and other substances that are released during inflammatory and allergic responses.	**B.** Antagonist
______	**3.** Long, slender extension of a neuron (nerve cell) that conducts electrical impulses away from the nerve cell body to adjacent cells.	**C.** Aorta
______	**4.** The chromosomes that do not carry the genes that determine sex.	**D.** Aortic valve
______	**5.** Imaginary line joining the positive and negative electrodes of a lead; also the second cervical vertebra.	**E.** Appendicular skeleton
______	**6.** The portion of the skeleton made up of the skull, thoracic cage, and vertebral column.	**F.** Aqueous humor
______	**7.** The area of the brain between the spinal cord and cerebrum that contains the midbrain, pons, and medulla; it controls functions that are necessary for life, such as breathing.	**G.** Arytenoid cartilages
______	**8.** Soft tissue that fills the inside of bones and is the site of production of red blood cells, platelets, and most white blood cells.	**H.** Astigmatism
______	**9.** A layer of tightly adhered cells that protects the brain and spinal cord from exposure to medications, toxins, and infectious particles.	**I.** Atlas
______	**10.** The ability of cardiac pacemaker cells to initiate an electrical impulse spontaneously without being stimulated by another source (such as a nerve).	**J.** Atrioventricular node
______	**11.** A group of cells that conduct an electrical impulse through the heart; located in the floor of the right atrium immediately behind the tricuspid valve and near the opening of the coronary sinus.	**K.** Automaticity
______	**12.** A molecule that blocks the ability of a given chemical to bind to its receptor, preventing a biologic response.	**L.** Autosomes
______	**13.** A prominence of the sternum that indicates the point where the second rib joins the sternum; also called the sternal angle or manubriosternal junction.	**M.** Axial skeleton
______	**14.** Watery fluid filling the anterior eye cavity; the quantity determines the intraocular pressure, which is critical to sight.	**N.** Axis
______	**15.** The portion of the skeletal system made up of the upper extremities, shoulder girdle, pelvic girdle, and lower extremities.	**O.** Axon
______	**16.** The semilunar valve that regulates blood flow from the left ventricle to the aorta.	**P.** Baroreceptors
______	**17.** The principal artery leaving the left side of the heart and carrying freshly oxygenated blood to the body; the largest artery in the body.	**Q.** Basophils
______	**18.** The first cervical vertebra (C1), which provides support for the head.	**R.** Blood-brain barrier
______	**19.** A condition where parts of the image are out of focus and others are in focus; caused by irregularities in the shape of the eye lens.	**S.** Bone marrow
______	**20.** Six paired cartilages stacked on top of each other in the larynx.	**T.** Brainstem

Part III

Match each of the definitions in the left column to the appropriate term in the right column.

		Definition	Term
O	**1.**	A thin, flap-like structure that allows air to pass into the trachea but prevents food and liquid from entering.	**A.** Depolarization
______	**2.**	A leukocyte that may play a role following infection in various areas in the body.	**B.** Dermatome
______	**3.**	Substances designed to speed up the rate of specific biochemical reactions.	**C.** Diaphragm
______	**4.**	The layer of the serous pericardium that lies closely against the heart; also called the visceral pericardium.	**D.** Diaphysis
______	**5.**	Glands that have no ducts and secrete chemicals directly into tissue fluid or blood.	**E.** Diastole
______	**6.**	Salt or acid substances that become ionic conductors when dissolved in a solvent (such as water); chemicals dissolved in the blood.	**F.** Diencephalon
______	**7.**	The outermost of the three meninges that enclose the brain and spinal cord; the toughest meningeal layer.	**G.** Diffusion
______	**8.**	The thin membrane lining the inside of the heart.	**H.** Dura mater
______	**9.**	Glands that secrete chemicals into ducts that open onto a surface for elimination.	**I.** Electrolytes
______	**10.**	The passive part of the breathing process, in which the diaphragm and the intercostal muscles relax, forcing air out of the lungs.	**J.** Endocardium
______	**11.**	The ability of cardiac muscle cells to respond to an electrical, chemical, or mechanical stimulus.	**K.** Endocrine glands
______	**12.**	A branch of the internal auditory canal that connects the middle ear to the oropharynx.	**L.** Enzymes
______	**13.**	A hormone released from the ovaries that stimulates the uterine lining during the menstrual cycle.	**M.** Eosinophil
______	**14.**	The rapid movement of electrolytes across a cell membrane in response to an action potential, which changes the overall charge of the cell; the main catalyst for muscle contractions and neural transmissions.	**N.** Epicardium
______	**15.**	The area of the skin supplied by a specific sensory spinal nerve.	**O.** Epiglottis
______	**16.**	The portion of the brain between the brainstem and the cerebrum; contains the epithalamus, thalamus, hypothalamus, and subthalamus.	**P.** Estrogen
______	**17.**	The process of particles moving from an area of higher concentration to an area of lower concentration along a concentration gradient until equilibrium is achieved.	**Q.** Eustachian tube
______	**18.**	The shaft of a long bone.	**R.** Excitability
______	**19.**	The large skeletal muscle that plays a major role in breathing and separates the chest cavity from the abdominal cavity.	**S.** Exhalation
______	**20.**	The phase of the cardiac cycle in which the atria and ventricles relax between contractions and blood enters these chambers.	**T.** Exocrine glands

Part IV

Match the following types of epithelial tissue with their function and/or location in the human body.

		Tissue	Function/Location
______	**1.**	Simple squamous	**A.** Distensibility, protection of the inner urinary bladder lining
______	**2.**	Simple cuboidal	**B.** Protection of the outer layer of the skin
______	**3.**	Simple columnar	**C.** Protection of gland ducts, pancreas, and salivary glands
______	**4.**	Pseudostratified columnar	**D.** Absorption and secretion in the kidney tubule linings
______	**5.**	Stratified squamous	**E.** Protection and secretion in part of male urethra and parts of pharynx
______	**6.**	Stratified cuboidal	**F.** Secretion in the endocrine, salivary, and sweat glands
______	**7.**	Stratified columnar	**G.** Movement of mucus, protection and secretion in respiratory passage linings
______	**8.**	Transitional	**H.** Diffusion, filtration, osmosis, covering of surfaces in air sacs of lungs and blood vessels
______	**9.**	Glandular	**I.** Absorption, protection, and secretion in the intestine, stomach, and uterine lining

Multiple Choice

Read each item carefully, and then select the best response.

D 1. All of the cells in the body, with the exception of the __________, have between a hundred and a few thousand organelles called __________, which are the powerhouses of the cell.

- A. white blood cells; lysosomes
- B. red blood cells; Golgi apparatus
- C. white blood cells; endoplasmic reticulum
- D. red blood cells; mitochondria

B 2. The movement of a solvent from an area of low solute concentration to one of high concentration through a selectively permeable membrane is called:

- A. facilitated diffusion.
- B. osmosis.
- C. active transport.
- D. differentiation.

C 3. There are 230 joints in the human body. The most complex joints, which allow free movement and are surrounded by an outer layer of ligaments forming a capsule, are called the:

- A. fibrous joints.
- B. cartilaginous joints.
- C. synovial joints.
- D. immovable joints.

C 4. The kidneys are found in which body cavity?

- A. Thoracic
- B. Abdominal
- C. Retroperitoneal
- D. Pelvic

_____ 5. The proximal end of the humerus articulates with the:

- A. clavicle.
- B. glenoid fossa.
- C. scapula.
- D. acromion process.

_____ 6. The neurotransmitter that stimulates skeletal muscle to contract is called:

- A. sarcoplasmic reticulum.
- B. myosin.
- C. actin.
- D. acetylcholine.

_____ 7. The muscle group located in the anterior femur is called the:

- A. gastrocnemius.
- B. rectus abdominis.
- C. quadriceps.
- D. triceps.

_____ 8. The muscle group that points the toes away from the head is called the:

- A. gastrocnemius.
- B. rectus abdominis.
- C. tibialis anterior.
- D. pectoralis.

_____ **9.** The heart valve that separates the left atrium from the left ventricle is called the __________ valve and is a __________ valve.

A. semilunar; tricuspid
B. pulmonic; bicuspid
C. mitral; bicuspid
D. aortic; tricuspid

_____ **10.** What percentage of the blood is made up of plasma?

A. 0.9%
B. 25%
C. 45%
D. 55%

_____ **11.** Of the following vessels, which is designed to withstand the highest pressures of any vessel in the body?

A. Common carotid artery
B. Ascending aorta
C. Brachial artery
D. Inferior vena cava

_____ **12.** The specialized portion of the venous system that drains blood from the stomach, intestines, and spleen is called the:

A. hepatic portal system.
B. lymphatic system.
C. abdominal aortic aneurism.
D. renal residual circulation.

_____ **13.** What percentage of the plasma is water?

A. 26%
B. 48%
C. 72%
D. 92%

_____ **14.** Which of the following substances found in the plasma of the blood is NOT considered a protein?

A. Albumin
B. Sodium bicarbonate
C. Globulin
D. Fibrinogen

_____ **15.** The occipital lobe of the brain is responsible for:

A. hearing, smell, and language.
B. vision and storage of visual memories.
C. basic emotions and basic reflexes, such as chewing.
D. judgment and predicting the consequences of actions.

_____ **16.** Which portion of the brain is responsible for emotions, temperature control, and interface with the endocrine system?

A. Occipital lobe
B. Temporal lobe
C. Prefrontal area
D. Diencephalon

_____ **17.** The fifth cranial nerve is called the:

A. optic nerve.
B. oculomotor nerve.
C. vagus nerve.
D. trigeminal nerve.

_____ **18.** The ninth cranial nerve is called the:

A. oculomotor nerve.
B. glossopharyngeal nerve.
C. facial nerve.
D. abducens nerve.

_____ **19.** The cranial nerve that is responsible for the sense of hearing and balance is the __________ cranial nerve.

A. 3rd
B. 8th
C. 9th
D. 10th

_____ **20.** When a patient has __________, the eyes may be oriented correctly, but one fails to send adequate signals to the vision center, causing a loss of depth perception and poor-quality images.

A. strabismus
B. amblyopia
C. macular degeneration
D. a blind spot

Fill in the Blank

Read each item carefully, and then complete the statement by filling in the missing word(s).

1. The __________ is a large, solid organ that takes up most of the area immediately beneath the diaphragm. The __________ is an outpouching from the bile ducts that serves as a reservoir and concentrating organ for __________ produced in the liver.

2. The __________ __________ is the major hollow organ of the abdomen whose cells produce enzymes and mucus to aid in digestion. The __________ __________ consists of the cecum, the __________, and the rectum.

3. The __________ system is made up of various glands located throughout the body. These glands release __________ such as insulin into the bloodstream. The major __________ glands include the pituitary, thyroid, and adrenal glands. The major __________ glands include the sweat glands, which secrete outside the body.

4. Let's review the pituitary gland hormones. The __________ hormone increases the size and division rate of body cells. The __________-stimulating hormone controls the thyroid gland hormone secretion. The sex cell hormone that aids in the release of female egg cells is called the __________ hormone. The hormone __________ is designed to contract the uterine wall muscles as well as __________ milk–secreting gland muscles.

5. Let's review the functions of the female reproductive organs. The female reproductive organ that produces oocytes and sex hormones is(are) the __________. The __________ __________ transport secondary oocytes in the direction of the uterus so that fertilization can occur normally. The muscular organ in which implantation, __________ formation, and fetal development occur is the uterus. The uterine secretions are transported to the outside of the female's body by the __________. The __________ __________ protects and encloses the female's external reproductive organs, and the __________ __________ protects the openings of the vagina and the urethra, which are contained in the __________.

Labeling

1. Bones of the skull
Label the names of the bones in the cranium.

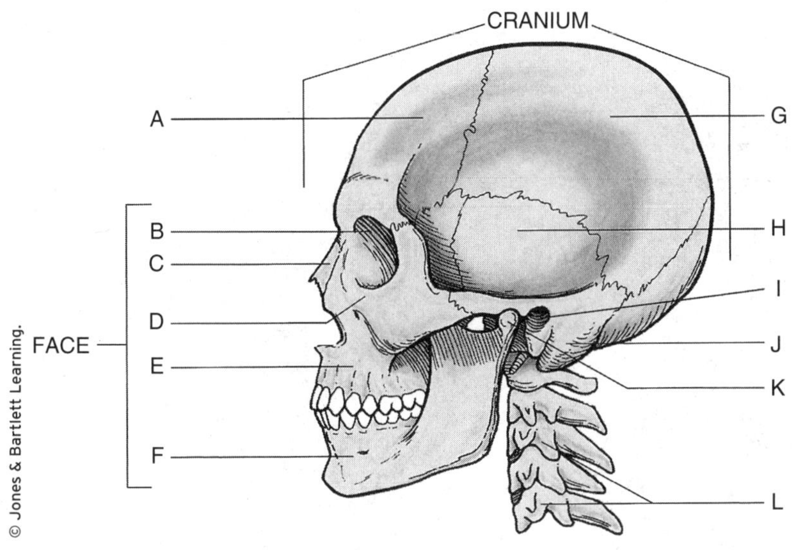

A. ______________________

B. ______________________

C. ______________________

D. ______________________

E. ______________________

F. ______________________

G. ______________________

H. ______________________

I. ______________________

J. ______________________

K. ______________________

L. ______________________

2. Lower extremity
Label the names of the principal parts of the lower extremity.

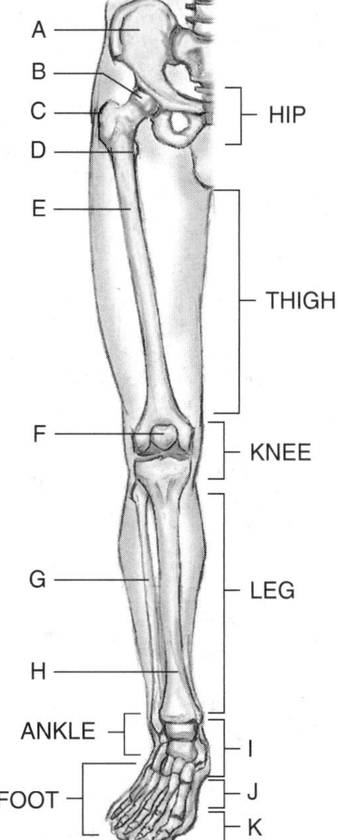

A. ______________________

B. ______________________

C. ______________________

D. ______________________

E. ______________________

F. ______________________

G. ______________________

H. ______________________

I. ______________________

J. ______________________

K. ______________________

3. Respiratory system

Label the names of the structures in the respiratory system.

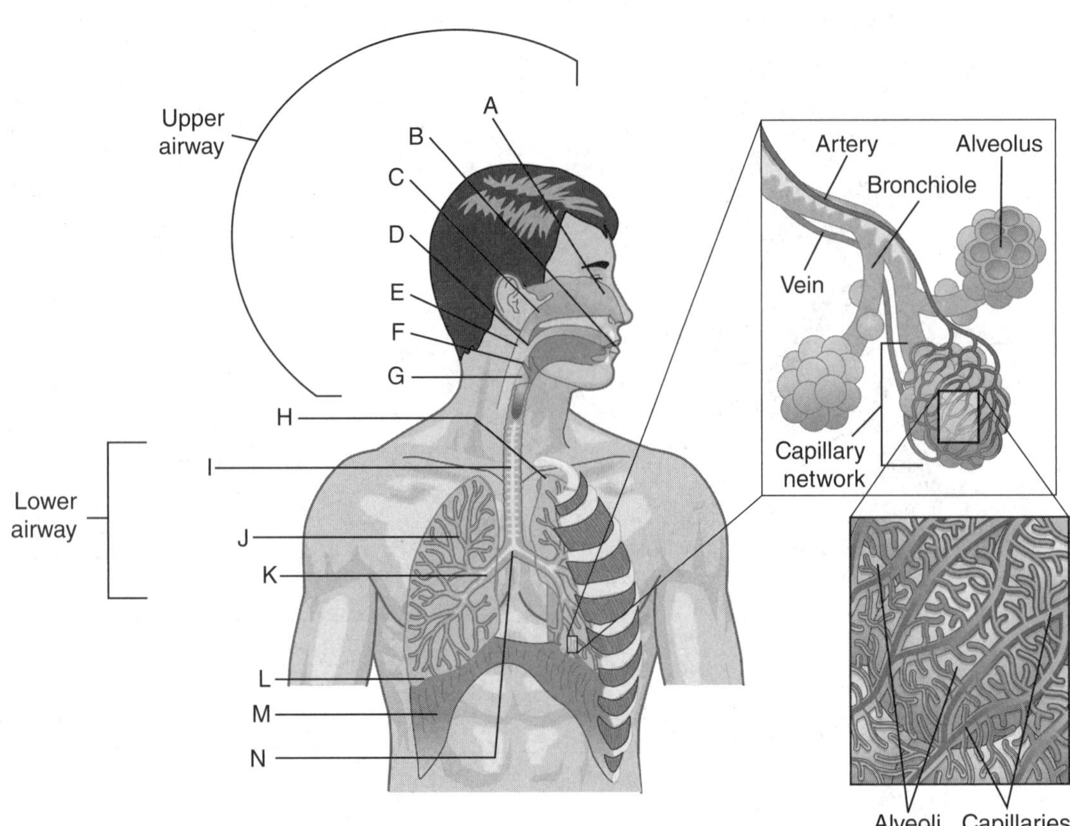

A. ______________________________

B. ______________________________

C. ______________________________

D. ______________________________

E. ______________________________

F. ______________________________

G. ______________________________

H. ______________________________

I. ______________________________

J. ______________________________

K. ______________________________

L. ______________________________

M. ______________________________

N. ______________________________

True/False

If you believe the statement to be more true than false, write the letter "T" in the space provided. If you believe the statement to be more false than true, write the letter "F."

_____ **1.** Parasympathetic stimulation can cause constriction of the pupil.

_____ **2.** Sympathetic stimulation can cause secretion of the hormone adrenalin.

_____ **3.** Parasympathetic stimulation can cause increased urination.

_____ **4.** Sympathetic stimulation causes increased emptying of the colon.

_____ **5.** Parasympathetic stimulation speeds up the heart.

_____ **6.** Sympathetic stimulation constricts the bronchioles.

_____ **7.** Parasympathetic stimulation increases the secretion of saliva.

_____ **8.** Sympathetic stimulation stops the secretion of the parotid gland.

_____ **9.** Parasympathetic stimulation increases the motility of the small intestines.

_____ **10.** The sympathetic division of the autonomic nervous system is responsible for the "rest and digest" reaction.

_____ **11.** The distal end of the radius articulates the irregularly shaped carpal bones of the wrist.

_____ **12.** The carpometacarpal joint of the thumb is a gliding joint.

_____ **13.** A plexus is an area where the spinal nerves come together and transmit their impulses to areas of the body through a common nerve.

_____ **14.** Four types of proteins make up myofilaments.

_____ **15.** The limbic system is responsible for fluid elimination in the body.

CHAPTER 9

Pathophysiology

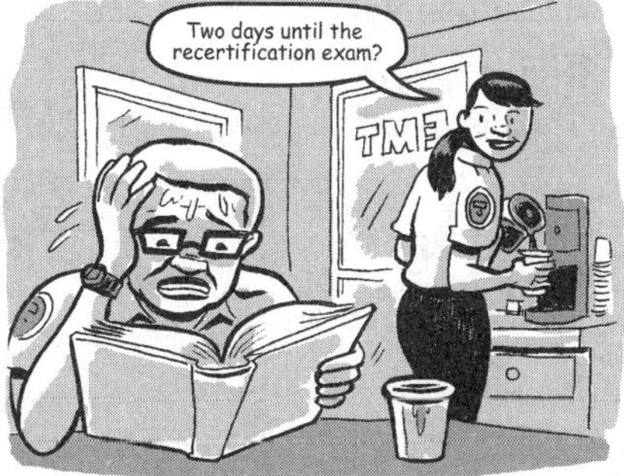

Excessive output can rapidly upset homeostasis; for example, severe perspiration, no matter what the reason, can cause excessive water loss and dehydration.

Matching

Part I

Match each of the definitions in the left column to the appropriate term in the right column.

______	**1.** Antibodies directed against the person's own proteins.	**A.** Acidosis
______	**2.** The production of antibodies or T cells that work against the tissues of a person's body, producing autoimmune disease or a hypersensitivity reaction.	**B.** Acquired immunity
______	**3.** A pattern of inheritance that involves genes that are located on autosomes or the nonsex chromosomes. Inheritance of only one copy of a particular form of a gene is needed to show the trait.	**C.** Activation
______	**4.** A pattern of inheritance that involves genes located on autosomes or the nonsex chromosomes. Inheritance of two copies of a particular form of a gene is needed to show the trait.	**D.** Adhesion
______	**5.** A severe hypersensitivity reaction that involves bronchoconstriction and cardiovascular collapse.	**E.** Alcoholic ketoacidosis
______	**6.** The growth of new blood vessels.	**F.** Alkalosis
______	**7.** A protein secreted by certain immune cells that bind antigens to make them more visible to the immune system.	**G.** Allergen
______	**8.** A foreign substance recognized by the immune system.	**H.** Allergy
______	**9.** Normal, genetically programmed cell death.	**I.** Anaphylactic shock
______	**10.** A chronic inflammatory lower airway condition resulting in intermittent wheezing and excess mucus production.	**J.** Angiogenesis
______	**11.** A decrease in cell size due to a loss of subcellular components.	**K.** Antibody
______	**12.** An allergic tendency.	**L.** Antigen
______	**13.** An increase in extracellular H^+ ions; a blood pH of less than 7.35.	**M.** Apoptosis
______	**14.** The metabolic acidotic state that manifests because of the inadequate nutritional habits associated with chronic alcohol abuse. The liver and body experience inadequate fuel reserves of glycogen and, therefore, have to switch to fatty acid metabolism.	**N.** Asthma
______	**15.** The attachment of polymorphonuclear neutrophils to endothelial cells, mediated by selectins and integrins.	**O.** Atopic
______	**16.** Mediators of inflammation trigger the appearance of molecules known as selectins and integrins on the surfaces of endothelial cells and polymorphonuclear neutrophils, respectively.	**P.** Atrophy

	Definition	Term
______	**17.** The immunity that occurs when the body is exposed to a foreign substance or disease and produces antibodies to the invader.	**Q.** Autoantibodies
______	**18.** A decrease is extracellular H^+ ions; a blood pH greater than 7.45.	**R.** Autoimmunity
______	**19.** Any substance that causes a hypersensitivity reaction.	**S.** Autosomal dominant
______	**20.** A hypersensitivity reaction to the presence of an agent (allergen) that is intrinsically harmless.	**T.** Autosomal recessive

Part II

Match each of the definitions in the left column to the appropriate term in the right column.

	Definition	Term
______	**1.** A group of plasma proteins whose function is to do one of three things: attract leukocytes to sites of inflammation, activate leukocytes, and directly destroy cells.	**A.** Carpopedal spasm
______	**2.** The system that forms blood clots in the body and facilitates repairs to the vascular tree.	**B.** Cell-mediated immunity
______	**3.** The movement of additional white blood cells to an area of inflammation in response to the release of chemical mediators, such as neutrophils, injured tissue, and monocytes.	**C.** Central shock
______	**4.** Components of the activated complement system that attract leukocytes from the circulation to help fight infections.	**D.** Chemotaxins
______	**5.** A type of shock caused by central pump failure, including cardiogenic shock and obstructive shock.	**E.** Chemotaxis
______	**6.** An inherited disease in which the body absorbs more iron than it needs and stores it in the liver, kidneys, and pancreas.	**F.** Coagulation system
______	**7.** A type of T lymphocyte that is involved in cell-mediated and antibody-mediated immune responses. It secretes cytokines that stimulate the B cells and other T cells.	**G.** Complement system
______	**8.** A substance that normally does not stimulate an immune response but can be combined with an antigen and at a later point initiate an antibody response.	**H.** Cytokines
______	**9.** A reaction of bacteria to a Gram stain in which the bacteria retain the dark purple stain; these types of bacteria have thick cell walls composed of many layers.	**I.** Distributive shock
______	**10.** A whitish, filamentous protein formed by the action of thrombin on fibrinogen; the protein that polymerizes (bonds) to form the fibrous component of a blood clot.	**J.** Dysplasia
______	**11.** Swelling caused by excessive fluid trapped in the body tissues.	**K.** Edema
______	**12.** An alteration in the size, shape, and organization of cells.	**L.** Fibrin
______	**13.** The type of shock caused by widespread dilation of the resistance vessels (small arterioles), the capacitance vessels (small venules), or both.	**M.** Fibrinolysis cascade
______	**14.** The products of cells that affect the function of other cells.	**N.** Free radicals
______	**15.** A reaction of bacteria to a Gram stain in which the bacteria do not retain the dark purple stain; these types of bacteria have cell walls that consist largely of lipids and have pathogenic qualities that make them especially problematic for humans.	**O.** General adaptation syndrome
______	**16.** A three-stage description of the body's short- and long-term reactions to stress.	**P.** Gram-negative
______	**17.** A molecule that is missing one electron in its outer shell.	**Q.** Gram-positive
______	**18.** The breakdown of fibrin in blood clots and the prevention of the polymerization of fibrin into new clots.	**R.** Hapten

______	**19.** A contorted position of the hand or foot in which the fingers or toes flex in a claw-like manner; may result from hyperventilation or hypocalcemia.	**S.** Helper T cells
______	**20.** The immune process by which T-cell lymphocytes recognize antigens and then secrete cytokines (specifically lymphokines) that attract other cells or stimulate the production of cytotoxic cells that kill the infected cells.	**T.** Hemochromatosis

Part III

Match each of the definitions in the left column to the appropriate term in the right column.

______	**1.** An abnormal condition in which some part of the body's immune system is inadequate, and consequently, resistance to infectious disease is decreased.	**A.** Hyponatremia
______	**2.** The body system that includes all of the structures and processes designated to mount a defense against foreign substances and disease-causing agents.	**B.** Hypoperfusion
______	**3.** The body's defense reaction to any substance that is recognized as foreign.	**C.** Hypophosphatemia
______	**4.** A condition that occurs when the circulating blood volume is inadequate to deliver adequate oxygen and nutrients to the body.	**D.** Hypothalamic-pituitary-adrenal axis
______	**5.** A major part of the neuroendocrine system that controls reactions to stress. It is the mechanism for a set of interactions among glands, hormones, and parts of the midbrain that mediate the general adaptation syndrome.	**E.** Hypovolemic shock
______	**6.** An elevated white blood cell count, often due to inflammation.	**F.** Immune response
______	**7.** Anaerobic cellular respiration due to hypoperfusion of tissues and organs.	**G.** Immune system
______	**8.** A group of polypeptides that mediate inflammatory responses by stimulating visceral smooth muscle and relaxing vascular smooth muscle to produce vasodilation.	**H.** Immunodeficiency
______	**9.** Acidic by-products of fat metabolism.	**I.** Immunogen
______	**10.** An acidotic state created by the production of ketones via fat metabolism.	**J.** Immunoglobulins
______	**11.** The formation of antibodies or T cells that are directed against antigens or another person's cells.	**K.** Incidence
______	**12.** A serum sodium level that is less than or equal to 135 mEq/L.	**L.** Inflammatory response
______	**13.** A condition that occurs when the level of tissue perfusion decreases below that needed to maintain normal cellular functions.	**M.** Interferon
______	**14.** A decreased serum phosphate level.	**N.** Interleukins
______	**15.** An antigen that is capable of generating an immune response.	**O.** Isoimmunity
______	**16.** Antibodies secreted by the B cells.	**P.** Ketoacidosis
______	**17.** The number of new cases of a disease in a population.	**Q.** Ketones
______	**18.** Chemical substances that attract white blood cells to the sites of injury and bacterial invasions.	**R.** Kinin system
______	**19.** A protein produced by cells in response to viral invasion that is released into the bloodstream or intercellular fluid to induce healthy cells to manufacture an enzyme that counters the infection.	**S.** Lactic acidosis
______	**20.** A reaction by tissues of the body to irritation or injury, characterized by pain, swelling, redness, and heat.	**T.** Leukocytosis

Multiple Choice

Read each item carefully, and then select the best response.

_____ **1.** When a patient hyperventilates and has carpopedal spasm, this reaction is a result of a developing:
- **A.** metabolic acidosis.
- **B.** respiratory alkalosis.
- **C.** metabolic alkalosis.
- **D.** respiratory acidosis.

_____ **2.** An increase in the size of cells caused by the synthesis of more subcellular components, which in turn leads to an increase in tissue and organ size, is called:
- **A.** hypertrophy.
- **B.** hyperplasia.
- **C.** dysplasia.
- **D.** metaplasia.

_____ **3.** Long-duration exercise in the heat, causing excessive sweating, may lead to life-threatening deficits in:
- **A.** phosphate.
- **B.** calcium.
- **C.** sodium.
- **D.** magnesium.

_____ **4.** When examining rates of disease, which of the following terms refers to the number of cases in a particular population?
- **A.** Incidence
- **B.** Prevalence
- **C.** Distribution
- **D.** Tendency

_____ **5.** Normal serum level of potassium should be:
- **A.** 1.3 to 2.1 mEq/L.
- **B.** 3.5 to 5.0 mEq/L.
- **C.** 8.2 to 10.2 mg/dL.
- **D.** 136 to 142 mEq/L.

_____ **6.** Which of the following is caused by autosomal dominant inheritance (where a person needs to inherit only one copy of the particular form of the gene to show the trait)?
- **A.** Sickle cell anemia
- **B.** Attached earlobe
- **C.** Tay-Sachs disease
- **D.** Freckles

_____ **7.** Individuals who suffer from long QT syndrome are at risk for all of the following, EXCEPT:
- **A.** ventricular dysrhythmias.
- **B.** palpitations.
- **C.** torsades de pointes.
- **D.** atrial fibrillation.

_____ **8.** Chronic obstructive pulmonary disease (COPD) gradually destroys lung tissue and inhibits oxygen and carbon dioxide exchange, eventually resulting in:
- **A.** respiratory alkalosis.
- **B.** respiratory acidosis.
- **C.** metabolic alkalosis.
- **D.** metabolic acidosis.

_____ **9.** Central shock consists of which two types of shock?
A. Hypovolemic and distributive
B. Cardiogenic and distributive
C. Cardiogenic and obstructive
D. Hypovolemic and obstructive

_____ **10.** Normal cell death is referred to as:
A. necrosis.
B. gangrene.
C. apoptosis.
D. liquefaction.

_____ **11.** Which of the following is NOT considered a neuromuscular disease?
A. Multiple sclerosis
B. Muscular dystrophy
C. Huntington disease
D. Gout

_____ **12.** The disease-causing ability of a microorganism is referred to as:
A. toxicity.
B. inflammation.
C. virulence.
D. pyrogen.

_____ **13.** Of the following, which is NOT an example of a cause of metabolic acidosis?
A. Gastrointestinal losses
B. Excessive water intake
C. Lactic acidosis
D. Aspirin overdose

_____ **14.** The major intracellular cation that is crucial to many cell functions is:
A. potassium.
B. calcium.
C. phosphate.
D. sodium.

_____ **15.** The total body water found in an infant is approximately_____of the infant's total weight.
A. 50%
B. 60%
C. 70%
D. 80%

Fill in the Blank

Read each item carefully, and then complete the statement by filling in the missing word(s).

1. Perfusion is defined as the delivery of _________ and _________ and ________ of wastes from cells, organs, and _________ by the _________ system.

2. Cardiogenic ________ occurs when the ________ cannot circulate enough ________ to maintain adequate peripheral _________ delivery.

3. Obstructive ________ occurs when blood _______ becomes ________ in the heart or great vessels.

4. Two types of _______ shock—__________ and endogenous—are possible, depending on where ______ loss occurs.

5. Anaphylactic shock occurs when histamine and other ________ proteins are _________ on exposure to a(n) ___________.

6. __________ is an elevated potassium level.

7. The molecules that modulate the changes in pH are called __________.

8. Normal cell death is called __________.

9. __________ __________ __________ __________ is a progressive condition usually characterized by concurrent failure of several organs, such as the lungs, liver, and kidneys.

10. __________ are lipopolysaccharides that are part of the cell walls of gram-negative bacteria. They cause inflammation, fever, and chills.

Labeling

1. Type I allergic reaction
Fill in the missing words that describe a type I allergic reaction.

A. ____

B. ____

C. ____

D. ____

E. ____

F. ____

G. ____

H. ____

I. ____

J. ____

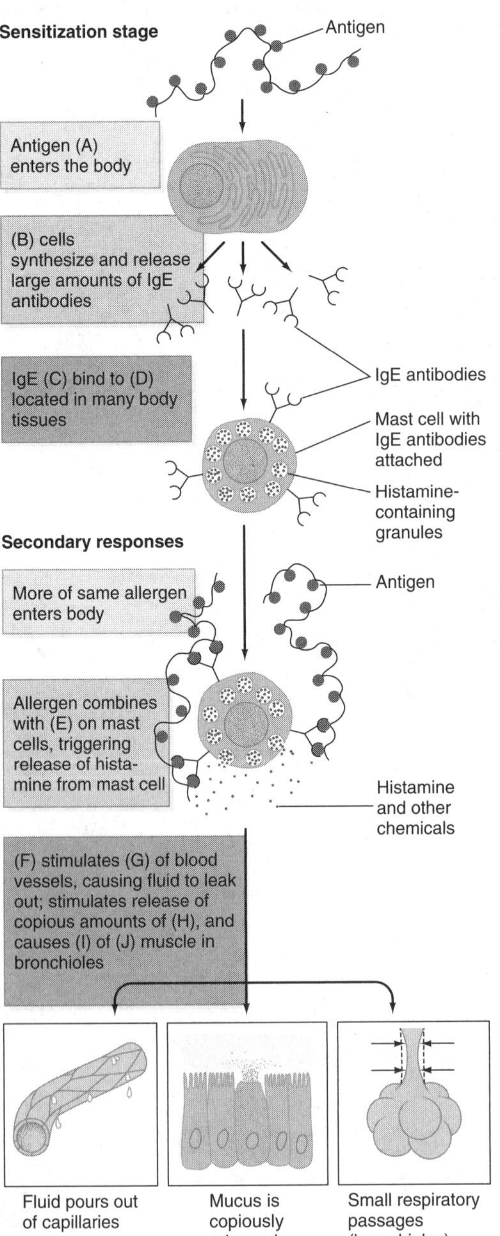

Identify

After reading the following case study, list the chief complaint, vital signs, and pertinent patient history.

You respond to a call to an assisted living manor for a 78-year-old man who is having difficulty breathing. Upon arrival, you find the patient sitting forward in a dining room chair with his "elbows out." He is looking rather distressed. You walk up to his table, introduce yourself, and ask what's wrong. The patient responds, with what appears to be great difficulty, "I... can't... breathe." Your partner starts to obtain vital signs as you place the patient on a non-rebreathing mask.

You obtain the history from the patient and the staff of the facility. The symptoms started about 30 minutes ago, with shortness of breath and coughing. The night nurse's aide tells you the patient said he was chilled, was sweaty, and felt warm. His temperature was taken before your arrival and was recorded on the chart as 102.5°F. The medical record states he has COPD, with a 40-year history of smoking two packs of cigarettes per day. Your partner tells you that respirations are 28 breaths/min and shallow, the pulse is 90 beats/min with occasional irregular beats, blood pressure (BP) is 160/90 mm Hg, and oxygen saturation is 90%.

You and your partner decide to place the patient on continuous positive airway pressure (CPAP) to assist his breathing. Just before you place the mask, the patient starts to cough and brings up blood-tinged sputum. You prepare the patient and transport. He is hospitalized for a week with a diagnosis of pneumonia before being placed in a nursing home.

1. Chief complaint:

___

___

2. Vital signs:

___

___

3. Pertinent patient history:

___

___

4. What was your presumptive diagnosis?

___

___

Ambulance Calls

The following case scenarios provide an opportunity to explore the concerns associated with patient management and paramedic care. Read each scenario, and then answer each question.

1. While on a call for a patient with chest pain, you are taking the SAMPLE history, and the patient tells you he is taking an angiotensin-converting enzyme (ACE) inhibitor for hypertension. Your partner has placed the patient on the electrocardiogram (ECG) monitor and informs you that there is a peaked T wave and a wide QRS complex with tachycardia.

   a. What do you suspect is the life-threatening emergency that is being identified on the ECG?

   ___

   ___

   b. Which drug should be considered as the first-line medication for this condition?

   ___

   ___

2. Approximately 500,000 people living in the United States are believed to have Crohn disease. When a person has an acute episode, he or she may call emergency medical services (EMS).
   a. Crohn disease is a disorder of which body system?

   ____

   ____

   b. Which symptoms would you expect a patient with Crohn disease to have?

   ____

   ____

3. It is not uncommon to encounter an elderly patient who has Alzheimer disease as an underlying problem. What are some of the factors that might affect your ability to get a good SAMPLE history and provide care for a patient with Alzheimer disease?

   ____

   ____

   ____

True/False

If you believe the statement to be more true than false, write the letter "T" in the space provided. If you believe the statement to be more false than true, write the letter "F."

______ 1. Plasma cells are white blood cells (WBCs) that develop from B cells.

______ 2. Helper B cells phagocytize bacteria.

______ 3. Acquired immunity is also called native immunity.

______ 4. The primary immune response takes place during the first exposure to an antibody.

______ 5. Cell-mediated immunity is characterized by the formation of a population of lymphocytes that can destroy foreign material.

______ 6. With autosomal recessive inheritance, a person must inherit only one copy of a particular form of a gene to show that trait.

______ 7. Distributive shock occurs when blood flow becomes blocked in the great vessels.

______ 8. Acquired immunity is a highly specific, inducible, discriminatory, and unforgetting method by which armies of cells respond to an immune stimulant.

______ 9. Type 1 diabetes is considered an autoimmune disease.

______ 10. The immune system includes all structures and processes associated with the body's defense against foreign substances and disease-causing agents.

______ 11. Myasthenia gravis is a chronic systemic disease that affects the body's lymphatic system.

______ 12. When hemoglobin is broken down, the iron in this molecule is recycled.

______ 13. Iron is transported in blood by transferrin.

______ 14. The disease sickle cell anemia causes pancreatic failure and mucus buildup in the lungs.

______ 15. Small masses of uric acid or calcium salts that form in the urinary system are called kidney stones.

Short Answer

Complete this section with short written answers using the space provided.

1. Allergens that can cause hypersensitivity reactions include:

   a. ____________________

   b. ____________________

   c. ____________________

   d. ____________________

   e. ____________________

   f. ____________________

2. Cellular injury can result from various causes. List five causes.

   a. ____________________

   b. ____________________

   c. ____________________

   d. ____________________

   e. ____________________

3. List seven common respiratory diseases that may be caused by environmental pollutants, viruses, or bacteria.

   a. ____________________

   b. ____________________

   c. ____________________

   d. ____________________

   e. ____________________

   f. ____________________

   g. ____________________

4. List four conditions for which you should always consider syncope to be caused by a life-threatening dysrhythmia until proved otherwise.

   a. ____________________

   b. ____________________

   c. ____________________

   d. ____________________

5. The goal of the cellular component of the acute inflammatory response is for the inflammatory cells (polymorphonuclear neutrophils) to arrive at the site in the tissue where they are needed. The process involves two major stages: intravascular phase and extravascular phase. During the later phase, leukocytes travel to the inflammation site and kill organisms. Name the five events in this sequence.

a. ____________________

b. ____________________

c. ____________________

d. ____________________

e. ____________________

6. What are the three stages of the general adaptation syndrome?

a. ____________________

b. ____________________

c. ____________________

Fill in the Table

Fill in the missing parts of the table on shock.

Signs and Symptoms of Compensated and Decompensated Hypoperfusion	
Compensated	**Decompensated**
Agitation, anxiety, restlessness	Altered mental status (verbal to unresponsive)
Sense of impending doom	____________________
____________________	____________________
Clammy (cool, moist) skin	Thready or absent peripheral pulses
____________________	Ashen, mottled, or cyanotic skin
Shortness of breath	____________________
____________________	____________________
Delayed capillary refill time in infants and children	Impending cardiac arrest
____________________	
Normal BP	

CHAPTER 10

Life Span Development

Prior to administering nitroglycerin, always ask the patient if he has used erectile dysfunction medication.

Matching

Part I

Match each of the definitions in the left column to the appropriate term in the right column.

_____ **1.** People who are 1 month to 1 year of age.

_____ **2.** People who are 61 years of age or older.

_____ **3.** The average amount of years a person can be expected to live.

_____ **4.** People who are 41 to 60 years of age.

_____ **5.** The cessation of menstruation, which begins in a woman's late 40s or early 50s and marks the end of the reproductive years.

_____ **6.** A female's first menstrual period.

_____ **7.** A parenting style that balances parental authority with the child's freedom by setting and enforcing rules but also allowing the child to have some freedom.

_____ **8.** Trauma resulting from increased pressure—for example, from too much pressure in the lungs.

_____ **9.** The formation of a close, personal relationship.

_____ **10.** Increased carbon dioxide levels in the bloodstream.

_____ **11.** Structures located on either end of an infant's bone that aid in lengthening bones as the child grows.

_____ **12.** Areas where the infant's skull has not fused together; usually disappear at approximately 18 months of age; also called soft spots.

_____ **13.** People who are 13 to 17 years of age.

_____ **14.** A swelling or enlargement of part of a blood vessel, resulting from weakening of the vessel wall.

_____ **15.** A bond between an infant and the parent/caregiver in which the infant is repeatedly rejected and develops an isolated lifestyle that does not depend on the support and care of others.

_____ **16.** The second phase of an infant's response to a situational crisis; characterized by monotonous wailing.

_____ **17.** A type of reasoning in which a child looks for approval from peers and society.

_____ **18.** People who are 18 to 40 years of age.

_____ **19.** A parenting style that demands absolute obedience.

_____ **20.** A disorder in which cholesterol and calcium build up inside the walls of the blood vessels, forming plaque, which eventually leads to partial or complete blockage of blood flow.

A. Adolescents
B. Aneurysm
C. Anxious avoidant attachment
D. Atherosclerosis
E. Authoritarian
F. Authoritative
G. Barotrauma
H. Bonding
I. Conventional reasoning
J. Despair phase
K. Early adults
L. Fontanelles
M. Growth plates
N. Hypercapnia
O. Infants
P. Late adults
Q. Life expectancy
R. Menarche
S. Menopause
T. Middle adults

Part II

Match each of the definitions in the left column to the appropriate term in the right column.

_____ 1. An instructional technique that builds on what has already been learned.
_____ 2. People who are 6 to 12 years of age.
_____ 3. A bond between an infant and the parent/caregiver in which the infant understands that parents/caregivers will be responsive to his or her needs and provide care when help is needed.
_____ 4. A person's perception of himself or herself.
_____ 5. A parenting style in which the parent does not impose many rules, if any, on the child; two subcategories include indifferent and indulgent.
_____ 6. A type of reasoning in which a child bases decisions on his or her conscience.
_____ 7. A type of reasoning in which a child acts almost purely to avoid punishment and to get what he or she wants.
_____ 8. People who are 3 to 5 years of age.
_____ 9. In the context of infant behavior, the final phase of an infant's response to a situational crisis; characterized by apathy and boredom.
_____ 10. A phrase that refers to a stage of development from birth to approximately 18 months of age, during which infants gain the trust of their parents and/or caregivers if their world is planned, organized, and routine.
_____ 11. People who are 1 to 3 years of age.
_____ 12. The theory that a person's mental function declines in the last 5 years of life.
_____ 13. An infant reflex that occurs when something is placed in the infant's palm; the infant grasps the object.
_____ 14. The basic filtering units of the kidneys.
_____ 15. An infant reflex in which, when caught off guard, the infant opens his or her arms wide.
_____ 16. An infant reflex that occurs when something touches an infant's cheek, and the infant instinctively turns his or her head toward the touch.
_____ 17. An infant's initial response to a situational crisis; characterized by loud crying.
_____ 18. A crisis caused by a specific set of circumstances.
_____ 19. How a person feels about himself or herself and how he or she fits in with peers.
_____ 20. An infant reflex in which the infant starts sucking when his or her lips are stroked.

A. Moro reflex
B. Nephrons
C. Palmar grasp
D. Permissive
E. Postconventional reasoning
F. Preconventional reasoning
G. Preschoolers
H. Protest phase
I. Rooting reflex
J. Scaffolding
K. School-age children
L. Secure attachment
M. Self-concept
N. Self-esteem
O. Situational crisis
P. Sucking reflex
Q. Terminal drop hypothesis
R. Toddlers
S. Trust and mistrust
T. Withdrawal

Multiple Choice

Read each item carefully, and then select the best response.

_____ 1. When a newborn's cheek is touched, he or she turns toward the touch. This is called the __________ reflex.

A. Moro
B. palmar
C. sucking
D. rooting

_____ **2.** The tidal volume of an infant starts at __________ mL/kg.

A. 4 to 6
B. 6 to 8
C. 8 to 12
D. 12 to 14

_____ **3.** Which of the infant's fontanelles can be used as a possible indicator of dehydration if sunken?

A. Posterior
B. Mastoid
C. Sphenoidal
D. Anterior

_____ **4.** At approximately what age does an infant start to become afraid of strangers?

A. 2 months
B. 7 months
C. 9 months
D. 1 year

_____ **5.** The filtration function of the kidneys declines by __________ between 20 and 90 years of age.

A. less than 25%
B. about 25%
C. about 50%
D. about 75%

_____ **6.** Bleeding can empty into voids in the older adult brain, resulting in which type of hemorrhage?

A. Meningeal
B. Epidural
C. Ventricular
D. Subdural

_____ **7.** In the 5 years preceding death, mental function is presumed to decline, a theory referred to as the:

A. terminal drop hypothesis.
B. organic dementia hypothesis.
C. geriatric shrinkage syndrome.
D. end-of-life physiopsych decline.

_____ **8.** In late adults, the vital capacity of the lungs decreases, and residual volume increases. The effect can produce which of the following conditions?

A. Hypercapnia
B. Hypocarbia
C. Hypoxia
D. Hyperoxygenation

_____ **9.** Which one of the following is NOT a usual response of the cardiovascular system in late adults?

A. Decrease in heart rate
B. Cardiac output that matches demand
C. Increase in systolic blood pressure
D. Partial blockage of blood flow

_____ **10.** School-age children learn various types of reasoning in their development. Which of the following is a type of reasoning they learn?

A. Cognitive
B. Distributive
C. Conventional
D. Affective

Fill in the Blank

Read each item carefully, and then complete the statement by filling in the missing word(s).

1. A full-term infant usually weighs approximately __________ pounds at birth. After birth, infants usually lose __________% to __________% of their birth weight due to the loss of __________ in the first week.

2. A(n) __________ __________ occurs when an object is placed in the infant's palm.

3. An infant's __________ allow the head to be molded when the newborn passes through the birth canal.

4. __________ __________, located on either end of the infant's bones, aid in the lengthening of a child's bones.

5. __________, or the formation of a close, personal relationship, is usually based on a secure attachment.

6. __________ and __________ refer to a stage of development from birth to about 18 months of age. Most infants desire that their world be planned, organized, and routine

7. Atherosclerosis can contribute to the development of a(n) __________, or weakening and bulging of a blood vessel wall.

8. In late adults, blood flow in the __________ (membranes that connect organs to the abdominal wall) may drop by as much as 50%.

9. In the 5 years preceding death, mental function is presumed to decline. This is a theory referred to as the __________ __________ __________.

10. In late adults, the size of the airway (______________), and the surface area of the alveoli (__________________).

Labeling

Label the four fontanelles of the infant's head.

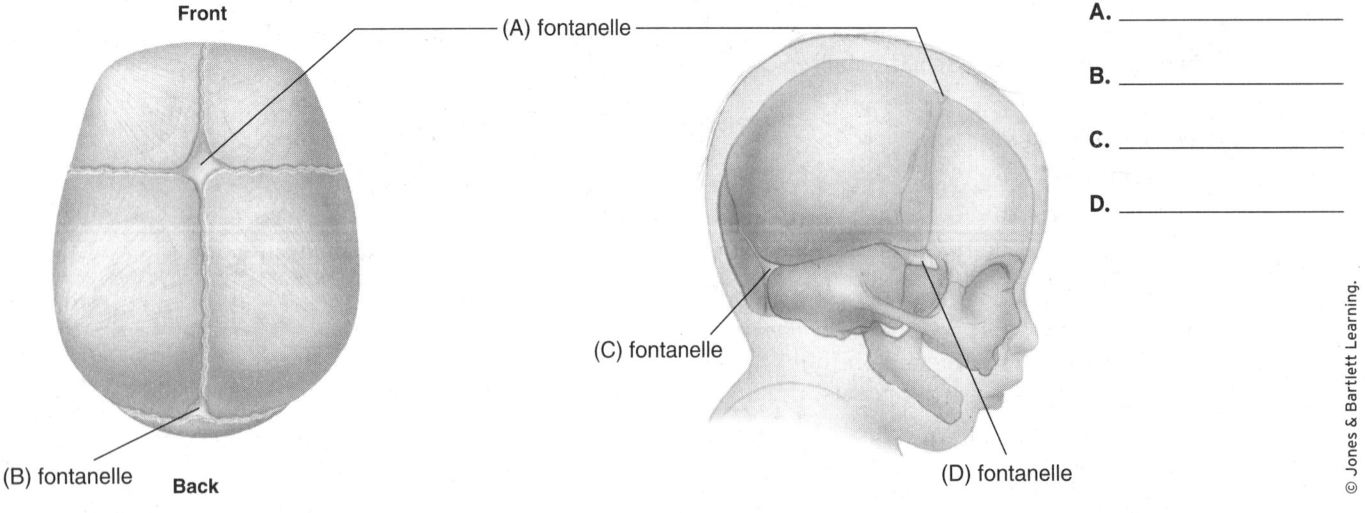

Identify

Read the following case study, and then list the chief complaint, vital signs, and SAMPLE history.

A call to an assisted living facility brings you to a 75-year-old woman who tripped on a chair and fell while walking from the living room to the kitchen. When you enter the apartment, the patient tells you she fell and has a great deal of pain in her hip. You gently palpate the injured area, and the patient yells. You take a set of vital signs and find a pulse of 90 beats/min and thready, respirations of 24 breaths/min and shallow, and blood pressure of 100/70 mm Hg. The SAMPLE history identifies an externally rotated foot and discoloration of the hip on the same side. The patient reports no allergies and is on several medications for congestive heart failure. She had a heart attack last year, and she has a two-pack-a-day history of smoking for more than 30 years but stopped smoking about 5 years ago. She ate breakfast 3 hours ago. You place the patient on an electrocardiogram (ECG) monitor, establish an IV, and package her for transport.

1. Chief complaint:

____

____

2. Vital signs:

____

____

3. SAMPLE history:

____

____

Ambulance Calls

The following case scenarios provide an opportunity to explore the concerns associated with patient management and paramedic care. Read each scenario, and then answer each question.

1. Your unit is dispatched to a call for an infant with a seizure. The response time is 5 minutes, and when you enter the residence, you find a distraught mother who is very anxious. The seizure seems to have stopped, but you understand the importance of an immediate primary survey (the MS–ABC Priority Plan). You immediately notice that the child has good color except for a little cyanosis of the fingers. The child is actively breathing, and the rate is adequate. Your partner starts to administer blow-by oxygen, and you examine the child quickly from head to toe to make sure there is no external bleeding or signs of trauma. The child is starting to respond and become more active. You prepare for transport and decide the child is stable and alert enough that the neurologic status can be assessed. Which reflexes would you check, and how would you test them? What are considered to be the appropriate responses from the infant? Fill in the following table.

Reflex	How to Test	Appropriate Response

2. A call to an assisted living facility finds a 75-year-old woman sitting with her partner and complaining of general body weakness. You approach the patient but have trouble communicating with her, and while doing the SAMPLE history, you have trouble getting necessary information from her. You decide that when asking about her past medical history, you should ask about individual body systems because this might help to identify the current problem.

a. What are some of the communication issues you might have encountered while taking the history of this patient?

____

____

____

____

b. What are some possible concerns you are thinking of while attempting to obtain the past medical history?

______

______

______

______

3. You receive a call to the residence of a 16-year-old girl with a chief complaint of abdominal pain. The girl is lying on the couch in the living room; her mother and a girlfriend are also in the room. Your partner is a man who is taking the lead on the assessment and SAMPLE history. While doing the SAMPLE history, he asks the patient if there is a possibility she is pregnant. She immediately and emphatically answers no. He then decides that he should palpate the abdomen and immediately proceeds to do so, with little explanation. The patient seems embarrassed. You realize that you need to package the patient and transport.

a. Which consideration should your partner have taken into account before questioning this patient about the possibility of pregnancy?

______

______

______

______

b. Is there a more appropriate way to handle the physical exam of the abdomen?

______

______

______

______

True/False

If you believe the statement to be more true than false, write the letter "T" in the space provided. If you believe the statement to be more false than true, write the letter "F."

______ **1.** An infant's ventilations that are too forceful can result in barotrauma.

______ **2.** The rooting reflex occurs when an infant's lips are stroked.

______ **3.** If the posterior fontanelle is sunken, the infant is most likely dehydrated.

______ **4.** Anxious avoidant attachment is observed in infants who are repeatedly rejected.

______ **5.** A toddler is at the critical age in human development to learn various types of reasoning.

______ **6.** Cardiac function declines with age consequent to anatomic and physiologic changes largely related to atherosclerosis.

______ **7.** In late adults, the vital capacity of the lungs decreases, and stagnant air remains in the alveoli and hampers gas exchange, which can produce hypercapnia.

______ **8.** In late adults, there is a surge of increased mental functioning in the last few years of life.

______ **9.** Age-related shrinkage creates a void between the brain and outermost layer of the meninges.

______ **10.** The number of nephrons in the kidneys increases between the ages of 30 and 80.

Short Answer

Complete this section with short written answers using the space provided.

1. Infants are born with certain reflexes and responses that can assist you in the neurologic assessment of an infant. Name four of these reflexes.

 a. ______

 b. ______

 c. ______

 d. ______

2. Cardiac function declines with age largely as a result of atherosclerosis. This disorder, which commonly affects coronary vessels, results from the formation of plaque. Which two substances are responsible for the buildup of plaque?

 a. ______

 b. ______

3. Loss of which mechanisms in the respiratory system of the late adult makes aspiration and obstruction more likely?

 a. ______

 b. ______

 c. ______

 d. ______

 e. ______

4. Late adults have sensory changes that can affect mobility and safety. Which sensory changes occur in this age group?

 a. ______

 b. ______

 c. ______

 d. ______

 e. ______

 f. ______

 g. ______

5. Colds often develop in toddlers and preschool-age children and may manifest as which types of infections?

 a. ______

 b. ______

6. Playing games is the way that toddlers learn. What can a child of this age learn from play?

 a. ______

 b. ______

 c. ______

7. In the late elderly, the vital capacity of the lungs decreases. Name three factors that contribute to this decline.

d. ______________________________

e. ______________________________

f. ______________________________

Fill in the Table

Fill in the missing parts of the tables.

1. Subtle changes occur during adolescence; one change is the development of secondary sexual characteristics. Fill in the table with these characteristics.

Male Characteristics	Female Characteristics

2. Fill in the table with the appropriate noticeable characteristics for various ages in the infant's development.

Psychosocial Characteristics at Various Ages

Age (in months)	Noticeable Characteristics
2	Recognizes familiar faces; (A) ______________
3	Brings objects to the mouth; (B) ______________
4	Reaches out to people; drools
5	Sleeps through the night; (C) ______________
6	Teething begins; (D) ______________
7	Afraid of strangers; (E) ______________
8	Responds to "no"; sits upright alone; plays peek-a-boo
9	Pulls himself or herself up; (F) ______________
10	Responds to his or her name; crawls efficiently
11	(G) ______________; ______________
12	Knows his or her name; can walk

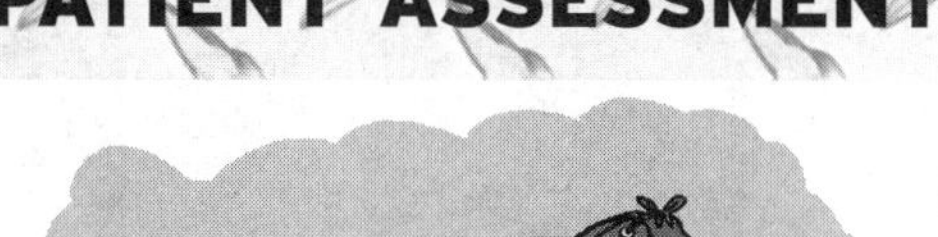

PATIENT ASSESSMENT

CHAPTER 11

Patient Assessment

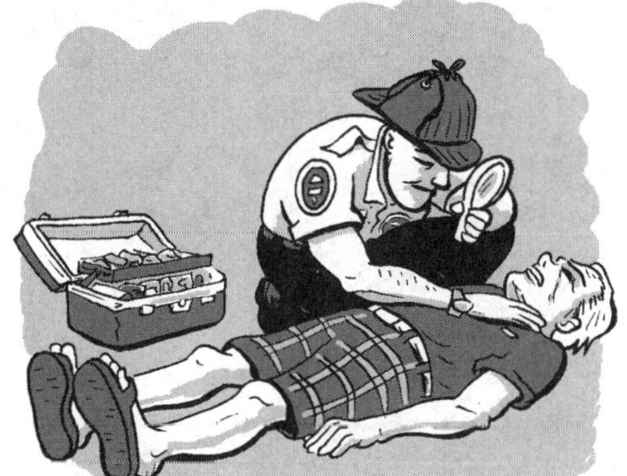

Being good at patient assessment is a lot like being a good detective

Matching

Part I

Match each of the definitions in the left column to the appropriate term in the right column.

______	**1.**	An acute confusional state characterized by global impairment of thinking, perception, judgment, and memory.	**A.** Anisocoria
______	**2.**	Double vision.	**B.** Aphasia
______	**3.**	Localized bruising or collection of blood within or under the skin.	**C.** Ascites
______	**4.**	A crackling, grating, or grinding sound often heard when fragments of broken bones rub together.	**D.** Aspiration
______	**5.**	An abnormal whooshing sound heard over the heart that indicates turbulent blood flow around a cardiac valve.	**E.** Battle sign
______	**6.**	A blotchy pattern on the skin; a typical finding in states of severe protracted hypoperfusion and shock.	**F.** Beck triad
______	**7.**	Outward curve of the thoracic spine.	**G.** Bronchial sounds
______	**8.**	Wet rattling, bubbling, or crackling lung sounds indicative of fluid in the small airways; also known as rales.	**H.** Bruit
______	**9.**	Ear wax.	**I.** Cerumen
______	**10.**	Unequal pupils with a difference greater than 1 mm.	**J.** Crackles
______	**11.**	A language impairment that affects the production or understanding of speech and the ability to read or write.	**K.** Crepitus
______	**12.**	The entry of fluids or solids into the trachea, bronchi, and lungs; the act of drawing material in or out by suction.	**L.** Delirium
______	**13.**	Abnormal accumulation of fluid in the peritoneal cavity; typically signals liver failure.	**M.** Diplopia
______	**14.**	Sounds related to blood pressure measurement that are heard by stethoscope.	**N.** Ecchymosis
______	**15.**	Looking at the patient, either in general or at a specific area (ie, a patient's overall appearance from the doorway versus looking specifically at the chest wall for abnormalities/deformities).	**O.** Guarding
______	**16.**	Related to a side effect or complication of medications or other medical treatment.	**P.** Iatrogenic
______	**17.**	Contraction of the abdominal muscles indicating peritoneal irritation.	**Q.** Inspection
______	**18.**	Sideways curvature of the spine.	**R.** Korotkoff sounds
______	**19.**	Involuntary motor responses to specific sensory stimuli, such as a tap on the knee or stroking the eyelash.	**S.** Kyphosis

______	**20.** The perception of the position and movement of the body or limbs.	**T.** Mottling
______	**21.** Physical touching for the purpose of obtaining information (ie, to detect tenderness).	**U.** Murmur
______	**22.** An abnormal whooshing sound of turbulent blood flow moving through a narrowed artery; usually heard in the carotid arteries.	**V.** Palpation
______	**23.** Hollow, tubular, lower-pitched sounds heard over the trachea.	**W.** Proprioception
______	**24.** The combination of a narrowed pulse pressure, muffled heart tones, and jugular venous distention (JVD) associated with cardiac tamponade; usually caused by penetrating chest trauma.	**X.** Reflexes
______	**25.** Bruising over the mastoid process, which may indicate a basilar skull fracture; also known as retroauricular ecchymosis or raccoon eyes.	**Y.** Scoliosis

Part II

During your EMT course, you learned many assessment findings. In the paramedic program, you will broaden your knowledge of assessment findings and learn their diagnostic significance so that you can come to a presumptive diagnosis. Using the knowledge you already have at this point, try to match each of the signs listed to the right with the phrase that best describes its possible diagnostic significance or presumptive diagnosis. (Note: More than one sign may have the same diagnostic significance.)

______	**1.** Narcotics overdose	**A.** Ecchymosis (discoloration) around the eyes
______	**2.** Cardiac arrest	**B.** Fruity (acetone) odor to the breath
______	**3.** Heart failure	**C.** Stridor on inspiration
______	**4.** Skull fracture	**D.** Pitting edema of both ankles
______	**5.** Stroke	**E.** Paralysis of upward gaze
______	**6.** Hypoxemia	**F.** Muffled heart sounds
______	**7.** Respiratory distress	**G.** Battle sign (discoloration of mastoid area)
______	**8.** Shock	**H.** Patient lies very still; cries out when stretcher is jarred
______	**9.** Diabetic ketoacidosis	**I.** Pinpoint pupils
______	**10.** Spinal cord injury	**J.** Cyanosis of the lips
______	**11.** Increased right ventricular pressure	**K.** Capillary refill takes 5 seconds
______	**12.** Laryngeal edema	**L.** Restlessness
______	**13.** Pelvic fracture	**M.** Absent pulse
______	**14.** Fluid/blood in the pericardium	**N.** Retraction of the suprasternal muscles
______	**15.** Intra-abdominal bleeding	**O.** Jugular veins distended to 10 cm when the patient is sitting
______	**16.** Peritonitis	**P.** Crackling sensation in the skin over the chest
______	**17.** Fracture of the orbit (eye socket in the skull)	**Q.** Distended, bruised abdomen in trauma victim
______	**18.** Pneumothorax	**R.** Pain on compression of the iliac crests
		S. Priapism
		T. No movement or sensation in the right arm or leg
		U. S_3 gallop (heart sound)
		V. Clear fluid draining from the ear

Part III

For each of the following patients, indicate whether their signs and/or symptoms classify them as sick or not sick.

S—Sick (life-threatening) NS—Not sick

______ **1.** 18-month-old boy who is limp and dusky blue in the face

______ **2.** 54-year-old woman with diffuse abdominal pain

______ **3.** 43-year-old man with confusion, sweating, and left arm pain

______ **4.** 22-year-old woman with rapid breathing and tingling in arms and feet

______ **5.** 4-year-old girl who is crying and has pain in her ear

______ **6.** 75-year-old man who is unable to speak or answer questions

______ **7.** 66-year-old woman who is unresponsive and breathing deeply and rapidly

______ **8.** 36-year-old woman who is depressed and does not want to talk

Multiple Choice

Read each item carefully, and then select the best response.

______ **1.** When responding to a call, a paramedic's demeanor and appearance should be all of the following, EXCEPT:
- **A.** clean.
- **B.** overbearing.
- **C.** positive.
- **D.** efficient.

______ **2.** Which of the following statements/questions would be considered a facilitation communication technique?
- **A.** That's all the information I need.
- **B.** You don't have to tell me if you don't want to.
- **C.** Can you think of anything else about his medical history?
- **D.** Can you narrow down his history to just the past few months?

______ **3.** Which communication technique is NOT helpful in a stressful situation?
- **A.** Confrontation
- **B.** Facilitation
- **C.** Empathetic response
- **D.** Clarification

______ **4.** What should the thinking paramedic do when faced with a possible physical abuse situation?
- **A.** Document.
- **B.** Gather evidence in a paper bag.
- **C.** Accuse the abuser to try to get the real story.
- **D.** Call for law enforcement before leaving the scene.

______ **5.** When a patient has a period of silence during a call, it should make you:
- **A.** begin to ask more questions.
- **B.** realize that the patient may not trust you, prompting you to respect the silence.
- **C.** look for a reason the patient is not talking, such as a change in condition.
- **D.** look for a weapon on the patient.

______ **6.** Your patient will not quit talking! Which of the following is NOT a reason for chattiness?
- **A.** The patient is on methamphetamine.
- **B.** The patient is very nervous.
- **C.** The patient has had several cups of coffee.
- **D.** All of the above can lead to chattiness.

______ **7.** You are dealing with a very angry young man who is being arrested for driving while intoxicated (DWI). He has a broken leg and arm, and you are transporting him to the hospital. What is the best way to treat this situation?
- **A.** Make sure you strap him down tight to the backboard so that he cannot get away.
- **B.** Tell him that if he does not calm down, you will give him a medication to calm him down.
- **C.** Treat him as you would any patient, and keep your anger and comments to yourself.
- **D.** Yell back at him, and let him know that you are the boss and will not tolerate this in the back of your squad.

______ **8.** Which of the following statements describes behavior that is NOT correct when interacting with a blind person?
- **A.** Always put things back exactly where you picked them up from.
- **B.** Speak very, very slowly and clearly.
- **C.** Announce your identity and reason for being there.
- **D.** Let the person know where you are and where you are going at all times during transport.

______ **9.** Which of the following signs and symptoms is NOT a sign of depression?
A. Feeling of high energy
B. Irritability
C. Eating disruptions
D. Pain with no source

______ **10.** What is a good thing to remember when asking for history from family members?
A. They will always know the patient's history.
B. They will be aware of drug or alcohol use.
C. You are not at liberty to share the patient's condition with them.
D. You will be able to give them an update on the patient once they reach the hospital.

______ **11.** While assessing a trauma patient, you press down lightly on the abdomen. This technique is called:
A. inspection.
B. percussion.
C. auscultation.
D. palpation.

______ **12.** Which of the following statements is NOT true regarding the use of a pulse oximeter?
A. It measures only the percentage of hemoglobin saturation.
B. It can help determine the patient's heart rhythm.
C. A cold person can have a false reading.
D. A hypotensive patient can have a false reading.

______ **13.** What is essential in getting an accurate blood pressure reading?
A. Using the right cuff size
B. Not having any clothing on the arm
C. Having the arm perfectly straight
D. The age of the patient

______ **14.** When assessing a patient's mental status, "P" on the AVPU scale stands for which of the following?
A. Pupil size
B. Pallor of the skin
C. Painful stimuli
D. Presence

______ **15.** Clubbing of the fingertips is possibly caused by which of the following conditions?
A. Bacterial endocarditis
B. Systemic illness
C. Chronic respiratory disease
D. Cirrhosis of the liver

______ **16.** An elderly woman who was walking across the living room reports that she felt and heard a "pop" in her hip, and then she fell to the floor. You think that there is a possibility she has a broken hip. Which process has happened to create this injury?
A. Pathologic fracture
B. Physiologic fracture
C. Psychogenic fracture
D. Psychical fracture

______ **17.** In assessing a patient's spine, you find an exaggerated inward curve of the lumbar area. This is known as:
A. kyphosis.
B. lordosis.
C. the Cullen sign.
D. dislocation of the lumbar spine.

_____ **18.** You are auscultating a patient's carotid arteries and hear a "whooshing." You are hearing bruit, which indicates:
- **A.** a heart murmur.
- **B.** turbulent blood flow around a cardiac valve.
- **C.** turbulent blood flow in the carotid arteries.
- **D.** reduced blood flow around a cardiac valve.

_____ **19.** When checking the cranial nerve IV, you will be checking for which of the following?
- **A.** Hearing and balance
- **B.** Smell
- **C.** Visual acuity
- **D.** Eye movements

_____ **20.** You are assessing a patient and notice cyanotic patches on the lower extremities. This finding is known as __________, and it is seen in severe states of shock and hypoperfusion.
- **A.** tenting
- **B.** turgor
- **C.** mottling
- **D.** crepitus

_____ **21.** The scene size-up component of the patient assessment includes all of the following, EXCEPT:
- **A.** focused assessment.
- **B.** mechanism of injury (MOI).
- **C.** requesting additional resources.
- **D.** scene safety.

_____ **22.** During the primary survey, the paramedic must:
- **A.** treat medical and trauma patients differently.
- **B.** determine the SAMPLE history.
- **C.** identify priority patients.
- **D.** obtain baseline vital signs.

_____ **23.** Which of the following standard precautions may be appropriate during the scene size-up and examination of a patient found lying on the kitchen floor for about a week?
- **A.** Gloves
- **B.** Gowns
- **C.** N95 masks
- **D.** All of the above

_____ **24.** When on a scene where people act aggressively or appear to be threatening, it is best for the paramedic to:
- **A.** consider retreating to the ambulance until the scene is secure.
- **B.** explain that you are there to help and do not intend any harm to the patient.
- **C.** explain that you are not law enforcement.
- **D.** begin acting authoritarian and aggressive toward the instigators.

_____ **25.** The most time-sensitive and important aspect of the patient assessment, where life threats are detected and quickly treated, is considered the:
- **A.** primary survey.
- **B.** focused assessment.
- **C.** secondary assessment.
- **D.** general impression.

_____ **26.** Which of the following is considered a "priority patient"?
- **A.** A pregnant patient involved in a low-speed motor vehicle crash without any complications
- **B.** A large multiple-casualty incident with a patient in cardiac arrest
- **C.** A patient who does not pass the "look test," giving a poor general impression
- **D.** A bystander who witnessed the event and is traumatized by what he saw

______ **27.** Evaluating an unresponsive medical patient requires you, the paramedic, to rely on which of the following?
- **A.** A head-to-toe physical exam
- **B.** The presence of a medical identification tag
- **C.** The bystander or family information
- **D.** All of the above

______ **28.** The rapid trauma exam is generally completed:
- **A.** on all patients entrapped in a vehicle.
- **B.** on any patient who does not have a readily identifiable medical problem.
- **C.** before all life threats have been identified and treated.
- **D.** prior to conducting a secondary assessment on the patient.

______ **29.** Which of the following patients typically requires a head-to-toe exam?
- **A.** A man with a minor laceration obtained while cutting vegetables in the kitchen.
- **B.** An athlete who was kicked in the shin while playing soccer.
- **C.** An intoxicated bar patron who fell off a stool and struck his head.
- **D.** A baseball catcher struck in the face while wearing his protective mask.

______ **30.** When assessing a patient's airway status, it is often helpful to do which of the following?
- **A.** Think from the simple to the complex.
- **B.** Intubate the patient quickly to manage the airway definitively.
- **C.** Alter your assessment based on the patient's age.
- **D.** Always open an unconscious patient's airway with a head tilt–chin lift maneuver.

Labeling

Label the following diagram with the missing terms.

1. Nine regions of the abdomen

A. ______________________

B. ______________________

C. ______________________

D. ______________________

E. ______________________

F. ______________________

G. ______________________

H. ______________________

I. ______________________

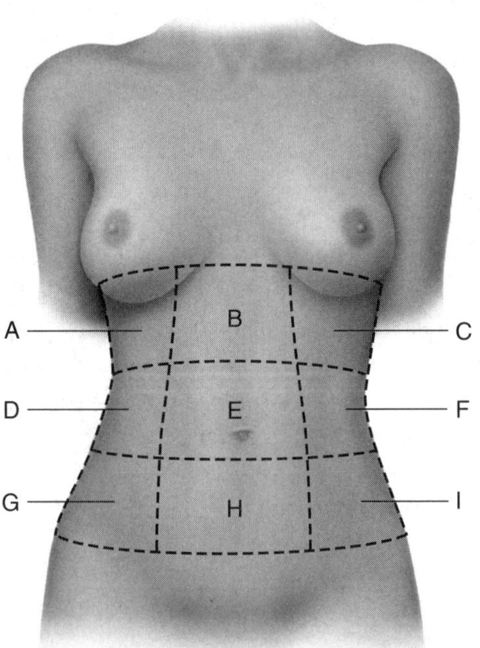

Fill in the Blank

Read each item carefully, and then complete the statement by filling in the missing word(s).

1. You will make your __________ __________ based on the patient's chief complaint, vital signs, and history.
2. The first step in making an approach to a patient is to __________ __________.
3. Once you have established the patient's chief complaint, you will want to check into the history of the __________ __________.
4. When using a translator to help interview your patient, be aware that medical terms and __________ often do not translate well.
5. You respond to a patient who is deaf. When communicating with the patient, you should orient yourself to be in __________-__________-__________ position with him or her.
6. __________ is described as one step further than sympathy.
7. When talking with a patient, you pause to consider something significant that you have just been told before proceeding. This technique is known as __________.
8. The federal law abbreviated as__________ governs the disclosure of patient information.
9. Always review transfer information before transferring a patient to a new facility so that you know the patient's __________ __________.
10. During your history taking, ensure the questions you ask are __________-appropriate and __________-appropriate.

Ambulance Calls

The following case scenarios provide an opportunity to explore the concerns associated with patient management and paramedic care. Read each scenario, and then answer each question.

1. You are called to the crash scene pictured here.

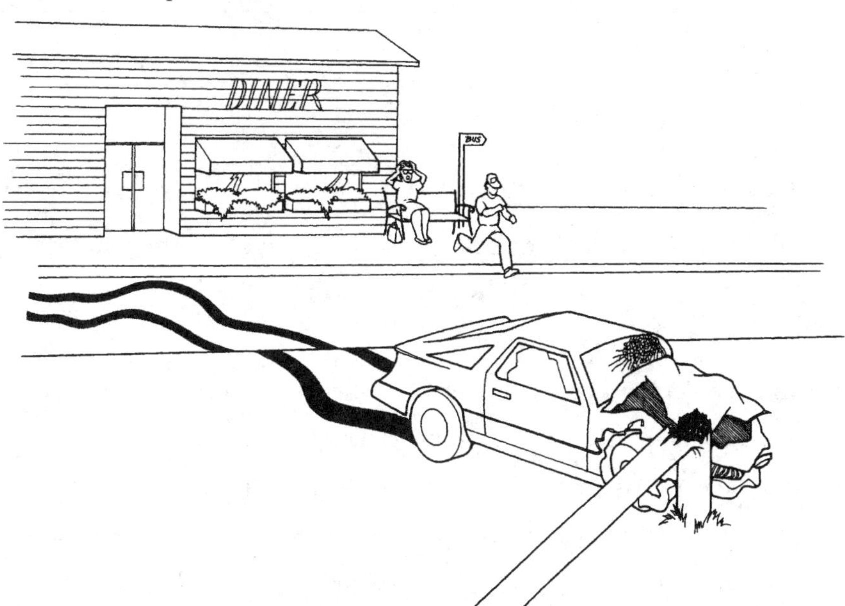

a. List four potential sources of information about what happened to the patient or about his medical background.

(1)____

(2)____

(3)____

(4)____

b. List five pieces of information you can derive simply from observing the scene.

(1)____

(2)____

(3)____

(4)____

(5)____

c. List four reasons why it is necessary to take a history from the driver of the car.

(1)____

(2)____

(3)____

(4)____

d. Before you start taking the history, however, you need to take some preliminary steps. List them.

(1)____

(2)____

(3)____

(4)____

(5)____

True/False

If you believe the statement to be more true than false, write the letter "T" in the space provided. If you believe the statement to be more false than true, write the letter "F."

______ **1.** Being able to think and perform well under pressure is a big part of being a good paramedic.

______ **2.** Patients will always be honest when it comes to their sexual history.

______ **3.** You will always be able to tell who is a heavy user of alcohol.

______ **4.** Patients sometimes need a few seconds to gather their thoughts and answer your questions.

______ **5.** Law enforcement should be called for *every* hostile patient.

______ **6.** You should check blood glucose on every patient who has an altered mental status.

______ **7.** Patients may suffer trauma because of a medical problem or their current health status.

______ **8.** You should be able to make your field diagnosis based on the patient's chief complaint.

_____ **9.** Using "pet names" with a patient will put the person at ease.

_____ **10.** The clarification communication technique is used when trying to clear up a vague history.

_____ **11.** Children do not become dehydrated as fast as adults do.

_____ **12.** Delirium is associated with an acute, sudden change in mental status.

_____ **13.** Aphasia is difficulty speaking, which is common in patients who have experienced cardiovascular disease or a stroke.

_____ **14.** The Babinski reflex is a normal finding in an older adult.

_____ **15.** When assessing a limb for signs of venous obstruction or insufficiency, you should check for edema and mild erythema.

_____ **16.** You should always assess a pulse in three different places on the foot.

_____ **17.** To assess a shoulder dislocation, you should be in front of the patient and looking down at both shoulders.

_____ **18.** Female and male genitalia should be assessed in a limited and discreet fashion.

_____ **19.** Right-sided heart failure is a common cause of JVD.

_____ **20.** You must have a stethoscope for evaluating blood pressure (BP).

Short Answer

Complete this section with short written answers using the space provided.

1. A male patient's chief complaint is "pain in my gut."

a. List six questions you would ask in eliciting the history of the present illness.

(1) _______________

(2) _______________

(3) _______________

(4) _______________

(5) _______________

(6) _______________

b. List four questions you would ask about his other medical history.

(1) _______________

(2) _______________

(3) _______________

(4) _______________

2. Taking the history of a patient requires excellent communications skills. List five communications techniques used by the paramedic in the field.

a. _______________

b. _______________

c. _______________

d. ____________________

e. ____________________

3. You are called to the scene of a multiple-vehicle crash on the interstate highway. As you approach the scene, you begin making your size-up. List four questions you need to answer in making your size-up of the collision scene.

a. ____________________

b. ____________________

c. ____________________

d. ____________________

4. Patient assessment consists largely of detective work—searching for and interpreting clues to form a picture of the patient's problem. At the scene of an incident or, for that matter, in the patient's home, there may be several sources of information about the patient. List four potential sources of information about the patient and what has happened to him or her.

a. ____________________

b. ____________________

c. ____________________

d. ____________________

Fill in the Blank

Fill in the missing parts of the tables.

1. When testing the cranial nerves, a number of simple maneuvers can be employed to determine the presence and degree of disability. Fill in the following table to indicate what to test for disability in the cranial nerves.

Tests for Disability in Cranial Nerves	
Cranial Nerve	**Test**
I	
II	
III	
IV	
V	
VI	
VII	
VIII	
IX, X	
XI	
XII	

2. In the secondary assessment physical exam of a patient with multisystem trauma, you must look for very specific clues to specific injuries. Fill in the following table to indicate what you will be looking for in particular as you examine each part of the body.

Body Region	What I Will Be Looking for in Particular
Head	
Neck	
Chest	
Abdomen	
Extremities	
Back/buttocks	

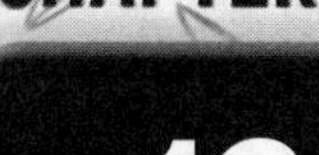

Chapter 12 Critical Thinking and Clinical Decision Making

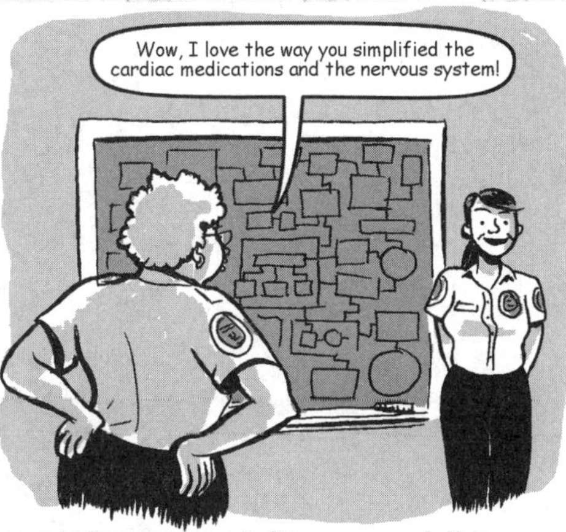

Matching

Part I

For each of the following scenarios, decide if you would follow protocols or use independent decisions.

A. Follow protocols B. Use independent decisions

_____ 1. An 86-year-old woman with facial droop and slurred speech

_____ 2. A 14-year-old boy, unconscious, who is trapped in a drain pipe

_____ 3. A diabetic woman with low blood glucose

_____ 4. A 57-year-old man with "classic ischemic" chest pain

_____ 5. A crop-duster crash with a conscious pilot who is yelling for help

_____ 6. A school where a person has shot several students

_____ 7. An allergic reaction to a bee sting in a 12-year-old girl

_____ 8. A motor vehicle crash where the car is smoking and appears to be on fire

_____ 9. A 20-year-old basketball player in cardiac arrest during a game

_____ 10. A man who is stuck inside a grain elevator and is being pulled under the grain

Part II

Match each of the definitions in the left column to the appropriate term in the right column.

_____	1. Vague or unclear aspects of medicine.	A. Affect
_____	2. Blindly following a protocol or algorithm without thinking about what is being done and whether it is working.	B. Comorbidity
_____	3. The patient's emotional state as reflected in the patient's physical behavior.	C. Concept formation
_____	4. The existence of two or more chronic diseases or conditions in a patient.	D. Cookbook medicine
_____	5. Focusing on or considering only one aspect of a situation without first taking into account all possibilities.	E. Medical ambiguity
_____	6. Pattern of understanding based on the initially obtained information; the first stage of the critical thinking process n prehospital care.	F. Tunnel vision

Multiple Choice

Read each item carefully, and then select the best response.

_____ **1.** __________ is processing the information presented by the patient you are treating.
A. Gathering
B. Evaluating
C. Synthesizing
D. Thinking

_____ **2.** Which of the following items is NOT included in the concept-formation process?
A. Smell
B. Sample history
C. Hearing
D. Seeing

_____ **3.** What is the second stage of critical thinking?
A. Application of principle
B. Reflection in action
C. Concept formation
D. Data interpretation

_____ **4.** What does *reflection in action* mean?
A. A call review of the run you just completed
B. Checking your interventions as you apply them to your patient
C. Stopping before you apply the intervention to make sure you are doing the right thing
D. Checking the protocols prior to doing anything

_____ **5.** Which of the following is NOT one of the "Six Rs" discussed in the chapter?
A. Read the scene.
B. Read the protocols.
C. Read the patient.
D. React.

_____ **6.** You respond to a patient's home for a report of chest pain. You are determining the chief complaint and taking the baseline vital signs. In which of the "Six Rs" are you working right now?
A. Reading the scene
B. Reacting
C. Reevaluating
D. Reading the patient

_____ **7.** When responding to a critical patient, why is it best to use a mental checklist?
A. So that you do not forget to take vital signs
B. So that you always follow your protocols
C. To facilitate better thinking on the scene
D. So that you will never be sued

_____ **8.** Which of the following is NOT used in synthesizing the patient's information?
A. Patient history
B. Patient allergies
C. Current complaints
D. Previous diseases

_____ **9.** Which of the following adult patients would be considered to have a serious condition?
A. Acute presentation of a first-time event
B. Acute presentation of a chronic event
C. Patient with small lacerations
D. Partial-thickness burns to an extremity, with less than 5% of body surface area (BSA) burned

______ **10.** What is the "third cornerstone" of effective paramedic practice?

A. Development and implementation of a patient care plan
B. Having the ability to think and work under pressure
C. Having the ability to use judgment and make independent decisions
D. Having the ability to gather, evaluate, and synthesize information

Fill in the Blank

Read each item carefully, and then complete the statement by filling in the missing word(s).

1. By taking a SAMPLE history and baseline vital signs, you are __________ information about the patient that will be used to assess and evaluate the patient and help form your treatment plan.
2. Your care plan for your patient is almost always defined by your __________.
3. Your final cornerstone of practicing as a paramedic is to __________ and __________ under pressure.
4. The process of gathering information by smell, sight, hearing, and touch is known as __________ __________.
5. Patients with major multisystem trauma, acute chronic conditions, and devastating single-system trauma would be examples of patients with critical__________ __________.
6. Once you have assessed the patient and begin treatment, you are using a(n) __________ __________.
7. Some of the primary elements involved in __________ the scene are evaluating the overall safety of the situation, the environmental conditions, the immediate surroundings, access and egress issues, and the MOI.
8. When dealing with a critical patient, you take vital signs three or more times. The readings allow you to assess __________.

Identify

After reading the following case study, list the chief complaint, vital signs, and any pertinent negatives.

It is 1600 hours, and you have been called to a residence for a woman who is not feeling well. When you arrive, you find a 56-year-old woman with a general feeling of malaise. You begin talking with her to gather some information while your partner takes baseline vital signs. During your SAMPLE history, you find out that she has diabetes. Your partner tests her blood glucose level, and it is 110 mg/dL. The patient states that she is very careful because of her illness. Her blood pressure (BP) is 160/100 mm Hg, and her pulse is 92 beats/min and regular, with normal sinus rhythm showing on the ECG monitor, but she is showing a little ST-segment depression. You ask her if she has ever had a heart attack, and she says no. Her Spo_2 is 97% on room air, all lung fields are clear, and she is breathing at 18 breaths/min. The patient's skin is warm and dry, and her pupils are PERRLA (Pupils Equal, Round, and Reactive to Light and Accommodation). She says she has been feeling this way for a few days and is so tired that she hasn't been able to do anything. She was afraid something major might be wrong with her, so she decided to give 9-1-1 a call. You tell the woman that she might have had a cardiac event and that you want to take her in. You apply oxygen by non-rebreathing mask at 15 L/min, start an IV at a to-keep-open (TKO) drip, and give her some nitroglycerin paste to bring down the BP en route. You take a 12-lead electrocardiogram (ECG) en route and transport her to the local emergency department (ED). The nitroglycerin brings the BP down to 120/70 mm Hg. All other vital signs stay the same. Later, you learn she has had a small myocardial infarction (MI), but because of her diabetes, she never had the classic signs.

1. Chief complaint:

____

____

____

2. Vital signs:

3. Pertinent negatives:

Ambulance Calls

The following case scenario provides an opportunity to explore the concerns associated with patient management and paramedic care. Read the scenario, and then answer each question.

1. You are on a rural squad, with no regional trauma center nearby. You are dispatched to an elementary school for a child who has fallen out of a tree. The school is reporting that the child is still on the ground outside on the playground. When you arrive, you find a 9-year-old girl sitting up. You ask your partner to take cervical spine precautions while you start your primary survey. The teacher says she was approximately 15 feet up when she fell. You note a large broken branch about 7 feet off the ground, and the teacher says that the child hit that branch on the way down on her left side and then landed on her head on the hard dirt. The child is unable to tell you her name and is confused about where she is and the day of the week. After finding no obvious life threats during the primary survey, you proceed with a rapid trauma exam because of the significant mechanism of injury (MOI). You decide she is a critical patient because of the MOI and call for Life Flight to take her to the regional trauma center. Your partner applies an extrication collar, and you carefully place her on a long backboard. You apply supplemental oxygen by nonrebreathing mask at 15 L/min. Your partner takes baseline vital signs that reveal a BP of 130/80 mm Hg, pulse of 52 beats/min, and respirations at 6 breaths/min. Lung sounds are clear. The patient responds only to painful stimuli at this point, and her Spo_2 is 88%. Her pupils are unequal, with the left pupil much larger than the right. The patient begins to gag and vomit. You suction all secretions, place an oropharyngeal airway, and start to assist her ventilations with the bag-mask device. Your partner gets an IV started as the helicopter is landing. The patient no longer has a gag reflex, so the flight medics insert an advanced airway. The Life Flight crew loads her and takes off, heading for the regional trauma center. Later, you learn that the girl died in the operating room (OR) as a result of massive head injury.

a. What is your first clue that this patient should be treated as a critical patient?

b. Under which type of consent can you transport this child without her parents' permission?

c. What do your baseline vital signs suggest for this patient?

d. What is your first concern with the patient, and how can you manage that concern?

____

____

____

2. You are traveling to Grandma's house for what you anticipate will be a wonderful Thanksgiving dinner. Traffic slows and comes to a stop. Knowing what you do about traffic and collisions, you pull out your primary survey kit and head up the road. A minivan loaded with people has crossed left of the center line and hit a car with another family in it. There are people everywhere—some trying to help patients from the vehicles and others just standing around. The 9-1-1 system has already been called, but you can't hear any sirens yet because you are about 20 miles from any town. You realize there are critical patients trapped in the van, and the Jaws of Life will be needed to extricate those patients.

a. How do you identify yourself and gain control of this scene?

____

____

____

b. Which type of equipment will you need at this scene?

____

____

____

c. Will you begin any type of treatment before help arrives?

____

____

____

True/False

If you believe the statement to be more true than false, write the letter "T" in the space provided. If you believe the statement to be more false than true, write the letter "F."

______ **1.** The first cornerstone of your practice is having the ability to gather, evaluate, and synthesize information on the scene.

______ **2.** Once you have evaluated the information you obtained from the scene, the patient, or a bystander and have determined which information is valid or invalid, you need to process—or synthesize—this information.

______ **3.** Protocols, standing orders, and patient care algorithms will address every patient for the paramedic and give a clear, defined path to treatment.

______ **4.** The patient who presents with an acute presentation of a new medical condition is considered a patient with a critical life threat.

______ **5.** The second stage of critical thinking is concept formation.

______ **6.** Reflection in action is the process of reassessing the patient.

______ **7.** When you identify a patient with medical ambiguity, it means that you have pinpointed the cause of the patient's medical problem.

______ **8.** When reading the scene, you are looking for information that is available only at the scene.

Short Answer

Complete this section with short written answers using the space provided.

1. Discuss the use of the "Six Rs" when responding to a routine call.
   - **a.** Read the scene:
   - **b.** Read the patient:
   - **c.** React:
   - **d.** Reevaluate:
   - **e.** Revise the plan:
   - **f.** Review your performance:

2. When using the cornerstone principles of critical thinking, discuss the differences in gathering information, evaluating information, and synthesizing.

CHAPTER 13

Principles of Pharmacology

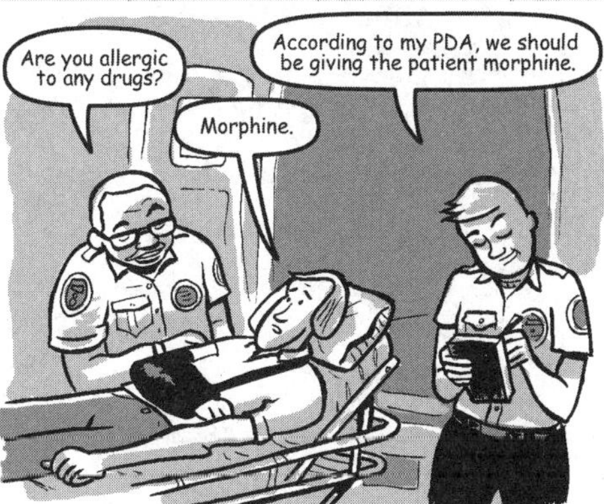

Do not administer a medication to which the patient has an allergy!

Matching

Part I

Listed here are medications that are considered controlled substances. Write the schedule, I to V, for the example given.

_____ 1. Hydrocodone (Vicodin)

_____ 2. Narcotic cough medicines

_____ 3. Heroin

_____ 4. Fentanyl (Sublimaze)

_____ 5. Diazepam (Valium)

_____ 6. Lorazepam (Ativan)

_____ 7. High abuse potential and no recognized medical purpose

_____ 8. High abuse potential and legitimate medical purpose

_____ 9. Cocaine

_____ 10. Codeine

Part II

Match each of the definitions in the left column to the appropriate term in the right column.

_____ 1. Medications that bind with heavy metals in the body and create a compound that can be eliminated; used in cases of ingestion or poisoning.

_____ 2. Widening of the bronchial tubes.

_____ 3. Narrowing of the bronchial tubes.

_____ 4. A process with four possible effects on a medication absorbed into the body: (1) an inactive substance can become active, capable of producing desired or unwanted clinical effects; (2) an active medication can be changed into another active medication; (3) an active medication can be completely or partially inactivated; or (4) a medication can be transformed into a substance (active or inactive) that is easier for the body to eliminate.

_____ 5. A term used to describe paralytic agents that act at the neuromuscular junction by binding with nicotinic receptors on muscles, causing fasciculations and preventing additional activation by acetylcholine.

_____ 6. Medications that temporarily bind with cellular receptor sites, displacing agonist chemicals.

A. Absolute refractory period

B. Absorption

C. Acetylcholinesterase

D. Active metabolite

E. Active transport

F. Adverse effect

______	**7.** The grouping to which a medication belongs. Medications are grouped according to their characteristics, traits, or primary components.	**G.**	Affinity
______	**8.** A term used to describe the fibers in the parasympathetic nervous system that release a chemical called acetylcholine.	**H.**	Agonist medications
______	**9.** The percentage of the unchanged medication that reaches systemic circulation.	**I.**	Analgesia
______	**10.** The state in which cardiac cells are at rest, waiting for the generation of a spontaneous impulse from within.	**J.**	Anaphylaxis
______	**11.** The medications used to kill or suppress the growth of microorganisms.	**K.**	Anesthetic
______	**12.** The medications used to treat fungal infections.	**L.**	Antagonist medications
______	**13.** The early phase of cardiac repolarization, in which the heart muscle cannot be stimulated to depolarize; also known as the effective refractory period.	**M.**	Antibiotics
______	**14.** The process by which the molecules of a substance are moved from the site of entry or administration into the systemic circulation.	**N.**	Antifungals
______	**15.** An enzyme that breaks down acetylcholine.	**O.**	Antimicrobials
______	**16.** A medication that has undergone biotransformation and is able to alter a cellular process or body function.	**P.**	Automaticity
______	**17.** The medications used to fight infection by killing the microorganisms or preventing their multiplication to allow the body's immune system to overcome them.	**Q.**	Bioavailability
______	**18.** The group of medications that prevent endogenous or exogenous agonist chemicals from reaching cell receptor sites and initiating or altering a particular cellular activity.	**R.**	Biotransformation
______	**19.** A medication that causes the inability to feel sensation.	**S.**	Bronchoconstriction
______	**20.** An extreme systemic form of an allergic reaction involving two or more body systems.	**T.**	Bronchodilation
______	**21.** The process of molecules binding with carrier proteins when energy is used to move the molecules against a concentration gradient.	**U.**	Chelating agents
______	**22.** Abnormal or harmful effect to an organism caused by exposure to a chemical; it is indicated by some result, such as death, a change in food or water consumption, altered body and organ weights, altered enzyme levels, or visible illness.	**V.**	Cholinergic
______	**23.** The ability of a medication to bind with a particular receptor site.	**W.**	Class
______	**24.** The state of being insensible to pain while still conscious.	**X.**	Competitive antagonists
______	**25.** The group of medications that initiate or alter a cellular activity by attaching to receptor sites, prompting a cellular response.	**Y.**	Competitive depolarizing

Part III

Match each of the definitions in the left column to the appropriate term in the right column.

______	**1.** Use of hydrostatic pressure to force water or dissolved particles through a semipermeable membrane.	**A.**	Dependence
______	**2.** The process in which the rate of elimination is directly influenced by plasma levels of a substance.	**B.**	Depolarization
______	**3.** The alteration of a medication via metabolism within the gastrointestinal tract before it reaches the systemic circulation.	**C.**	Depressant
______	**4.** An unusual tolerance to the therapeutic and adverse clinical effects of a medication or chemical.	**D.**	Digitalis preparation
______	**5.** The time needed in an average person for metabolism or elimination of 50% of a substance in the plasma.	**E.**	Distribution
______	**6.** The physical, behavioral, or emotional need for a medication or chemical to maintain "normal" physiologic function.	**F.**	Diuretic

_____ **7.** The process of discharging resting cardiac muscle fibers by an electric impulse that causes them to contract.

_____ **8.** A chemical or medication that decreases the performance of the central nervous system or sympathetic nervous system.

_____ **9.** A drug used in the treatment of heart failure and certain atrial dysrhythmias.

_____ **10.** The movement and transportation of a medication throughout the bloodstream to tissues and cells and, ultimately, to its target receptor.

_____ **11.** Brief, uncoordinated, visible twitching of small muscle groups; may be caused by the administration of a depolarizing neuromuscular blocking agent (namely, succinylcholine).

_____ **12.** The process of medication molecules binding with carrier proteins when no energy is expended.

_____ **13.** Seepage of blood and medication into the tissue surrounding the blood vessel.

_____ **14.** Originating outside the organism (body).

_____ **15.** Originating from within the organism (body).

_____ **16.** A chemical that increases urinary output.

_____ **17.** A graphic illustration of the response of a drug according to the dose administered.

_____ **18.** The specified amount of a medication to be given at specific intervals.

_____ **19.** The process in which a mechanism reducing available cell receptors for a particular medication results in tolerance.

_____ **20.** A substance that has some therapeutic effect (such as reducing inflammation, fighting bacteria, or producing euphoria) when given in the appropriate circumstances and in the appropriate dose.

_____ **21.** In a pharmacologic context, the removal of a medication or its by-products from the body.

_____ **22.** In a pharmacologic context, the ability of a medication to produce the desired effect.

_____ **23.** Sites of generation of electrical impulses other than normal pacemaker cells.

_____ **24.** In a pharmacologic context, the time a medication concentration can be expected to remain above the minimum level needed to provide the intended action.

_____ **25.** Pertaining to voluntary muscle movements that are distorted or impaired because of abnormal muscle tone.

G. Dose-response curve
H. Dosing
I. Down-regulation
J. Drug
K. Duration
L. Dystonic
M. Ectopic foci
N. Efficacy
O. Elimination
P. Endogenous
Q. Exogenous
R. Extravasation
S. Facilitated diffusion
T. Fasciculation
U. Filtration
V. First-order elimination
W. First-pass effect
X. Habituation
Y. Half-life

Multiple Choice

Read each item carefully, and then select the best response.

_____ **1.** The nonproprietary name is a general name for a drug and is not manufacturer specific. What is another name for nonproprietary drugs?

A. Chemical
B. Generic
C. Trade
D. Official

_____ **2.** What was the first US federal law, legislated in 1906, aimed at protecting the public from mislabeled and harmful drugs?

A. Food, Drug, and Cosmetic Act
B. Harrison Narcotic Act
C. Pure Food and Drug Act
D. Narcotic Control Act

_____ **3.** Which US government agency has jurisdiction over approving new medications?
- **A.** Food and Drug Administration
- **B.** Centers for Disease Control and Prevention
- **C.** Drug Enforcement Administration
- **D.** Federal Trade Commission

_____ **4.** What is the medication interaction that is utilized when the emergency department (ED) physician considers administering some ethanol to a patient who has been poisoned due to drinking ethylene glycol (antifreeze)?
- **A.** Altered absorption
- **B.** Drug antagonism
- **C.** Altered metabolism
- **D.** Neutralization

_____ **5.** The formulation in which a medication is surrounded by a wax-like material that dissolves in a body cavity is called a(n):
- **A.** capsule.
- **B.** suppository.
- **C.** powder.
- **D.** inhaler.

_____ **6.** Which of the following forms of medication is dissolved or suspended in liquid intended for oral consumption?
- **A.** Suppository
- **B.** Inhaler/spray
- **C.** Drop
- **D.** Liquid

_____ **7.** What is the name given to the small particles of medication designed to be dissolved or mixed into a solution or liquid?
- **A.** Tablet
- **B.** Powder
- **C.** Pill
- **D.** Pulvule

_____ **8.** Which receptor sites would have an agonist effect of insulin secretion, uterine relaxation, and bronchiole relaxation?
- **A.** Alpha-1
- **B.** Alpha-2
- **C.** Beta-1
- **D.** Beta-2

_____ **9.** Certain medications are known to have decreased efficacy or potency when taken repeatedly by a patient. This state is known as:
- **A.** synergy.
- **B.** biotransformation.
- **C.** tolerance.
- **D.** reabsorption.

_____ **10.** Medications become distributed into each of the following types of body substances, EXCEPT:
- **A.** oils.
- **B.** lipids.
- **C.** water.
- **D.** proteins.

_____ **11.** The *most basic* concern regarding medication storage is:
- **A.** ample supply.
- **B.** need for refrigeration.
- **C.** integrity of the container.
- **D.** double-locked cabinetry.

_____ **12.** Medications can become unsafe to use if exposed to each of the following, EXCEPT:
- **A.** direct sunlight.
- **B.** extreme heat.
- **C.** IV solutions.
- **D.** extreme cold.

_____ **13.** If there is positive evidence of human fetal risk for a certain medication, but the benefits from use in pregnant women may be acceptable despite the risk, this specific medication is given a pregnancy category of:
- **A.** A.
- **B.** B.
- **C.** C.
- **D.** D.

_____ **14.** Unmatched blood is almost always which of the following?
- **A.** Type AB, Rh positive
- **B.** Type O, Rh negative
- **C.** Type A, Rh negative
- **D.** Type O, Rh positive

Fill in the Blank

Read each item carefully, and then complete the statement by filling in the missing word(s).

1. A medication's __________ are the reasons or conditions for which the medication is given.
2. Two medications can bind together in the body, creating an inactive substance. This process is referred to as __________.
3. Opiate __________ medication reverses the effects of opioid drugs.
4. When the effect of one medication is greatly enhanced by the presence of another medication, which does not have the ability to produce the same effect, this state is referred to as __________.
5. An agonist that produces vasoconstriction of arteries and veins is called a(n) __________ receptor.
6. An agonist that stimulates bronchus and bronchiole relaxation, as well as insulin secretion and uterine relaxation, is called a(n) __________ receptor.
7. __________ medications cause the kidneys to remove excess amounts of salt and water from the body.
8. Medications that reduce heart rate and blood pressure are called __________ agents.
9. __________ __________ are drugs that decrease the heart rate and improve contractility.
10. Drugs that decrease inflammation and are immunosuppressants are called __________.

Identify

Read the following case study, then list the chief complaint, vital signs, and pertinent negatives.

You are called to a private residence for a 65-year-old woman who has general body weakness. Upon arrival, you find a woman sitting on her couch in the living room. When you ask what the problem is, she tells you that she has heart palpitations. She does not appear to be in distress. Her husband tells you that his wife went to the doctor yesterday for a checkup, and she seemed to be doing okay.

You check the patient's vital signs and find that the pulse is 60 beats/min, regular and weak; respirations are slightly labored at 22 breaths/min; blood pressure (BP) is 90/60 mm Hg; and Spo_2 is 97%. While your partner starts an IV, you listen to the patient's lung sounds, perform a 12-lead electrocardiogram (ECG), and get a SAMPLE history. You observe that the patient seems pale. She tells you that she has no pain or nausea and that she is on medication for hypertension and gastric reflux. She was put on a new medication yesterday for her gastric reflux and an additional medication for her blood pressure. She has had no hospitalizations and has been in relatively good health. The patient was watching TV when her symptoms started.

According to her husband, it is time for the patient's afternoon medications, but you think that she should wait until she gets to the hospital, a 15-minute transport time, and discuss them with the doctor before taking these medications. You transport the patient and reassess her vital signs en route.

1. Chief complaint:

____

____

2. Vital signs:

____

____

3. Pertinent negatives:

____

____

Ambulance Calls

The following case scenarios provide an opportunity to explore the concerns associated with patient management and paramedic care. Read each scenario, and then answer each question.

1. You are on the scene where a 58-year-old man is reporting substernal chest pain rated as 8 out of 10 that came on while he was shoveling snow. You have placed the patient on supplemental oxygen and administered aspirin, and your partner is obtaining vital signs and a 12-lead ECG. You obtain lung sounds and administer nitroglycerin, which has no effect. The patient is now reporting 10 out of 10 for pain. His BP is 160/100 mm Hg, so you decide to administer 5 mg of morphine. The 10 rights for medication administration run through your head as you prepare the drug for administration. What are the 10 rights, and how do they apply?

   a. ______________________________

   b. ______________________________

   c. ______________________________

   d. ______________________________

   e. ______________________________

   f. ______________________________

   g. ______________________________

   h. ______________________________

   i. ______________________________

   j. ______________________________

2. Many medications undergo some degree of chemical change by the body, known as biotransformation. What are the four possible effects that this process may have on how a medication is absorbed into the body?

   a. ______________________________

   b. ______________________________

   c. ______________________________

   d. ______________________________

3. Very young and very old patients may present with factors that can affect the actions of medications that are administered in the prehospital setting. Which factors should the paramedic consider when providing care to the young and the old, including additional factors that may need to be considered if the patient has underlying medical conditions?

a. ______________________________

b. ______________________________

c. ______________________________

d. ______________________________

e. ______________________________

f. ______________________________

True/False

If you believe the statement to be more true than false, write the letter "T" in the space provided. If you believe the statement to be more false than true, write the letter "F."

_____ 1. The general, nonproprietary name for a drug is its official name.

_____ 2. Schedule V drugs have the highest abuse potential and a propensity for severe dependency.

_____ 3. The changes in pharmacokinetics in geriatric patients are comparable to those observed in young children.

_____ 4. The rate of elimination of a medication is directly influenced by the plasma levels of the substance.

_____ 5. Patients at extremes of age are disproportionately prone to paradoxical medication reactions.

_____ 6. Diuretic medications can help improve the effects of sickle cell disease.

_____ 7. In the cardiac muscle cell, during phases 0, 1, 2, and 3, no additional depolarization may occur because of external stimuli.

_____ 8. Idiosyncrasy is an abnormal reaction by a person to a medication to which most other people do not react.

_____ 9. An unusual tolerance to the therapeutic and adverse clinical effects of a medication or chemical is known as synergism.

_____ 10. Promethazine (Phenergan) is an antidysrhythmic medication taken by cardiac patients.

_____ 11. Disposal of partially used or damaged controlled substances requires verification by an appropriate witness.

_____ 12. Whole blood transfusions are no longer used clinically in the United States.

_____ 13. If studies in animals or humans have demonstrated fetal abnormalities, making the drug contraindicated in women who are pregnant, this is a pregnancy category X drug.

Short Answer

Complete this section with short written answers using the space provided.

1. The medical director of your emergency medical services (EMS) agency announces that a new medication will be introduced into the agency's protocols. As part of an in-service program to learn about this new drug, you are given the pharmaceutical company's drug profile to review. What are the three different names for the medication that will be listed in this literature?

a. ______________________________

b. ______________________________

c. ______________________________

2. What are the components of a drug profile?

a. ______________________________

b. ______________________________

c. ______________________________

d. ______________________________

e. ______________________________

f. ______________________________

g. ______________________________

h. ______________________________

i. ______________________________

j. ______________________________

k. ______________________________

l. ______________________________

3. The Institute for Safe Medication Practices (ISMP) has developed a list of error-prone medication abbreviations. List five potential errors, and explain how they can be avoided.

a. ______________________________

b. ______________________________

c. ______________________________

d. ______________________________

e. ______________________________

4. List eight common adverse effects of medications.

a. ______________________________

b. ______________________________

c. ______________________________

d. ______________________________

e. ______________________________

f. ______________________________

g. ______________________________

h. ______________________________

5. For each of the following medication descriptions, write the medication class next to the common indications or purpose.

a. Treat or prevent nausea and vomiting: __________

b. Decrease gastrointestinal (GI) motility; alter GI secretion activity: __________

c. Treat bacterial infection: __________

d. Neutralize excess acids present in the stomach: __________

e. Block histamine receptors; dry mucous membranes; inhibit immune response in allergic reactions: __________

f. Reduce heart rate and blood pressure: __________

g. Treat anxiety and seizures; provide sedation: __________

h. Decrease inflammation; immunosuppressant: __________

i. Dissolve clots present in blood vessels or vascular access devices: __________

j. Replace hormones; improve bone density that has decreased due to aging and hormone loss: __________

k. Relieve pain and relieve or suppress cough: __________

l. Increase blood pressure, heart rate, and cardiac output; constrict blood vessels: __________

Fill in the Blank

Fill in the missing parts of the tables.

Veins Used During Intraosseous (IO) Infusion	
Intraosseous Site	**Vein**
Proximal tibia	__________
Femur	__________
__________	Great saphenous vein
__________	Axillary vein
Manubrium (sternum)	__________

Gastrointestinal Medication Absorption	
Factor	**Medication Absorption**
__________	Ability of medication to pass through the GI tract into the bloodstream
__________	Perfusion of the GI system (may be decreased during systemic trauma or shock)
__________	Injury or bleeding in the GI system (both can alter GI motility, decreasing the time that oral medications can be absorbed)

Sources of Medications	
Source	**Examples**
__________	Atropine, aspirin, digoxin, morphine
__________	Heparin, antivenom, thyroid preparations, insulin
__________	Streptokinase, numerous antibiotics
__________	Iron, magnesium sulfate, lithium, phosphorus, calcium

CHAPTER 14

Medication Administration

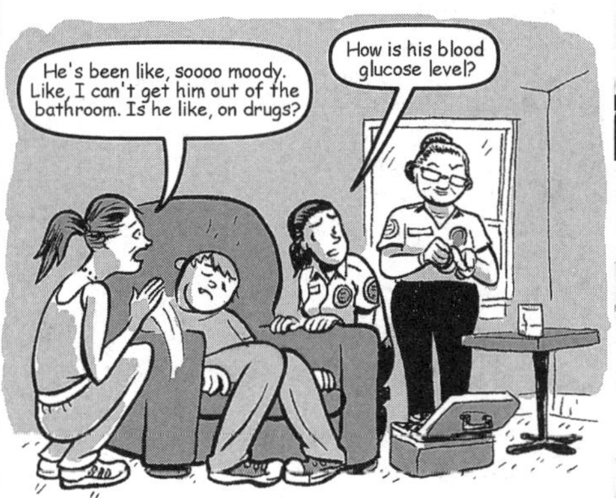

Matching

Part I

In choosing a medication, selecting the route of administration relates to the medication's onset of action. For each of the following, match the onset of action with the route of administration:

_____ **1.** Intramuscular injection
_____ **2.** Nasal mucosal atomization (MAD)
_____ **3.** Endotracheal
_____ **4.** Intraosseous
_____ **5.** Sublingual
_____ **6.** Inhalation
_____ **7.** Intravenous

A. 30–60 seconds
B. 2–3 minutes
C. 3–5 minutes
D. 10–20 minutes

Part II

Match each of the definitions in the left column to the appropriate term in the right column.

_____ **1.** The amount of a drug that the physician orders for the patient.
_____ **2.** Solutions that contain molecules (usually proteins) that are too large to pass out of the capillary membranes and, therefore, remain in the vascular compartment.
_____ **3.** Chemicals used to cleanse an area before performing an invasive procedure, such as starting an IV line; not toxic to living tissues; examples include isopropyl alcohol and iodine.
_____ **4.** Pertaining to the ear.
_____ **5.** The anterior aspect of the elbow.
_____ **6.** Small glass containers that are sealed and the contents sterilized.
_____ **7.** Tubing that connects to the IV bag access port and the catheter to deliver IV fluid.
_____ **8.** A sealed hub on an administration set designed for sterile access to the IV fluid.
_____ **9.** A condition in which a needle is reinserted into the catheter, and it slices through the catheter, creating a free-floating segment.
_____ **10.** The body's natural blood-clotting mechanism.
_____ **11.** The internal diameter of an IV catheter or needle.
_____ **12.** The area of the administration set in which fluid accumulates so that the tubing remains filled with fluid.

A. Access port
B. Administration set
C. Ampules
D. Antecubital
E. Antiseptics
F. Aural
G. Bolus
H. Bone Injection Gun (BIG)
I. Buccal
J. Catheter shear
K. Colloid solutions
L. Desired dose

_____ **13.** A solution (usually water or normal saline) used for diluting a medication. — **M.** Diluent

_____ **14.** Injecting sterile water or saline from one vial into another vial containing a powdered form of a drug. — **N.** Drip chamber

_____ **15.** Medication administration that involves the medication passing through a portion of the gastrointestinal tract. — **O.** Drug reconstitution

_____ **16.** Large neck vein that is lateral to the carotid artery. — **P.** Enteral medications

_____ **17.** The area of an IV catheter that fills with blood to help indicate when a vein is cannulated. — **Q.** External jugular (EJ) vein

_____ **18.** Between the cheek and gums. — **R.** Flash chamber

_____ **19.** A spring-loaded device that is used for inserting an intraosseous needle into the proximal tibia in adult and pediatric patients. — **S.** Gauge

_____ **20.** A term used to describe "in one mass"; in medication administration, a single dose given by the intravenous or intraosseous route, which may be a small or large quantity of the drug. — **T.** Hemostasis

Part III

Match each of the definitions in the left column to the appropriate term in the right column.

_____ **1.** A pressurized canister that delivers a specific dose of a medication; commonly used for beta-agonist bronchodilators. — **A.** Hypotonic solution

_____ **2.** A type of surgical drain often used as a constricting band. — **B.** Implanted vascular access device

_____ **3.** A device for producing a fine spray or mist that is used to deliver inhaled medications. — **C.** Infiltration

_____ **4.** A reaction characterized by an abrupt temperature elevation with severe chills, backache, headache, weakness, nausea, and vomiting; a potential complication of intravenous or intraosseous therapy. — **D.** Infusion pump

_____ **5.** A solution of 0.9% sodium chloride; an isotonic crystalloid. — **E.** Inhalation

_____ **6.** Blockage, usually of a tubular structure such as a blood vessel or IV catheter. — **F.** Intradermal

_____ **7.** The ability to influence the movement of water across a semipermeable membrane. — **G.** Intranasal

_____ **8.** Feature of an IV catheter that allows it to appear on a radiograph. — **H.** Intraosseous (IO) space

_____ **9.** A Teflon catheter inserted over a hollow needle. — **I.** Intravenous (IV) therapy

_____ **10.** A solution that has a lower concentration of sodium than does the cell; the increased osmotic pressure lets water flow into the cell, causing it to swell and possibly burst. — **J.** Isotonic crystalloids

_____ **11.** The escape of fluid into the surrounding tissue; the result of vein perforation during IV cannulation. — **K.** Isotonic solution

_____ **12.** Devices that are implanted in surgery and sutured under the skin, for the purpose of long-term medication administration, total parenteral nutrition, chemotherapy, blood product administration, or venous blood sampling. — **L.** Metered-dose inhaler (MDI)

_____ **13.** A mechanical device that infuses a precise intravenous volume programmed by the clinician. — **M.** Nebulizer

_____ **14.** The layer of the dermis, just beneath the epidermis, a medication delivery route. — **N.** Normal saline

_____ **15.** Breathing into the lungs; a medication delivery route. — **O.** Occlusion

_____ **16.** A solution that has the same concentration of sodium as does the cell; in this case, water does not shift, and no change in cell shape occurs. — **P.** Osmolarity

_____ **17.** Intravenous solutions that do not cause a fluid shift into or out of the cell; examples include normal saline and lactated Ringer solutions. — **Q.** Over-the-needle catheter

_____ 18. Cannulation of a vein with an IV catheter to access the patient's vascular system. — R. Penrose drain

_____ 19. The spongy cancellous bone of the epiphyses and the medullary cavity of the diaphysis, collectively. — S. Pyrogenic reaction

_____ 20. Within the nose. — T. Radiopaque

Multiple Choice

Read each item carefully, and then select the best response.

_____ **1.** When the patient needs fluid infusion and there are no obvious IV sites available, most emergency medical services (EMS) systems utilize the _______________ IO site.

A. FASTR for the humeral
B. FAST-1 for the sternal
C. BIG for the proximal tibial
D. venous cutdown

_____ **2.** When necessary, medications can be administered via the endotracheal (ET) route. The mnemonic _________ helps the paramedic remember which medications are acceptable.

A. SOAP
B. CBERNE
C. LEAN
D. MEDS

_____ **3.** Which of the following solutions is the best choice for administration, in the prehospital setting, when the patient needs to have body fluids replaced?

A. Hypertonic
B. Hypotonic
C. Colloid
D. Crystalloid

_____ **4.** Which administration set will allow for administration of 60 gtt/mL?

A. Blood tubing
B. Microdrip set
C. Macrodrip set
D. Volutrol administration set

_____ **5.** When inserting an IV catheter, the bevel should be:

A. facing down.
B. facing up.
C. pointed to the side.
D. rolled as you insert it.

_____ **6.** After starting an IV on a patient, which of the following is NOT necessary to document?

A. The site of the IV
B. The gauge of the needle used
C. The patient's pain scale when you started the IV
D. The type of fluid you are using

_____ **7.** There are many potential complications with an IV site; __________ means there is an inflammation of the vein.

A. thrombophlebitis
B. hematoma
C. occlusion
D. vein irritation

_____ **8.** If a sternal IO is used in your EMS system, consideration should be made to review the _____________ IO device for this application.

A. BIG
B. FASTR
C. EZ-IO
D. Jamshidi needle

_____ **9.** When taking a blood sample in the field, what is the green-topped tube used for?

A. Determining the patient's blood type
B. Checking glucose and electrolyte levels
C. Determining how long it takes for the patient's blood to clot
D. Checking for alcohol and drugs in the blood system

_____ **10.** Which of the following is an example of an antiseptic?

A. Virex
B. Iodine
C. Cidex
D. Microcide

_____ **11.** Which medication route is usually the fastest and most commonly used in the prehospital setting?

A. Intradermal
B. Subcutaneous
C. Intramuscular
D. Intravenous

_____ **12.** A(n) __________ is a breakable sterile glass container that carries a single dose of medication.

A. vial
B. ampule
C. mix-o-vial
D. prefill

_____ **13.** A(n)__________ injection is given at a 90° angle.

A. subcutaneous
B. intravascular
C. intramuscular
D. bolus

_____ **14.** Which of the following medications is NOT given by the intranasal route?

A. Naloxone
B. Fentanyl
C. Nitroglycerin
D. Glucagon

_____ **15.** How much normal saline should you use as a flush after administering a medication through a gastric tube?

A. 15 to 30 mL
B. 30 to 60 mL
C. 60 to 75 mL
D. You do not use normal saline for a flush.

_____ **16.** Which tool uses the principles of crew resource management by requiring a process for verification for every medication?

A. FMEA
B. CRM
C. MACC
D. MADD

______ 17. When using the Medication Administration Cross-Check tool, after the first provider who is going to administer the drug clearly states the dose, drug name, route, rate, and reason, the second provider should state:

A. contraindications.

B. quantity.

C. volume

D. "Ready."

______ 18. Of the following medication routes, which has the slowest onset of action of absorption?

A. Intraosseous

B. Inhalation

C. Oral

D. Intramuscular injection

______ 19. When a patient takes a medication by the __________ route, it is administered between the cheek and the gums.

A. sublingual

B. transdermal

C. aural

D. buccal

______ 20. Which of the following measures will NOT help prevent thrombophlebitis?

A. Always wear gloves when you are performing a venipuncture.

B. Anchor the catheter and tubing securely to prevent movement in the vein.

C. Apply a warm pressure bandage on the extremity into which the catheter is inserted.

D. Use a povidone-iodine preparation to scrub the skin.

Fill in the Blank

Read each item carefully, and then complete the statement by filling in the missing word(s).

1. An intravenous solution that contains large molecules such as proteins is a(n) __________.

2. An intravenous solution that does not contain large molecules such as proteins is a(n) __________. One example of such a solution is normal __________.

3. When two solutions of different solute concentration are placed on either side of a semipermeable membrane, the more concentrated solution is said to be __________ with respect to the less concentrated solution. Conversely, the less concentrated solution is considered __________ with respect to the more concentrated solution. If the two solutions have the same concentration, they are said to be __________. Thus, for example, 4% saline is __________ with respect to serum; Ringer solution is __________ with respect to serum; and half normal saline (0.45% NaCl) is __________ with respect to serum.

4. When two solutions of different solute concentrations are placed on either side of a semipermeable membrane, water will move from the solution of __________ solute concentration to the solution of __________ solute concentration. The process by which water migrates in that fashion is called __________.

5. The signs and symptoms of circulatory overload include __________, jugular vein distention, and __________.

Labeling

Label the common sites for intramuscular injections.

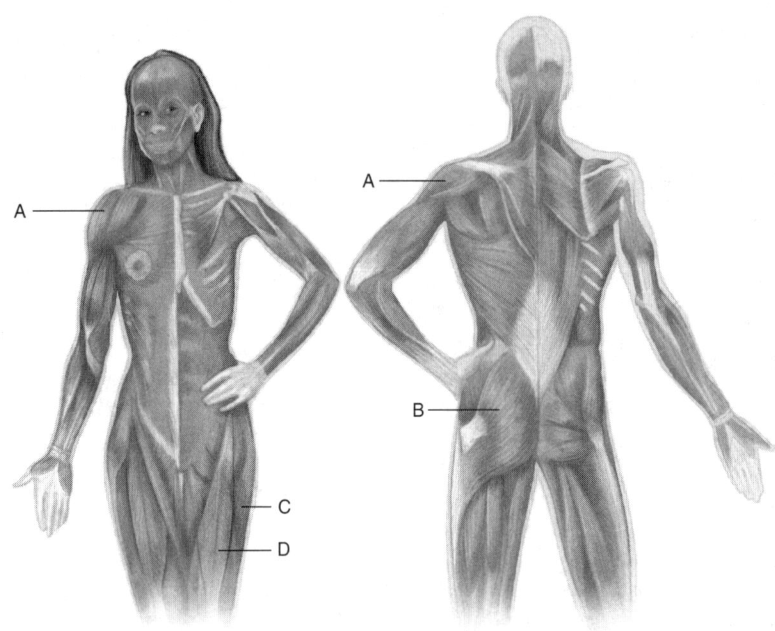

Ambulance Calls

All of the patients described in the following scenarios are experiencing a problem related to their intravenous therapy. Identify the problem in each case, and explain what you will do to manage it.

1. The patient is a 59-year-old man with severe chest pain on whom you have started a "keep-open" IV. It is a long way to the hospital, and about 10 minutes into the transport, he starts complaining of breathing difficulty. You notice that his respirations have become more rapid, and when you listen to his chest, you can hear crackling (rales) sounds. Meanwhile, you suddenly notice that the liter bag of IV fluid is empty.
   a. What is the patient's problem?

   ____

   ____

   ____

   b. What are you going to do about it?

   ____

   ____

   ____

2. You have started an IV on a frail old woman. After a few minutes, you notice that the IV is infusing more and more slowly. You open the clamp wide, but that does not help. You lower the IV bag below the stretcher; there is no blood return into the tubing. Then you check the IV site. There seems to be a lump in the skin, and the skin feels quite cool.
   a. What is the patient's problem?

   ____

   ____

   ____

b. What are you going to do about it?

______

______

______

c. What other problems might cause an IV to slow down or stop?

______

______

______

3. You are starting an IV near the wrist of a petite 22-year-old woman. When the IV catheter enters the vessel, bright red blood comes spurting back onto your face shield.

a. What is the patient's problem?

______

______

______

b. What are you going to do about it?

______

______

______

4. You are transporting a patient between hospitals. The patient has an IV already running (it was started earlier in the day by the paramedics who brought the patient to the first hospital). The patient complains of pain at the IV site, and you notice that it is red, hot, and swollen.

a. What is the patient's problem?

______

______

______

b. What are you going to do about it?

______

______

______

c. How could this problem have been prevented?

(1)______

(2)______

(3)______

(4)______

5. A driver is found conscious but very restless. He keeps asking you, "Can't you give me some water? I'm so thirsty—please give me something to drink." His skin is cold and sweaty. You do not see any external signs of serious injury.

a. Do you think this patient has been seriously injured? Explain the reasons for your answer.

____

____

____

b. You decide to start an IV with lactated Ringer solution, which is a __________ (colloid or crystalloid?) solution. Your protocol calls for administering 200 mL/h in these circumstances. You have an administration set that delivers 10 gtt/mL. To set the infusion rate to deliver 200 mL/h, you will need to set the drops per minute at __________ gtt/min. (Show your calculations.)

c. A few minutes after you adjust the IV rate, you notice that the IV has slowed down to the point that it is hardly flowing at all. List the five steps you would take to try to identify and solve the problem with the IV.

(1)____

(2)____

(3)____

(4)____

(5)____

True/False

If you believe the statement to be more true than false, write the letter "T" in the space provided. If you believe the statement to be more false than true, write the letter "F."

______ **1.** MDIs are more reliable than nebulizers for administering beta-agonist medications.

______ **2.** "Where sodium goes, water follows."

______ **3.** Calcium is the primary buffer in body fluids.

______ **4.** A peripheral inserted central catheter (PICC) line is considered a non-tunneling device for long-term use.

______ **5.** The region between the cheek and gums is highly vascular.

______ **6.** Nitroglycerin, estrogen, and nicotine are examples of medications that are administered by the intramuscular (IM) route.

______ **7.** A healthy person will lose up to 1 L of fluid a day as a result of urine output and exhalation.

______ **8.** Lactated Ringer or normal saline is used for patients who have lost a large amount of blood in the field.

______ **9.** A crystalloid solution can carry oxygen to the cells.

______ **10.** A macrodrip administration set delivers 10 or 15 gtt/mL.

______ **11.** A good thing to do when starting an IV is to work down, in case you miss the first attempt.

______ **12.** A butterfly catheter has a Teflon catheter over the hollow needle.

______ **13.** You should always have the bevel to the side when starting an IV.

______ **14.** When changing an IV bag, you must start all over with the process and restart the IV.

_____ **15.** When an IV infiltrates, you will notice edema at the catheter site.

_____ **16.** When you have cannulated an artery, you must pull the catheter out and apply direct pressure for at least 5 minutes.

_____ **17.** A healthy adult can handle only 1 to 2 extra liters of fluid.

_____ **18.** A red-topped tube is used to determine the blood type of a patient.

_____ **19.** An IO infusion is easier to use, so it should be used as much as possible for the pediatric patient.

_____ **20.** When placing an IO needle, you should feel two "pops."

_____ **21.** The basic unit of weight in the metric system is the gram.

_____ **22.** One pound is equal to 2.2 kg.

_____ **23.** The desired dose is what is ordered to give to the patient.

_____ **24.** Dopamine is delivered to the patient in micrograms.

_____ **25.** The use of Luer-lock IV tubing helps to minimize risks during medication administration.

Short Answer

Complete this section with short written answers using the space provided.

1. Name three ways to make the vein "stand up" so that it is easier to see.

a. ______________________________

b. ______________________________

c. ______________________________

2. List the five things that are a *must* when documenting the IV.

a. ______________________________

b. ______________________________

c. ______________________________

d. ______________________________

e. ______________________________

3. There are seven local reactions that can happen when starting an IV. List three complications and their signs and symptoms.

a. ______________________________

b. ______________________________

c. ______________________________

4. List the six points of information you should document when you administer a medication to a patient.

a. ______________________________

b. ______________________________

c. ______________________________

d. ______________________________

e. ______________________________

f. ______________________________

Fill in the Table

Fill in the missing parts of the table.

Route of Administration	Where in the Body the Medication Goes
Enteral	1.
Oral	2.
Intradermal	3.
Percutaneous	4.
Sublingual	5.
Endotracheal	6.
Buccal	7.
Transdermal	8.
Intramuscular	9.
Rectal	10.
Parenteral	11.
Subcutaneous	12.
Intravenous	13.
Ocular	14.
Aural	15.
Inhalation	16.
Intranasal	17.

Problem Solving

Practice your calculation skills by solving the following math problems.

1. You have started an IV on a bakery worker suffering from heat exhaustion. The physician instructs you to run normal saline by IV at 200 mL/h. Your bag of saline is a 1,000-mL bag. Your administration set delivers 10 gtt/mL. At what rate (how many drops per minute) do you have to run the infusion to give 200 mL/h? (Show your calculations.)

2. You have started a "keep-open" IV with a microdrip infusion set (which delivers 60 gtt/mL). Your instructions are to run the IV at 30 mL/h. At what rate (how many drops per minute) should you set the flow? (Show your calculations.)

3. You are ordered to give a lidocaine drip at a rate of 2 mg/min. You have the following on hand:
   - A vial containing 50 mL of 4% lidocaine
   - A 500-mL bag of D_5W
   - A microdrip administration set that delivers 60 gtt/mL

   a. How many grams of lidocaine are in the vial? __________ g (Show your calculations.)

   b. When you add the contents of the vial to the IV bag, what will be the concentration of lidocaine in the IV bag? __________ mg/mL (Show your calculations.)

   c. How many milliliters per minute (mL/min) will the patient have to receive to get the dosage ordered (2 mg/min)? __________ mL/min (Show your calculations.)

   d. How many drops per minute (gtt/min) is that equivalent to? __________ gtt/min (Show your calculations.)

4. Convert 12 g to milligrams: 12 g × __________ = __________ mg

5. Convert 156 lb to kilograms: 156 lb ÷ __________ = __________ kg (round up)

6. Now use the second method to estimate the patient's weight in kilograms. The patient weighs 135 lb.

   Step 1: Divide the patient's weight by 2: __________ ÷ 2 = __________

   Step 2: Take the total from step 1 and multiply it by 10%: __________ × 0.10 = __________ (round up)

   * Remember to round the percentage number for easier subtraction. __________

   Step 3: Take the total of step 1 and subtract the rounded percentage. __________ – __________ = __________ patient's weight in kilograms; once again, you may need to round up to __________. What weight would you use for the patient? __________ kg

7. You are ordered to give a patient 6 mg of morphine. The morphine comes in 10 mg/mL. How much will you give? ________ mL

8. You are ordered to give 2 mg of diazepam (Valium). Your vial contains 20 mg in 10 mL. What is the concentration on hand? ________ mg/mL
How many mL will you give? ________ mL

9. You are ordered to deliver 10 mcg/kg/min of dopamine for an 80-kg patient. You have mixed 800 mg of dopamine into a 500-mL bag of normal saline. Show your calculations for the following.
   a. What is the desired dose? ________ mcg/min
   b. Determine the dose on hand.________ mg/mL
   c. Convert the mg from answer (b) to mcg. ________ mcg/mL
   d. Determine the amount of volume to infuse per minute. Use the desired dose to calculate this volume. ________ mL/min
   e. Determine how many drops/min will deliver the desired dose, using a microdrip set (60 gtt/mL). ________ gtt/min

10. Fill in the following tables so that each row will contain different ways of representing the same values.

Microgram (mcg)	Milligram (mg)	Gram (g)	Kilogram (kg)
500	0.5	0.0005	0.0000005
________	________	1.0	________
________	________	________	1.0
________	1.0	________	________
1.0	________	________	________
________	800.0	________	________
15.0	________	________	________

Milliliter (mL)	Deciliter (dL)	Liter (L)
5,000.0	50.0	5.0
1.0	________	________
10.0	________	________
________	________	1.0
250.0	________	0.25

11. Fill in the blanks in the calculations, changing the patient's weight from pounds to kilograms using the "10% trick." Compare your answers using the formula:

patient's weight (lb) ÷ 2.2 = patient's weight (kg)

Patient's Weight (lb)	Patient's Weight (lb) ÷ 2	Weight (lb) ÷ 2 × 10%	Subtract Your 10% from the Weight ÷ 2	Patient's Weight in Kilograms (kg)	Patient's Weight in lb ÷ 2.2 = Patient's Weight in Kilograms (kg)
60	60 ÷ 2 = 30	30 × 10% = 3	30 − 3 = 27	27	27.27
16	________	________	________	________	________
138	________	________	________	________	________
8	________	________	________	________	________
250	________	________	________	________	________
36	________	________	________	________	________
82	________	________	________	________	________
180	________	________	________	________	________
330	________	________	________	________	________

12. Volume conversions: Fill in the blanks indicating the amount of medication found in each bag of normal saline (NS), assuming the concentration is the same in each bag. Follow the example in the first row of the table:

1,000 mL NS	500 mL NS	250 mL NS	100 mL NS	50 mL NS
100 g	50 g	25 g	10 g	5 g
________	800 g	________	________	________
________	________	250 g	________	________
________	________	________	4 g	________
________	50 g	________	________	________

13. Determine the number of milliliters of fluid infused over 1 minute to the patient by filling in the following blanks.

a. 60-gtt admin set infused 120 gtt/min = __________ mL/min

b. 15-gtt admin set infused 120 gtt/min = __________ mL/min

c. 30-gtt admin set infused 120 gtt/min = __________ mL/min

14. Convert the following temperatures from degrees Fahrenheit (°F) to degrees Celsius (°C) by completing the following table. Follow the example in the third row.
This table is based on the formula (°F – 32) × 0.555 = °C.

Temperature in °F	°F – 32	(°F - 32) × 0.555	Temperature in °C
32			
95.0			
98.6	98.6 - 32 = 66.6	66.6 × 0.555 = 36.96	36.96 (approximately 37)
101.0			
104.0			

15. Determine how much medication is prescribed for the patient by body weight by filling in the following table.

Desired Dose	Patient's Weight in Pounds (lb)	Patient's Weight in Kilograms (kg)	Medication Administered
1 mg/kg lidocaine	90	90 ÷ 2.2 = 40.9 kg (≈ 41 kg)	41 kg × 1 mg lidocaine = 41 mg lidocaine to administer
0.2 mg/kg atropine	30		
0.05 mg/kg lorazepam	180		
30 mg/kg methylprednisolone	220		
15 mg/kg phenobarbital	12		

16. Calculate the volume of normal saline needed to administer to the following trauma patients. Base your calculations on volumes replaced at 20 mL/kg of patient body weight.

Patient's Weight in Pounds (lb)	Patient's Weight in Kilograms: Weight in lb ÷ 2.2 = Weight in kg (or Use the "10% Trick")	Volume to be Infused with First Bolus at 20 mL/kg
60		
80		
100		
125		
150		
175		
190		
220		
300		

17. Find the weight of the following medications in 1 mL of solution.

a. 100 mg/10 mL lidocaine = __________ mg/1 mL lidocaine

b. 1 mg/10 mL epinephrine = __________ mg/1 mL epinephrine

c. 40 mg/14 mL furosemide = __________ mg/1 mL furosemide

d. 6 mg/2 mL adenosine = __________ mg/1 mL adenosine

e. 20 mg/5 mL diazepam = __________ mg/1 mL diazepam

f. 10 mg/5 mL naloxone = __________ mg/1 mL naloxone

g. 2 mg/5 mL albuterol = __________ mg/1 mL albuterol

h. 150 mg/3 mL amiodarone = __________ mg/1 mL amiodarone

i. 25 g/125 mL activated charcoal = __________ g/1 mL activated charcoal = __________ mg/1 mL activated charcoal

18. Find the weight of the following medications in 1 mL of solution.
Follow this example:

50% dextrose = 50 g/100 mL = 0.5 g/1 mL

a. 1% xylocaine

b. 10% dextrose

c. 0.5% albuterol

d. 10% calcium chloride

e. 50% magnesium sulfate

f. 5% Alupent

g. 0.9% sodium chloride

19. Determine the amount of dopamine in micrograms (mcg) per milliliter when 800 mg of dopamine is added to the following bags of normal saline (NS). (Note: 1 mg = 1,000 mcg)

a. 800 mg dopamine is added to a 500-mL bag NS = __________ mcg/mL
b. 800 mg dopamine is added to a 250-mL bag NS = __________ mcg/mL
c. 800 mg dopamine is added to a 1,000-mL bag NS = __________ mcg/mL
d. 800 mg dopamine is added to a 100-mL bag NS = __________ mcg/mL

20. Medical control has directed you to administer the correct dosage of medication for your patient (desired dose). The concentration available to you is listed for each calculation. Determine the volume of medication you will administer for each order.

Desired dose in mg ÷ concentration in mg/mL = volume to administer

a. You are ordered to give 15 mg labetalol. You have a vial with 100 mg/20 mL solution in stock.

b. You are ordered to give 3 mg haloperidol. You have a 1-mL ampule containing 5 mg of medication.

c. You are directed to administer 750 mg calcium chloride. You have a bottle containing 1,000 mg of medication in 10 mL of solution.

CHAPTER 15

Airway Management

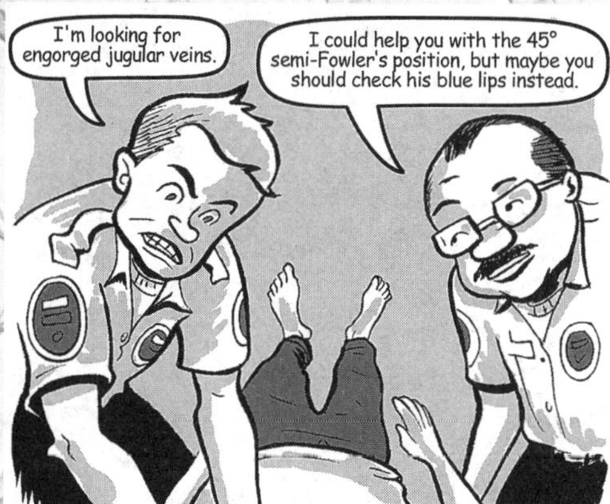

Matching

Part I

For each of the following definitions, insert the letter of the appropriate term on the line provided.

	Definition	Term
______	**1.** A gradually increasing rate and depth of respirations followed by a gradual decrease with intermittent periods of apnea; associated with brainstem insult.	**A.** Abdominal thrust maneuver
______	**2.** The backward, upward, and rightward pressure used during intubation to improve the laryngoscopic view of the glottis opening and vocal cords; also called external laryngoscopic view of the glottis opening and vocal cords; also called external laryngeal manipulation.	**B.** Accessory muscles
______	**3.** Irregular pattern, rate, and depth of respirations with intermittent periods of apnea; resulting from increased intracranial pressure.	**C.** Agonal gasps
______	**4.** Prolonged gasping inspirations followed by extremely short, ineffective expirations; associated with brainstem insult.	**D.** Anoxia
______	**5.** The continued alveolar uptake of oxygen, even when the patient is apneic; can be facilitated by administering oxygen via nasal cannula during intubation.	**E.** Apneic oxygenation
______	**6.** An inability to remember events after the onset of amnesia.	**F.** Apneustic respirations
______	**7.** A medication that distorts perception of sight and sound and induces a feeling of detachment from environment and self.	**G.** Bimanual laryngoscopy
______	**8.** An automatic reaction when something touches an area deep in the oral cavity that helps protect the lower airway from aspiration.	**H.** Biot (ataxic) respirations
______	**9.** A leaf-shaped cartilaginous structure that closes over the trachea during swallowing.	**I.** BURP maneuver
______	**10.** The breath sounds produced as fluid-filled alveoli pop open under increasing inspiratory pressure; can be fine or coarse; formerly called rales.	**J.** Cheyne-Stokes respirations
______	**11.** A surgical procedure in which the larynx is removed.	**K.** Crackles
______	**12.** A decrease in arterial oxygen level.	**L.** Dissociative anesthetic
______	**13.** An approximation of the extent of bronchoconstriction; used to determine whether therapy (such as with inhaled bronchodilators) is effective.	**M.** Epiglottis
______	**14.** Drugs that paralyze skeletal muscles; used in emergency situations to facilitate intubation; also called neuromuscular blocking agents.	**N.** Gag reflex
______	**15.** A device that measures oxygen saturation level.	**O.** Hypoxemia
______	**16.** Forcing of air into the lungs.	**P.** Laryngectomy
______	**17.** In the context of the airway, the resultant orifice of a tracheostomy that connects the trachea to the outside air; located in the midline of the anterior part of the neck.	**Q.** Orotracheal intubation

______	**18.** A continuous, low-pitched sound, which indicates the presence of mucus or fluid in the larger lower airways.	**R.** Orthopnea
______	**19.** Insertion of an endotracheal tube into the trachea through the mouth.	**S.** Paralytics
______	**20.** Positional dyspnea.	**T.** Peak expiratory flow
______	**21.** An absence of oxygen.	**U.** Positive pressure ventilation
______	**22.** Slow, shallow, irregular respirations or occasional gasping breaths that result from cerebral anoxia.	**V.** Pulse oximeter
______	**23.** Abdominal thrusts performed to relieve a foreign body airway obstruction.	**W.** Rhonchi
______	**24.** The muscles not normally used during normal breathing, which include the sternocleidomastoid muscles of the neck and the chest and abdominal muscles.	**X.** Stoma

Part II

Nasotracheal intubation is an excellent technique for establishing control over the airway under select circumstances. In other circumstances, it is preferable to insert the tracheal tube through the mouth; and in yet other limited circumstances, it may be necessary to establish an airway surgically, by cricothyrotomy. For each of the following patients, indicate which of the following intubation methods is preferred.

N Blind nasotracheal intubation is the preferred technique.

T Endotracheal intubation is the preferred technique.

C Cricothyrotomy is the preferred technique.

______ **1.** A 65-year-old man in cardiac arrest.

______ **2.** A 28-year-old woman with complete airway obstruction from laryngeal edema.

______ **3.** A 26-year-old vehicle-collision victim with clear fluid draining from his nose and left ear.

______ **4.** An 18-year-old woman in a coma from a drug overdose.

______ **5.** A 48-year-old man extricated from a wrecked car; he is unconscious and has an injury to the back of his head.

______ **6.** A 58-year-old man with pulmonary edema, who has been taking warfarin (Coumadin; an anticoagulant drug) ever since his heart attack last year.

______ **7.** A 6-year-old boy who choked on a piece of meat.

______ **8.** A 52-year-old woman who was given succinylcholine (a paralyzing drug) prior to an intubation attempt; the attempt failed, and afterward, it became impossible to maintain her airway by manual methods.

Part III

For each of the following patients, indicate the most appropriate device for administering supplemental oxygen. (Note: You may use any of the items once, more than once, or not at all.)

______	**1.** A 63-year-old man in severe respiratory distress from acute pulmonary edema.	**A.** Nasal cannula
______	**2.** A 56-year-old man complaining of crushing chest pain.	**B.** Nonrebreathing mask
______	**3.** A car-crash victim in cardiac arrest; you are doing one-rescuer cardiopulmonary resuscitation (CPR) because your partner is busy with another casualty.	**C.** Pocket mask (mouth-to-mask ventilation) with added supplemental oxygen
______	**4.** A 78-year-old woman who suddenly stopped speaking this morning and cannot move her left arm or left leg.	**D.** Bag-mask device with an oxygen reservoir
______	**5.** A 26-year-old man who has overdosed on heroin; he is unconscious and breathing shallowly at 6 breaths/min.	**E.** Flow-restricted, oxygen-powered ventilation device (manually triggered ventilation device)
______	**6.** A 26-year-old car-crash victim who was thrown forward against the steering wheel; he is coughing up blood, and his lips look rather blue.	**F.** Continuous positive airway pressure (CPAP)
______	**7.** A 48-year-old man who collapsed in the street; he is in cardiac arrest by the time you arrive.	
______	**8.** An unconscious 10-year-old boy who was rescued from a house fire.	

Multiple Choice

Read each item carefully, and then select the best response.

_____ **1.** What is the leaf-shaped structure that prevents food and liquid from getting into the larynx during swallowing?

A. Vallecula
B. Uvula
C. Epiglottis
D. Pharynx

_____ **2.** Which of the following is the MOST common cause of a partial airway obstruction?

A. The tongue
B. Food
C. Blood
D. Vomitus

_____ **3.** What is the preferred device to deliver supplemental oxygen to the patient who is breathing and has an Spo_2 of 93%?

A. Nasal cannula
B. Bag-mask device
C. Simple face mask
D. Nonrebreathing mask

_____ **4.** What is the MOST definitive way to control the airway in an unconscious patient?

A. Bag-mask device
B. Endotracheal tube
C. Oral airway adjunct
D. Head tilt–chin lift maneuver

_____ **5.** In which position should the patient's head be placed when preparing to intubate with a Combitube?

A. Flexed forward
B. Neutral position
C. Hyperextended back
D. Slightly to the right

_____ **6.** Which medication is the only depolarizing neuromuscular blocking agent that is used in the field?

A. Vecuronium bromide
B. Pancuronium bromide
C. Rocuronium bromide
D. Succinylcholine chloride

_____ **7.** How much sterile saline should you have ready when you are performing a needle cricothyrotomy?

A. 3 mL
B. 5 mL
C. 7 mL
D. 10 mL

_____ **8.** The commonly used mnemonic __________ is used to guide assessment of the difficult airway.

A. SAMPLE
B. ISTAT
C. LEMON
D. CBARR

_____ **9.** The clinical finding in which the systolic blood pressure drops more than 10 mm Hg during inhalation is called:

A. intercostal stimulation.
B. vagus nerve stimulation.
C. pulsus paradoxus.
D. asymmetric movement.

______ **10.** Which abnormal respiratory pattern do you see in the patient with ketoacidosis?

A. Cheyne-Stokes
B. Agonal
C. Biot
D. Kussmaul

______ **11.** What is the major advantage of a multilumen airway device?

A. It fits all patients, from pediatric to adult.
B. It prevents all aspiration.
C. It cannot be placed improperly.
D. It always provides 100% oxygen to the patient.

______ **12.** Which of the following is NOT a complication of placing a multilumen airway device?

A. Vomiting
B. Unrecognized displacement of the tube
C. Esophageal trauma
D. Hyperventilation

______ **13.** How much air should inflate the proximal balloon on the Combitube?

A. 15 mL
B. 25 mL
C. 100 mL
D. 150 mL

______ **14.** When should you use a laryngeal mask airway (LMA) in the field?

A. When the patient cannot be intubated, as an alternative to the bag-mask device (alone)
B. When the patient is morbidly obese and has a difficult airway
C. When the patient has heart failure and is unconscious
D. When the patient is less than 5 feet tall and needs attention to the airway

______ **15.** Using the Mallampati classification to predict the relative difficulty of an intubation, if the posterior pharynx cannot be seen, but the base of the uvula is exposed, it is a Class:

A. I.
B. II.
C. III.
D. IV.

______ **16.** Complications of the King LT airway may include each of the following, EXCEPT:

A. possible hypoventilation.
B. a herniated diaphragm.
C. vomiting.
D. laryngospasm.

______ **17.** Typical rapid sequence intubation (RSI) protocols for a hemodynamically stable patient would include:

A. immediate sedation.
B. half the succinylcholine dose.
C. preoxygenation for 2 to 3 minutes.
D. administering a polarizing paralytic agent.

______ **18.** Of the following neuromuscular blocking agents, which has the shortest duration of action?

A. Vecuronium
B. Rocuronium
C. Pancuronium
D. Succinylcholine

______ **19.** Which sedative used in airway management is considered a dissociative anesthetic?

A. Diazepam
B. Ketamine
C. Fentanyl
D. Etomidate

______ **20.** Tracheobronchial suctioning requires:

A. a rescue airway in place.
B. surgical jelly.
C. a stoma in place.
D. strict attention to sterile technique.

Fill in the Blank

Read each item carefully, and then complete the statement by filling in the missing word(s).

1. The principal hazard associated with intubation is __________. That hazard can be minimized by __________.
2. For tracheal intubation to proceed smoothly, it is essential to position the patient correctly to bring the trachea into alignment with the mouth and pharynx. To do so, you need to place the patient in the __________ position.
3. An intubation attempt should take no longer than __________ seconds.
4. The ________ features an integral _______ _______, a gastric access _________ that allows for passage of a 12-Fr __________ tube, a supplemental oxygen inlet port to facilitate passive oxygenation, and a(n) __________ strap to secure in position.
5. Foreign body airway obstructions are sometimes the result of decreased airway reflexes, sometimes caused by alcohol consumption or by __________.
6. When you suction the airway, a nonrigid catheter is called a(n) __________ or __________-__________ catheter, but the rigid tip is called a(n) __________-__________ catheter.
7. The _________ on the video laryngoscope is located on the ________ end of the device. You will be unable to obtain a view of the ________ anatomy if the camera becomes ________ by secretions.
8. You should always adequately __________ a patient before you intubate.
9. The King LT airway should not be used in patients with a(n) __________ __________ __________, patients with known esophageal disease, or patients who have ingested a(n) __________ substance.
10. When examining the patient's airway with the mouth wide open, you note that the posterior pharynx is __________ __________. This is considered a Class II in the __________ classification.

Labeling

Label the following diagram with the correct terms.

1. Parts of the larynx

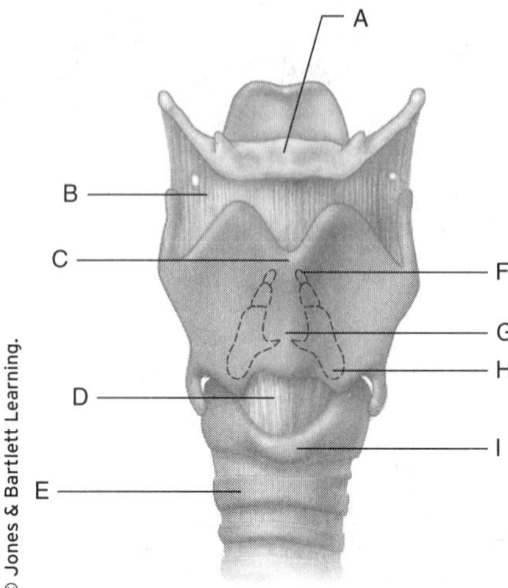

A. ____________________

B. ____________________

C. ____________________

D. ____________________

E. ____________________

F. ____________________

G. ____________________

H. ____________________

I. ____________________

Identify

In the following case study, list the chief complaint, vital signs, and pertinent negatives.

You are called to the high school for a teenager choking. When you arrive, you are directed to a 14-year-old boy who was walking down the hallway when someone scared him from behind. He was chewing on a small cap of a pen when this happened and has sucked the cap into his airway. He is seated in the tripod position and is cyanotic around the lips. You immediately assess that he is breathing because with each breath he makes a whistling noise. A teacher performed the Heimlich maneuver (abdominal thrusts) on him in the hallway initially, and he can at least draw a small breath in. Your partner applies a nonrebreathing mask at 15 L/min. The patient's respirations are 28 breaths/min and shallow. He has decreased lung sounds on the right side and clear sounds on the left. His heart rate is 98 beats/min and regular and his blood pressure (BP) is 128/86 mm Hg. His skin is cyanotic in the face and fingertips and is cool. His oxygen saturation is 90%, and he is a little confused. Because the patient is conscious and you know the cap is in the lungs, and because of the sounds in the lung fields, you position the boy on the cot, sitting up, with oxygen running, and take off for the hospital. You run the unit at Priority 1 (lights and siren) to the emergency department (ED). Later, you learn that the patient had to be taken into surgery to remove the cap.

1. Chief complaint:

____

____

2. Vital signs:

____

____

3. Pertinent negatives:

____

____

Complete the Patient Care Report (PCR)

Reread the incident scenario in the "Identify" section, and then complete the following PCR. Feel free to create the times and numbers, as well as the date of the incident.

EMS Patient Care Report (PCR)			
Date:	Incident No.:	Nature of Call:	Location:

Dispatched:	En Route:	At Scene:	Transport:	At Hospital:	In Service:

Patient Information	
Age: Sex: Weight (in kg [lb]):	Allergies: Medications: Past Medical History: Chief Complaint:

Vital Signs				
Time:	BP:	Pulse:	Respirations:	SpO_2:
Time:	BP:	Pulse:	Respirations:	SpO_2:
Time:	BP:	Pulse:	Respirations:	SpO_2:

EMS Treatment (circle all that apply)				
Oxygen @ ______ L/min via (circle one): NC NRM Bag-mask device		Assisted Ventilation	Airway Adjunct	CPR
Defibrillation	Bleeding Control	Bandaging	Splinting	Other:

Narrative

Ambulance Calls

The following case scenarios provide an opportunity to explore the concerns associated with patient management and paramedic care. Read each scenario, and then answer each question.

1. You finish a call and return to Joe's Steak 'n' Lobster Shack, where you were having dinner when a previous emergency arose. You hope that they haven't already fed your sirloin to the dog. Happily, Joe has kept your steak waiting for you, and he whips it into the microwave to rewarm it. At last, the steak is back in front of you, along with a generous order of fries. You lift your knife and fork to dig in when, out of the corner of your eye, you see a strange pantomime occurring two tables away. A middle-aged man in a business suit suddenly pushes himself away from the table, clutches his neck, and lurches to his feet. He staggers a few paces and then pitches to the floor—all in complete silence.

a. The man is showing signs of:

(1) food poisoning.

(2) choking.

(3) strep throat.

(4) anaphylaxis.

(5) hysteria.

b. Which treatment is needed?

(1) Pump out his stomach.

(2) Give him manual thrusts.

(3) Have him gargle with saltwater.

(4) Give epinephrine 1 mg/mL (1:1,000), 0.5 mL subcutaneously.

(5) Give diazepam (Valium), 10 mg IM.

2. You are having a barbecue in the backyard one Sunday. The beer has been flowing freely, and everyone is in a jolly mood. You tell a funny story, and everyone present starts laughing uproariously, including one of your friends who had just taken a big bite out of his hot dog. Suddenly, he starts coughing violently. His face gets very red.

a. At that point, you should take which of the following actions?

(1) Tilt his head back and attempt to ventilate.

(2) Perform a quick finger sweep to remove accessible obstructing material.

(3) Give manual thrusts.

(4) Reach into his throat with the barbecue tongs and try to snare the hot dog.

(5) Encourage him to keep coughing.

b. That course of action does not seem to help. Your friend becomes completely silent, and his face turns a dusky gray as he struggles to breathe. What should you do now?

(1) Tilt his head back and attempt to ventilate.

(2) Perform a quick finger sweep to remove accessible obstructing material.

(3) Do the Heimlich maneuver (abdominal thrusts).

(4) Reach into his throat with the barbecue tongs and try to snare the hot dog.

(5) Encourage him to keep coughing.

c. Your friend collapses, unconscious, to the ground. List the next four steps you would take.

(1)____

(2)____

(3)____

(4)____

d. Meanwhile, an ambulance has arrived (someone had the sense to call 9-1-1), and a couple of paramedics come stampeding through your flower garden carrying what looks like all the equipment from their rig. Now that you have equipment available, which steps will be taken?

(1)____

(2)____

(3)____

(4)____

3. You are struggling to intubate a 30-year-old male bodybuilder who collapsed while working out at the local health club. You found him in cardiac arrest, and high-quality CPR is in progress. Despite the fact that you have positioned him just as the textbook instructs, you cannot seem to bring his vocal cords into view; they remain hidden just above your laryngoscope blade.

a. To bring the cords into view, you ask your partner to perform the __________ __________, which is __________, __________, __________ pressure on the larynx.

b. That maneuver seems helpful in bringing the vocal cords into view. Another tool that can be useful is the __________ __________ __________, which facilitates entry into the glottis opening and enables you to feel the ridges of the tracheal wall.

c. You finally manage to insert the endotracheal (ET) tube. After confirming proper placement, you secure it with a commercial tube restraint. List some of the specifics you should document on your PCR concerning this intubation.

(1)____

(2)____

(3)____

(4)____

4. You are attempting a blind nasotracheal intubation on a 60-kg 24-year-old female who took an overdose of sleeping pills. You have succeeded in advancing the tip of the ET tube just beyond the oropharynx.

a. As you continue to advance the tube, how can you tell whether the tip is moving toward the glottis (as opposed to the esophagus)?

(1)____

(2)____

(3)____

b. As you are advancing the tube, you become aware that the bleeps from the cardiac monitor are getting further apart. What has happened?

____

____

____

c. What should you do about it?

(1)______________________________

(2)______________________________

(3)______________________________

5. You are involved in a search-and-rescue mission to find a 43-year-old male hiker lost in the woods. At last you find him, sitting down, propped against a tree. He tells you that he experienced severe chest pain and could not go on. Because there is a strong possibility that he is experiencing an acute myocardial infarction (AMI), you and your partner will have to carry him the 40-minute walk back to the ambulance. You hook the patient to supplemental oxygen via nasal cannula at a flow rate of 5 L/min. You notice that the pressure gauge on your E cylinder is reading 800 psi.

a. How long will the oxygen in the E cylinder last?

____

____

b. Will that be long enough to get the patient back to the ambulance? (Show your calculations.)

____

____

6. You are sitting at the movies on your night off when you notice someone a few rows ahead of you suddenly slump over. You leap like a gazelle over several rows of seats to reach the person's side, and you discover that he has stopped breathing. You drag him into an aisle and start mouth-to-mouth ventilation with the barrier device you usually carry in your jacket. How can you tell if you are actually getting air into his lungs?

(1)______________________________

(2)______________________________

(3)______________________________

7. As you continue mouth-to-mouth ventilation on the patient described in question 6, you reflect that you would like to avoid causing gastric distention because you would prefer not to deal with the mess that might follow.

a. What can you do, that is noninvasive, to minimize gastric distention during artificial ventilation?

(1)______________________________

(2)______________________________

(3)______________________________

b. Despite your best efforts, you notice that the man's belly is starting to get enlarged. What else should you do (that may be considered invasive)?

____

____

____

8. After your experience in the movie theater, you promise yourself that you will never go anywhere without a pocket mask, or barrier shield, in your pocket, not only to make things more pleasant for yourself, but also because these devices have several advantages over other methods of giving artificial ventilation. List four specific advantages of a pocket mask.

(1)__________

(2)__________

(3)__________

(4)__________

9. A 53-year-old man calls for an ambulance because of shortness of breath. You find him in severe respiratory distress, with foam bubbling out of his mouth. Your examination reveals signs of heart failure (a condition in which fluid backs up into the lungs and interferes with gas exchange).

a. The patient's pulse oximeter reading when you first arrive shows an oxygen saturation (Spo_2) of 86%. That reading is:

(1) normal for the patient's age.

(2) abnormally high.

(3) abnormally low.

(4) probably an artifact.

b. Which measure should you take immediately?

____

c. You treat the patient according to your protocol for heart failure, and his condition improves markedly. Now the Spo_2 reading is 96%. You move the patient to a stretcher and bring him out to the ambulance for transport. When you have him loaded in the ambulance, you notice that the Spo_2 is now reading 85%. The patient, however, still looks comfortable and is not in any respiratory distress, so you conclude that the reading on the pulse oximeter must be an error. List three of the possible causes of the erroneous reading in this patient:

(1)__________

(2)__________

(3)__________

10. You are attempting a blind nasotracheal intubation on an unconscious patient who took an overdose of sleeping pills. When you think you have the tracheal tube in place, you check the end-tidal carbon dioxide monitor that you've snapped onto the tracheal tube. Its color is purple, indicating that the air being exhaled through the tube contains less than 0.5% carbon dioxide.

a. What can you conclude from that reading?

____

____

b. Which actions should you take?

____

____

11. You are at the scene of a two car collision. A passenger riding in a car #2 is breathing quietly at 12 breaths/min, taking in 500 mL of air with each breath.

a. What effect do you expect that change in minute volume to have on the patient's arterial P_{CO_2}?

____

b. That, in turn, will cause the patient's pH to __________ (rise or fall?).

c. The resulting derangement in his acid–base balance is called a __________ (respiratory or metabolic?) __________ (acidosis or alkalosis?).

d. Which treatment is required?

____

12. Now it's on to a cardiac arrest in a fourth-floor walk-up apartment. You grab the jump kit and the handiest D cylinder from the ambulance while your partner takes the drug box and monitor/defibrillator, and you sprint up the four flights of stairs to the patient's apartment. While your partner starts CPR chest compressions, you "crack" the oxygen cylinder, hook up the oxygen to a bag-mask device, and open the flow control to 10 L/min. As you do so, you notice that the reading on the pressure gauge is 900 psi. How much time do you have before you need to switch to a fresh cylinder? __________ minutes (The cylinder constant for a D cylinder is 0.16. Show your calculations.)

____

____

____

13. A 34-year-old man has been injured in a road collision in which his head apparently struck the windshield with some force. When you first reach the scene, the patient is unconscious. He is breathing 8 breaths/min, inhaling approximately 500 mL of air with each breath.

a. We can conclude that the patient's arterial P_{CO_2} will tend to __________ (increase or decrease?), so his pH will __________ (increase or decrease?). The net effect will be an acid–base disorder called a __________ (respiratory or metabolic?) __________ (acidosis or alkalosis?). The way you can help correct that abnormality is to ____.

14. The laboratory calls down another blood gas report. "You'd better check on this guy," the lab technician says. "His P_{O_2} is only 48 mm Hg." As you sprint off to alert the doctor about the blood gas results, you review in your mind the conditions that can cause hypoxemia.

a. List six conditions that can cause respiratory distress and inadequate ventilation.

(1)____

(2)____

(3)____

(4)____

(5)____

(6)____

b. What is the treatment for hypoxemia?

____

____

True/False

If you believe the statement to be more true than false, write the letter "T" in the space provided. If you believe the statement to be more false than true, write the letter "F."

_____ **1.** Any patient who is to be suctioned should first be preoxygenated.

_____ **2.** You should not suction while inserting the catheter.

_____ **3.** Suction a stoma for only 2 minutes at a time.

_____ **4.** A tonsil-tip catheter is a good choice for suctioning the oropharynx.

_____ **5.** The Cobra PLA is contraindicated with massive oral cavity trauma.

_____ **6.** The physical act of moving air into and out of the lungs is oxygenation.

_____ **7.** The exchange of oxygen and carbon dioxide in the alveoli and the tissues of the body is called ventilation.

_____ **8.** A barrier to ventilation would include neuromuscular disease.

_____ **9.** Using the 3-3-2 rule, the mouth should be at least 3 fingerbreadths wide open. The space from the chin to the larynx should be 3 inches, and the distance to the stoma should be 2 fingerbreadths.

_____ **10.** If your patient weighs over 198 lb (>90 kg), you should use the yellow i-gel.

Short Answer

Complete this section with short written answers using the space provided.

1. Obstruction of the upper airway is an immediate threat to life. The upper airway may become obstructed in several ways. List four causes of upper airway obstruction, and put an asterisk beside the most common cause.

a. ______________________________

b. ______________________________

c. ______________________________

d. ______________________________

2. Endotracheal intubation has several advantages over other methods of airway control. List three advantages of endotracheal intubation.

a. ______________________________

b. ______________________________

c. ______________________________

3. Despite all its advantages, endotracheal intubation is not for all patients. Like every other medical procedure, it has specific indications. List three indications for endotracheal intubation.

a. ______________________________

b. ______________________________

c. ______________________________

4. Endotracheal intubation is not without potential complications. The most serious acute complications can, however, be avoided by meticulous attention to correct technique.

a. List a potential complication of endotracheal intubation.

____

b. How can it be avoided?

(1)___

(2)___

(3)___

(4)___

c. How can it be detected and corrected if it does occur?

(1)___

(2)___

(3)___

d. List another potential complication of endotracheal intubation.

___

e. How can it be avoided?

___

f. How can it be detected and corrected if it does occur?

___

___

5. In some emergency medical services (EMS) systems, paramedics are authorized to use paralyzing drugs to facilitate tracheal intubation. Although such drugs undoubtedly make life easier for the paramedic, they may make life quite precarious for the patient. What is the principal hazard of administering a neuromuscular blocking agent to a patient who needs to be intubated?

___

___

6. Oxygen is a drug, and like any other drug, it should be given when there are indications for its use. List five indications for administering supplemental oxygen to a patient.

a. ___

b. ___

c. ___

d. ___

e. ___

7. Sometimes the patient will "tell" you, through his or her symptoms and signs, that either the oxygenation, the ventilation, or both are insufficient—that is, the patient is suffering from acute respiratory insufficiency. List four signs of acute respiratory insufficiency.

a. ______________________________

b. ______________________________

c. ______________________________

d. ______________________________

8. Oxygen is stored in cylinders at pressures up to 2,000 psi, which means that oxygen cylinders have to be treated with respect. List six safety precautions that should be observed when using or storing oxygen cylinders.

a. ______________________________

b. ______________________________

c. ______________________________

d. ______________________________

e. ______________________________

f. ______________________________

9. List three ways of identifying someone in respiratory arrest.

a. ______________________________

b. ______________________________

c. ______________________________

10. A person who has suffered respiratory arrest will need __________ (assisted or artificial?) ventilation.

11. What is the difference between artificial and assisted ventilation?

____

____

12. What is the objective of any form of artificial ventilation?

____

____

13. List three situations in which information from pulse oximetry could be helpful to you in the field.

a. ______________________________

b. ______________________________

c. ______________________________

14. A car-crash victim who has sustained injury to the cervical spinal cord may develop weakness or paralysis of the respiratory muscles. If so, such a patient may not have the strength to inhale as deeply as he or she otherwise would. Thus, the patient's minute volume will __________ (increase or decrease?), leading to a(n) __________ in the arterial PCO_2.

Fill in the Table

Fill in the missing parts of the table.

1. In mastering the use of any given piece of equipment, it is essential to learn not only how to use the equipment but also when to use it (and when not to use it). Artificial airways can be enormously helpful when applied in the appropriate circumstances; they can be downright dangerous when used in inappropriate circumstances. Fill in the table to summarize the indications and contraindications for the oropharyngeal airway (OPA) and the nasopharyngeal airway (NPA).

	Oropharyngeal Airway	Nasopharyngeal Airway
Use for:		
Do not use for:		

2. Oxygen-delivery devices

Device	Flow Rate (L/min)	Oxygen Delivered (%)
Nasal cannula		
Nonrebreathing mask		
Bag-mask device with reservoir		

3. Airway adjuncts can be very helpful in ensuring a patent air passage, but one needs to use the right adjunct in the right situation. Fill in the following table to remind yourself what to use (and not to use) and when to use it.

Adjunct	Indicated for:	Do Not Use in:
Oropharyngeal airway		
Combitube		
LMA		
Endotracheal intubation		

CHAPTER 16

Respiratory Emergencies

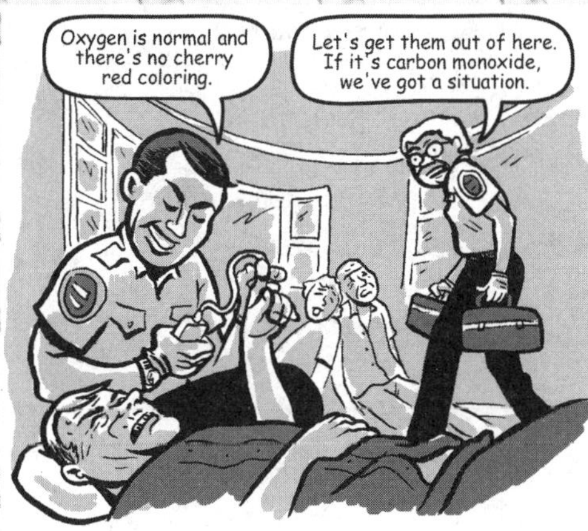

Matching

Part I

Match each of the items in the left column to the appropriate term in the right column.

______	**1.** A sitting position with the head elevated to 90 degrees.	**A.**	Adventitious
______	**2.** The infiltration of any tissue by air or gas; a chronic obstructive pulmonary disease characterized by distention of the alveoli and destructive changes in the lung parenchyma.	**B.**	Alveoli
______	**3.** The production of large amounts of urine by the kidney.	**C.**	Aspiration
______	**4.** A common disease of infancy and childhood caused by upper airway obstruction and characterized by stridor, hoarseness, and a barking cough.	**D.**	Atelectasis
______	**5.** Abnormal breath sounds that have a fine, crackling quality; previously called rales.	**E.**	Beta-2 agonist
______	**6.** Abnormal breath sounds or noises that occur in addition to the normal breath sounds; examples are crackles and wheezes.	**F.**	Botulism
______	**7.** The saclike units at the end of the bronchioles in which gas exchange takes place.	**G.**	Bronchospasm
______	**8.** The inhalation of anything other than breathable gases.	**H.**	Cape cyanosis
______	**9.** Collapse of the alveolar air spaces of the lungs.	**I.**	Carina
______	**10.** A pharmacologic agent that stimulates the beta-2 receptor sites found in smooth muscle; includes common bronchodilators such as albuterol and levalbuterol.	**J.**	Carpopedal spasm
______	**11.** An iron-containing protein with red blood cells that has the ability to combine with oxygen.	**K.**	Chronic bronchitis
______	**12.** A disease of unknown cause characterized by progressive paralysis moving from the feet to the head (ascending paralysis). If paralysis reaches the diaphragm, the patient may require respiratory support.	**L.**	Cor pulmonale
______	**13.** A mesh filter placed in the inferior vena cava to catch blood clots in patients who are at high risk of pulmonary embolus.	**M.**	Crackles
______	**14.** A ridgelike projection of tracheal cartilage located where the trachea bifurcates into the right and left mainstem bronchi.	**N.**	Croup
______	**15.** Deep cyanosis of the face and neck that extends across the chest and back; associated with little or no blood flow; a particularly ominous sign.	**O.**	Diuresis
______	**16.** Severe constriction of smooth muscle surrounding the bronchial tree.	**P.**	Emphysema

______	**17.** Heart disease that develops because of chronic lung disease and affects primarily the right side of the heart.	**Q.** Fowler position
______	**18.** A chronic inflammatory condition affecting the bronchi that is characterized by excessive mucus production as a result of overgrowth of the mucous glands in the airways.	**R.** Greenfield filter
______	**19.** Contorted positioning of the head or foot in which the fingers or toes flex in a clawlike manner; may be caused by hyperventilation.	**S.** Guillain-Barré syndrome
______	**20.** Poisoning characterized by severe muscle paralysis and usually caused by eating food containing botulinum toxin.	**T.** Hemoglobin

Part II

Match each of the items in the left column to the appropriate term in the right column.

______	**1.** Excessive accumulation of fluid in the pleural space.	**A.** Hemoptysis
______	**2.** Severe shortness of breath occurring suddenly at night after several hours of recumbency, as fluid pools in the lungs.	**B.** Hepatojugular reflux
______	**3.** The functional portions of a gland or solid organ.	**C.** Hyperoxia
______	**4.** Severe dyspnea experienced when recumbent that is relieved by sitting or standing up.	**D.** Hypoventilate
______	**5.** The sound of one note during wheezing caused by the vibration of a single bronchus.	**E.** Hypoxia
______	**6.** A dangerous condition in which the supply of oxygen to the tissues is reduced.	**F.** Hypoxic drive
______	**7.** To move inadequate volumes of air into the lungs.	**G.** Jugular venous distension
______	**8.** An excess of oxygen.	**H.** Kussmaul respirations
______	**9.** Engorgement of the jugular veins when the liver is gently pressed; this finding is specific to right-sided heart failure.	**I.** Laryngotracheo-bronchitis
______	**10.** Coughing up blood in the sputum.	**J.** Lung consolidation
______	**11.** Full of pus; having the character of pus.	**K.** Metastasis
______	**12.** A false membrane formed by a dead tissue layer; seen in the posterior pharynx of patients with diphtheria.	**L.** Monophonic
______	**13.** The sound of multiple notes during wheezing caused by the vibrations of multiple bronchi.	**M.** Orthopnea
______	**14.** The production of too many red blood cells over time, making the blood thick; a characteristic of people with chronic lung disease and chronic hypoxia.	**N.** Parenchyma
______	**15.** The transfer of a disease from one organ or part of the body to another that is not directly connected to the original site; often used to describe a cancer that has spread to another part of the body.	**O.** Paroxysmal nocturnal dyspnea
______	**16.** Firming of the lungs as a result of fluid accumulation.	**P.** Pleural effusion
______	**17.** Inflammation of the larynx, trachea, and bronchi.	**Q.** Polycythemia
______	**18.** A respiratory pattern characteristic of diabetic ketoacidosis with marked hyperpnea and tachypnea; represents the body's attempt to compensate for the acidosis.	**R.** Polyphonic
______	**19.** The visible bulging of the jugular veins when a patient is in a semi-Fowler or full-Fowler position; indicates inadequate blood movement through the heart and/or lungs.	**S.** Pseudo-membrane
______	**20.** A state in which the stimulus to breathe comes from a decrease in Pao_2, rather than from the normal stimulus of an increase in $Paco_2$.	**T.** Purulent

Multiple Choice

Read each item carefully, and then select the best response.

______ **1.** The ridgelike point at which the tracheal cartilage bifurcates is called the:
A. epiglottis.
B. carina.
C. larynx.
D. glottis.

______ **2.** In a pneumothorax, where is air trapped?
A. Inside the alveoli
B. In the nasopharynx
C. Between visceral and parietal pleurae
D. Between the alveoli

______ **3.** Which of the following substances are thin secretions in the airway that the body can eliminate by coughing?
A. Antitussives
B. Corticosteroids
C. Diuretics
D. Expectorants

______ **4.** Right-sided heart failure that has been caused by a chronic lung disease is known as:
A. Guillain-Barré syndrome.
B. polycythemia.
C. cor pulmonale.
D. atelectasis.

______ **5.** Which of the following breathing patterns is characterized by breathing that becomes faster and deeper until there is a period of apnea before the pattern begins again?
A. Cheyne-Stokes
B. Kussmaul
C. Cor pulmonale
D. Ataxic

______ **6.** What is another name for *rales*?
A. Rhonchus
B. Wheezing
C. Crackles
D. Death rattle

______ **7.** You respond to a patient who is having difficulty breathing. He is coughing up frothy sputum. What is the classic cause of frothy sputum?
A. Allergic reaction
B. Asthma attack
C. Heart failure
D. Acute myocardial infarction

______ **8.** Overdose, Lou Gehrig disease, and carbon dioxide narcosis are examples of conditions that affect ventilation through:
A. upper airway obstruction.
B. neuromuscular impairment.
C. chest wall impairment.
D. lower airway obstruction.

_____ 9. Which of the following is NOT used to treat asthma as defined in the asthma triad?
- A. Expectorant
- B. Corticosteroid
- C. Bronchodilator
- D. Hyperventilation

_____ 10. When the body attempts to compensate for acidosis through hyperventilation, this is called:
- A. Kussmaul respirations.
- B. botulism.
- C. Guillain-Barré syndrome.
- D. opioid overdose.

Fill in the Blank

Read each item carefully, and then complete the statement by filling in the missing word(s).

1. Alveolar collapse is known as __________.

2. ________ ________ dyspnea comes on in the middle of the night and may be a sign of _________ heart failure.

3. A surplus of red blood cells that the body makes as a result of a chronic lung disease is called __________.

4. Your patient has two or more ribs, broken in two or more places, that are inhibiting her breathing. In your radio report, you report this as a(n) __________ __________.

5. The medical term for shortness of breath is __________, and the medical term for blue-tinged skin caused by lack of oxygen is __________.

6. Being awakened by difficulty breathing during the night is known as __________ __________ __________.

7. __________ __________ are vibrations felt in the chest when a patient breathes.

8. There are __________ [number] lobes in the right lung and __________ [number] lobes in the left lung.

9. During inhalation, the _______ cartilage is drawn ________, and the area just above the sternal notch is pulled in if there is tracheal tugging.

10. Breathing in a way that allows patients to exhale slowly under controlled pressure is called __________-__________ __________.

Labeling

Label the following diagrams with the correct terms.

1. Respiratory patterns

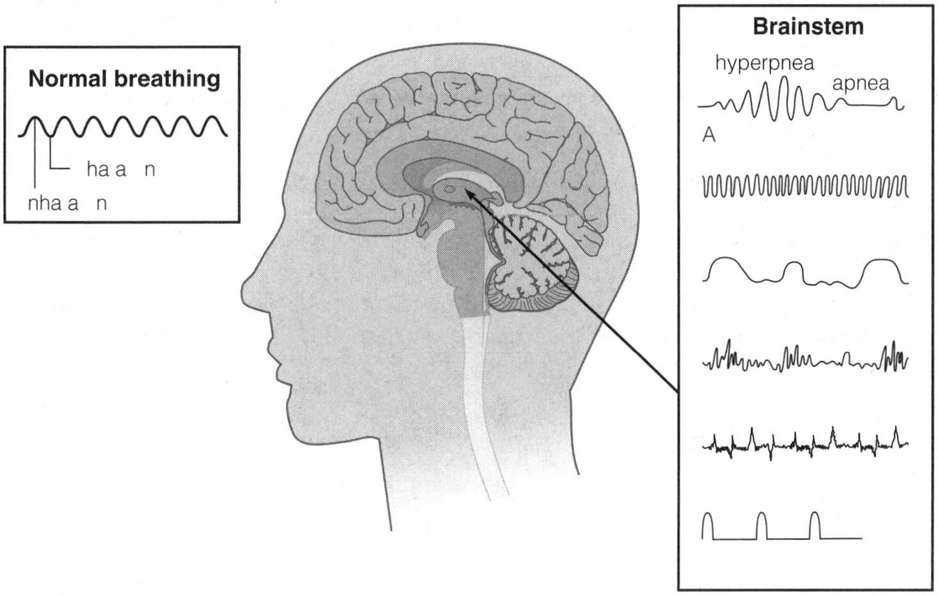

Normal breathing

ha a n

nha a n

Brainstem

hyperpnea

apnea

A

A. ____________________

B. ____________________

C. ____________________

D. ____________________

E. ____________________

F. ____________________

Identify

After reading the following case study, list the chief complaint, vital signs, and pertinent negatives.

You respond to a call for a baby not breathing. As you approach the home, a mother comes running out holding a 1-year-old boy, named Tommy. He is limp in her arms. You immediately jump out and take the child from her, get into the back of the unit, and lay him on the cot. The child is unconscious and blue, and he has no respirations. You begin the steps of cardiopulmonary resuscitation (CPR) by opening the airway and trying to give two breaths. Your partner has crawled into the back along with the mother and is trying to calm her down and help you at the same time. Using a pediatric bag-mask device, you give a breath and notice no chest rise and fall. You reposition the head and try again; once again, there is no rise and fall of the chest. You check the brachial artery and find a faint pulse. Your partner has pulled out the intubation kit and is ready to try to insert an advanced airway. As he looks for the tracheal tube, he reaches for the Magill forceps and suction. After suctioning and using the forceps, he removes a small plastic game piece from the boy. You immediately start to bag the child again with 100% supplemental oxygen. The child's chest rises now. His oxygen saturation is 64%, and the pulse is bradycardic at 46 beats/min. You are unable to get a blood pressure (BP). You manage respirations at one every 3 seconds. After a minute, the child is beginning to "pink up," his "sats" come up to 88%, and his heart rate is steadily climbing and at the moment is 92 beats/min. The child is regaining consciousness and begins to cry and fight you. He is now breathing on his own. His mother wants the child transported to be checked out. Your partner has a pediatric nonrebreathing mask ready with 100% supplemental oxygen. The mother holds the nonrebreathing mask while you strap the child into the special car seat designed for your stretcher and place the mother on the crew bench with the seat belt buckled. By the time you reach the emergency department (ED), little Tommy's heart rate is normal, and his oxygen saturation is 99%; his mother begins to cry with the realization of how close Tommy was to death.

1. Chief complaint:

____

____

2. Vital signs:

____

____

3. Pertinent negatives:

______

______

Ambulance Calls

The following case scenarios provide an opportunity to explore the concerns associated with patient management and paramedic care. Read each scenario, and then answer each question.

1. You are called to an office building for a "possible heart attack." On arriving, you are somewhat surprised to find that the patient is a clerical worker who looks about 22 years old—not at all like the usual heart attack patient. The woman looks pale and anxious, however, and complains of stabbing pains in her chest that came on "out of the blue." She also complains of a "funny tingly feeling in my lips." On examination, her pulse is 110 beats/min and regular, respirations are 30 breaths/min and unlabored, BP is 140/84 mm Hg, and Spo_2 is 93% without significant variation during the respiratory cycle. There are no abnormal physical findings except that the patient's hands look a bit odd, almost like claws.

a. What is the most probable diagnosis in this case?

______

______

______

b. Which steps will you take in managing this case?

(1)______

(2)______

(3)______

c. This woman's arterial Pco_2 is probably ______ (higher or lower?) than normal. Explain why.

______

______

2. You are called late one night to the Smith family residence for a "man who can't breathe." The patient's wife answers the door, quite distraught, and hurries you into the bedroom. She blurts out, "This is the worst it's ever been. I kept telling him to leave those cigarettes alone—the doctor's been saying the same thing—but do you think he listens? Might as well be talking to a brick wall."

In the bedroom, you find a heavy-set man about 65 years old sitting up at the edge of the bed in obvious respiratory distress. In fact, his "obvious" respiratory distress is obvious only if you know the signs of respiratory distress (increased work of breathing).

a. List eight signs of respiratory distress or increased work of breathing.

(1)______

(2)______

(3)______

(4)______

(5)______________________________

(6)______________________________

(7)______________________________

(8)______________________________

b. Which steps will you take at this point?

____

____

____

c. In due course, you learn that the patient called for an ambulance because he awoke from sleep unable to breathe. List seven questions you need to ask in taking his history.

(1)______________________________

(2)______________________________

(3)______________________________

(4)______________________________

(5)______________________________

(6)______________________________

(7)______________________________

d. As you proceed systematically through the secondary assessment of this man, you will be looking for some specific abnormalities at each step. In the following table, indicate what, in particular, you will be looking for as you examine each part of the body indicated.

Part of the Body	What I Am Looking for in Particular
General appearance	
Vital signs	
Head	
Neck	
Chest	
Abdomen	
Extremities	

e. In the course of the focused history, you learn that the patient has been a three-pack-per-day cigarette smoker for about 48 years. He "keeps a cough," but lately it has been worse than usual, and he has been bringing up a lot more sputum. His feet have also begun swelling, to the point that he can hardly get his shoes on. (Most of this you learn from the patient's wife; the patient is too short of breath to provide more than two or three words at a time.)

(1) This patient most likely has which of the following conditions?

(a) Pulmonary embolism

(b) Chronic obstructive pulmonary disease (COPD)

(c) Pneumonia

(d) Pickwickian syndrome

(e) Acute asthmatic attack

(2) How will you manage this patient?

____

____

____

____

3. A 56-year-old man calls for an ambulance because of severe dyspnea. His wife greets you at the door. She tells you, "My husband, he's a heart patient. Please get him to the hospital quickly. I think he's having another heart attack."

You find the patient in the living room, sitting in an armchair and in obvious distress. "Hit me like a ton of bricks," he gasps. "Not like the heart attack"—gasp—"Can't get air"—gasp—"Hurts to breathe."

On physical examination, his skin is cool and moist. Vital signs are as follows: pulse 120 beats/min and regular, respirations 32 breaths/min and shallow, BP 174/96 mm Hg, and Spo_2 of 94%. The neck veins look a bit distended, but otherwise there are no abnormal findings.

a. This patient is most likely suffering from which of the following conditions?

(1) Pulmonary embolism

(2) Decompensated COPD

(3) Pneumonia

(4) Pickwickian syndrome

(5) Acute asthmatic attack

b. Which steps will you take in managing this patient?

(1)______________________________

(2)______________________________

(3)______________________________

(4)______________________________

True/False

If you believe the statement to be more true than false, write the letter "T" in the space provided. If you believe the statement to be more false than true, write the letter "F."

_____ **1.** Right-sided heart failure because of chronic lung disease is known as cor pulmonale.

_____ **2.** The right lung has three lobes, whereas the left lung only has two lobes.

_____ **3.** Gas exchange happens only in the alveoli.

_____ **4.** Hiccups, yawns, and sighs are all forms of breathing patterns.

_____ **5.** Laying a patient flat will help the patient breathe better.

_____ **6.** Stridor is a result of a partial obstruction of the upper airway.

_____ **7.** A patient who is sitting in the tripod position (elbows out) and who can speak only in two- or three-word statements is a patient in distress.

_____ **8.** Patients who suffer from severe COPD often have jugular venous distention (JVD).

_____ **9.** The diaphragm of a stethoscope is for listening to high-pitched breath sounds.

_____ **10.** Pulse oximetry is a tool that can give false readings if the patient has a low hemoglobin level.

_____ **11.** An abnormal breathing pattern due to injury to the brainstem is central neurogenic hyperventilation.

_____ **12.** Acute pulmonary edema will sometimes present as a wheeze that sounds like an asthma attack.

_____ **13.** You should withhold high concentrations of oxygen for the patient who breathes with the hypoxic drive.

_____ **14.** An asthmatic who tells you he was previously intubated for his breathing difficulty is at increased risk of death.

_____ **15.** Anticholinergics have emerged as a central component in the management of COPD.

_____ **16.** If you use an aerosol nebulizer to deliver medication, you can expect the patient to benefit from 90% of the medication dose.

_____ **17.** Immediate, fast-acting medications used for bronchodilation are beta-1 agonists.

_____ **18.** When giving a corticosteroid as an IV bolus, you will see immediate results.

_____ **19.** Morphine should be used as the first-line vasodilator in the treatment of pulmonary edema.

_____ **20.** A continuous positive airway pressure (CPAP) machine cannot be used in the field.

Short Answer

Complete this section with short written answers using the space provided.

1. List four things that can cause a pulmonary embolism.

a. ____

b. ____

c. ____

d. ____

2. Discuss the clues to diagnosing a pulmonary embolism.

3. What are the contraindications to supplemental oxygen therapy?

4. Not every patient who presents with dyspnea and wheezing has bronchial asthma. List four other conditions that can produce wheezing.

a. _____

b. _____

c. _____

d. _____

5. Asthma is common in children, so it is important to be able to distinguish a mild asthmatic attack from one that is potentially life threatening. List at least five signs that an asthmatic attack is very severe and warrants urgent transport to the hospital.

a. _____

b. _____

c. _____

d. _____

e. _____

Fill in the Table

Provide the signs and symptoms of the various breathing patterns listed in the following table.

1. Breathing Patterns

Pattern	Comments
Agonal	__________ __________ that are widely spaced; usually represent __________ __________ __________ in a dying patient; occasional agonal gasp not unusual in patients with no pulse; not actually considered a form of breathing
Apneustic	Characterized by a(n) __________ __________ __________ (sometimes called "__________ breathing"); follows damage to the __________ __________ in the brain; an ominous sign of severe __________ __________
Ataxic	Chaotically irregular respirations that indicate __________ brain injury or __________ __________
Biot respirations	Irregular pattern, __________, and depth of respirations, characterized by intermittent patterns of __________; indicates severe brain injury or __________ herniation
Bradypnea	Unusually __________ respirations
Central neurogenic hyperventilation	Tachypneic __________; rapid and deep respirations caused by __________ __________ __________ or direct __________ __________; drives __________ __________ level down and __________ up, resulting in respiratory __________
Cheyne-Stokes respirations	__________-__________ breathing with a period of __________ between cycles; not considered ominous unless grossly __________ or occurs in a patient with brain __________
Cough	Forced exhalation against a closed __________; an airway-clearing maneuver; also seen when __________ __________ irritate the airways; controlled by the cough center in the brain (__________ medications work on the cough center to reduce this sometimes annoying physiologic response)
Eupnea	__________ breathing
Hiccup	Spasmodic contraction of the __________, causing short __________ with a characteristic sound; sometimes seen in cases of diaphragmatic (or __________) nerve irritation from __________ __________ __________, ulcer disease, or __________ __________
Hyperpnea	Abnormally __________ rate and depth of breathing; seen in various __________ or chemical disorders, including overdose with certain drugs
Hypopnea	Abnormally __________ rate and depth of breathing
Kussmaul respirations	The same pattern as in __________ __________ __________, but caused by the body's response to metabolic __________, attempting to rid itself of blood __________ via the lungs; seen in diabetic __________; accompanied by a(n) __________ (acetone) breath odor and, usually, __________ and dry mouth and lips
Sighing	Periodically taking a very deep breath of about __________ the normal volume; forces open __________ that routinely close from time to time
Tachypnea	Unusually __________ breathing; does not reflect __________ of respiration and does not mean a patient is __________ (breathing too rapidly and deeply, resulting in a lowered __________ __________ level); often involves moving only small volumes of air, or __________ (much like a panting dog)
Yawning	Seems beneficial in the same manner as __________

Complete the Patient Care Report (PCR)

Read the incident scenario in the "Identify" exercise, and then complete the following PCR.

EMS Patient Care Report (PCR)					
Date:	Incident No.:	Nature of Call:		Location:	
Dispatched:	En Route:	At Scene:	Transport:	At Hospital:	In Service:

Patient Information	
Age: Sex: Weight (in kg [lb]):	Allergies: Medications: Past Medical History: Chief Complaint:

Vital Signs				
Time:	BP:	Pulse:	Respirations:	SpO_2:
Time:	BP:	Pulse:	Respirations:	SpO_2:
Time:	BP:	Pulse:	Respirations:	SpO_2:

EMS Treatment (circle all that apply)				
Oxygen @ ______ L/min via (circle one): NC NRM Bag-mask device		Assisted Ventilation	Airway Adjunct	CPR
Defibrillation	Bleeding Control	Bandaging	Splinting	Other:

Narrative

CHAPTER

17

Cardiovascular Emergencies

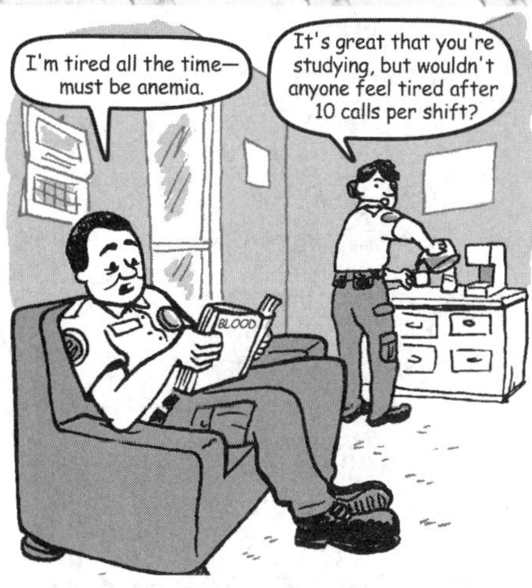

Welcome to the cardiac chapter of the workbook. Because of the length and the amount of material covered in this chapter, it has been divided into three parts to facilitate learning: Part 1 covers cardiac function; Part 2 addresses heart rhythms and the electrocardiogram (ECG), and Part 3 deals with putting it all together and practice ECG strips.

Part 1: Cardiac Function

Matching

Part I

Match each of the definitions in the left column to the appropriate term in the right column.

_____	**1.** An outpouching or bulge in the wall of a portion of the aorta, caused by weakening and dilation of the vessel wall; its rupture is life threatening.	**A.** Aberration
_____	**2.** A pathologic condition in which the thickening and stiffening of the arterial walls make the arteries less elastic.	**B.** Absolute refractory period
_____	**3.** The sudden pain that occurs when the oxygen supply to the myocardium is insufficient to meet demand, causing ischemic changes in the tissue.	**C.** Acute coronary syndromes
_____	**4.** The portion of the conduction system of the heart that consists of the AV node and the nonbranching portion of the bundle of His.	**D.** Agonal
_____	**5.** An accumulation of fat inside a blood vessel that narrows the diameter of the lumen.	**E.** Angina pectoris
_____	**6.** A mass of fatty tissue that gradually calcifies, hardening into an atheromatous plaque that infiltrates the arterial wall and diminishes its elasticity.	**F.** Aortic aneurysm
_____	**7.** A dysrhythmia in which every other complex is a premature complex, causing a normal-early beat-normal-early beat pattern; can be atrial, junctional, or ventricular.	**G.** Arteriosclerosis
_____	**8.** The classic trio of signs associated with cardiac tamponade: narrowed pulse pressure, muffled heart tones, and jugular vein distention.	**H.** Artifact
_____	**9.** Movement of the heart's QRS axis to the right or left of its normal position.	**I.** Asystole
_____	**10.** An intraventricular conduction disturbance involving impedance of electrical impulses from the bundle of His to the right or left bundle branch.	**J.** Atheroma
_____	**11.** Abnormal whooshing sounds indicating turbulent blood flow within a narrowed vessel; usually heard in the carotid arteries.	**K.** Atherosclerosis
_____	**12.** On an ECG, leads that contain both a positive pole and a negative pole; leads I, II, and III.	**L.** Atrioventricular junction
_____	**13.** A term describing the shape of the QRS complex in aberrantly conducted beats.	**M.** Axis deviation

______	14. The early phase of cardiac repolarization, wherein the heart muscle cannot be stimulated to depolarize; also known as the effective refractory period.	N.	Beck triad
______	15. A series of cardiac conditions caused by an abrupt reduction in coronary artery blood flow.	O.	Bigeminy
______	16. Pertaining to the period of dying.	P.	Bipolar leads
______	17. An artificial product; in cardiology, used to refer to noise or interference in an ECG tracing.	Q.	Bruits
______	18. The absence of ventricular contraction or electrical activity.	R.	Bundle branch block
______	19. Pathologic process characterized by progressive atherosclerotic narrowing and eventual obstruction of the coronary arteries.	S.	Cardiac cycle
______	20. The blood vessels that supply blood to the tissues of the heart.	T.	Cardiac tamponade
______	21. Leads that view geographically similar areas of the myocardium, such as leads II, III, and aVF; useful for localizing areas of ischemia.	U.	Claudication
______	22. The period from one cardiac contraction to the next; it includes both ventricular contraction (systole) and relaxation (diastole).	V.	Concordant precordial pattern
______	23. A pathologic condition characterized by restriction of cardiac contraction, falling cardiac output, and shock as a result of pericardial fluid accumulation.	W.	Contiguous leads
______	24. Pain, cramping, muscle tightness, fatigue, or weakness of the legs during physical activity as a result of increased oxygen demand by the muscle tissue of the legs, hips, and buttocks.	X.	Coronary arteries
______	25. An ECG pattern in which the QRS complexes are all in the same direction in the precordial leads as a result of improper lead placement, anterior wall myocardial infarction, ventricular tachycardia, or other variables.	Y.	Coronary artery disease

Part II

Match each of the definitions in the left column to the appropriate term in the right column.

______	1. Death of a localized area of tissue caused by ischemia.	A.	Couplet
______	2. Related to only the ventricles; produced by the ventricles.	B.	Delta wave
______	3. A syndrome that occurs when the heart is unable to pump powerfully enough or fast enough to empty its chambers; as a result, blood backs up into the systemic circuit, the pulmonary circuit, or both.	C.	Depolarization
______	4. Inflammation of the endocardium as a result of infection.	D.	Dissection
______	5. An impulse or rhythm that originates from a site other than the sinoatrial (SA) node.	E.	Dysrhythmias
______	6. Two consecutive (paired) premature ventricular complexes.	F.	Ectopic
______	7. The slurring of the upstroke of the first part of the QRS complex that occurs in Wolff-Parkinson-White syndrome.	G.	Endocarditis
______	8. The process of discharging resting cardiac muscle fibers by means of an electrical impulse that stimulates contraction.	H.	Fascicular block
______	9. The process by which the intimal and medial layers of a vessel separate after a tear occurs in an aneurysmal portion of the arterial wall; with each ventricular systole, a jet of blood is forced into the torn arterial wall, creating and propagating a false channel.	I.	Fibrinolytic therapy
______	10. Cardiac rhythm disturbances.	J.	First-degree AV block
______	11. Inflammation of the pericardial sac.	K.	Heart failure
______	12. The first wave of the ECG complex representing depolarization of the ventricles.	L.	Idioventricular
______	13. Having a common shape.	M.	Infarction
______	14. Arising from or pertaining to many foci or locations.	N.	Internodal pathways
______	15. The death of tissue, usually caused by a cessation of its blood supply.	O.	Ischemia
______	16. The baseline of the ECG, which is neither positive nor negative.	P.	Isoelectric line

______	**17.** Tissue anoxia caused by diminished blood flow, usually as a result of narrowing or occlusion of an artery.	**Q.** Left anterior descending artery
______	**18.** The three atrial pathways of electrical conduction that transmit impulses from the SA node to the atrioventricular (AV) node.	**R.** Left ventricular hypertrophy
______	**19.** A condition characterized by a QT interval exceeding approximately 0.45 seconds (450 milliseconds).	**S.** Long QT syndrome
______	**20.** A cardiac condition in which the left ventricle becomes enlarged, most often as a result of hypertension.	**T.** Monomorphic
______	**21.** One of the two branches of the left main coronary artery; these branches supply the left ventricle, interventricular septum, and part of the right ventricle.	**U.** Multifocal
______	**22.** Failure of the anterior or posterior fascicles of the heart to conduct electrical impulses because of disease or ischemia.	**V.** Myocarditis
______	**23.** The use of medications that act to dissolve blood clots.	**W.** Necrosis
______	**24.** A delay in the conduction of the depolarizing impulse from the SA node to the ventricles, prolonging the PR interval.	**X.** P wave
______	**25.** Inflammation of the myocardium.	**Y.** Pericarditis

Multiple Choice

Read each item carefully, and then select the best response.

______ **1.** The innermost smooth layer of the heart is called the:

- **A.** myocardium.
- **B.** endocardium.
- **C.** epicardium.
- **D.** pericardium.

______ **2.** During the ________ refractory period, cardiac cells are unable to respond to any stimulus.

- **A.** complete
- **B.** absolute
- **C.** relative
- **D.** nonessential

______ **3.** The normal dominant pacemaker for the heart is the:

- **A.** Purkinje fibers.
- **B.** AV node.
- **C.** bundle of His.
- **D.** SA node.

______ **4.** The ________ component of the ECG represents the depolarization of the ventricles.

- **A.** P wave
- **B.** QRS complex
- **C.** R-R interval
- **D.** T wave

______ **5.** The paramedic is palpating the radial pulse while listening to the apical pulse with a stethoscope. Which abnormality is he or she likely to find?

- **A.** Pulsus paradoxus
- **B.** Pulse deficit
- **C.** Pulsus alternans
- **D.** Pericardial friction rub

______ **6.** Of the following, which is NOT a cause of a cardiac dysrhythmia?

- **A.** Myocardial ischemia
- **B.** Cor pulmonale
- **C.** Hypoglycemia
- **D.** Increased vagal tone

_____ 7. An area of fat in the arteries that has calcified is known as a:
A. bruit.
B. phlebitis.
C. thrombophlebitis.
D. plaque.

_____ 8. In a 65-year-old man, a systolic blood pressure of __________ would indicate hypertension.
A. 120 mm Hg
B. 130 mm Hg
C. 140 mm Hg
D. 150 mm Hg

_____ 9. Which of the following symptoms is NOT associated with an acute myocardial infarction (AMI) or acute cardiac syndrome (ACS)?
A. Bulimia
B. Dizziness
C. Palpitations
D. Diaphoresis

_____ 10. The "M" in the mnemonic MONA stands for:
A. myocardium.
B. morphine.
C. management.
D. monitor.

Fill in the Blank

Read each item carefully, and then complete the statement by filling in the missing word(s).

1. Alternative routes of blood flow around the heart are known as __________ __________. These are used in case of a blockage.
2. The __________ valve prevents blood from flowing back into the left ventricle.
3. __________ leads refers to leads that view geographically similar areas of myocardium.
4. The __________ __________ consists of the blood vessels between the right ventricle and left atrium, which receive the output of the right side of the heart.
5. Early, ______ advanced airway management is essential for the patient whose cardiac arrest is the result of __________.
6. Because ______-________ AV block may occur with any _________ in which a(n) ______ wave precedes the ______, the rate associated with it is that of the underlying rhythm.
7. The ____________________ serves as the gatekeeper to the ventricles.
8. In right ________ hypertrophy the right ventricle becomes ________.
9. During the __________ __________ __________, the heart muscle will not contract because it is drained of all its energy.
10. Repolarization of the ventricles and atria will produce a(n) __________ __________ marking on an ECG.

Labeling

Label the following diagrams with the correct terms.

1. Coronary arteries

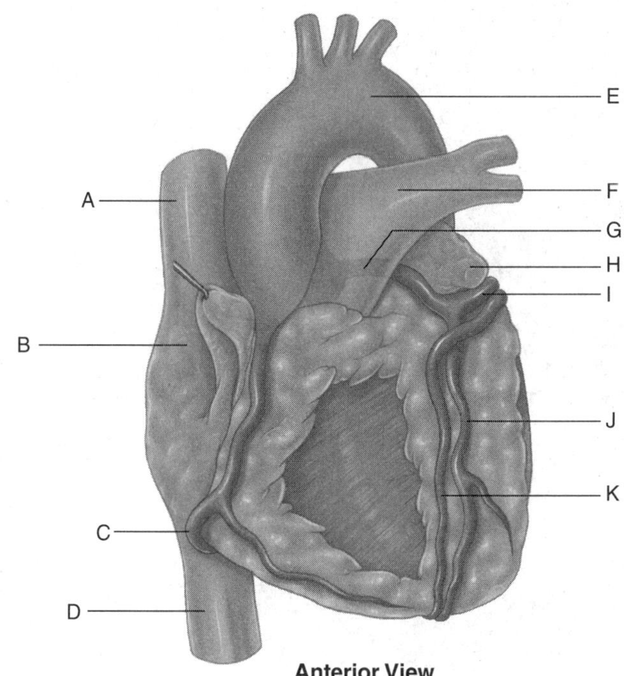

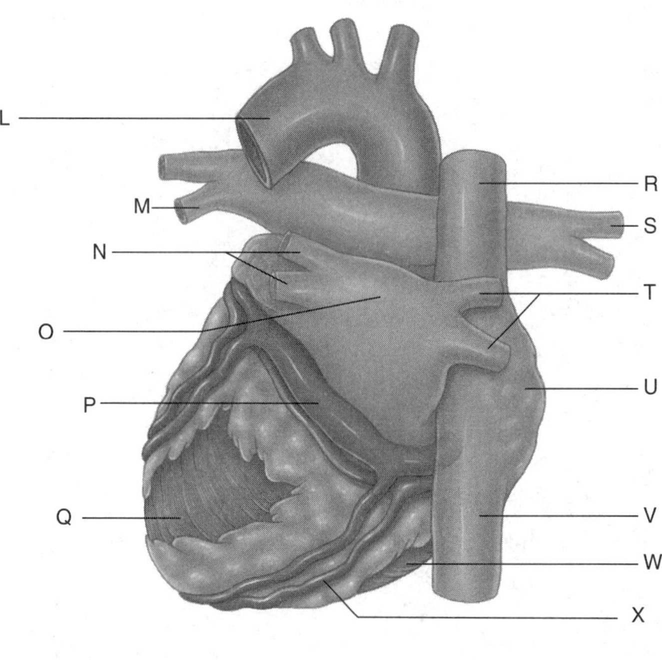

A. ______________________

B. ______________________

C. ______________________

D. ______________________

E. ______________________

F. ______________________

G. ______________________

H. ______________________

I. ______________________

J. ______________________

K. ______________________

L. ______________________

M. ______________________

N. ______________________

O. ______________________

P. ______________________

Q. ______________________

R. ______________________

S. ______________________

T. ______________________

U. ______________________

V. ______________________

W. ______________________

X. ______________________

2. Location of precordial leads

A. ______________________________

B. ______________________________

C. ______________________________

D. ______________________________

E. ______________________________

F. ______________________________

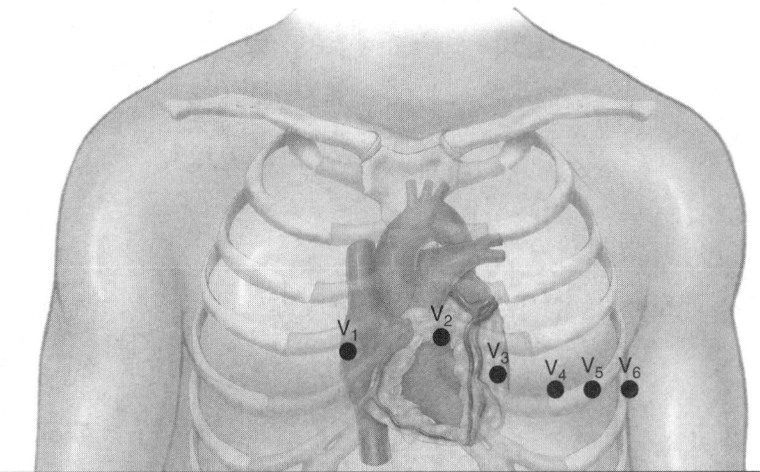

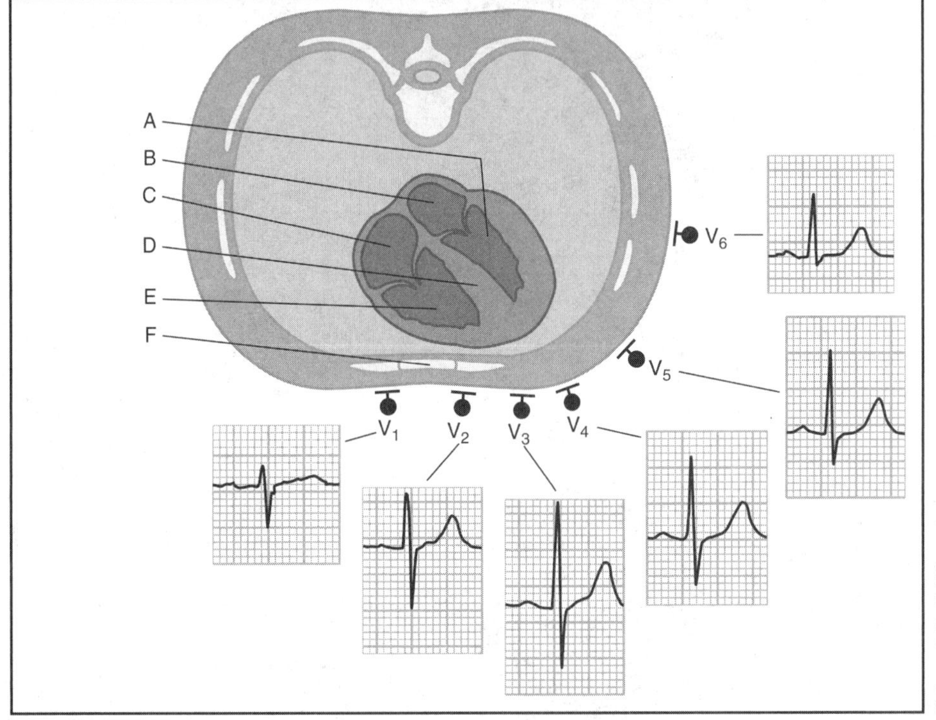

True/False

If you believe the statement to be more true than false, write the letter "T" in the space provided. If you believe the statement to be more false than true, write the letter "F."

______ **1.** Labetalol and nitroglycerin are drugs that can lower blood pressure.

______ **2.** The most characteristic physical finding with rupture of an abdominal aortic aneurysm (AAA) is decreased pedal pulse.

______ **3.** An ECG will be very helpful in diagnosing cardiac tamponade.

______ **4.** Management of left-sided heart failure should be to decrease preload.

______ **5.** Furosemide (Lasix) is a diuretic that always helps with left heart failure.

______ **6.** Percutaneous intervention can be used for a patient who does not qualify for fibrinolytic therapy.

______ **7.** Fibrinolytic therapy should begin within 2 hours after the AMI has occurred.

_____ **8.** Patients with diabetes experience incredible pain when suffering from ACS.

_____ **9.** The most common symptom of ACS is chest pain.

_____ **10.** Stable angina follows a recurrent pattern and usually occurs after exertion.

Fill in the Table

Fill in the missing parts of the table.

1. Role of electrolytes in cardiac function

Electrolyte	Role in Cardiac Function
_________	Flows into the cell to initiate depolarization
_________	Flows out of the cell to initiate _________ Decreased or increased levels of potassium result in the following: • _________ → increased myocardial irritability • _________ → decreased automaticity/conduction
_________	Has a major role in the depolarization of _________ cells (maintains depolarization) and in myocardial contractility (involved in contraction of heart muscle tissue) Decreased or increased levels of calcium result in the following: • _________ → decreased contractility and increased myocardial irritability • _________ → increased contractility
_________	Stabilizes the cell membrane; acts in concert with _________, and opposes the actions of calcium Decreased or increased levels of magnesium result in the following: • _________ → decreased conduction • _________ → increased myocardial irritability

Part 2: Heart Rhythms and the ECG

Matching

Part I

Match each of the items in the left column to the appropriate term in the right column.

_____	**1.** Where the "RA" (white) or "RL" (green) lead is traditionally placed by paramedics.	**A.** First-degree AV block
_____	**2.** Where the "LL" (red) lead is traditionally placed by paramedics.	**B.** Heart rate
_____	**3.** The point where the QRS complex ends and the ST segment begins.	**C.** Left lower chest
_____	**4.** Represents ventricular repolarization on an ECG.	**D.** T wave
_____	**5.** A regular rhythm, 60 to 100 beats/min.	**E.** Atrial flutter
_____	**6.** SA node pacemaker with a rate of 100 beats/min or more.	**F.** Tachycardia
_____	**7.** A rhythm in which the atria are contracting at a rate that is too fast for the ventricles to match.	**G.** Right upper shoulder
_____	**8.** When an impulse reaching the AV node is delayed and results in a PR interval longer than 0.20 seconds.	**H.** Wolff-Parkinson-White syndrome
_____	**9.** Rhythm that occurs when the ventricles take over at a rate of 20 to 40 beats/min.	**I.** J point
_____	**10.** A delta wave is an indication of this condition.	**J.** Idioventricular rhythm

Part II

Match each of the definitions in the left column to the appropriate term in the right column.

______ **1.** An inflammatory disease caused by streptococcal bacteria; the disease can cause mitral or aortic valve stenosis.

______ **2.** Dilation of the right atrium that occurs when returning venous pressure is elevated or pulmonary pressure is high.

______ **3.** Artery that provides oxygenated blood to the walls of the right atrium and ventricle, a portion of the inferior part of the left ventricle, and portions of the conduction system.

______ **4.** A condition in which the right side of the heart must work increasingly harder to pump blood into engorged pulmonary vessels; eventually, it is unable to keep up with the increased workload.

______ **5.** Treatment intended to facilitate the resumption of blood through a blocked vessel; therapy may be either procedural, such as cardiac catheterization, or pharmacologic, such as administration of a fibrinolytic agent.

______ **6.** A short period immediately after depolarization during which the myocytes have not yet repolarized and are unable to fire or conduct an impulse or have partially repolarized and may depolarize in response to an electrical stimulus.

______ **7.** Spread of an impulse through tissue already stimulated by that same impulse.

______ **8.** Mirror-image J-point, ST-segment, and T-wave changes seen on the ECG during ACS.

______ **9.** The use of a synchronized direct current electric shock to convert a tachydysrhythmia (such as supraventricular tachycardia) to a normal sinus rhythm.

______ **10.** A type of acute myocardial infarction in which the ischemic process affects only the inner layer of muscle.

______ **11.** Angina pectoris characterized by periodic pain with a predictable pattern.

______ **12.** The interval between the end of the QRS complex (the J point) and the beginning of the T wave; when there is significant myocardial ischemia or injury, it is often depressed or elevated with respect to the isoelectric line on the ECG.

______ **13.** The thick wall that separates the right and left sides of the heart.

______ **14.** A disease caused by the bacterium *Streptococcus pyogenes* and characterized by a sore throat, fever, rash, and "strawberry tongue."

______ **15.** The period between the onset of one QRS complex and the onset of the next QRS complex.

______ **16.** A cardiac condition in which the right ventricle becomes enlarged, usually as a result of pulmonary hypertension.

______ **17.** A single vector that represents the mean (or average) of all vectors created by the ventricles during depolarization.

______ **18.** A network of cardiac muscle fibers distributed throughout the inner surfaces of the ventricular walls that conducts the excitation impulse from the bundle branches to the ventricular myocardium.

______ **19.** An organized cardiac rhythm (other than ventricular tachycardia) on an ECG monitor that is not accompanied by any detectable pulse.

______ **20.** Obstruction in one or more pulmonary arteries by a solid, liquid, or gas that has swept through the right side of the heart into the lungs.

______ **21.** A sinus rhythm characterized by a heart rate greater than 100 beats/min.

______ **22.** A variation of cycling of a sinus rhythm that is often associated with respiratory cycle fluctuations; the rate increases during inspiration and decreases during expiration.

A. Pulmonary embolism
B. Pulseless electrical activity
C. Purkinje fibers
D. QRS axis
E. QRS complex
F. Reciprocal changes
G. Reentry
H. Refractory period
I. Reperfusion therapy
J. Rheumatic fever
K. Right atrial abnormality
L. Right coronary artery
M. Right ventricular failure
N. Right ventricular hypertrophy
O. R-R interval
P. Scarlet fever
Q. Septum
R. Sinoatrial node
S. Sinus bradycardia
T. Sinus dysrhythmia
U. Sinus tachycardia
V. ST segment

______	**23.** A sinus rhythm characterized by a heart rate of less than 60 beats/min.	**W.** Stable angina
______	**24.** The dominant pacemaker of the heart, located at the junction of the superior vena cava and the right atrium.	**X.** Subendocardial myocardial infarction
______	**25.** Deflection of the ECG produced by ventricular depolarization.	**Y.** Synchronized cardioversion

Multiple Choice

Read each item carefully, and then select the best response.

______ **1.** __________ is an electrolyte imbalance that causes very tall and pointed T waves.

A. Hypokalemia
B. Hyperkalemia
C. Hyperglycemia
D. Hypocalcemia

______ **2.** Lead __________ is NOT a limb lead.

A. I
B. aVR
C. aVF
D. V_2

______ **3.** During an AMI, the stage of injury appears as a(n) __________ on the ECG.

A. T-wave inversion
B. ST-segment depression
C. ST-segment elevation
D. spiked P wave

______ **4.** Lead V_5 is placed on the patient on the:

A. anterior axillary line.
B. midaxillary line.
C. fourth intercostal space.
D. left arm.

______ **5.** __________ is NOT a possible cause of pulseless electrical activity.

A. Hypovolemia
B. Hyperthermia
C. Cardiac tamponade
D. Pulmonary embolism

______ **6.** The signs and symptoms of sick sinus syndrome include all of the following, EXCEPT:

A. dizziness.
B. palpitation.
C. bounding pulse.
D. near-syncope.

______ **7.** When using an automated external defibrillator (AED) to administer a shock, for safety, do each of the following, EXCEPT:

A. ensure no one is touching the patient.
B. do not defibrillate someone who is touching metal.
C. place the defibrillation pad over the nitroglycerin patch.
D. if the patient has an implanted pacemaker, place the defibrillation pad below the device.

______ **8.** The correct term for the use of a defibrillator to end a dysrhythmia other than ventricular fibrillation (VF) or pulseless ventricular tachycardia (VT) is:

A. cardioversion.
B. transcutaneous cardiac pacing.
C. defibrillation.
D. conversion.

______ **9.** A genetic condition in which the myocardial wall becomes very thick is called:
- **A.** Brugada syndrome.
- **B.** hypertrophic cardiomyopathy.
- **C.** long Q-T syndrome.
- **D.** Prinzmetal angina.

______ **10.** One small box on the ECG strip represents __________ seconds.
- **A.** 0.04
- **B.** 0.40
- **C.** 0.02
- **D.** 0.20

Fill in the Blank

Read each item carefully, and then complete the statement by filling in the missing word(s).

1. __________ __________ occurs when the SA node fails to fire and initiate an impulse, which in turn eliminates an entire cardiac cycle. After the missed set, the normal function returns.

2. A tachycardic rhythm that begins in the pacemaker above the ventricles is known as a(n) __________ __________.

3. The SA node ceases to fire and the AV node (in the junction) takes over as the pacemaker; however, the rate is greater than 60 beats/min. This is called __________ __________ __________.

4. A(n) __________-__________ heart block occurs when no pulses move between the AV node and the ventricles. In such a case, the junctional or ventricular pacemaker runs the heart.

5. __________ __________ occurs when the entire heart begins to quiver without any organized contractions.

6. The pattern __________ occurs when there is a normal complex followed by a premature ventricular complex (PVC). This pattern repeats itself. If every third beat is a PVC, it is then called __________.

7. __________ occurs when the entire heart is at a standstill and there is no electrical activity.

8. A(n) __________ __________ is an indication of Wolff-Parkinson-White syndrome.

9. When a PVC comes from the same site, it is known as __________, but when the premature ventricular complexes come from different sites in the ventricles, the condition is known as __________.

10. The pacemaker is the SA node, but with a rate of less than 60 beats/min. This is called __________ __________.

True/False

If you believe the statement to be more true than false, write the letter "T" in the space provided. If you believe the statement to be more false than true, write the letter "F."

______ **1.** When performing an ECG, the electrodes should be attached to the leads prior to placing them on the patient's skin.

______ **2.** P waves indicate that the pacemaker for the heart is in the AV node.

______ **3.** The "6-second method" is the simplest, but not the most accurate, method for determining the heart rate when the rhythm is slow.

______ **4.** A heart rate of more than 100 beats/min is called tachycardia.

_____ 5. Wandering atrial pacemaker is most commonly seen in patients with diabetes.

_____ 6. Prehospital treatment of atrial fibrillation is common.

_____ 7. Mobitz type I occurs when each successive impulse is delayed a little longer, until finally one impulse is not able to continue.

_____ 8. The ventricles will take over as the pacemaker if the SA node fails.

_____ 9. Polymorphic VT is more serious than monomorphic VT.

_____ 10. An agonal rhythm will produce a pulse.

Short Answer

Complete this section with short written answers using the space provided.

1. Discuss the basic principles in placing electrodes on a patient's chest.

2. Explain the causes of the P wave, PR interval, QRS complex, and T wave.

3. Describe how a 12-lead ECG helps to "look" at the heart.

4. What should you do if you find a patient in cardiac arrest?

5. If you are able to terminate cardiopulmonary resuscitation (CPR) in the field, which steps should you and your medical director take before you implement your protocols to do so?

Part 3: Putting It All Together and Practice ECG Strips

Matching

Match the generic name with the trade name for the following drugs.

______	1. Amiodarone	A. Capoten
______	2. Metoprolol	B. Lopressor
______	3. Furosemide	C. Inderal
______	4. Digoxin	D. Coumadin
______	5. Captopril	E. Lasix
______	6. Propranolol	F. Lanoxin
______	7. Atorvastatin	G. Nitrostat
______	8. Warfarin	H. Lipitor
______	9. Verapamil	I. Cordarone
______	10. Nitroglycerin	J. Calan

Labeling

Label the following diagrams with the correct terms.

1. Electrical conduction system

A. ______________________

B. ______________________

C. ______________________

D. ______________________

E. ______________________

F. ______________________

G. ______________________

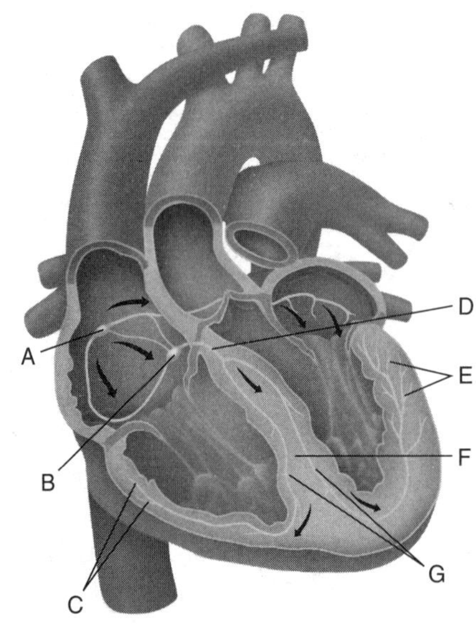

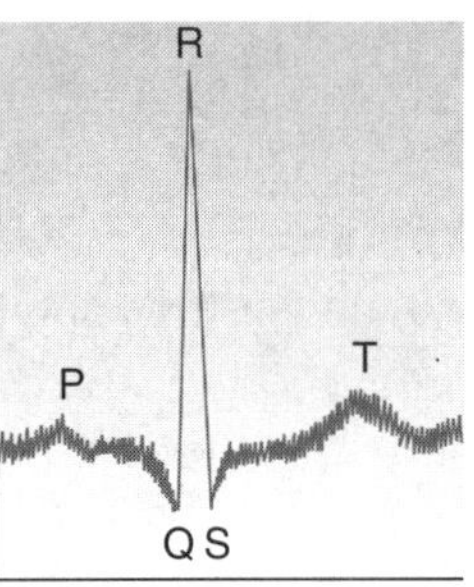

Fill in the Table

Fill in the missing parts of the table.

1. Components of the ECG

ECG Representation	Cardiac Event
P wave	Depolarization of the _____
PRI	Depolarization of the atria and delay at the ____ junction
QRS complex	Depolarization of the _____
ST segment	Period between ventricular depolarization and beginning of _____
T wave	Ventricular _____
R-R interval	Time between two _____ ventricular depolarizations

Ambulance Calls

Read each scenario, and then answer all the questions following the scenario.

1. You are called to see a 62-year-old man complaining of severe chest pain. He says that the pain came on an hour earlier and that it feels "like a thousand-pound weight on my chest." The patient is very restless and seems confused, so it is difficult to get much history. On physical examination, he is obviously in marked distress. His skin is pale and cold. His pulse is 82 beats/min and thready, respirations are 32 breaths/min and shallow, and blood pressure (BP) is 90/62 mm Hg. His oxygen saturation is 91% on room air.

   a. Identify the chief complaint and vital signs for this patient.

   Chief complaint:

   ____

   ____

   Vital signs:

   ____

   ____

   b. Which steps would you direct your partner to take at this time of the call?

   (1)______________________________

   (2)______________________________

   (3)______________________________

   (4)______________________________

   c. After your partner hooks up the monitor, you run a 3-lead ECG strip and see this:

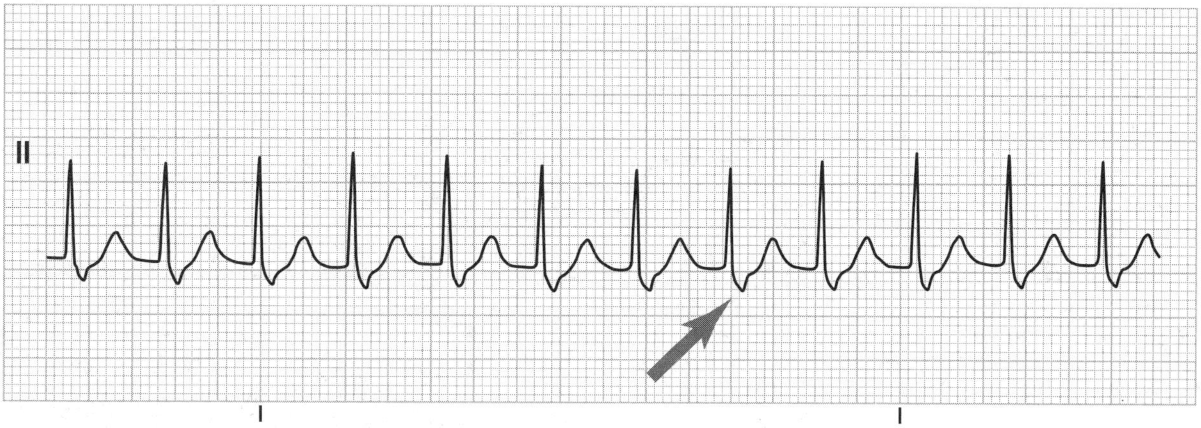

   II

   Reproduced from *Arrhythmia Recognition: The Art of Interpretation*, courtesy of Tomas B.

   (1) Is the rhythm regular? __________

   (2) What is the rate? __________

   (3) Are the P waves present or absent? __________

   (4) If present, is there a P wave before every QRS? __________

   (5) P-R interval: __________ seconds

   (6) QRS complex width: __________

   (7) T waves present or absent? Upright? __________

   (8) What is the name of this rhythm? __________

d. Which field diagnosis will you give this patient and why?

___

e. Which treatment will you provide for this patient?

___

2. You are called to see a patient whose chief complaint is dyspnea. He tells you in gasps that for several nights he has been waking up around 0200 hours unable to breathe. He has to get up and sit on the side of the bed to catch his breath. Tonight, sitting up has not helped. "Must be those cigarettes," he wheezes. He tells you that he "keeps a cough," but lately he has been bringing up much more sputum than usual. On physical examination, the patient is in obvious respiratory distress, coughing periodically. His lips look rather blue. His pulse is 102 beats/min and irregular. His respirations are 60 breaths/min and labored, and his BP is 170/94 mm Hg in both arms. His neck veins are distended to the angle of the jaw. His chest is a veritable symphony of crackles and wheezes, and his oxygen saturation is 86% on room air. There is a tender fullness in the right upper quadrant of his abdomen. Both feet are swollen well above the ankles.

a. Identify the chief complaint and vital signs for this patient.

Chief complaint:

Vital signs:

b. Which steps would you take at this point in the call?

(1)

(2)

(3)

(4)

c. What do you think the patient is experiencing?

d. What can you do to help this patient?

3. The family of a 76-year-old woman calls for an ambulance after the woman fainted while preparing Sunday dinner. The patient is lying on the sofa when you arrive. She is conscious but somewhat confused. She was unharmed in the fall. Your partner begins to take her vital signs as you try to get a history. The patient's pulse is 44 beats/min and regular,

respirations are 22 breaths/min and full, and oxygen saturation is 94%. She says that she is having some pain in her chest but cannot rate the pain because of her confusion. Her BP is 82/40 mm Hg, and her skin is cool. Her lungs are clear, and she seems to be in good health otherwise. She takes a daily vitamin.

a. Identify the chief complaint and vital signs for this patient.

Chief complaint:

____

____

Vital signs:

____

____

b. List at least four causes of syncopal episodes.

(1)____

(2)____

(3)____

(4)____

c. You hook up the monitor and see sinus bradycardia. What is your treatment for this patient now?

(1)____

(2)____

d. If pharmacologic therapies do not help, what else can you do to raise the heart rate in this patient?

____

____

____

4. A 64-year-old man calls for an ambulance because he has been "feeling poorly." His symptoms are not anything specific; they are nothing he can really pin down. He has just been feeling very weak and washed out for the last few days, so he thought perhaps he ought to go to the hospital and have a doctor take a look at him. There are no striking findings on physical exam except for an irregular heartbeat. The patient's pulse is about 76 beats/min but very irregular so that it is hard to count. His BP is 110/74 mm Hg on both arms. He has no significant history and has not been to a doctor except for a yearly checkup. His lungs are clear, and his oxygen saturation is 97%. His skin is a little cool. You hook up the heart monitor to take a quick peek, and this is what you see.

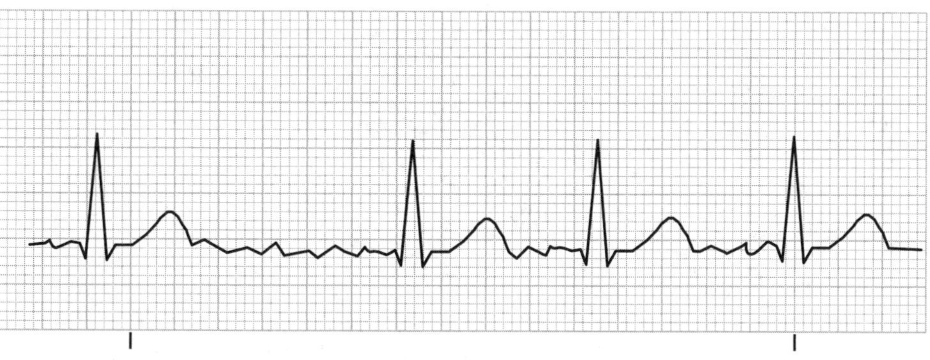

Reproduced from *Arrhythmia Recognition: The Art of Interpretation*, courtesy of Tomas B. Garcia, MD.

a. Identify the chief complaint and vital signs of this patient.
Chief complaint:

____

Vital signs:

____

____

b. Answer the following questions.

(1) Is the rhythm regular? __________

(2) What is the rate? __________

(3) Are the P waves present or absent? __________

(4) If present, is there a P before every QRS? __________

(5) Is there a QRS after every P? __________

(6) P-R interval: __________

(7) QRS complexes: __________ normal __________ abnormal

(8) Name of rhythm: __________

(9) Treatment: __________

5. You are taking a quick break at the emergency department (ED) after several hectic calls. You have made friends with the nurses, and they let you sit at the desk, where you can see the following heart monitors for different patients. Write the correct name of the rhythm on the line below the strip.

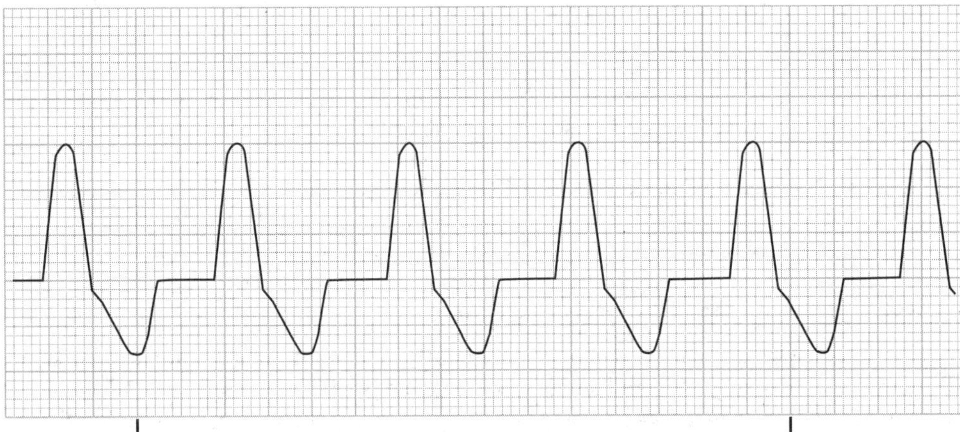

a. ____

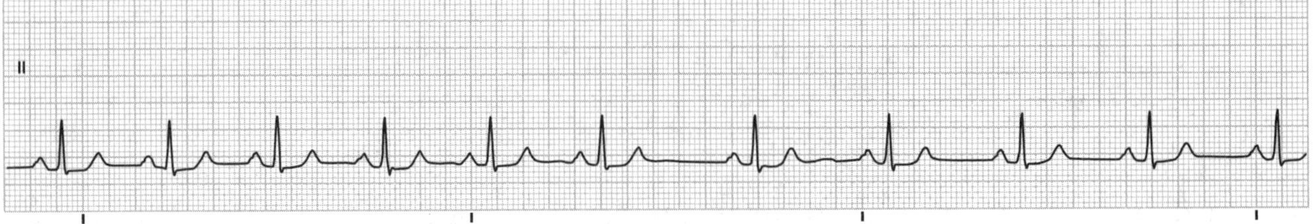

Reproduced from *Arrhythmia Recognition: The Art of Interpretation*, courtesy of Tomas B. Garcia, MD.

b. ____

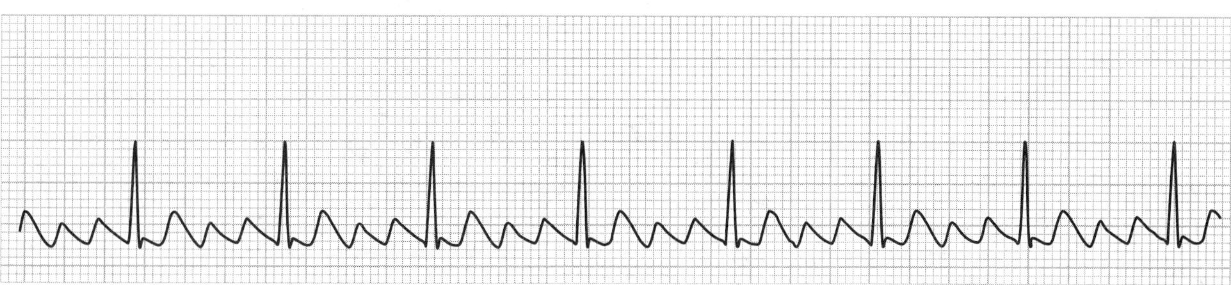

c. ______

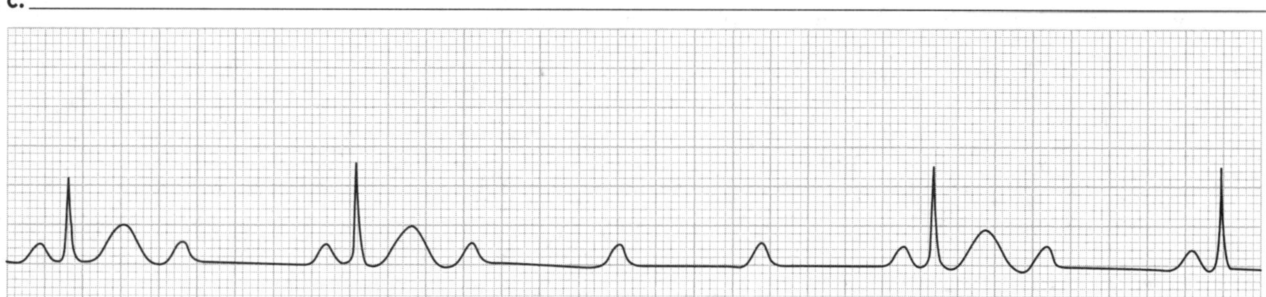

Reproduced from *Arrhythmia Recognition: The Art of Interpretation*, courtesy of Tomas B. Garcia, MD.

d. ______

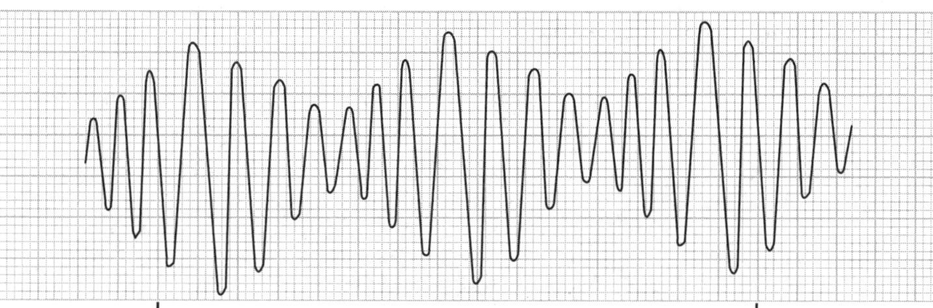

Reproduced from *Arrhythmia Recognition: The Art of Interpretation*, courtesy of Tomas B. Garcia, MD.

e. ______

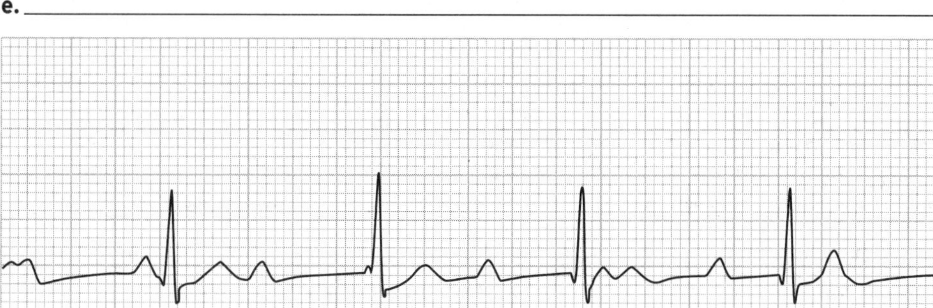

Reproduced from *Arrhythmia Recognition: The Art of Interpretation*, courtesy of Tomas B. Garcia, MD.

f. ______

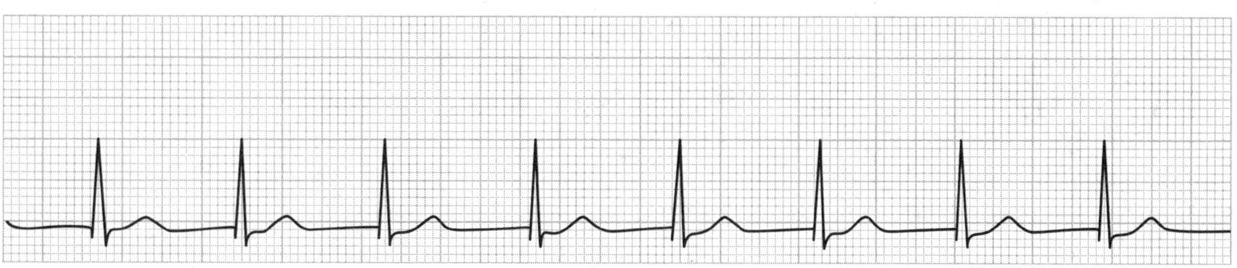

Reproduced from *Arrhythmia Recognition: The Art of Interpretation*, courtesy of Tomas B. Garcia, MD.

g. ______

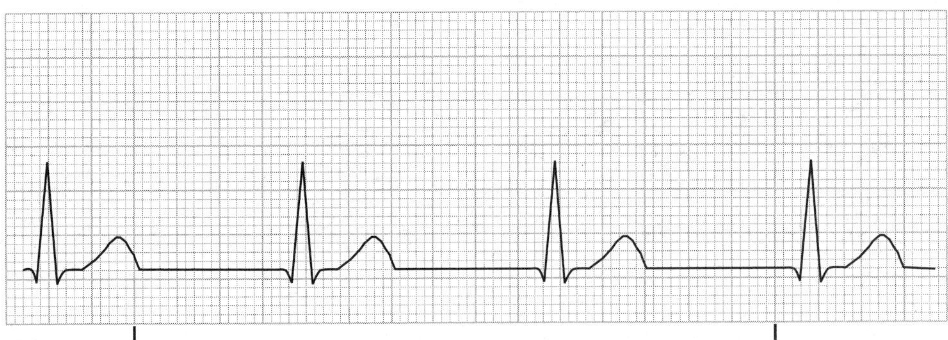

Reproduced from *Arrhythmia Recognition: The Art of Interpretation*, courtesy of Tomas B. Garcia, MD.

h. ______________________________

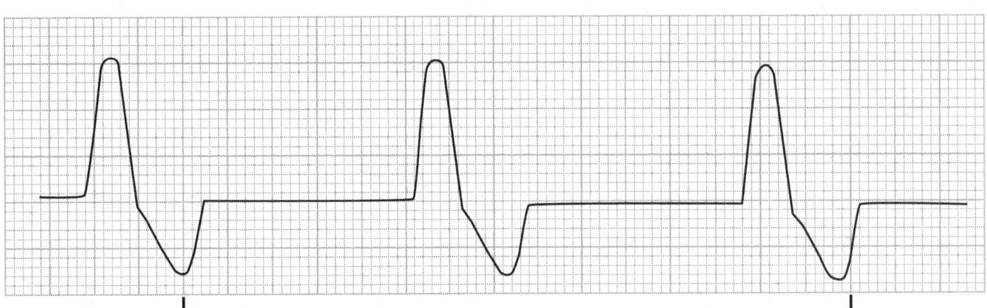

Modified from *Arrhythmia Recognition: The Art of Interpretation*, courtesy of Tomas B. Garcia, MD.

i. ______________________________

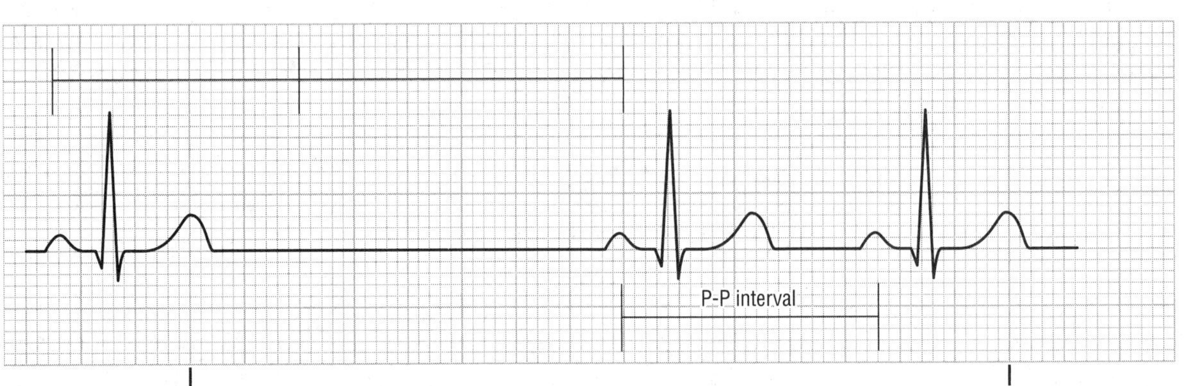

Reproduced from *Arrhythmia Recognition: The Art of Interpretation*, courtesy of Tomas B. Garcia, MD.

j. ______________________________

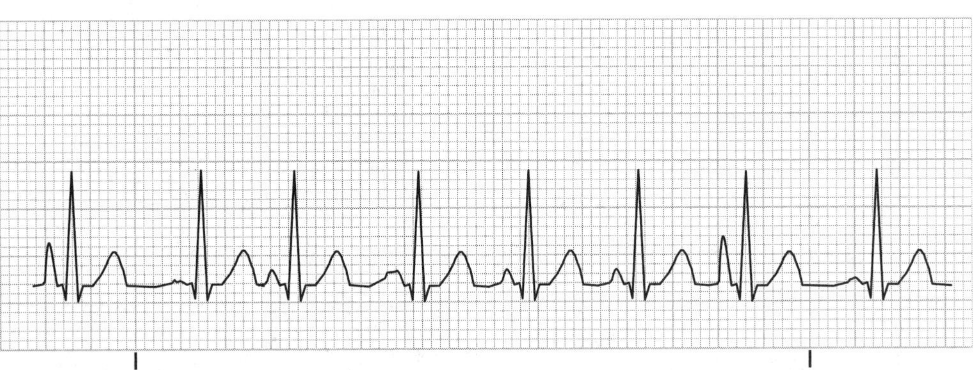

Reproduced from *Arrhythmia Recognition: The Art of Interpretation*, courtesy of Tomas B. Garcia, MD.

k. ______________________________

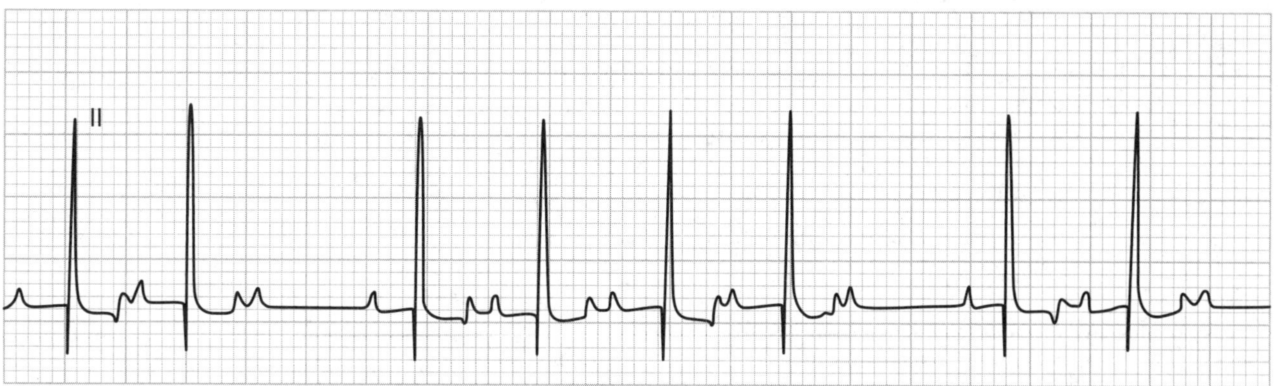

Reproduced from *Arrhythmia Recognition: The Art of Interpretation*, courtesy of Tomas B. Garcia, MD.

l. ____________________

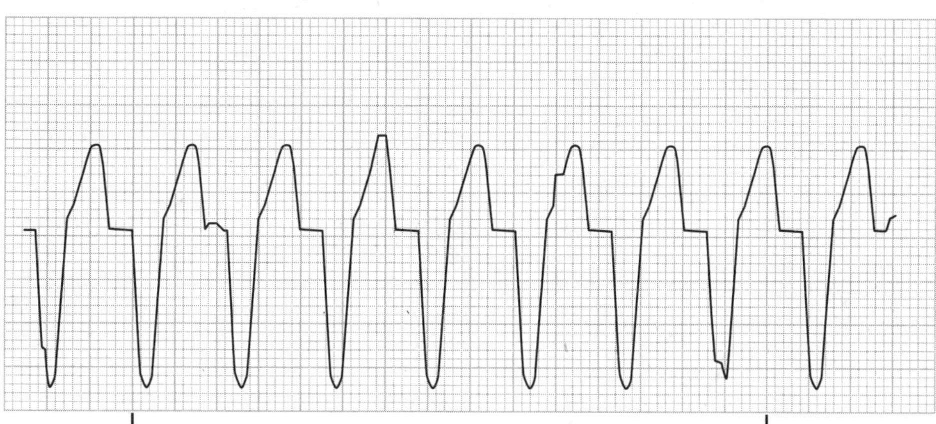

Reproduced from *Arrhythmia Recognition: The Art of Interpretation*, courtesy of Tomas B. Garcia, MD.

m. ____________________

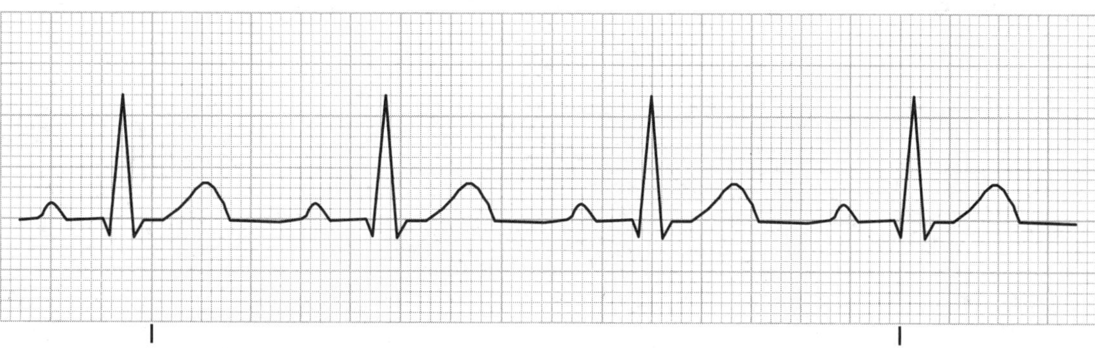

Reproduced from *Arrhythmia Recognition: The Art of Interpretation*, courtesy of Tomas B. Garcia, MD.

n. ____________________

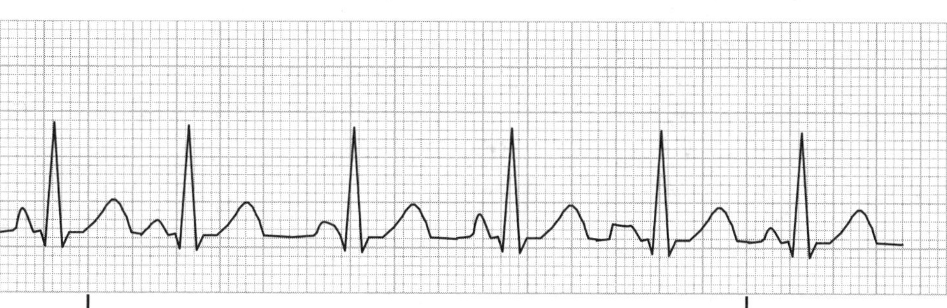

Reproduced from *Arrhythmia Recognition: The Art of Interpretation*, courtesy of Tomas B. Garcia, MD.

o. ____________________

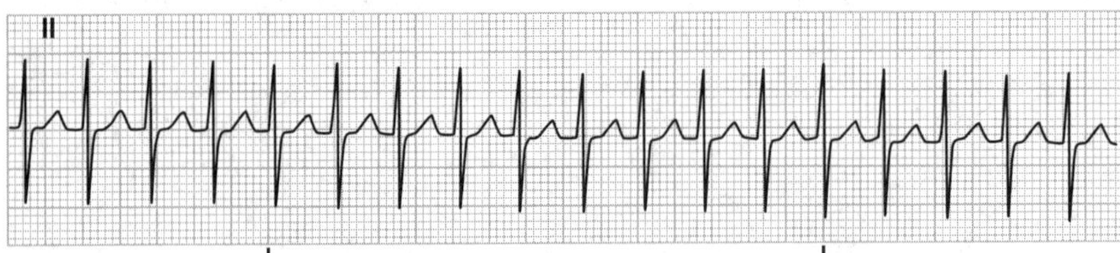

Reproduced from *Arrhythmia Recognition: The Art of Interpretation*, courtesy of Tomas B. Garcia, MD.

p. ____________________

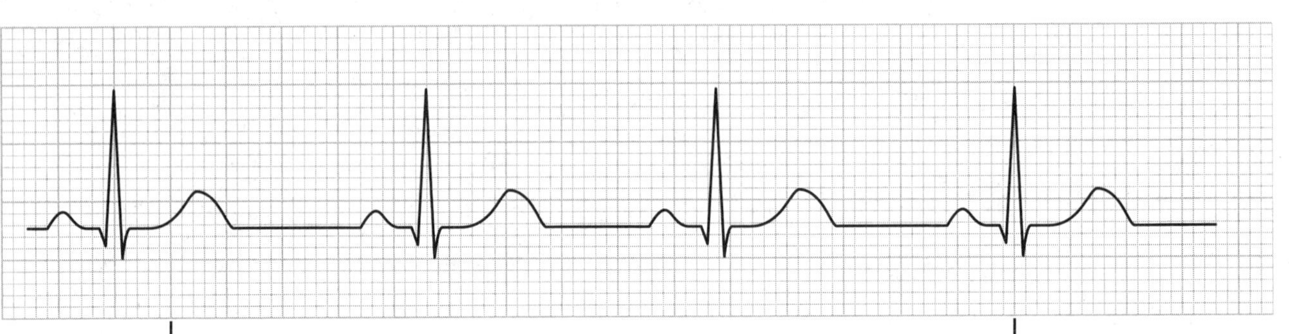

Reproduced from *Arrhythmia Recognition: The Art of Interpretation*, courtesy of Tomas B. Garcia, MD.

q. ____________________

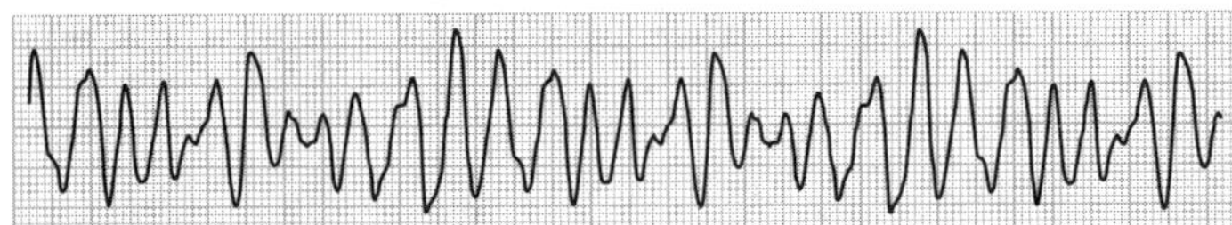

Reproduced from *Arrhythmia Recognition: The Art of Interpretation*, courtesy of Tomas B. Garcia, MD.

r. ____________________

6. The nurse hands you the following three strips and asks you if you can figure out which type of ectopic beat is present in each strip.

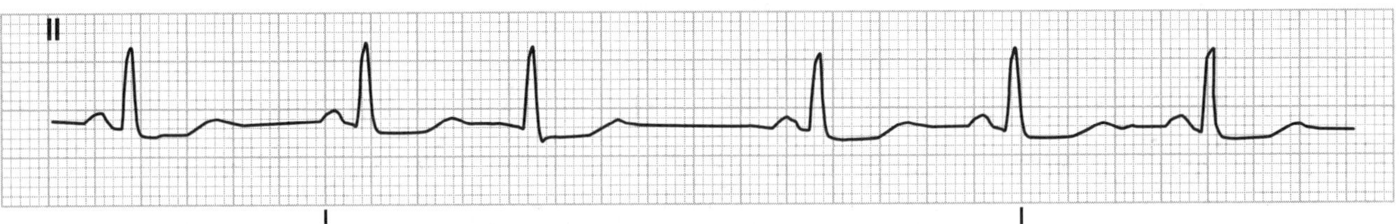

Reproduced from *Arrhythmia Recognition: The Art of Interpretation*, courtesy of Tomas B. Garcia, MD.

a. ____________________

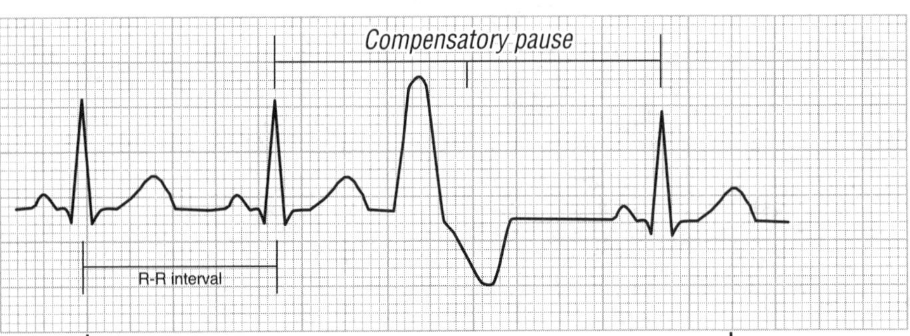

Modified from *Arrhythmia Recognition: The Art of Interpretation*, courtesy of Tomas B. Garcia, MD.

b. ____________________

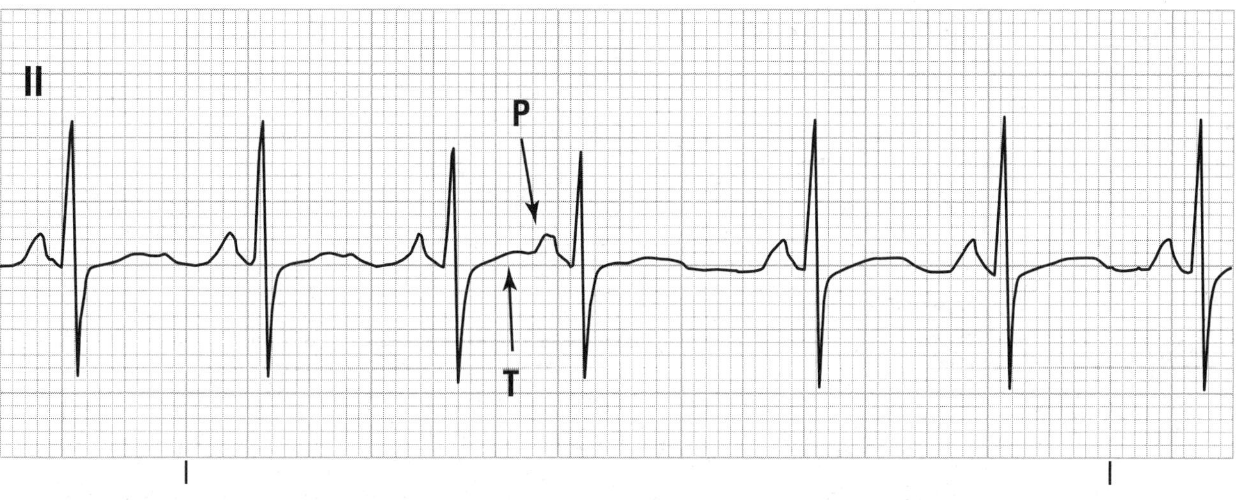

Reproduced from *Arrhythmia Recognition: The Art of Interpretation*, courtesy of Tomas B. Garcia, MD.

c. __________

Short Answer

1. How many seconds, or portions of a second, does a small box on an ECG graph paper represent? __________
2. How many small boxes does it take to make a large box on the ECG graph paper? __________
3. List the signs and symptoms that are present during a tachycardia that would make the patient "symptomatic" and a candidate for electric cardioversion.

   a. __________

   b. __________

   c. __________

   d. __________

   e. __________
4. What is the initial drug of choice when dealing with patients with a stable tachycardia and a regular rhythm that is not breaking with a trial of vagal maneuvers?

   ____
5. Which drug would be a consideration in a patient with a wide-complex stable tachycardia (ie, possible VT)?

   ____

   ____
6. You are faced with a patient who has a third-degree heart block and a heart rate of 48 beats/min. The patient shows signs of poor perfusion. After starting an IV, what would you do next?

   ____
7. List the initial correct dosage of medication in the following scenarios.
   a. Epinephrine in the care of a patient in cardiac arrest: __________
   b. Epinephrine for a conscious patient with a bradycardia and poor perfusion: __________
   c. Adenosine for a patient with stable, narrow, regular QRS tachycardia with pulses: __________
   d. Amiodarone for a patient with stable, wide-complex tachycardia or PVCs in salvos: __________

8. List the Hs and Ts that you should be thinking about during a cardiac arrest.

H ______________________	T ______________________
H ______________________	T ______________________
H ______________________	T ______________________
H ______________________	T ______________________
H ______________________	
H ______________________	

Problem Solving

Practice your calculation skills by solving the following math problems.

1. Suppose a person at rest has a heart rate of 72 beats/min and a stroke volume of 75 mL/beat. What is his cardiac output? __________ mL/min

2. Now that same person is running to catch a bus. His heart speeds up to 100 beats/min, and his stroke volume increases to 90 mL/beat. What is his cardiac output now? __________ mL/min

3. You often need to use your knowledge of anatomy, physiology, and pathophysiology to problem-solve situations you are presented with and arrive at a working field diagnosis. In this case, take the given signs or symptoms and quickly decide if the patient could have left- or right-sided heart failure. Place an L for left-sided and an R for right-sided heart failure before the following signs and symptoms.

a. ______ Dyspnea
b. ______ Jugular vein distention
c. ______ Swelling of the feet
d. ______ Crackles on auscultation
e. ______ Hepatomegaly
f. ______ Sacral edema
g. ______ Pink, frothy sputum

4. Find the MAP for the following blood pressures.

a. 160/94 mm Hg __________
b. 200/126 mm Hg __________
c. 148/86 mm Hg __________

Practice ECG Strips

Examine each of the following ECG strips, and state the rate, the rhythm, and the significant findings for each.

1.

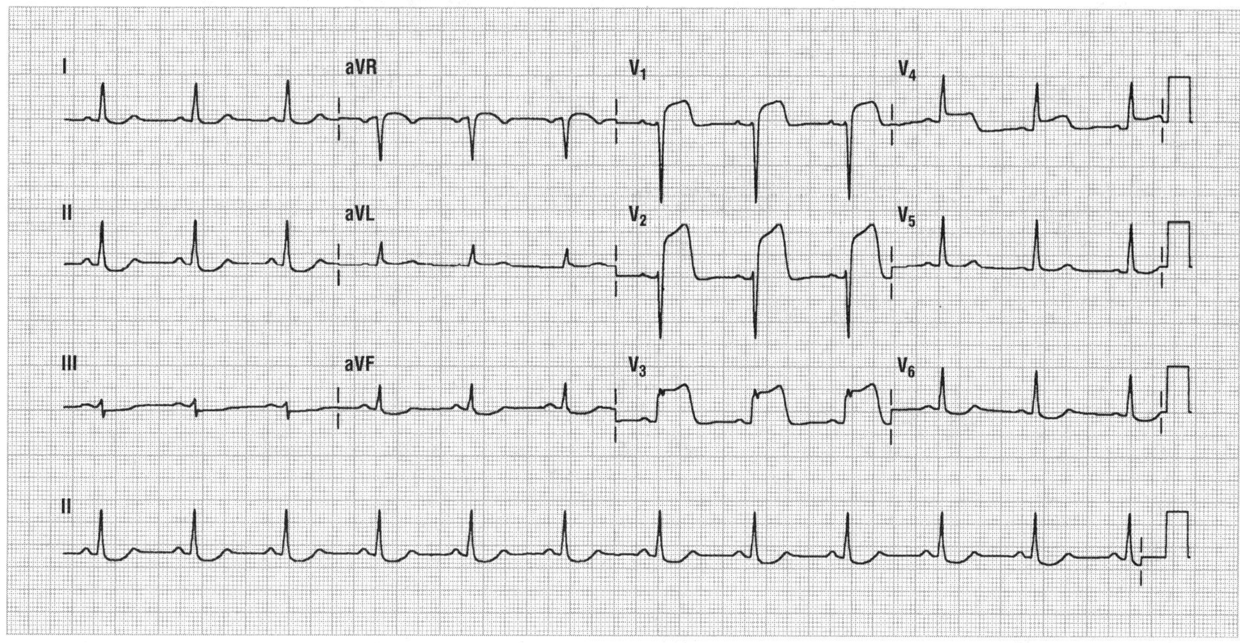

Reproduced from *12-Lead ECG: The Art of Interpretation*, courtesy of Tomas B. Garcia, MD.

Rate: __________

Rhythm: __________

Significant findings: ______________________________

2.

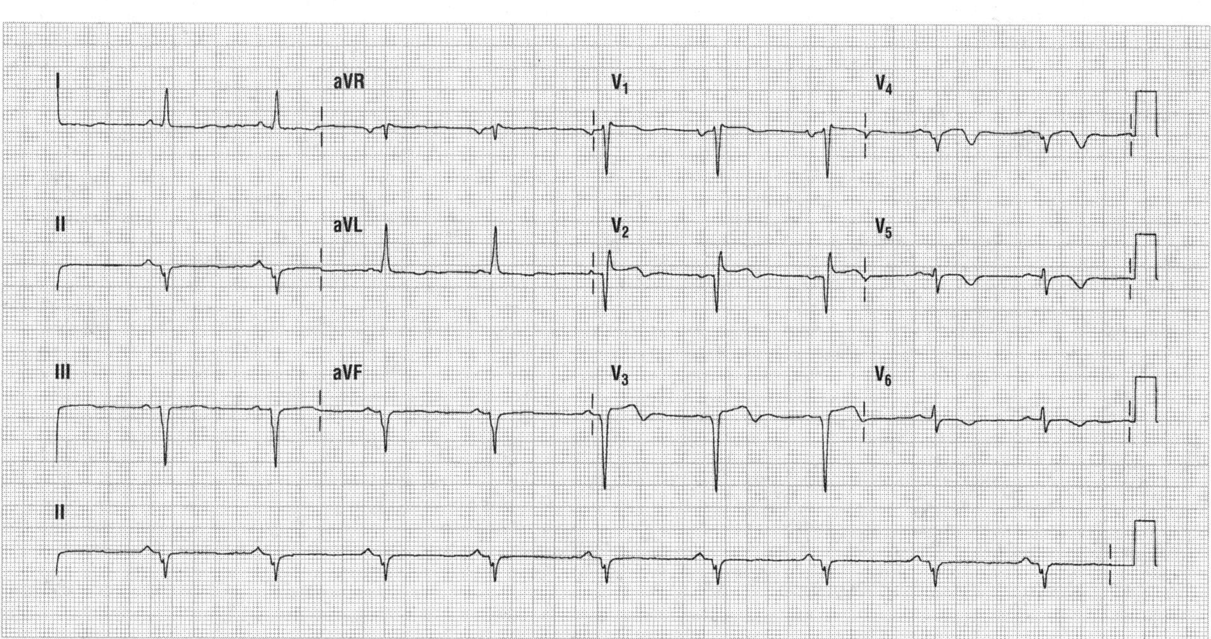

Reproduced from *12-Lead ECG: The Art of Interpretation*, courtesy of Tomas B. Garcia, MD.

Rate: __________

Rhythm: __________

Significant findings: ______________________________

3.

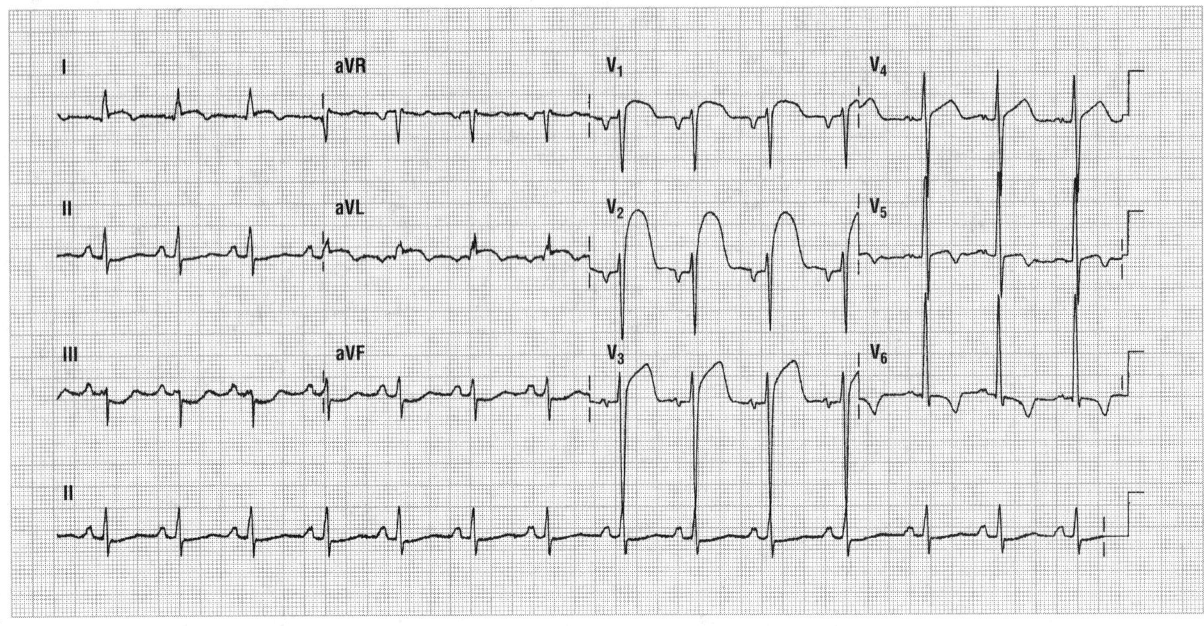

Reproduced from *12-Lead ECG: The Art of Interpretation*, courtesy of Tomas B. Garcia, MD.

Rate: __________

Rhythm: __________

Significant findings: ______________________________

4.

Reproduced from *12-Lead ECG: The Art of Interpretation*, courtesy of Tomas B. Garcia, MD.

Rate: __________

Rhythm: __________

Significant findings: ______________________________

5.

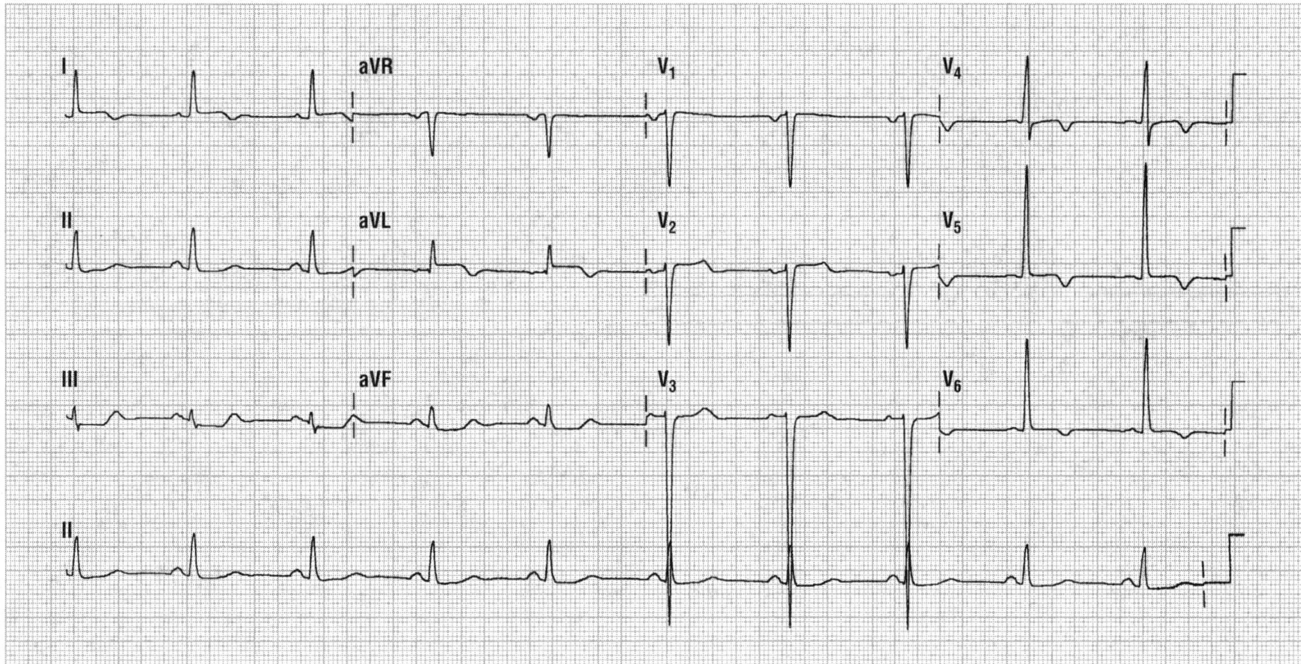

Reproduced from *12-Lead ECG: The Art of Interpretation*, courtesy of Tomas B. Garcia, MD.

Rate:

Rhythm:

Significant findings:

6.

Reproduced from *12-Lead ECG: The Art of Interpretation*, courtesy of Tomas B. Garcia, MD.

I aVR V1 V4
II aVL V2 V5
III aVF V3 V6
II

Rate:

Rhythm:

Significant findings:

7.

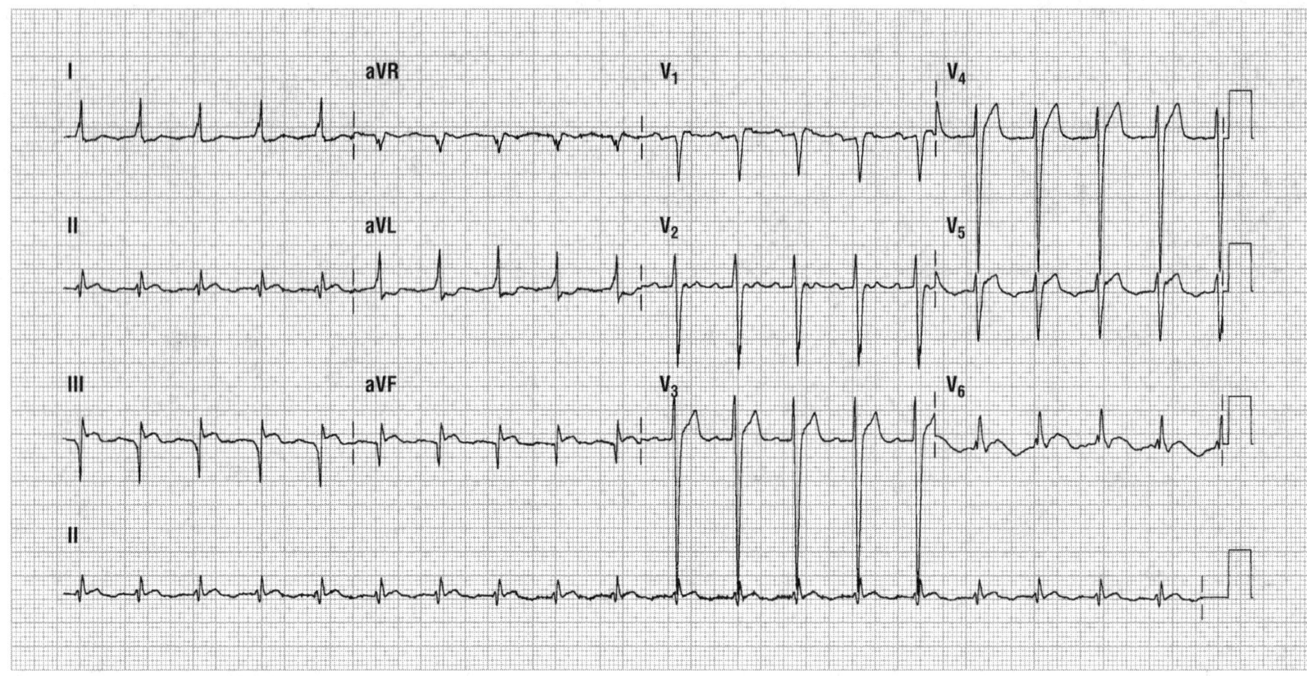

Reproduced from *12-Lead ECG: The Art of Interpretation*, courtesy of Tomas B. Garcia, MD.

Rate: __________

Rhythm: __________

Significant findings: ______________________________

8.

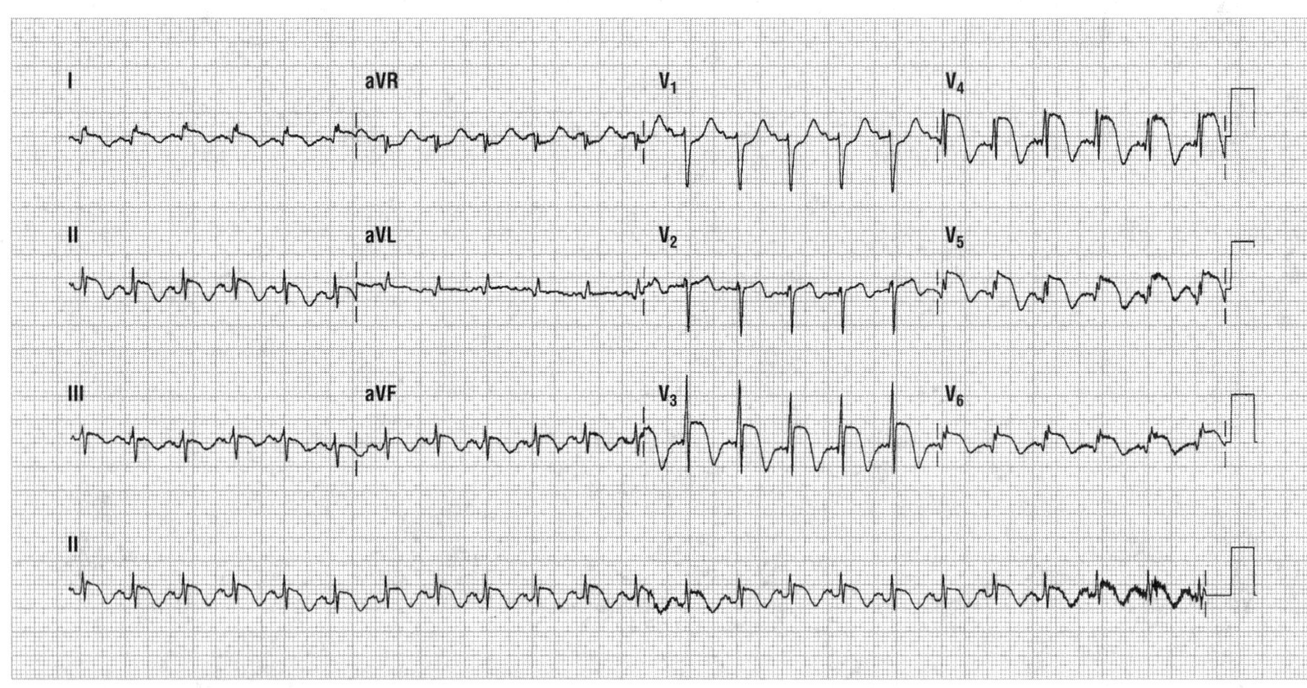

Reproduced from *12-Lead ECG: The Art of Interpretation*, courtesy of Tomas B. Garcia, MD.

Rate: __________

Rhythm: __________

Significant findings: ______________________________

9.

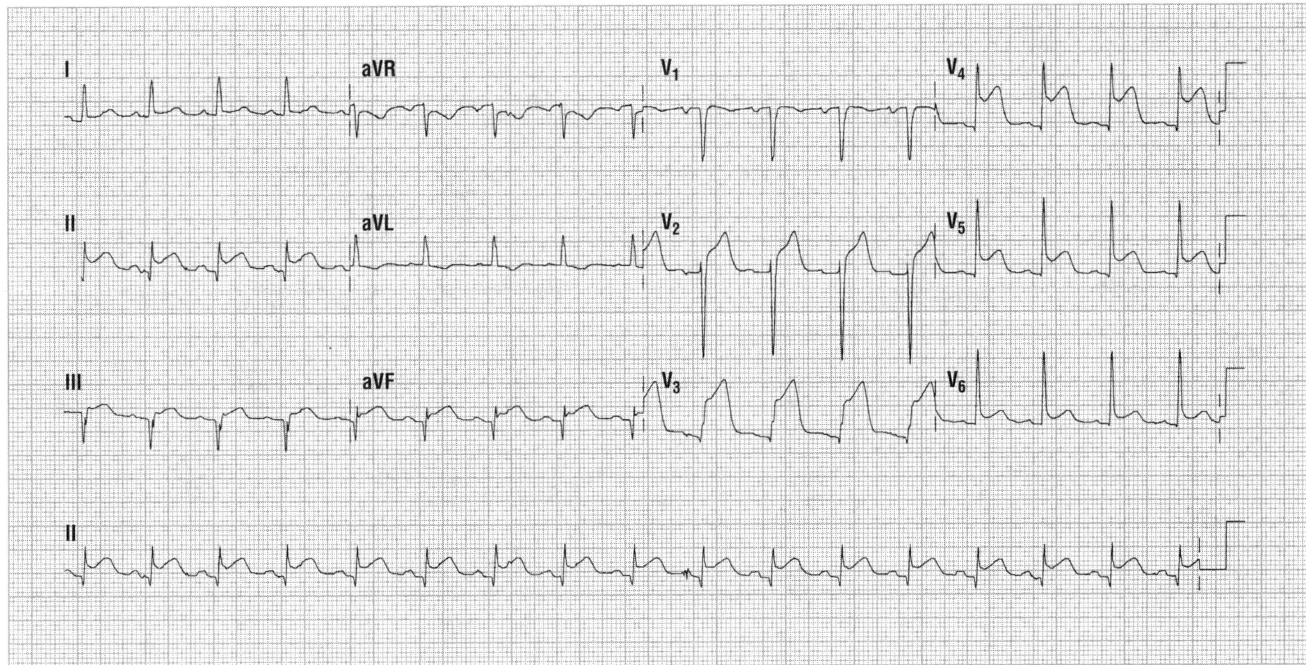

Reproduced from *12-Lead ECG: The Art of Interpretation*, courtesy of Tomas B. Garcia, MD.

Rate: __________

Rhythm: __________

Significant findings: ______________________________

10.

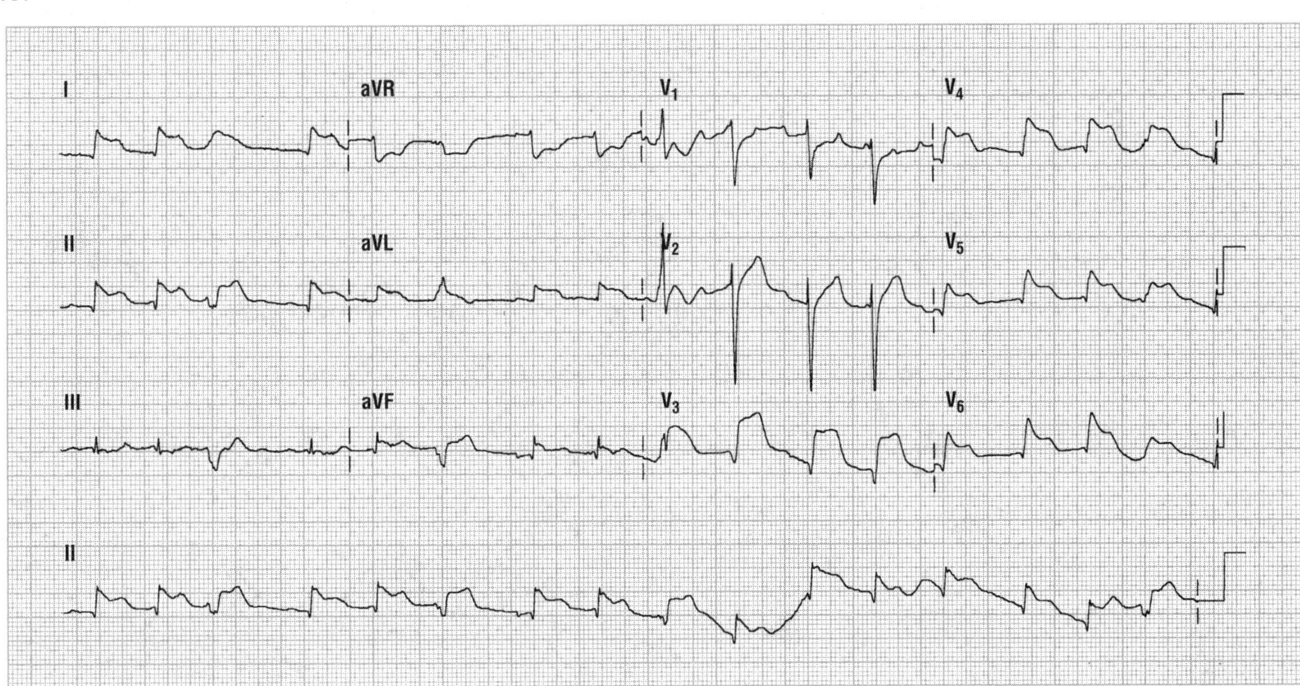

Reproduced from *12-Lead ECG: The Art of Interpretation*, courtesy of Tomas B. Garcia, MD.

Rate: __________

Rhythm: __________

Significant findings: ______________________________

11.

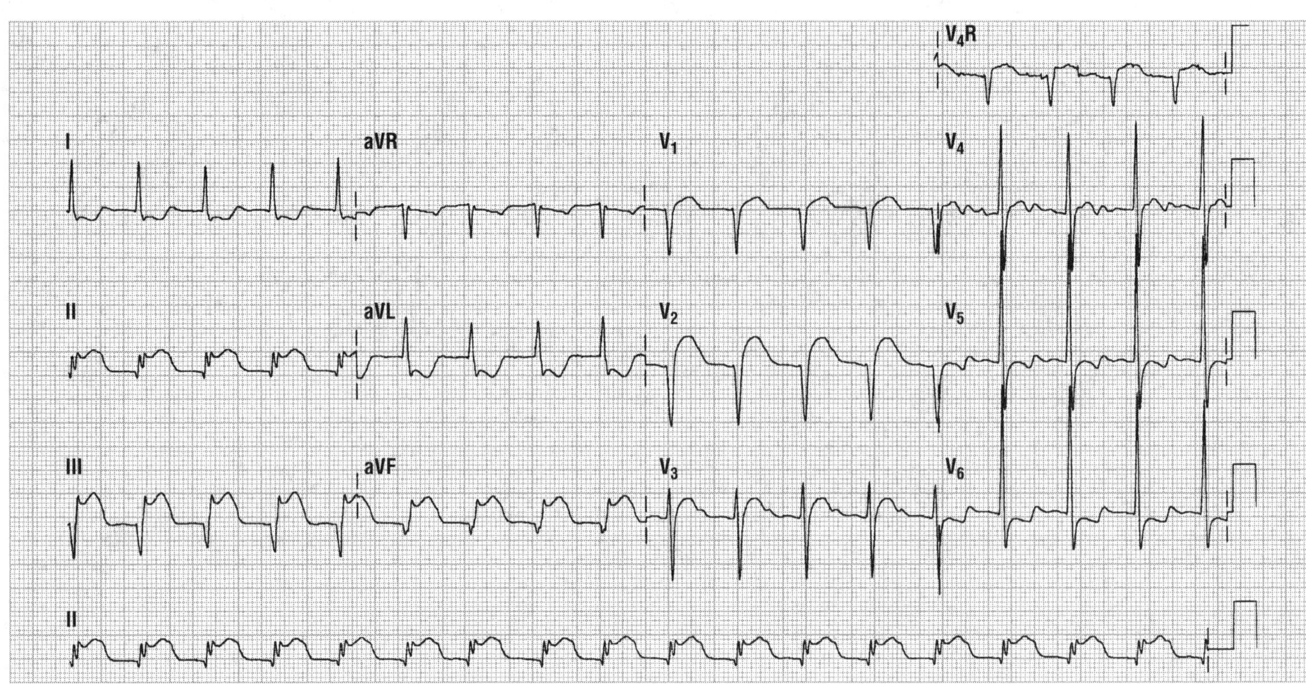

Reproduced from *12-Lead ECG: The Art of Interpretation*, courtesy of Tomas B. Garcia, MD.

Rate: ___________

Rhythm: ___________

Significant findings: _________________________________

12.

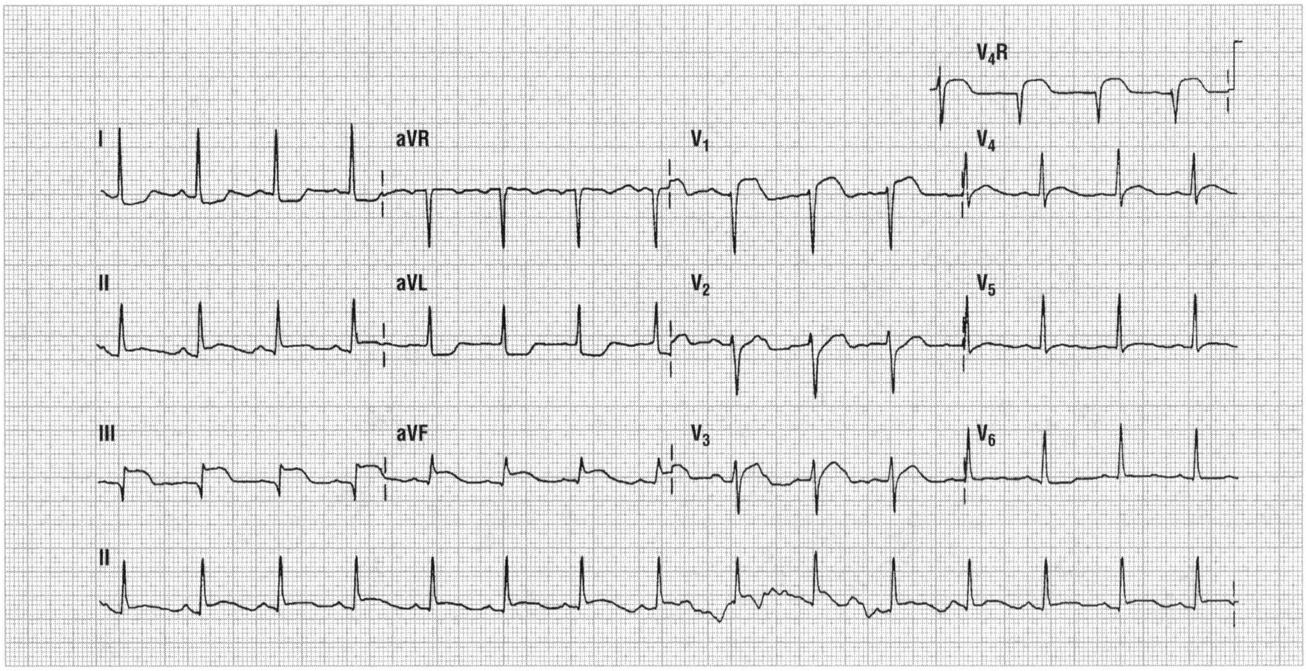

Reproduced from *12-Lead ECG: The Art of Interpretation*, courtesy of Tomas B. Garcia, MD.

Rate: ___________

Rhythm: ___________

Significant findings: _________________________________

13.

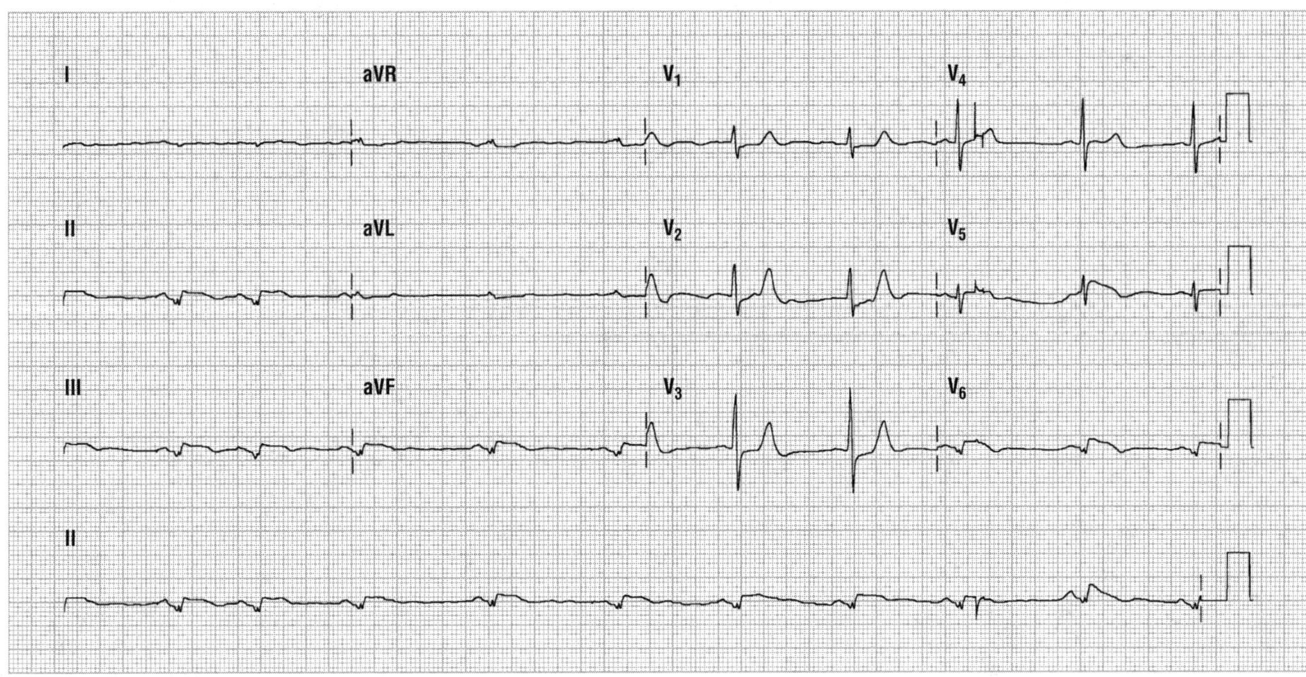

Reproduced from *12-Lead ECG: The Art of Interpretation*, courtesy of Tomas B. Garcia, MD.

Rate: ___________

Rhythm: ___________

Significant findings: ___________________________________

14.

Reproduced from *12-Lead ECG: The Art of Interpretation*, courtesy of Tomas B. Garcia, MD.

Rate: ___________

Rhythm: ___________

Significant findings: ___________________________________

15.

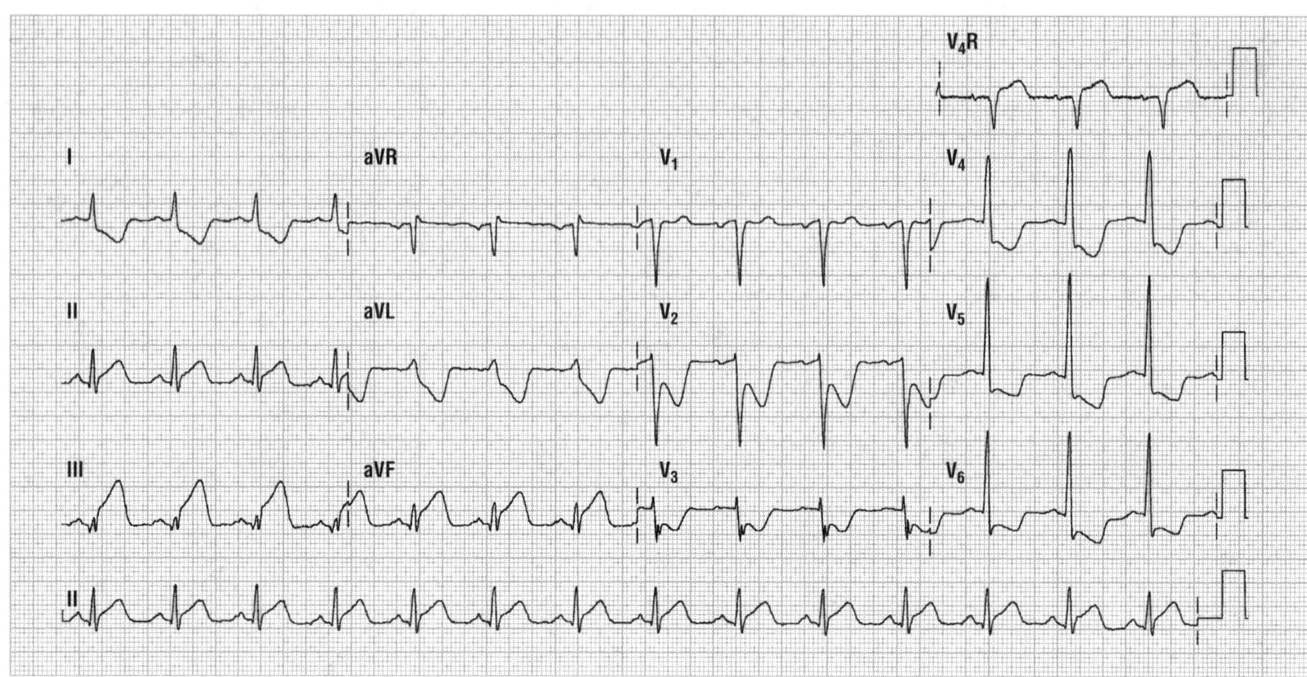

Reproduced from *12-Lead ECG: The Art of Interpretation*, courtesy of Tomas B. Garcia, MD.

Rate: __________

Rhythm: __________

Significant findings: ______________________________

16.

Reproduced from *12-Lead ECG: The Art of Interpretation*, courtesy of Tomas B. Garcia, MD.

Rate: __________

Rhythm: __________

Significant findings: ______________________________

17.

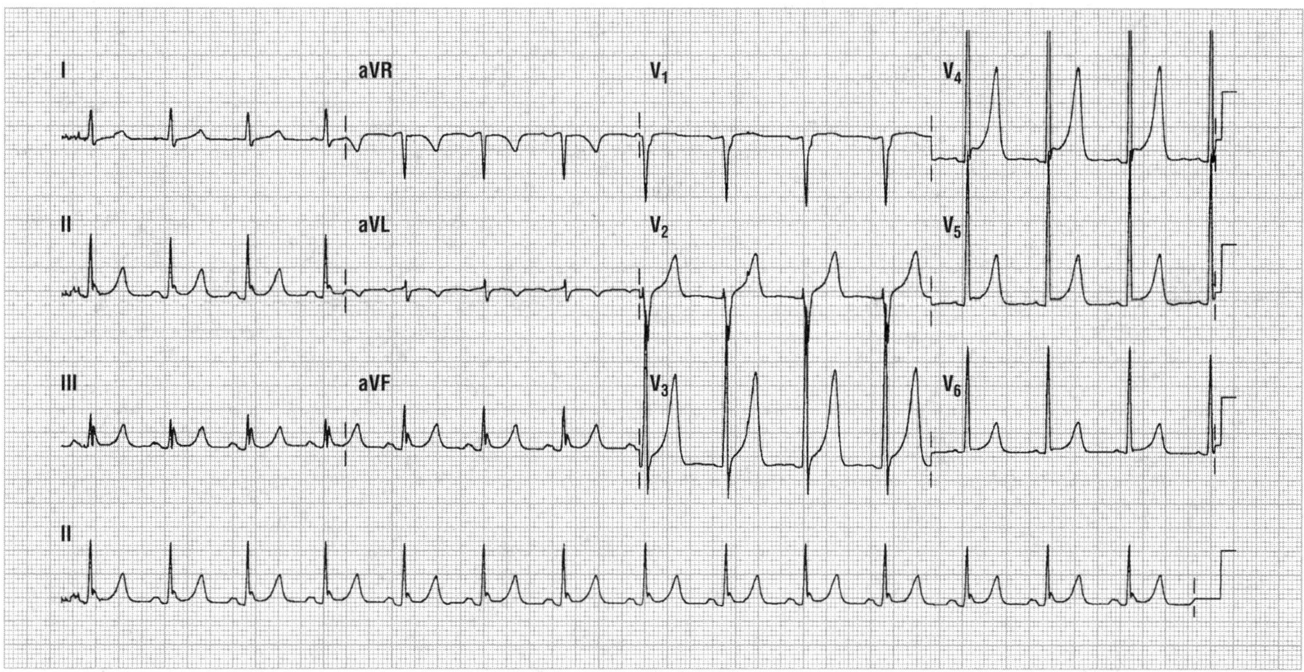

Reproduced from *12-Lead ECG: The Art of Interpretation*, courtesy of Tomas B. Garcia, MD.

Rate: __________

Rhythm: __________

Significant findings: ______________________________

18.

Rate: __________

Rhythm: __________

Significant findings: ______________________________

19.

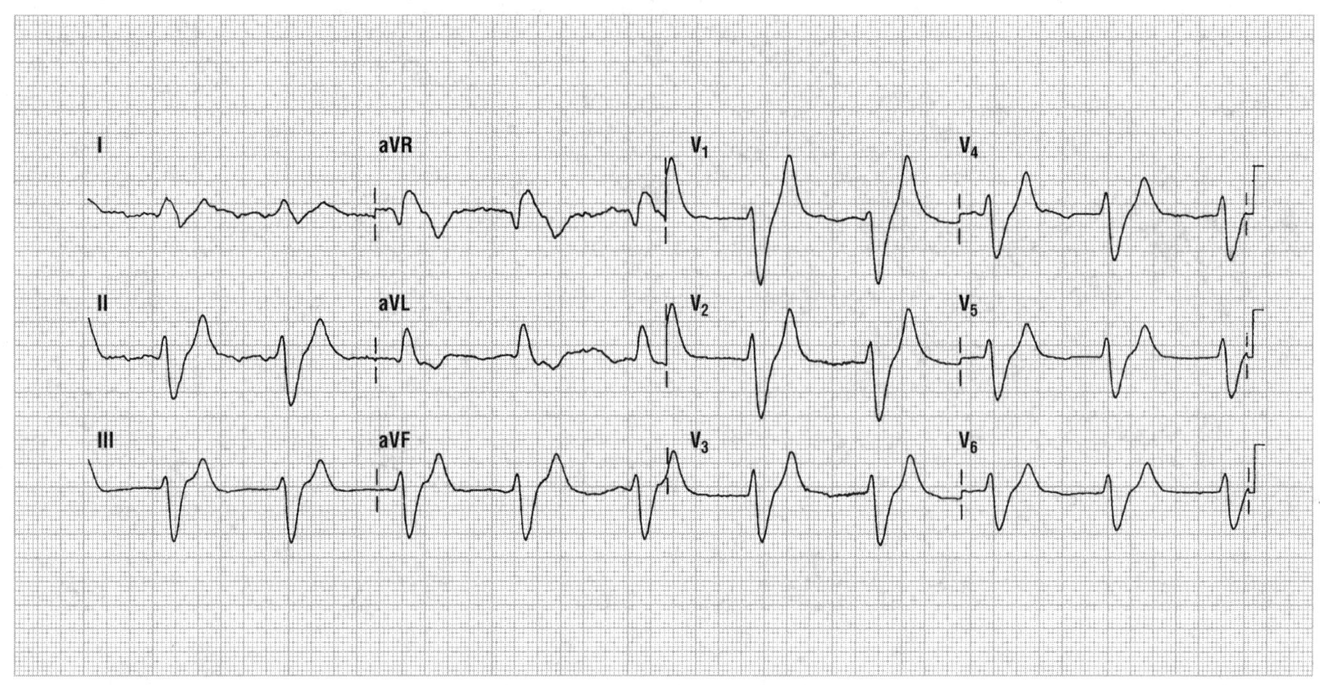

Reproduced from *12-Lead ECG: The Art of Interpretation*, courtesy of Tomas B. Garcia, MD.

Rate: __________

Rhythm: __________

Significant findings: ______________________________

20.

Reproduced from *12-Lead ECG: The Art of Interpretation*, courtesy of Tomas B. Garcia, MD.

Rate: __________

Rhythm: __________

Significant findings: ______________________________

Step on it. Dispatch says the patient has a migraine!
I guess you've had more than a few?

CHAPTER 18

Neurologic Emergencies

Matching

Part I

For each of the following items, indicate the letter that corresponds to each definition.

_____ **1.** A temporary paralysis of the facial nerve (cranial nerve VII), which controls the muscles on each side of the face.

_____ **2.** Sensations commonly experienced before a seizure or migraine headache occurs; may include visual changes in addition to hallucinations.

_____ **3.** Alteration in the ability to perform coordinated motions such as walking.

_____ **4.** Unequal pupils with a difference of greater than 1 mm.

_____ **5.** Paralysis of one side of the body.

_____ **6.** Weakness of one side of the body.

_____ **7.** Sensory stimulation that cannot be verified by others.

_____ **8.** A rare condition that begins as a sensation of weakness and tingling in the legs, moving to the arms and the thorax; the disorder can lead to paralysis within 2 weeks.

_____ **9.** The slow, progressive onset of disorientation, shortened attention span, and loss of cognitive function.

_____ **10.** Thoughts, ideas, or perceived abilities that have no basis in common reality.

_____ **11.** Abnormal flexion of the arms toward the chest with the toes pointed; this finding indicates lower cerebral damage.

_____ **12.** Abnormal extension of the arms with rotation of the wrists along with the toes pointed; this finding indicates brainstem damage.

_____ **13.** An area in the brain or spinal cord in which cells have been attacked, typically by an infectious agent. To prevent the spread of infection, the immune system "walls off" the area. Pus can collect.

_____ **14.** A progressive, organic condition in which neurons in the brain die, causing dementia.

_____ **15.** A condition that strikes the voluntary motor neurons, causing their death. The disease is characterized by fatigue and general weakness of muscle groups; eventually the patient becomes unable to walk, eat, or speak; also known as Lou Gehrig disease.

_____ **16.** Lack of feeling within a body part.

_____ **17.** A protective movement that results in blinking, moving the head posteriorly, and pupillary constriction.

A. Abscess
B. Alzheimer disease
C. Amyotrophic lateral sclerosis
D. Anesthesia
E. Anisocoria
F. Ataxia
G. Aura
H. Bell palsy
I. Bradykinesia
J. Clonic activity
K. Coma
L. Common reality
M. Corneal reflex
N. Decerebrate posturing
O. Decorticate posturing
P. Delusions
Q. Dementia

______	18. Sensory stimulation that can be verified by others.	R. Dystonia
______	19. A state in which a person does not respond to either verbal or painful stimuli.	S. Endotoxin
______	20. Type of seizure movement involving the contraction and relaxation of muscle groups.	T. Exotoxin
______	21. Patterns of walking or ambulating.	U. Gait
______	22. The slowing down of voluntary body movements; found in patients with Parkinson disease.	V. Guillain-Barré syndrome
______	23. A toxin released by some bacteria when they die.	W. Hallucinations
______	24. A toxin secreted by living cells to aid in the death and digestion of other cells.	X. Hemiparesis
______	25. Contractions of body into bizarre positions.	Y. Hemiplegia

Part II

For each of the following items, indicate the letter that corresponds to each definition.

______	1. A tumor.	A. Hemorrhagic stroke
______	2. Involuntary jerking motions of the body.	B. Idiopathic
______	3. A condition in which the body generates antibodies against its own acetylcholine receptors, causing muscle weakness, often in the face.	C. Intention tremor
______	4. An autoimmune condition in which the body attacks the myelin that insulates the brain and spinal cord, causing scarring.	D. Ischemic stroke
______	5. The process by which cells from a malignant neoplasm break away from the site of origin, such as the lung, and move through the bloodstream or lymphatic system to other body sites, such as the brain.	E. Jacksonian march
______	6. A tremor that occurs when the body part is not in motion.	F. Limbic system
______	7. Prolapse of a body part; often refers to drooping of the eyelid.	G. Metastasis
______	8. Breaking with common reality and existing mainly within an internal world.	H. Multiple sclerosis
______	9. Rotation of the lower arms in a palms-down manner.	I. Myasthenia gravis
______	10. An early sign or symptom that occurs before a disease or condition fully appears (eg, dizziness before fainting).	J. Myoclonus
______	11. A group of conditions in which the nerves that exit the spinal cord are damaged, distorting signals to or from the brain. One type is caused by diabetes; peripheral nerves are damaged as the blood glucose level rises, resulting in lack of sensation, numbness, burning, pain, paresthesia, and muscle weakness.	K. Neoplasm
______	12. A neurologic condition in which the portion of the brain responsible for production of dopamine has been damaged or overused, resulting in tremors.	L. Nystagmus
______	13. Sensation of tingling or numbness in a body part.	M. Paresthesia
	14. Involuntary, rhythmic shaking of the eyes.	N. Parkinson disease
______	15. Structures within the cerebrum and diencephalon that influence emotions, motivation, mood, and sensations of pain and pleasure.	O. Peripheral neuropathy
______	16. The wavelike movement of a seizure from a point of focus to other areas of the brain.	P. Poliomyelitis
______	17. One of the two main types of stroke, also called an occlusive stroke; occurs when blood flow to a particular part of the brain is cut off by a blockage such as a blood clot, within an artery.	Q. Postictal
______	18. A tremor that occurs when trying to accomplish a task.	R. Post-polio syndrome

______	**19.** Of no known cause.	**S.** Postural tremor
______	**20.** One of the two main types of stroke; occurs as a result of bleeding inside the brain.	**T.** Posturing
______	**21.** Abnormal body positioning that indicates damage to the brain.	**U.** Prodrome
______	**22.** A tremor that occurs as the person holds a body part still.	**V.** Pronation
______	**23.** The death of nerve fibers as a late consequence of poliomyelitis; characterized by swallowing difficulties, weakness, fatigue, and breathing problems.	**W.** Psychosis
______	**24.** A now-rare viral infection that attacks and destroys nerve axons, especially motor axons; the disease can cause weakness, paralysis, and respiratory arrest.	**X.** Ptosis
______	**25.** The period after a seizure in which the brain is reorganizing activity.	**Y.** Rest tremor

Multiple Choice

Read each item carefully, and then select the best response.

______ **1.** The nervous system is responsible for all of the following functions, EXCEPT:
- **A.** pulse rate.
- **B.** blood pressure.
- **C.** breathing.
- **D.** heart rhythm.

______ **2.** What area of the brain acts as a relay center to filter and prioritize the information that you need for conscious thought?
- **A.** Pons
- **B.** Medulla oblongata
- **C.** Diencephalon
- **D.** Mid stem

______ **3.** Which of the following acts as "insulation" around the axon?
- **A.** Myelin
- **B.** Neuron
- **C.** Diencephalon
- **D.** Neurotransmitter

______ **4.** When the brain receives too much oxygen, it can cause increased intracranial pressure (ICP). What happens to the cerebral arteries during this time?
- **A.** They vasodilate.
- **B.** They vasoconstrict.
- **C.** They leak blood.
- **D.** They remain normal.

______ **5.** You respond to a collision in which a woman has been thrown from a vehicle. She is unconscious; her arms are curled to her chest, and her toes are pointed. How would you describe her position?
- **A.** Trismus posture
- **B.** Decerebrate posture
- **C.** Decorticate posture
- **D.** Pronation posture

______ **6.** Pupils may be changed by many different things. Which of the following does NOT change the shape of a patient's pupils?
- **A.** Drugs
- **B.** Trauma
- **C.** Seizure
- **D.** Increased ICP

_____ **7.** You are treating a 22-year-old male who is having a seizure. At this time, he is still except for his left arm, which is rocking back and forth in a rhythmic motion. What is the correct term for this activity?

A. Clonic activity
B. Tonic activity
C. Intension tremors
D. Paresthesia

_____ **8.** Which subdivision of the brain is responsible for judgment and prediction of the consequences of actions?

A. Occipital
B. Temporal
C. Frontal
D. Limbic system

_____ **9.** Your patient suffers from an autoimmune disorder in which the body attacks the myelin sheath. What is this called?

A. Dystonia
B. Parkinson disease
C. Trigeminal neuralgia
D. Multiple sclerosis

_____ **10.** What is the correct term for a temporary paralysis of the seventh cranial nerve?

A. Guillain-Barré syndrome
B. Bell palsy
C. Poliomyelitis
D. Myasthenia gravis

Labeling

Label the following diagrams with the correct terms.

1. Pupil responses

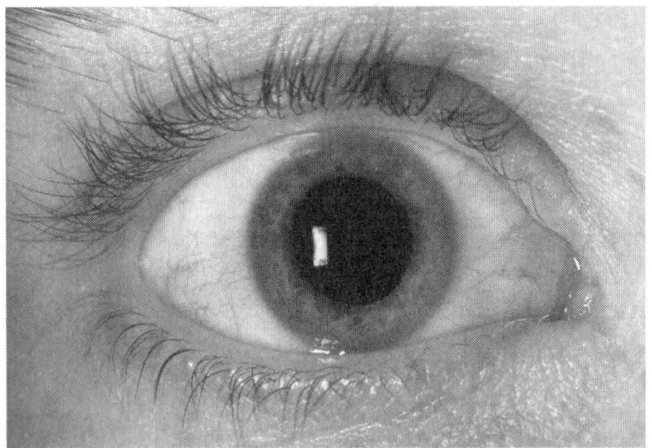

1. ______________________________

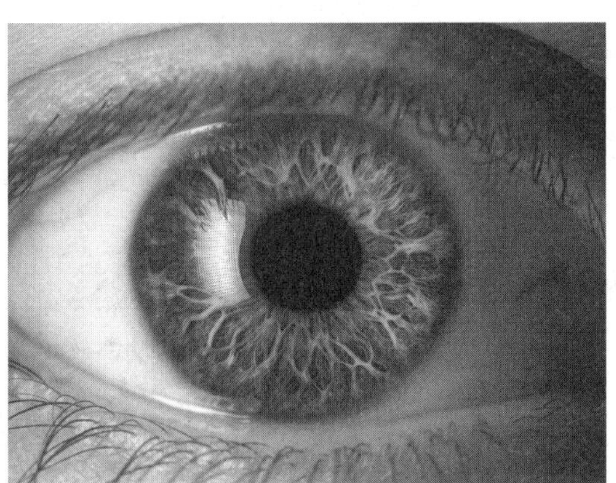

2. ______________________________

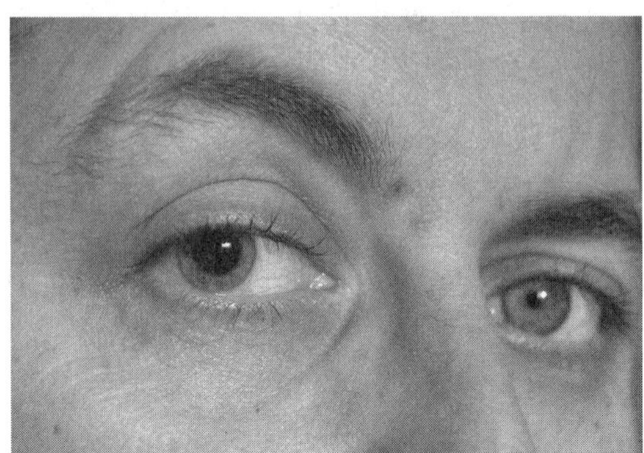

3. ______________________________

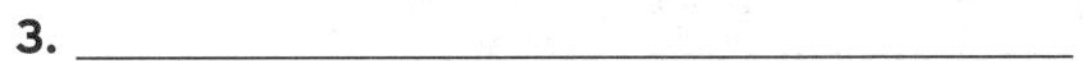

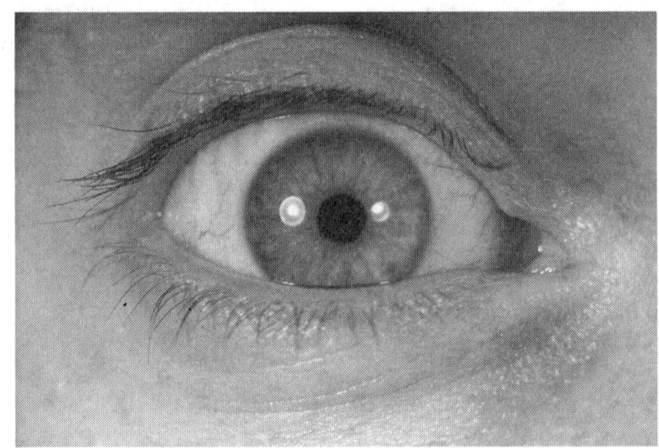

4. ______________________________

A. Normal
B. Constricted (pinpoint)
C. Dilated
D. Unequal

Fill in the Blank

Read each item carefully, and then complete the statement by filling in the missing word(s).

1. A neurotransmitter is a chemical released into a(n) ________ that helps make the connection between one _______ and another.

2. ______________ respirations are gradually _________ and decreases in respirations with periods of ________.

3. When gram-negative bacteria die inside our body, they release a protein that is called a(n) __________.

4. The skull is filled with three substances: the __________, __________, and __________ __________.

5. When a patient has increased ICP, the heart rate and respiratory rate will __________, and the blood pressure (BP) will __________.

6. Kussmaul respirations are ___________ tachypnea and __________.

7. ___________ activity is a rigid contracted _________ posture.

8. __________ is the fuel for our brain. A normal reading is __________ mg/dL.

9. There are two types of strokes: __________ and __________.

10. There are two types of generalized seizures: __________ and __________.

Identify

After reading the following case study, list the chief complaint, vital signs, and pertinent negatives.

You are called to a middle-class home for a 32-year-old man. He is alert and can answer all your questions. His main complaint is general weakness; he is unable to stand or squeeze your hands. His symptoms started this morning around 0900 hours and have intensified over the last 6 hours. He is having visual disturbances and doesn't want to open his eyes because the double vision he is experiencing is making him nauseous. You begin your assessment with vital signs and a SAMPLE history. His blood pressure (BP) is 128/76 mm Hg, and his pulse is 84 beats/min and regular. He has no allergies and takes no medications. His lungs are clear, and his oxygen saturation is 95% on room air. Because you are still not sure what is going on and his SpO_2 is borderline, you place him on a nasal cannula at 4 L/min. Blood glucose check is 112 mg/dL, and he had a light lunch of a sandwich and soup around noon. He has no history of any illness and appears to be a very healthy individual. You question him about sustaining any trauma, and he denies that he has suffered any in the last year. He does not have a headache or any pain anywhere in his body. He has no signs of any infections. You and your partner have spent a lot of time on scene looking for clues as to what is happening to him. One thing you are both sure of is that he needs to be seen at the emergency department (ED). You provide supportive care and start an IV line as a medication line in case the patient happens to get worse. Later, you check in on the patient and find out they are leaning toward a diagnosis of multiple sclerosis.

1. Chief complaint:

____

____

2. Vital signs:

____

____

3. Pertinent negatives:

____

____

Complete the Patient Care Report (PCR)

Read the incident scenario in the "Identify" exercise, and then complete the following PCR.

EMS Patient Care Report (PCR)					
Date:	Incident No.:	Nature of Call:	Location:		
Dispatched:	En Route:	At Scene:	Transport:	At Hospital:	In Service:
Patient Information					
Age: Sex: Weight (in kg [lb]):			Allergies: Medications: Past Medical History: Chief Complaint:		
Vital Signs					
Time:	BP:	Pulse:	Respirations:	SpO_2:	
Time:	BP:	Pulse:	Respirations:	SpO_2:	
Time:	BP:	Pulse:	Respirations:	SpO_2:	
EMS Treatment (circle all that apply)					
Oxygen @ ______ L/min via (circle one): NC NRM Bag-mask device	Assisted Ventilation	Airway Adjunct	CPR		
Defibrillation	Bleeding Control	Bandaging	Splinting	Other:	
Narrative					

Ambulance Calls

The following case scenarios provide an opportunity to explore the concerns associated with patient management and paramedic care. Read each scenario, and then answer each question.

1. You receive a call for a patient having seizures. This time it is one of the city's homeless whom the police found lying in an alley. He is having a generalized motor seizure when you arrive. It lasts about 3 minutes and then subsides. You quickly open the airway by jaw lift, start supplemental oxygen, and prepare to start an IV line, but before you can do so, the patient has another generalized motor seizure that lasts about 3 minutes.

   a. Urgent treatment measures will take priority over the secondary assessment. When you do get around to examining this patient, what will you look for in particular?

   (1)________________________________

   (2)________________________________

   (3)________________________________

   (4)________________________________

   (5)________________________________

   (6)________________________________

   (7)________________________________

   (8)________________________________

   (9)________________________________

   (10)________________________________

   b. List the steps in the prehospital management of this patient.

   (1)________________________________

   (2)________________________________

   (3)________________________________

   (4)________________________________

   c. What medication is given in the field for repeated seizures? (You may need to refer to the Emergency Medications appendix.)

   ____

   ____

   (1) What are the contraindications to this medication?

   ____

   ____

   (2) What is the correct dosage in the present situation, and how is it administered?

   ____

   ____

   (3) What possible adverse side effects might occur when administering this medicine?

   ____

   ____

2. You are called to the home of a 68-year-old woman for a "possible stroke." Arriving at the scene, you are greeted at the door by the woman's daughter. "I phoned and phoned all morning," she says, "and when no one answered, I figured I'd better come and check. I found Mother lying in the bathroom." You proceed to the bathroom, where you find the patient lying on the floor. She is conscious but does not seem to be able to answer your questions—she just makes garbled noises. Her skin is warm and dry. Her vital signs are a pulse of 70 beats/min and slightly irregular, respirations of 20 breaths/min and unlabored, and a BP of 190/120 mm Hg. During the physical exam, you find no evidence of head injury, but the woman's face looks a bit lopsided, and tears are streaming down. The pupils are 4 mm, equal, and reactive. The gag reflex is absent. The right arm and right leg are flaccid. There is no evidence of injury.

a. Do you think the patient is right-handed or left-handed? __________
How did you reach that conclusion?

____

____

b. List the steps in treating this patient.

(1)____

(2)____

(3)____

(4)____

(5)____

(6)____

3. You are called to a department store where a woman who appears to be about 60 years old has been found unconscious in the ladies' restroom.

a. List nine possible causes of coma.

(1)____

(2)____

(3)____

(4)____

(5)____

(6)____

(7)____

(8)____

(9)____

b. Now list eight things you would do to manage this comatose woman.

(1)____

(2)____

(3)____

(4)____

(5)____

(6)____

(7)____

(8)____

True/False

If you believe the statement to be more true than false, write the letter "T" in the space provided. If you believe the statement to be more false than true, write the letter "F."

______ **1.** The peripheral nervous system is responsible for conducting nerve impulses between the brain and the body.

______ **2.** Normal CPP is 70 to 90 mmHg.

______ **3.** The respiratory pattern that involves extreme tachypnea and hyperpnea is called Cheyne-Stokes.

______ **4.** The medical term for cancer is neoplasm.

______ **5.** The respiratory pattern that involves rapid, regular, deep respirations is called hyperpnea.

______ **6.** The average MAP is 100 to 120 mm Hg.

______ **7.** Trismus may result from head trauma, cerebral hypoxia, and seizures.

______ **8.** When you assess a stroke patient, you can ask the person to smile. This will show if the patient has ptosis.

______ **9.** By stimulating the cough or gag reflex in a patient, you can decrease ICP.

______ **10.** Syncope is caused by a brief interruption in cerebral blood flow.

______ **11.** Hyperglycemic patients do not need any fluid, so you must make sure to give less than 100 mL of fluid.

______ **12.** The Cincinnati Prehospital Stroke Scale uses a six-part criteria scale to assess for a stroke.

______ **13.** A little over one-third of the patients who have a transient ischemic attack (TIA) will have a stroke soon after the initial event.

______ **14.** An aura will usually precede a generalized (grand mal) seizure.

Short Answer

Complete this section with short written answers using the space provided.

1. Define the following vocabulary words:

a. Hemiparesis

____

____

b. Pseudoseizures

____

____

2. Over the course of a week of ambulance runs, you have found two patients in a coma. You don't have any information about either of them except for the medications found at the scene or on the patient's person. Nonetheless, based on those medications and assessment, you can make an educated guess at least as to each patient's underlying illnesses. For each of the comatose patients whose medications are listed here, indicate the most probable underlying illness(es).
   a. Patient 1 is carrying phenobarbital (Luminal) and phenytoin (Dilantin) in her purse.

   Probable underlying illness(es): ________________________________

   b. Patient 2 is carrying insulin.

   Probable underlying illness: ________________________________

Fill in the Table

Fill in the missing parts of the table.

1. Fill in the table with the missing types of dystonias.

Type	Presentation
	Most common form of focal dystonia; intermittent, patterned, repetitive, spasmodic motion of the head in a twisting, flexing, extending, or tilting manner; can involve more than one motion type
	Deviation of the eyes in any direction, usually with eyes strained toward the top of the head
	Forceful contractions of the face, which can involve the tongue darting in and out of the mouth
Blepharospasm	
	Slow, writhing motions commonly involving the face and distal extremities
	Cramping of the hands, elbows, and arms (eg, graphospasm [writer's cramp])
	Quick, jerky, irregular, and unpredictable movements; often found in the face, arms, and hands
Spasmodic dysphonia	

2. Complete the following list of common causes of seizures.

Birth anomaly
Hypertension during pregnancy (eclampsia)
Idiopathic (of no known cause)
Systematic infection

3. Fill in the names of the cranial nerves.

Cranial Nerve	Function
I. ______________	Smell
II. ______________	Vision
III. ______________	Movement of the eye, pupil, and eyelid
IV. ______________	Movement of the eye
V. ______________	Chewing Pain Temperature Touch of the mouth and face
VI. ______________	Movement of the eye
VII. ______________	Movement of the face Tears Salivation and taste
VII. ______________	Hearing and balance
IX. ______________	Swallowing, taste, and sensation in the mouth and pharynx
X. ______________	Sensation and movement of the pharynx, larynx, thorax, and gastrointestinal (GI) system
XI. ______________	Movement of the head and shoulders
XII. ______________	Movement of the tongue

Problem Solving

Read the following scenario, and then list the portions of the scenario under the correct stroke scale or stroke screen.

You respond to a 69-year-old woman. Her daughter is waiting at the door for you when you arrive. Dispatch information said that the woman might be having a stroke. You enter the room to find "Betty" sitting in her recliner with her feet up. She acknowledges your entrance. "Hi, Mrs. Smith, my name is Jake Johnson, and my partner is Julie Barnes. We are paramedics, and I am here at the request of your daughter. Can you tell me what is wrong today?" Mrs. Smith responds by telling you that her name is Betty, and she doesn't think anything is wrong with her. Her daughter is always fussing over her. You tell Betty that is because her daughter loves her and say that if Betty loves her daughter, she should be smiling about all the attention. Betty does respond with a smile, but the right side of her face doesn't respond as well as the left. Julie asks permission to do a set of vital signs, and Betty says to go right ahead. Julie gets a BP of 136/82 mm Hg, a pulse of 86 beats/min and regular, oxygen saturation of 97% on room air, and respirations of 18 breaths/min. Lung sounds are clear. She checks Betty's blood glucose, which is 110 mg/dL. During this time, you ask Betty to say "You can't teach an old dog new tricks." However, Betty can't seem to get the sentence out very clearly. You proceed by having Betty squeeze both your hands at the same time. Her grip strength is about half strength in the right arm. You then ask her to close her eyes and hold both arms up straight. When she does this, her right arm drifts downward. You then ask Betty and her daughter how long she has been having these symptoms. Betty's daughter says that she had no problems this morning when she was up fixing breakfast at 0800, but she says she began to notice a few minor things around 1100, which is when she decided to call 9-1-1. You take a SAMPLE history and find that Betty has never had any medical problems at all; she takes only a vitamin every morning. Both you and Julie feel she should be seen in the ED, and Betty agrees to go with you. You prepare to take Betty in.

You and Julie did a great job using both the Cincinnati Prehospital Stroke Scale and the Los Angles Prehospital Stroke Screen Assessments. Write the portions of the preceding scenario under the correct assessments. Remember, the same action might be on both assessments.

1. Cincinnati Prehospital Stroke Scale

a. ______________________________

b. ______________________________

c. ______________________________

2. Los Angles Prehospital Stroke Screen
   a. ______________________________
   b. ______________________________
   c. ______________________________
   d. ______________________________
   e. ______________________________
   f. ______________________________
   g. ______________________________
   h. ______________________________

CHAPTER 19

Diseases of the Eyes, Ears, Nose, and Throat

Can you tell me what is wrong?

Maybe we should ask how Mr. Smith likes to communicate?

Can you hear me now?

Matching

Match each of the items in the left column to the appropriate definition in the right column.

_____	**1.** Swelling and inflammation of the larynx that is associated with hoarseness or loss of voice.	**A.** Anisocoria
_____	**2.** Irritation and swelling in the inner ear that produces a loss of balance and possibly tinnitus, dizziness, loss of hearing, nausea, and vomiting.	**B.** Battle sign
_____	**3.** Inflammation of the iris; also called anterior uveitis.	**C.** Cataract
_____	**4.** A red, tender lump in the eyelid or at the lid margin; commonly known as a stye.	**D.** Cerebrospinal rhinorrhea
_____	**5.** A group of conditions that lead to increased intraocular pressure, causing damage to the optic nerve; a leading cause of blindness.	**E.** Cerumen
_____	**6.** A condition that presents as white lesions on the tongue and inner cheeks, caused by the fungus *Candida albicans*; also called thrush.	**F.** Chalazion
_____	**7.** Either of the second cranial nerves that enter the eyeball posteriorly; through the optic foramen.	**G.** Conjunctivitis
_____	**8.** A device used to examine the fundus of the eye.	**H.** Dental abscess
_____	**9.** Third cranial nerve; it innervates the muscles that cause motion of the eyeballs and upper eyelids.	**I.** Dentalgia
_____	**10.** An inner ear disorder in which endolymphatic rupture creates increased pressure in the cochlear duct, which then leads to damage to the organ of Corti and the semicircular canal; symptoms include severe vertigo, tinnitus, and sensorineural hearing loss.	**J.** Diabetic retinopathy
_____	**11.** A condition in which the pupils are not of equal size.	**K.** Dysconjugate gaze
_____	**12.** Bruising over the mastoid bone behind the ear, commonly seen following a basilar skull fracture; also called retroauricular ecchymosis.	**L.** Dysphagia
_____	**13.** A clouding of the lens of the eye that is normally a result of aging.	**M.** Epiglottitis
_____	**14.** Cerebrospinal fluid drainage from the nose.	**N.** Epistaxis
_____	**15.** Earwax.	**O.** Glaucoma
_____	**16.** A type of cellulitis that occurs on the floor of the mouth under the tongue; it is caused by bacteria from an infected tooth root (tooth abscess) or mouth injury.	**P.** Hordeolum
_____	**17.** A condition associated with diabetes, in which the small blood vessels of the retina are affected; it can eventually lead to blindness.	**Q.** Iritis
_____	**18.** Paralysis of gaze or lack of coordination between the movements of the two eyes.	**R.** Labyrinthitis
_____	**19.** Pain when swallowing.	**S.** Laryngitis

_____	**20.** An inflammation of the epiglottis.	**T.** Ludwig angina
_____	**21.** Nosebleed.	**U.** Meniere disease
_____	**22.** Toothache.	**V.** Oculomotor nerve
_____	**23.** A collection of pus that forms in the gums, facial tissue, bones, and/or neck.	**W.** Ophthalmoscope
_____	**24.** An inflammation of the conjunctivae of the eye that usually is caused by bacteria, viruses, allergies, or foreign bodies; it should be considered highly contagious. Also called pinkeye.	**X.** Optic nerve
_____	**25.** A small, swollen bump or pustule on the external eyelid, which arises when the eyelid's oil glands or ducts become blocked.	**Y.** Oral candidiasis

Multiple Choice

Read each item carefully, and then select the best response.

_____ **1.** The nerve that innervates the muscles that cause motion of the eyeballs and upper eyelids, as well as constriction of the pupil, is the _____________ nerve.

A. optic
B. oculomotor
C. trigeminal
D. vagus

_____ **2.** The __________ chamber of the globe is filled with __________ humor, which is a clear, watery fluid.

A. anterior; vitreous
B. anterior; aqueous
C. posterior; vitreous
D. posterior; aqueous

_____ **3.** Symptoms that may indicate a serious ocular condition include all of the following, EXCEPT:

A. visual loss.
B. double vision.
C. lack of eye pain.
D. a foreign body sensation.

_____ **4.** Physical exam of the eyes includes assessment of the visible ocular structures, including:

A. globes.
B. corneas.
C. eyelids.
D. All of the above

_____ **5.** A group of conditions that leads to increased intraocular pressure and that is one of the leading causes of blindness is:

A. hyphema.
B. retinal detachment.
C. glaucoma.
D. papilledema.

_____ **6.** When examining the eyes, ocular motility involves checking for:

A. peripheral vision.
B. dysconjugate gaze.
C. orbital rim.
D. visual acuity.

_____ **7.** Of the following components of the ear, which is NOT in the middle ear?

A. Tympanic membrane
B. Ossicles
C. Cochlea
D. Malleus

______ **8.** The feeling of vertigo or loss of balance after an ear infection or upper respiratory infection is MOST likely attributable to:
- **A.** impacted cerumen.
- **B.** Meniere disease.
- **C.** otitis.
- **D.** labyrinthitis.

______ **9.** An inner ear disorder that usually affects adults and in which there is ultimately damage to the organ of Corti and the semicircular canal is:
- **A.** Meniere disease.
- **B.** labyrinthitis.
- **C.** perforated tympanic membrane.
- **D.** barotrauma.

______ **10.** You are treating a 10-year-old boy who has the chills, difficulty opening his mouth, and pain with opening of the mouth. He denies any trauma, although he appears to have facial swelling and is drooling and speaking with a muffled voice. What is MOST likely his condition?
- **A.** Tonsillitis
- **B.** Peritonsillar abscess
- **C.** Pharyngitis
- **D.** Tracheitis

______ **11.** All of the following are considered medical conditions of the ear, EXCEPT:
- **A.** impacted cerumen.
- **B.** labyrinthitis.
- **C.** glaucoma.
- **D.** Meniere disease.

______ **12.** Which of the following is a specific medical problem related to the nose?
- **A.** Dentalgia
- **B.** Thrush
- **C.** Otitis
- **D.** Sinusitis

Labeling

Label the following diagrams with the correct terms.

1. Structures of the eye

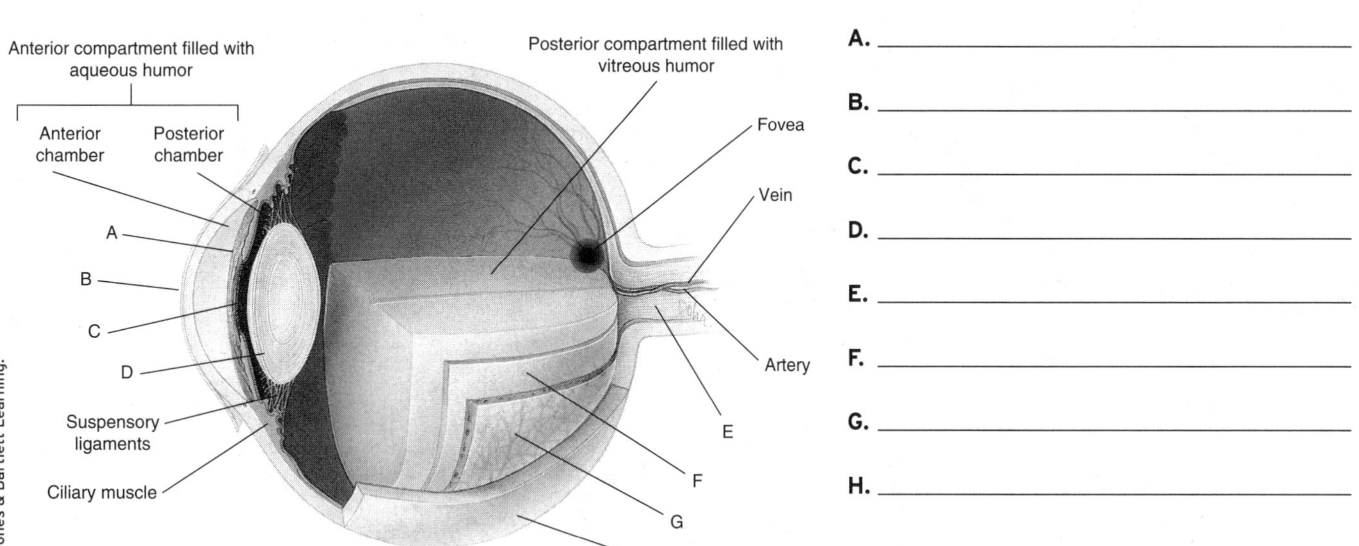

A. ______________________

B. ______________________

C. ______________________

D. ______________________

E. ______________________

F. ______________________

G. ______________________

H. ______________________

2. Structures of the ear

A. ______________________________

B. ______________________________

C. ______________________________

D. ______________________________

E. ______________________________

F. ______________________________

G. ______________________________

H. ______________________________

I. ______________________________

3. Structure of a tooth

A. ______________________________

B. ______________________________

C. ______________________________

D. ______________________________

E. ______________________________

Fill in the Blank

Read each item carefully, and then complete the statement by filling in the missing word(s).

1. Assess the __________ for ecchymosis, __________, lacerations, and any abnormalities.

2. You may encounter patients who wear _______ ______. In general, if the eye is injured, you should not attempt to ________ contact lenses because you may further aggravate the injury.

3. Practitioners may use a(n) __________ to perform a thorough _______ exam.

4. __________, also known as "pinkeye," is a condition in which the __________ becomes inflamed and red.

5. A(n) ________ is a small, usually ________ lump or _______ on the external eyelid that appears red and swollen.

6. In ____________ glaucoma, the aqueous fluid drains too _________.

Identify

After reading the following case studies, list the chief complaint, vital signs, and pertinent negatives.

1. "Medic 620, respond Priority One for a 43-year-old female patient with dizziness. Patient is now conscious and alert." As you enter the apartment, you determine that the scene seems to be safe, and there is only one patient, so you have enough help at this point. The patient is found sitting in a chair in the kitchen. She appears pale and diaphoretic, and you notice that she is drooling. You and your partner lift her off the chair and lay her on the floor, which you have covered with a blanket. Her skin color slightly improves, as does her level of consciousness (LOC). You immediately place the patient on high-flow supplemental oxygen and begin your primary survey. You already have formed your general impression and realize that the patient is suffering from a fever. Her vital signs are a respiratory rate of 20 breaths/min, a pulse oximetry of 89%, a pulse rate (lying flat) of 118 beats/min and regular, and a blood pressure (BP) of 98/P mm Hg. She is complaining of pain when she swallows, which made her nervous, so she asked her husband to call EMS. She denies any loss of consciousness or any pain to her head, chest, or abdomen.

a. Chief complaint:

____

____

b. Vital signs:

____

____

c. Pertinent negatives:

____

____

2. You are dispatched to a reported "nosebleed." On arrival, you find a 78-year-old man standing in the bathroom, spitting blood into the sink. His daughter states that he has been bleeding for hours, and they were not able to stop the nosebleed. She said he is starting to get dizzy and has lost a lot of blood. She also mentions that he is on a "blood thinner" since he had a "mini-stroke" 5 years ago. He has not eaten all day because this nosebleed has been occupying most of his attention. His mental status is alert, and you obtain the following vital signs: respirations of 20 breaths/min and regular, pulse rate of 108 beats/min and irregular, BP of 170/102 mm Hg, and Spo_2 of 95%. You check his blood glucose, and it is 110 mg/dL. He states he has a headache and that his doctor told him he has an ECG of A-fib normally. He denies any trauma or shortness of breath. You make an attempt to control the bleeding and prepare to transport him to the hospital.

a. Chief complaint:

____

____

b. Vital signs:

c. Pertinent negatives:

Ambulance Calls

The following case scenarios provide an opportunity to explore the concerns associated with patient management and paramedic care. Read each scenario, and then answer each question.

1. You are assessing and treating a conscious, alert 17-year-old boy who was playing baseball in a high school league when he was struck in the right eye with a wild pitch. He is in extreme pain and may have sustained blunt trauma to the globe of the eye. Upon examination of his eye and interviewing the patient, you conclude that he may have sustained a corneal abrasion.

a. What are five of the signs and symptoms you are likely to find in this patient?

b. Your patient denies any other previous medical history, he is not on any medications, and he states he has an allergy to sulfa medications. His vital signs are respiratory rate of 20 breaths/min and regular, pulse of 110 beats/min and regular, BP of 120/78 mm Hg, and SpO_2 of 98%. What would be the appropriate treatment for this patient?

2. You are treating a 15-year-old boy whose parent called the ambulance to their home after an accident in their backyard. Your patient states that his eye is burning up. He says he splashed concentrated chlorine into his left eye when he was pouring the chemical into their in-ground pool.

a. What would your prehospital treatment for this patient include?

True/False

If you believe the statement to be more true than false, write the letter "T" in the space provided. If you believe the statement to be more false than true, write the letter "F."

______ 1. Nasal foreign bodies are usually not visible in the anterior nares.

______ 2. Certain medications can cause rhinitis.

______ 3. Sinusitis occurs when drainage from one or more of the sinuses becomes disrupted.

______ 4. Esophageal disorders can also affect the throat.

______ 5. The symptoms of vertigo and tinnitus are common with Meniere disease.

______ 6. A toothache is also referred to as dentalgia.

______ 7. When bacteria growth spreads directly from the cavity into the gums or facial tissue, this can cause a dental abscess.

______ 8. Thrush is also called oral candidiasis.

______ 9. Oral candidiasis is caused by a virus and is not curable

______ 10. Epiglottitis is most commonly found in pediatric patients aged 4 to 9 years.

CHAPTER 20

Abdominal and Gastrointestinal Emergencies

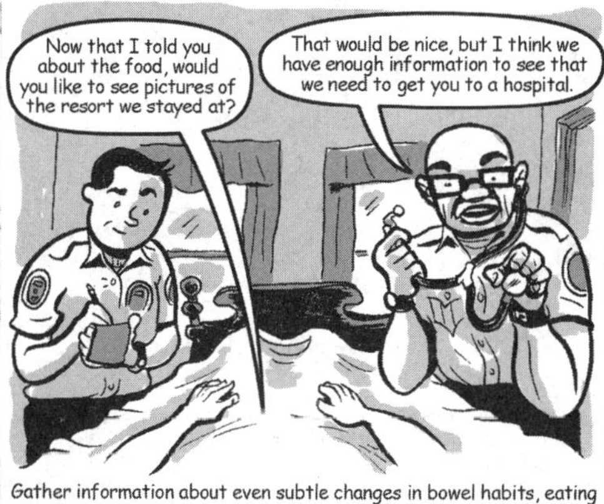

Gather information about even subtle changes in bowel habits, eating habits, new foods, travel, new medications, or low-grade fevers.

Matching

Part I

Match each of the items in the left column to the appropriate definition in the right column.

_____	**1.** A weak area in the colon that begins to have small outcroppings that turn into pouches.	**A.** Acholic stools
_____	**2.** Inflammation of pouches in the colon; these pouches form as a result of difficulty moving feces through the colon. Bacteria can become trapped in the pouches, leading to inflammation and infection.	**B.** Acute abdomen
_____	**3.** The mechanical and chemical breakdown of the large molecules in food into small molecules that can be absorbed in the gastrointestinal tract and converted to energy for cellular function.	**C.** Acute gastroenteritis
_____	**4.** Liquid stool.	**D.** Anal fissures
_____	**5.** A pre-ulcerative state where the stomach is inflamed, but erosions have not yet occurred.	**E.** Appendicitis
_____	**6.** An abnormal connection between two cavities.	**F.** Ascites
_____	**7.** Smelling of feces.	**G.** Biliary tract disorders
_____	**8.** Dilated blood vessels of the esophagus, commonly caused by difficulty in blood flow through the liver; the presence of these can lead to vessel rupture.	**H.** Boerhaave syndrome
_____	**9.** A bowel sound characterized by increased activity within the bowel; also called hyperperistalsis.	**I.** Borborygmi
_____	**10.** Forceful vomiting that results in a tear in the esophagus that extends entirely through the esophageal wall, creating a hole.	**J.** Cholangitis
_____	**10.** A group of disorders that involve inflammation of the gallbladder; these include cholangitis, cholelithiasis, cholecystitis, and acalculous cholecystitis.	**K.** Cholelithiasis
_____	**12.** Abdominal edema typically signaling liver failure.	**L.** Cholecystitis
_____	**13.** A condition of sudden onset of pain within the abdomen, usually indicating peritonitis; demands immediate medical or surgical treatment.	**M.** Cirrhosis
_____	**14.** Light, clay-colored stools indicative of liver failure.	**N.** Crohn disease
_____	**15.** Inflammation of the ileum and possibly other portions of the gastrointestinal tract, in which the immune system attacks portions of the intestinal walls, causing them to become scarred, narrowed, stiff, and weakened.	**O.** Diarrhea
_____	**16.** Early failure of the liver; characterized by portal hypertension, coagulation deficiencies, and diminished detoxification.	**P.** Digestion

______	**17.** An inflammation of the esophagus.	**Q.** Diverticulitis
______	**18.** The region of the abdomen directly inferior to the xiphoid process and superior to the umbilicus.	**R.** Diverticulum
______	**19.** Insertion of a flexible fiber-optic tube into the esophagus to visualize, remove, or repair damaged or diseased tissue.	**S.** Endoscopy
______	**20.** A family of conditions that revolve around a central theme of infection with fever, abdominal pain, diarrhea, nausea, and vomiting.	**T.** Epigastric
______	**21.** Linear tears to the mucosal lining in and near the anus, possibly caused by the passage of large, hard stools; a cause of lower gastrointestinal (GI) bleeding.	**U.** Esophagitis
______	**22.** Inflammation of the appendix.	**V.** Esophagogastric varices
______	**23.** Inflammation of the gallbladder.	**W.** Feculent
______	**24.** The presence of stones within the gallbladder.	**X.** Fistula
______	**25.** Inflammation of the bile duct.	**Y.** Gastritis

Part II

Match each of the items in the left column to the appropriate definition in the right column.

______	**1.** Dark, tarry, malodorous stools caused by upper gastrointestinal bleeding.	**A.** Gastroesophageal reflux disease
______	**2.** A condition in which the junction between the esophagus and the stomach tears, causing severe bleeding and, potentially, death.	**B.** Hematemesis
______	**3.** The sphincter between the esophagus and the stomach; controls the amount of food that moves up the esophagus; also called the cardiac sphincter.	**C.** Hematochezia
______	**4.** A condition in which patients have abdominal pain and changes in their bowel habits; generally, the pain and accompanying changes in bowel habits must be present for at least 3 days a month for at least 3 months to be considered this disease.	**D.** Hepatic encephalopathy
______	**5.** Increased pressure in the portal veins; caused by the inability of blood to flow normally through the liver; can lead to rupture of these vessels.	**E.** Hepatitis
______	**6.** Inflammation of the peritoneum, the protective membrane that lines the abdominal and pelvic cavities.	**F.** Hernia
______	**7.** A disease in which the mucous lining of the stomach and duodenum have been eroded, allowing the acid to eat into these organs.	**G.** Hiatal hernia
______	**8.** Pain caused by inflammation of the parietal peritoneum that is generally described as steady, aching, and aggravated by movement.	**H.** Hyperperistalsis
______	**9.** A condition in which the sphincter between the esophagus and the stomach opens, allowing stomach acid to move superiorly; can cause a burning sensation within the chest (heartburn); also called acid reflux disease.	**I.** Hypoperistalsis
______	**10.** Vomit with blood; can either look like coffee grounds, or contain bright red blood, indicating active bleeding.	**J.** Icteric
______	**11.** The passage of stool in which bright red blood can be distinguished; caused by lower GI bleeding.	**K.** Incarcerated
______	**12.** Impairment of brain function resulting from failure of the liver.	**L.** Incisional
______	**13.** Inflammation of the liver, usually caused by a virus, that causes fever, loss of appetite, jaundice, fatigue, and altered liver function.	**M.** Inflammatory bowel disease
______	**14.** Telescoping of the intestines into themselves.	**N.** Intussusception
______	**15.** Chronic inflammation of all or part of the gastrointestinal tract.	**O.** Irritable bowel syndrome
______	**16.** Inflammation of the pancreas.	**P.** Lower esophageal sphincter

_____	**17.** A mass of tissue produced by abnormal cell growth and division that may be malignant (cancerous) or benign.	**Q.** Mallory-Weiss syndrome
_____	**18.** An interruption of the blood supply to the mesentery.	**R.** Melena
_____	**19.** A type of hernia in which intestinal contents herniate through an incision, for example, after abdominal surgery.	**S.** Mesenteric ischemia
_____	**20.** A type of hernia in which an organ is trapped in the new location; most commonly obstructs the bowel.	**T.** Neoplasm
_____	**21.** Yellowish coloration of the conjunctiva (the whites of the eyes) caused by the buildup of bilirubin in the blood during liver failure.	**U.** Pancreatitis
_____	**22.** The protrusion of a loop of an organ or tissue through an abnormal body opening.	**V.** Parietal pain
_____	**23.** A protrusion of a portion of the stomach through the diaphragm.	**W.** Peptic ulcer disease
_____	**24.** Increased activity within the bowel; also called borborygmi.	**X.** Peritonitis
_____	**25.** Decreased activity in the bowel.	**Y.** Portal hypertension

Multiple Choice

Read each item carefully, and then select the best response.

_____ **1.** A 45-year-old woman calls for an ambulance because of "burning" epigastric pain of several hours' duration. She says that yesterday she noticed her bowel movement was "black as pitch," and about an hour ago she vomited some "stuff that looked like coffee grounds." She also feels quite dizzy. She takes no medications except Mylanta (alumina/magnesia/simethicone) "for my heartburn." On physical examination, she looks pale and anxious, and she sits leaning forward. Her skin is cold and sweaty. Her pulse is 140 beats/min and regular; her respirations are 20 breaths/min and slightly labored; her blood pressure (BP) is 90/60 mm Hg. Her abdomen is diffusely tender, especially over the epigastrium. There is guarding but no real rigidity. Peripheral pulses are intact. This patient's findings are most consistent with which of the following conditions?

- **A.** Peptic ulcer disease
- **B.** Diverticulitis
- **C.** Mesenteric ischemia
- **D.** A leaking abdominal aortic aneurysm

_____ **2.** A 70-year-old woman calls for an ambulance because of abdominal pain of 4 hours' duration. "I just knew I shouldn't have eaten all that rich, fatty food," she says. "It never agrees with me. Oh, I hate to cause everyone so much bother." And she starts to cry. On questioning, she says she had some diarrhea, but it didn't relieve the pain. Her past medical history is notable for two previous acute myocardial infarctions. On physical examination, the woman appears to be in considerable distress. Pulse is 108 beats/min and slightly irregular; respirations are 20 breaths/min and shallow; BP is 160/100 mm Hg in both arms. The chest is clear. The patient has a positive Murphy sign. This patient most likely has which of the following conditions?

- **A.** Peptic ulcer disease
- **B.** Diverticulitis
- **C.** Cholecystitis
- **D.** A leaking abdominal aortic aneurysm

_____ **3.** A 52-year-old woman called for an ambulance because of severe abdominal pain. She says the pain started a couple of days ago as a kind of steady ache (she points to the left lower quadrant), and it just kept getting worse and worse. Now her whole abdomen hurts. It's been 2 days since she had a bowel movement, and that one may have had some blood in it. On physical examination, the patient is in obvious distress. She lies very still on the stretcher and cries out with pain when your partner accidentally bumps the stretcher. Her pulse is 128 beats/min and regular; respirations are 28 breaths/min and shallow; BP is 150/80 mm Hg. The abdomen is slightly distended, and it does not move with respiration. On palpation, it feels like a slab of concrete. The pedal pulses are equal. You are told that the patient has a history of underlying thrombotic disease. This patient's findings are most consistent with which of the following conditions?

- **A.** Peptic ulcer disease
- **B.** Diverticulitis
- **C.** Mesenteric ischemia
- **D.** A leaking abdominal aortic aneurysm

_____ **4.** A 30-year-old man contacts calls 9-1-1 and states he has severe abdominal pain in the lower right quadrant. He states a history of rectal bleeding, diarrhea, arthritis, and fever. He further states episodic periods of similar symptoms. This patient's findings are most consistent with which of the following conditions?

A. Peptic ulcer disease
B. Diverticulitis
C. Crohn disease
D. A leaking abdominal aortic aneurysm

_____ **5.** Pain that originates in the abdomen and causes pain in a distant location as a result of similar paths for the peripheral nerves of the abdomen and the distant location is considered __________ pain.

A. referred
B. parietal
C. somatic
D. rebound

_____ **6.** On arrival, you discover that your patient is a 28-year-old woman complaining of severe vomiting. She explains that she is in the first trimester of pregnancy and has been suffering from morning sickness. Her vomiting is so severe that she is now vomiting blood. She most likely has which of the following conditions?

A. Peptic ulcer disease
B. Hemorrhoids
C. Pancreatitis
D. Mallory-Weiss syndrome

_____ **7.** The proper treatment for esophageal varices includes:

A. narcotic pain relief.
B. treatment with 5% dextrose and water.
C. fluid resuscitation.
D. placement of a laryngeal mask airway (LMA) to prevent aspiration.

_____ **8.** Pain that is difficult to localize and is described as a burning, cramping, gnawing, or aching is called __________ pain.

A. referred
B. visceral
C. somatic
D. parietal

_____ **9.** You receive an emergency call for a conscious, alert 26-year-old man with a sudden onset of severe abdominal pain. He is complaining of an associated fever, nausea, and vomiting. The pain appears isolated to the right lower quadrant (RLQ). Your patient most likely has which of the following conditions?

A. Hypovolemia
B. Inflammation of the interstitial lining
C. Esophageal varices
D. Appendicitis

_____ **10.** Which of the following would NOT cause a bowel obstruction?

A. Paralysis of the intestines
B. An immune attack against the GI tract
C. Infection
D. Kidney disease

Fill in the Blank

Read each item carefully, and then complete the statement by filling in the missing word(s).

1. When patients have ______________________, any drug that is given may remain active within the body for __________ than anticipated.
2. Chronic consumption of __________ or __________ may increase the acidity in the stomach beyond the limits of the protective __________ layer.
3. The __________ vein transports __________ blood from the GI tract directly to the liver for processing of the nutrients that have been __________.
4. The medication ketorolac (Toradol) is a(n) ____________ and, therefore, does not tend to cause ___________ and respiratory depression.
5. People who are __________ are more likely to have a poor outcome from __________-__________ illness.
6. Most peptic ulcers are the result of infection of the stomach with __________ __________. Another major cause is chronic use of __________ anti-inflammatory drugs.
7. __________ __________ __________ involve inflammation of the gallbladder.
8. Ulcerative __________ is caused by inflammation of the colon.
9. __________ __________ is a disease of the young; most patients are between 15 and 30 years of age. It occurs with equal incidence in men and women. There is a strong __________ component to this disease.
10. The presentation of appendicitis can be divided into the following three stages: __________, __________, and __________.

Labeling

Label the following diagrams with the correct terms.

1. Normal versus hiatal hernia

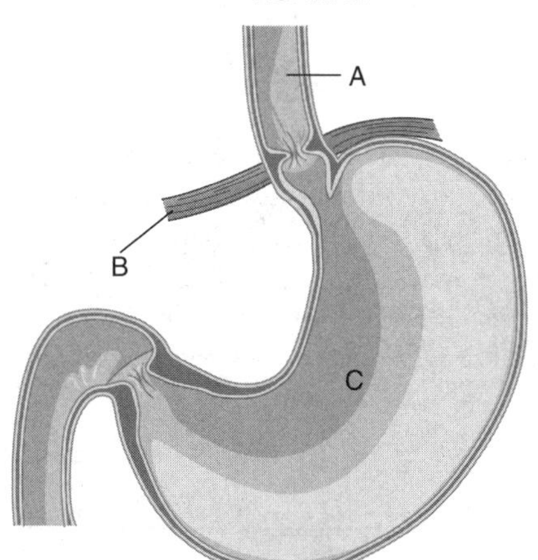

Normal:

A. ____

B. ____

C. ____

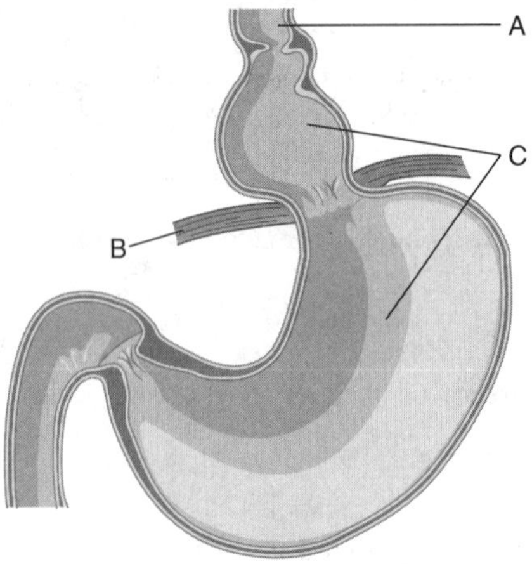

HIATAL HERNIA

A

C

B

Hiatal hernia:

A. ______________________________

B. ______________________________

C. ______________________________

2. Common locations of abdominal hernias

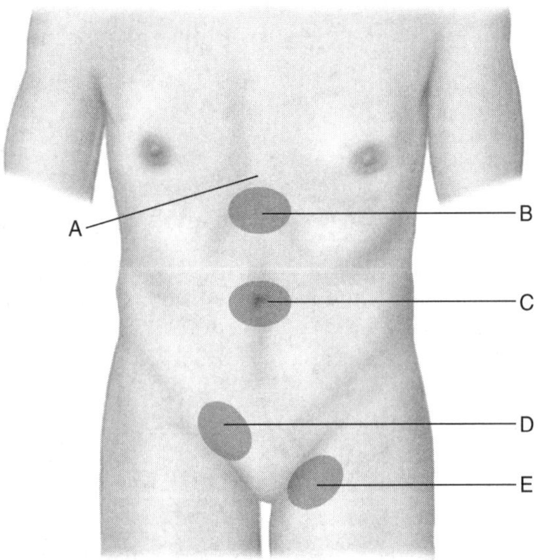

A

B

C

D

E

A. ______________________________

B. ______________________________

C. ______________________________

D. ______________________________

E. ______________________________

Identify

In the following case studies, list the chief complaint, vital signs, and pertinent negatives.

1. "Medic 640, respond Priority One for a 63-year-old male patient, near syncope. Patient is now conscious and alert." As you enter the apartment, you recognize the odor. It smells as though the patient has melena stools. Your paramedic instructor was right; it's an unforgettable smell even for a brand-new, inexperienced paramedic. The patient is found to be sitting on the commode in the bathroom. He appears ashen, diaphoretic, and barely able to sit up. You and your partner lift him off the commode and lay him on the floor, which you have covered with towels. His skin color slightly improves, and his level of consciousness (LOC) improves as well. You immediately place the patient on high-flow supplemental oxygen and begin your primary survey. You already have formed your general impression and realize that the patient is suffering from a GI bleed. His vital signs are a pulse oximetry of 89%, a pulse rate (lying flat) of 118 beats/min, and BP of 88/P mm Hg. His abdomen is slightly distended. The patient tells you that he has an extensive history of rectal bleeding.

a. Chief complaint:

____

____

b. Vital signs:

____

____

c. Pertinent negatives:

____

____

2. You are dispatched to a reported "man down." On arrival, you find law enforcement standing next to a man who presents as very unkempt. He has an empty bottle of Wild Irish something in his hands. You assume that this is a street person. Regardless of your feelings, you understand the importance of remaining professional. Law enforcement explains that the patient is highly intoxicated, is a danger to himself, and needs to be transported to a detox unit. You begin to assess the patient and decide that he looks much older than his real age of 42. Assessment reveals a male patient with an odor of ETOH and urine. He is conscious and alert but slurring his words. He is mostly cooperative. The patient has icteric sclera and right upper quadrant (RUQ) pain on palpation. His blood glucose is 110 mg/dL. His oxygen saturation level is 94%, pulse rate is 104 beats/min and regular, and BP is 142/86 mm Hg. His skin is jaundiced but cool and dry. He has equal bilateral motor neurologic function to all extremities. His lungs are essentially clear and equal bilaterally. The patient has slightly delayed capillary refill. He has sinus tachycardia on the monitor and appears to have had several bowel movements that appear to have been alcoholic in nature. The patient denies any recent injury or falls. He's not a very good historian.

a. Chief complaint:

____

____

b. Vital signs:

____

____

c. Pertinent negatives:

____

____

3. It's New Year's Eve, and your patient is a 45-year-old slightly overweight woman. She is complaining of severe RUQ pain. She states that she knows better than to eat fatty foods, but after all, it's New Year's Eve. She is in pain that she describes as "worse than childbirth." She is slightly nauseated and complains of gas pains. She denies any recent injury or trauma. She states a history of gallbladder disease that is usually controlled by diet. But tonight the pain is "unbearable." She further states that tonight's episode is consistent with other bouts of gallbladder attack. She says that after tonight she is going to "finally have it taken out." Her vital signs are as follows: Her pulse is 92 beats/min, strong and regular. She has equal bilateral radial pulses. The abdomen is tender in the RUQ. Her oxygen saturation is 99%. Electrocardiogram (ECG) reveals sinus rhythm. Capillary refill is normal. Skin color is normal, and skin is warm and slightly diaphoretic. Your patient is crying for pain relief.

a. Chief complaint:

____

____

b. Vital signs:

____

____

c. Pertinent negatives:

____

____

Ambulance Calls

The following case scenarios provide an opportunity to explore the concerns associated with patient management and paramedic care. Read each scenario, and then answer each question.

1. You are assessing and treating a conscious, alert 23-year-old man with a sudden severe onset of periumbilical pain that migrates to the right lower quadrant. He states that he can't find a position of comfort and feels slightly nauseated and febrile.

a. What is your initial impression of this patient's presentation?

____

____

b. Your patient denies any other previous medical history, he is not on any medications, and he denies allergies to medications. His vital signs would be considered within normal limits. How would you treat this patient?

(1)____

(2)____

(3)____

(4)____

(5)____

(6)____

c. Your patient is very nauseated and is vomiting frequently. You have a choice of the following standing-order medications in your drug box: ondansetron (Zofran), diphenhydramine (Benadryl), hydroxyzine (Vistaril), and promethazine (Phenergan). List the cautions of each.

(1) Ondansetron (Zofran):

____

____

(2) Diphenhydramine (Benadryl):

____

____

(3) Hydroxyzine (Vistaril):

____

____

(4) Promethazine (Phenergan):

____

____

2. Your patient presents with a history of esophageal varices. He is vomiting copious amounts of undigested blood. What would your prehospital treatment for this patient include?

a. ______________________________

b. ______________________________

c. ______________________________

d. ______________________________

3. You respond to a call for a 76-year-old woman with a possible bowel obstruction. In the prehospital setting, there might not be much you can do to treat this particular patient. List the general treatment guidelines for patients with GI disease.

a. ______________________________

b. ______________________________

c. ______________________________

d. ______________________________

e. ______________________________

f. ______________________________

g. ______________________________

True/False

If you believe the statement to be more true than false, write the letter "T" in the space provided. If you believe the statement to be more false than true, write the letter "F."

______ 1. Promethazine is a drug for managing patients with nausea and vomiting.

______ 2. Ulcerative colitis presents with a chronic complaint of abdominal pain, often in the lower right area. This pain corresponds to the location of the ileum. Rectal bleeding, weight loss, and diarrhea are some symptoms of this condition.

______ 3. All types of severe liver damage will lead to liver failure.

______ 4. Patients with peptic ulcers experience a classic sequence of burning or gnawing pain in the stomach that subsides or diminishes immediately after eating and then reemerges 2 to 3 hours later.

______ 5. Deep palpation can help you discern some of the organs and structures in the cavity and requires a level of technique usually employed in the prehospital setting.

______ 6. Pain is often an unimportant finding with GI patients. The patient's complaint of pain is something that a paramedic must learn to expect.

______ 7. The major presenting problems from GI diseases typically result in pain, hypovolemia, and infection.

______ 8. True absent bowel sounds, which are characterized by no sounds heard for 2 minutes, are typically not practical to discover in the prehospital setting.

______ 9. The foul-smelling stools that accompany GI emergencies are to be expected.

______ 10. Orthostatic vital signs are only relevant when dealing with abdominal trauma.

Short Answer

Complete this section with short written answers using the space provided.

1. Define the following vocabulary words:

a. Borborygmi:

____

____

b. Cholecystitis:

____

____

c. Scaphoid:

____

____

d. Mallory-Weiss syndrome:

____

____

2. A 15-year-old girl complains of sharp pain in the right lower quadrant. The pain is made worse by coughing or moving around. The spot she points to is the spot that is most tender to palpation. She lies very still, with her right leg flexed at the hip and knee.

   a. What type of abdominal pain is this?

   ____

   b. What mechanism is most likely to produce this type of pain?

   ____

   c. Describe the causes of this type of pain.

   ____

3. Your patient is complaining of pain localized to the right upper abdomen. The patient describes the pain as sharp and as the worst pain he's ever felt. He also states that he is nauseous and has vomited several times. Physical exam reveals fever, tachycardia, hypotension, and muscle spasms in the extremities.

   a. What type of abdominal pain is this?

   ____

   b. When does this type of pain usually occur?

   ____

Fill in the Table

Fill in the missing parts of the table.

1. In the course of a busy week (is there any other kind?), you have several calls for patients with abdominal pain. Each time you have to evaluate a different story and a different set of physical findings. Among the findings in the patients you cared for were those listed here. For each finding, explain its clinical significance.

Finding	What the Finding Tells Me
Coffee-ground vomitus	
Melena	
Tenting of the skin	
Patient very still	

CHAPTER

21

Genitourinary and Renal Emergencies

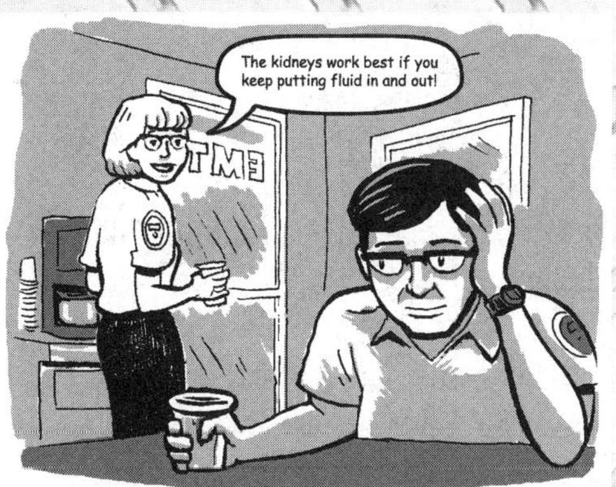

According to the National Institutes of Health, there are more than 600,000 emergency department visits for renal calculi.

Matching

Part I

Match each of the items in the left column to the appropriate term in the right column.

_____	**1.** A double-layered cup with the inner layer infiltrating and surrounding the capillaries of the glomerulus.	**A.** Acute kidney injury
_____	**2.** A condition that results from bacteria entering the skin of the scrotum or perineum, causing infection and subsequent necrosis of the subcutaneal tissue and muscle in the scrotum.	**B.** Air embolism
_____	**3.** A surgically created connection between an artery and a vein, usually in the arm, for dialysis access.	**C.** Anuria
_____	**4.** An infection that causes inflammation of the epididymis along the posterior border of the testis; a possible complication of male urinary tract infection.	**D.** Arteriovenous graft
_____	**5.** A condition in which the kidneys are unable to function, and toxic waste materials build up in the patient's blood; occurs after acute or chronic kidney injury.	**E.** Azotemia
_____	**6.** The U-shaped portion of the renal tubule that extends from the proximal to the distal convoluted tubule; concentrates the filtrate and converts it to urine.	**F.** Benign prostate hypertrophy
_____	**7.** Solid crystalline masses formed in the kidney, resulting from an excess of insoluble salts or uric acid crystallizing in the urine; may become trapped anywhere along the urinary tract.	**G.** Chronic kidney disease
_____	**8.** Solid, bean-shaped organs housed in the retroperitoneal space that filter blood and excrete body wastes in the form of urine.	**H.** Disequilibrium syndrome
_____	**9.** A type of acute kidney injury characterized by damage in the kidney itself. Often caused by immune-mediated diseases, prerenal acute kidney injury, toxins, heavy metals, some medications, or some organic compounds.	**I.** Distal convoluted tubule
_____	**10.** A chronic inflammation of the interstitial cells surrounding the nephrons.	**J.** End-stage renal disease
_____	**11.** The presence of blood in the urine.	**K.** Epididymitis
_____	**12.** Connects with the kidney's collecting tubules.	**L.** Fistula
_____	**13.** A condition characterized by nausea, vomiting, headache, and confusion, which results when, as a consequence of dialysis, water initially shifts from the bloodstream into the cerebrospinal fluid, mildly increasing intracranial pressure (ICP).	**M.** Fournier gangrene

______	14. Progressive and irreversible inadequate kidney function caused by the prostate gland.	N. Glomerular (Bowman) capsule
______	15. Age-related nonmalignant enlargement of the prostate gland.	O. Hematuria
______	16. A sudden decrease in filtration through the glomeruli.	P. Interstitial nephritis
______	17. The presence of air in the venous circulation, which forms a gas bubble that can block the outflow of blood from the right ventricle to the lung; can lead to cardiac arrest, shock, or other life-threatening complications.	Q. Intrarenal acute kidney injury
______	18. A complete cessation of urine production.	R. Kidneys
______	19. A surgical connection between an artery and a vein.	S. Kidney stones
______	20. Increased nitrogenous wastes in the blood.	T. Loop of Henle

Part II

Match each of the items in the left column to the appropriate term in the right column.

______	1. A pair of thick-walled, hollow tubes that transport urine from the kidneys to the bladder.	A. Nephrons
______	2. A hollow tubular structure that drains urine from the bladder, expelling it from the body.	B. Oliguria
______	3. A hollow muscular sac in the midline of the lower abdominal area that stores urine until it is released from the body.	C. Orchitis
______	4. The inability to control the release of urine from the bladder.	D. Paraphimosis
______	5. A connection between the arterial and venous system in which no gas exchange occurs.	E. Phimosis
______	6. Twisting of the testicle on the spermatic cord, from which it is suspended; associated with scrotal pain and swelling, and is a medical emergency.	F. Postrenal acute kidney injury
______	7. The presence of excessive amounts of urea and other waste products in the blood.	G. Prerenal acute kidney injury
______	8. A powdery buildup of uric acid, especially on the skin of the face.	H. Priapism
______	9. A technique for filtering the blood of its toxic wastes, removing excess fluids, and restoring the normal balance of electrolytes.	I. Prostatitis
______	10. An upper urinary tract infection in which the kidneys are involved.	J. Proximal convoluted tubule
______	11. One of the two complex sections of the nephron: includes an enlargement at the end called the glomerular capsule.	K. Pyelonephritis
______	12. Inflammation of the prostate gland.	L. Renal dialysis
______	13. A condition that results when the foreskin is retracted over the glans penis and becomes entrapped; constriction of the glans causes it to swell even further.	M. Shunt
______	14. A complication of a male urinary tract infection in which one or both testes become infected, enlarged, and tender, causing pain and swelling in the scrotum.	N. Testicular torsion
______	15. Urine output of less than 500 mL/day.	O. Uremia
______	16. The structural and functional units of the kidney that form urine, composed of the glomerulus, the glomerular (Bowman) capsule, the proximal convoluted tubule, the loop of Henle, and the distal convoluted tubule.	P. Uremic frost
______	17. Inability to retract the distal foreskin over the glans penis.	Q. Ureters
______	18. A type of acute kidney injury caused by obstruction of urine flow from the kidneys, commonly caused by a blockage of the urethra by an enlarged prostate gland, blood clots, or strictures.	R. Urethra

_____	**19.** A type of acute kidney injury that is caused by hypoperfusion of the kidneys, resulting from hypovolemia (hemorrhage, dehydration), trauma, shock, sepsis, and heart failure (secondary to myocardial infarction); often reversible if the underlying condition can be found and perfusion restored to the kidney.	**S.** Urinary bladder
_____	**20.** A painful, tender, persistent erection of the penis; can result from spinal cord injury; erectile dysfunction drugs, or sickle cell disease.	**T.** Urinary incontinence

Multiple Choice

Read each item carefully, and then select the best response.

_____ **1.** Which of the following is NOT considered part of the urinary system?
- **A.** Ureters
- **B.** Kidney
- **C.** Liver
- **D.** Bladder

_____ **2.** Excessive amounts of urea and other waste products cause a condition called:
- **A.** hypoxia.
- **B.** sepsis.
- **C.** uremia.
- **D.** hypovolemia.

_____ **3.** Inflammation of the kidney linings is caused by:
- **A.** sepsis.
- **B.** urinary tract infection.
- **C.** uremia.
- **D.** hypoxia.

_____ **4.** Treatment options for kidney stones include each of the following, EXCEPT:
- **A.** extracorporeal lithotripsy.
- **B.** cystoscopy with stent placement.
- **C.** smooth muscle constriction.
- **D.** percutaneous nephrostomy tube.

_____ **5.** What is the most common composition of kidney stones?
- **A.** Calcium
- **B.** Salt
- **C.** Glucose
- **D.** Fat

_____ **6.** When a patient is suffering pain from a kidney stone, it is important to remember that the greater the pain, the:
- **A.** lower the BP and pulse will be.
- **B.** higher the BP and pulse will be.
- **C.** higher the BP will be and the lower the pulse will be.
- **D.** lower the BP will be and the higher the pulse will be.

_____ **7.** What is the name of the condition when urine output stops completely?
- **A.** Oliguria
- **B.** Uremia
- **C.** Anuria
- **D.** Hematuria

_____ **8.** When reading an electrocardiogram (ECG), what is a classic finding of hyperkalemia?
- **A.** Peaked T waves
- **B.** Inverted T waves
- **C.** Atrial flutter
- **D.** No T waves at all

______ **9.** Which of the following is NOT a sign of air embolism caused by a loose dialysis system?
- **A.** Cyanosis
- **B.** Hypertension
- **C.** Hypotension
- **D.** Dyspnea

______ **10.** How should pain be managed in the 25-year-old man whom you suspect has a kidney stone?
- **A.** Conservatively administer low doses of Valium.
- **B.** Aggressively administer a narcotic analgesic with medical control's permission.
- **C.** Administer oxygen and acetylsalicylic acid (ASA).
- **D.** Withhold pain medications until arrival at the emergency department (ED).

Labeling

Label the following diagrams with the correct terms.

1. The urinary system

A. ______________________

B. ______________________

C. ______________________

D. ______________________

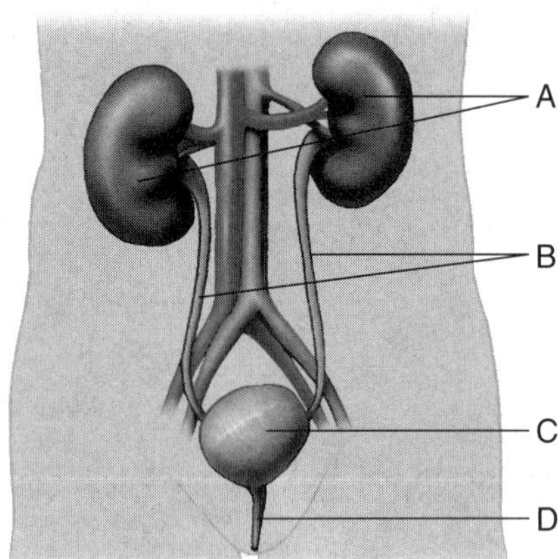

2. The four-quadrant system

A. ______________________

B. ______________________

C. ______________________

D. ______________________

E. ______________________

F. ______________________

G. ______________________

H. ______________________

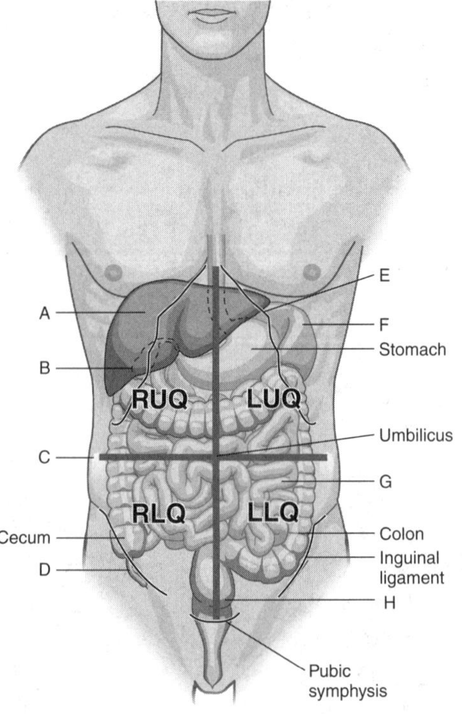

3. The nine-section system

A

Epigastric region

D

B

Peri-umbilical region

E

C

Hypogastric region

F

A. __________

B. __________

C. __________

D. __________

E. __________

F. __________

Fill in the Blank

Read each item carefully, and then complete the statement by filling in the missing word(s).

1. When managing a patient whose chief complaint is renal calculi, your focus should be on __________ and __________.
2. The kidneys' internal anatomy is divided into three regions: the __________, the __________, and the __________.
3. __________ __________ __________ is a sudden decrease in the rate of filtration through the glomeruli.
4. During __________, the patient's blood circulates through a dialysis machine that works the same way the patient's kidneys function.
5. __________ __________ occurs during dialysis and happens because of the water shifting from the bloodstream into the cerebrospinal fluid.
6. Leukemia and tumors, blunt penetrating trauma, cocaine abuse, and spinal cord injury can cause __________ in the male patient.
7. __________ pain is usually associated with hollow organs and presents with a crampy, aching pain deep within the body.
8. You should always monitor the patient's fluid imbalances, electrolyte abnormalities, and __________ function when dealing with an end-stage renal patient.

9. Treatment of kidney stones in the prehospital setting should revolve around __________ __________ for the patient.

10. Urinary tract infections usually occur in the __________ urinary tract.

Identify

After reading the following case study, list the chief complaint, vital signs, and pertinent negatives.

You're just about to hit the hay after a long day at the fire station. Unfortunately, Bill, the paramedic on duty, is not feeling very well, and so you have to fill in for him. He has had a crampy pain in his lower back all day, and he is worried he is coming down with the flu. At about 0100 hours, Bill wakes you and tells you something is really wrong. He is having pain in his lower quadrants, and he can't take it anymore. You give him a little ribbing about all the potato chips he has been eating and the gallons of sports drink he drinks each day. You tell him to go back to sleep. It is just an upset stomach. He tells you he is about to jump through his skin because it hurts so badly and asks you to get up and haul him to the ED. You decide that maybe Bill is having some problems, so you wake up the other emergency medical technician (EMT) and start an assessment on Bill. He is 47 years old, he is alert, and his oxygen saturation is 98%. You put him on a nasal cannula at 4 L/min just for good measure. Your partner takes his pulse, which is 104 beats/min, and the heart monitor shows a sinus tachycardia with no ectopy. BP is 148/94 mm Hg, respirations are 18 breaths/min, and all lung fields are clear. His skin is warm and dry, and he has a normal temperature. Not wanting to miss anything on Bill, you measure his blood glucose, which is 96 mg/dL. His pain is a 10 on a scale of 1 to 10, and he is really hurting. Bill doesn't smoke and, other than a fast-food diet, he keeps in good shape.

Both you and Bill are now suspecting a kidney stone. You start an IV line and give him a 500-mL bolus of normal saline on the way to the hospital. Medical direction agrees with you about the possibility of a stone and orders 5 mg morphine for the pain. Bill is feeling a lot better when you reach the ED. His pain is down to a 4 out of 10. You check back with him in the morning when you get off shift. He says that he passed a stone about 4 hours after you brought him in. They will run a few more tests, but he thinks he will be out of the hospital around noon. He is now swearing off sports drinks and promises water is his new buddy.

1. Chief complaint:

____

____

____

2. Vital signs:

____

____

____

3. Pertinent negatives:

____

____

____

Ambulance Calls

The following case scenarios provide an opportunity to explore the concerns associated with patient management and paramedic care. Read each scenario, and then answer each question.

1. A 52-year-old man complains of crampy abdominal pain that builds up to a peak, subsides, and then builds again. When you ask where the pain is, he points to the general area of the umbilicus, but when you palpate his abdomen, the part that is tender is in the left lower quadrant. He tells you that he has been vomiting nearly constantly since the pain started, about 6 hours ago.
   a. What type of abdominal pain is this?

____

____

____

b. What mechanism is most likely to produce this type of pain?

______

______

______

c. Describe the causes of this type of pain.

______

______

______

2. On the first hot day of the summer, a 35-year-old construction worker calls for an ambulance because of "excruciating" abdominal pain. He was hit in the back lower right quadrant by a steel beam that was being moved into place by a crane. It knocked him down, but he didn't want to appear hurt to his coworkers. So, after catching his breath, he went back to work. He has come home for lunch and now is hurting badly. His wife admits you to the house, where you find the patient in the bedroom, writhing about on the bed, tears rolling down his face. "I can't take it. I can't take it," he says. "Please give me something for the pain." His wife says that he came home from work complaining of back pain and then pain in his groin, and it just got worse and worse. He has been vomiting for the past hour or so. On physical examination, he is clearly in severe distress. His pulse is 124 beats/min and regular, respirations are 30 breaths/min, and BP is 160/80 mm Hg. There is some guarding in the abdomen and tenderness on the left side, but no rigidity. This patient's findings are most consistent with which of the following conditions? Please explain.

A. Peptic ulcer disease
B. Diverticulitis
C. Mesenteric ischemia
D. Leaking abdominal aortic aneurysm
E. Trauma to the kidneys
F. None of the above

______

______

______

3. The following ambulance calls involve dialysis patients. For each situation described, indicate what you think is the problem and what you would do about it.

a. A patient is due for dialysis today but says he feels "too weak and dizzy even to get out of bed." His ECG shows a rate of 40 beats/min; flattened P waves; wide QRS complexes; and tall, pointy T waves. You are 30 minutes from the hospital ED.

(1) What do you think is the problem?

______

(2) What steps will you take to manage the problem?

(a) ______
(b) ______
(c) ______
(d) ______
(e) ______

b. The patient just got home from a dialysis session at the local kidney center. He complains of a severe headache and nausea. He has vomited twice since getting home. On physical examination, he seems a little confused. His pulse is 56 beats/min and regular, respirations are 16 breaths/min, and BP is 180/102 mm Hg.
(1) What do you think is the problem?

____

True/False

If you believe the statement to be more true than false, write the letter "T" in the space provided. If you believe the statement to be more false than true, write the letter "F."

______ **1.** Prerenal acute kidney injury is caused by hyperperfusion of the kidneys.

______ **2.** Hyperkalemia presents with an inverted T wave on the ECG.

______ **3.** Chronic inflammation of the interstitial cells surrounding the nephrons can produce intrarenal acute kidney injury (IAKI).

______ **4.** Nephrons are the functioning units inside the kidney that form urine.

______ **5.** Patients with chronic kidney disease exhibit edema in the extremities and face.

______ **6.** In hemodialysis, the patient's blood circulates through a dialysis machine that functions as a normal liver.

______ **7.** Dialysis patients are more vulnerable to heart failure.

______ **8.** The female urethra is much shorter than the male urethra.

______ **9.** Men are more prone to urinary tract infections than women are because of the length of their urethra.

______ **10.** Prerenal acute kidney injury is caused by a lack of blood flow to the kidneys.

Short Answer

Complete this section with short written answers using the space provided.

1. Many patients with chronic kidney disease are kept alive by periodic hemodialysis. Although dialysis does remove toxic wastes from the blood and helps restore fluid and electrolyte balance, it does not by any means solve all the patient's problems. Patients maintained on long-term dialysis for chronic kidney disease are much more vulnerable than patients with normal kidneys. List five medical problems to which patients with chronic kidney disease, who are taking dialysis treatments, are more vulnerable:

a. ____

b. ____

c. ____

d. ____

e. ____

Fill in the Table

Fill in the missing parts of the table.

Signs and Symptoms of Acute Kidney Injury	
Type of Acute Kidney Injury	Signs and Symptoms
Prerenal	______________________
Intrarenal	______________________
Postrenal	______________________

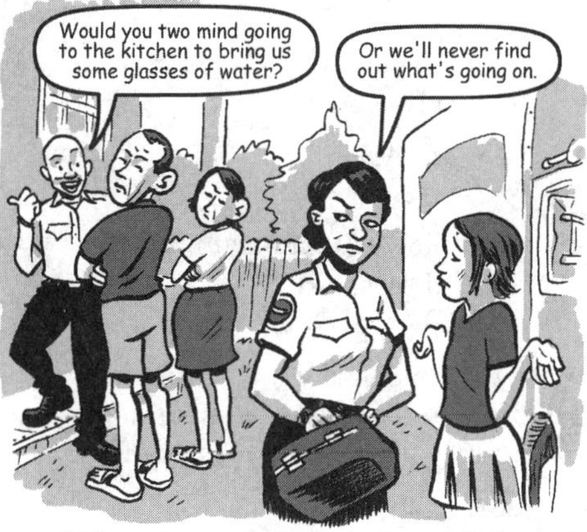

CHAPTER 22

Gynecologic Emergencies

Matching

Part I

Match each of the items in the left column to the appropriate term in the right column.

______	**1.** A pregnancy in which the fertilized oocyte implants somewhere other than the uterus.	**A.** Amenorrhea
______	**2.** Uterine bleeding that is abnormal in amount or frequency (more than every 21 days).	**B.** Bartholin glands
______	**3.** Infection caused by bacteria that travel from the perineum, through the genital tract, into the urethral opening; also called bladder infection.	**C.** Cervix
______	**4.** A small, cylindrical mass of erectile tissue and nerves located at the anterior junction of the labia minora, similar to the glans penis of the male.	**D.** Clitoris
______	**5.** A fluid-filled sac that forms on or within an ovary.	**E.** Cystitis
______	**6.** A rounded pad of fatty tissue that overlies the symphysis pubis and is anterior to the urethral and vaginal openings.	**F.** Dysfunctional uterine bleeding
______	**7.** Cyclical shedding of the endometrial lining from the uterine cavity.	**G.** Ectopic pregnancy
______	**8.** The period when a woman's reproductive cycle ceases; also called the female climacteric.	**H.** Embryo
______	**9.** The inner layer of the uterine wall.	**I.** Endometriosis
______	**10.** An inflammation of the endometrium that is often associated with a bacterial infection.	**J.** Endometritis
______	**11.** The presence of tissue outside the uterus that resembles the endometrium in both structure and function.	**K.** Endometrium
______	**12.** Fertilized egg.	**L.** Fallopian tube
______	**13.** The narrowest portion (lower third of the neck) of the uterus that opens into the vagina.	**M.** Hymen
______	**14.** The glands that secrete mucus for sexual lubrication.	**N.** Labia majora
______	**15.** Absence of menstruation.	**O.** Labia minora
______	**16.** The first menstrual cycle; the onset of menses.	**P.** Menarche
______	**17.** A pair of skin folds devoid of pubic hair that protects the vagina.	**Q.** Menopause
______	**18.** A pair of prominent, rounded folds of skin covered with pubic hair that protects the vagina.	**R.** Menstruation
______	**19.** A membrane that protects the vaginal orifice before first intercourse.	**S.** Mons pubis
______	**20.** The anatomic structure that connects each ovary with the uterus and provides a passageway for the ova.	**T.** Ovarian cyst

Part II

Match each of the items in the left column to the appropriate term in the right column.

______	1. The muscular, inverted, pear-shaped organ where the fetus grows.	A.	Ovarian torsion
______	2. A condition in which the uterus moves or drops into the vagina.	B.	Ovaries
______	3. An inflammation of the external vulva.	C.	Ovulation
______	4. An inflammation of the vagina.	D.	Pelvic inflammatory disease (PID)
______	5. An infection cause by the fungus *Candida albicans*, in which fungi overpopulate the vagina.	E.	Perineum
______	6. Any type of sexual contact or behavior that occurs without the explicit consent of the recipient.	F.	Pyelonephritis
______	7. A fluid-filled sac within the ovary that bursts from internal pressure.	G.	Rape
______	8. Nonconsensual oral, anal, or vaginal penetration of the victim by body parts or objects using force, threats of bodily harm, or taking advantage of a victim who is incapacitated or otherwise incapable of giving consent.	H.	Ruptured ovarian cyst
______	9. Kidney infection.	I.	Sexual assault
______	10. The genital canal in the female that serves as a passageway for the elimination of menstrual fluids, receives the penis during sexual intercourse, holds the spermatozoa before their passage into the uterus, and serves as the passageway for childbirth.	J.	Uterine prolapse
______	11. The area between the vaginal opening and the anus.	K.	Uterus
______	12. An infection of the female reproductive organs.	L.	Vagina
______	13. Midcycle release of an egg (ovum) during the menstrual cycle.	M.	Vaginal yeast infection
______	14. A pair of female reproductive organs that release eggs (ova) that, if fertilized, will develop into a fetus.	N.	Vaginitis
______	15. A painful condition in which the ovary becomes twisted.	O.	Vulvovaginitis

Multiple Choice

Read each item carefully, and then select the best response.

______ 1. How many days is the average "cycle" of a woman?

- A. 5 days
- B. 10 days
- C. 28 days
- D. 30 days

______ 2. What is the onset of the first menses called?

- A. Menopause
- B. Premenstrual syndrome
- C. Menstruation
- D. Menarche

______ 3. During an ectopic pregnancy, where do most eggs implant?

- A. In the uterus
- B. In the fallopian tube
- C. In the ovary
- D. In the cervical opening

______ 4. Which of the following is the most common cause of amenorrhea?

- A. Exercise
- B. Pregnancy
- C. A low body fat percentage
- D. Anorexia nervosa

_____ **5.** Which of the following is NOT one of the classic diagnostic triad for ectopic pregnancy?
- **A.** Vaginal bleeding
- **B.** Anxiety and decreased pulse pressure
- **C.** Amenorrhea
- **D.** Abdominal pain

_____ **6.** Which of the following is NOT considered a life-threatening gynecologic condition?
- **A.** Childbirth
- **B.** Ectopic pregnancy
- **C.** Tubo-ovarian abscess
- **D.** Ruptured ovarian cyst

_____ **7.** Each of the following drugs is considered a "club drug" and has been used to facilitate a sexual rape, EXCEPT:
- **A.** Rohypnol.
- **B.** GHB.
- **C.** naloxone.
- **D.** ketamine.

_____ **8.** Which of the following is a cause of an ectopic pregnancy?
- **A.** Pelvic inflammatory disease
- **B.** IUD use
- **C.** Pelvic surgery
- **D.** All of the above

_____ **9.** When dealing with a victim of sexual assault, which of the following statements is true?
- **A.** You should try to obtain as much information as possible about the assault.
- **B.** You should place the patient's articles in a paper bag.
- **C.** You should place the patient's articles in a plastic bag to preserve DNA.
- **D.** You should allow the patient time to wash himself or herself.

_____ **10.** Which condition involves the presence of tissue outside the uterus that resembles the endometrium in both structure and function?
- **A.** Ovarian cyst
- **B.** Ovarian torsion
- **C.** Endometriosis
- **D.** Endometritis

Labeling

Label the following diagrams with the correct terms.

1. Anatomy of the female genital tract and pelvis

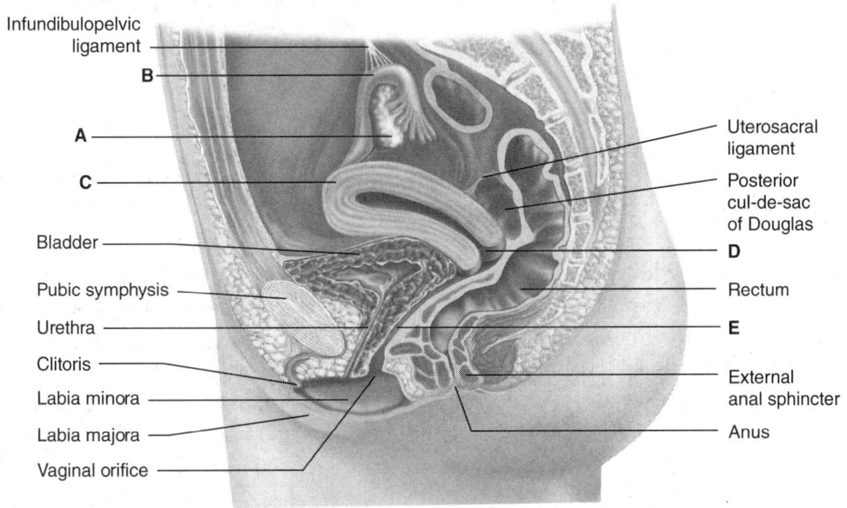

A. ______________________

B. ______________________

C. ______________________

D. ______________________

E. ______________________

2. Reproductive system with an ectopic pregnancy

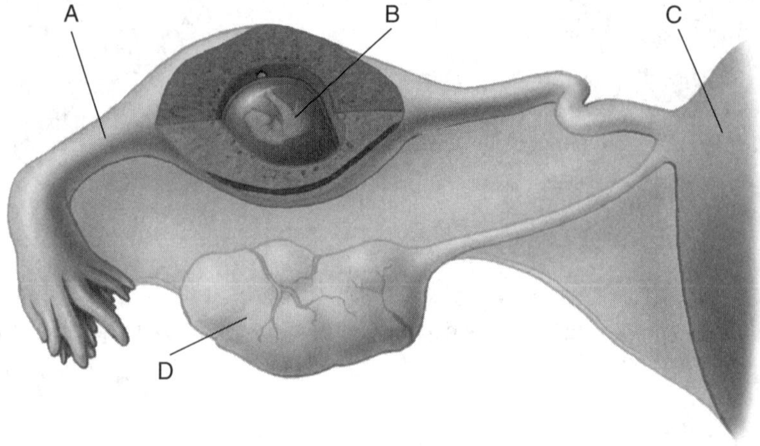

A. ______________________

B. ______________________

C. ______________________

D. ______________________

Fill in the Blank

Read each item carefully, and then complete the statement by filling in the missing word(s).

1. The lower portion of the birth canal is also called the __________.
2. In some cases, a(n) __________ __________ will completely cover the vaginal orifice.
3. The cessation of menses is known as __________.
4. __________ is cessation of ovarian function and of the menstrual cycle such that a woman is no longer able to bear children.
5. Endometrial tissue grows outside the uterus and causes __________.
6. In _________ pregnancy, bleeding usually occurs _______ the onset of pain.
7. __________ __________ is the first thing to ensure when called to a gynecologic emergency.
8. At all times, you should try to protect a patient's __________ when treating a gynecologic emergency.
9. __________ sign or __________ __________ sign may indicate internal bleeding.
10. __________ is usually caused by ________ that ascend from the _________ through the genital tract into the urethral opening.

Identify

Read the following case study, and then list the chief complaint, vital signs, and pertinent negatives.

Your unit has been called to the local high school for a young woman with severe abdominal pain. When you arrive, the 16-year-old patient, Lucy, is doubled up in pain. She is crying. You begin your primary survey (ABCDE) and apply supplemental oxygen via a nonrebreathing mask. Lucy rates her pain as 10 on a scale of 1 to 10. Your partner Abe begins with her baseline vital signs as you gather a personal history. Lucy's heart rate is 120 beats/min, her electrocardiogram (ECG) rhythm is sinus tachycardia, and her blood pressure (BP) is 140/92 mm Hg. Her oxygen saturation is 94%, and respirations are 20 breaths/min. Her skin is very warm, and her temperature is 102°F. Pupils are equal, round, and reactive to light and accommodation (PERRLA). Lung sounds are clear. The patient has no history of illness or trauma. She denies being sexually active yet. A physical examination reveals guarding of the abdomen. She has rebound tenderness, and her abdomen is distended. She says she is going to be sick and then begins to vomit. You believe that she is a load-and-go priority patient, so your partner gets an IV line started, and you load the patient quickly and get to the emergency department (ED) as quickly as possible.

1. Chief complaint:

2. Vital signs:

3. Pertinent negatives:

Ambulance Calls

The following case scenarios provide an opportunity to explore the concerns associated with patient management and paramedic care. Read each scenario, and then answer each question.

1. A 25-year-old woman calls for an ambulance because of abdominal pain. She says the pain started yesterday and has just gotten worse and worse. It is a "heavy," aching pain in the lower abdomen. This afternoon, she started having chills as well, and she threw up once. Her last menstrual period was 5 days ago and was normal. She uses an intrauterine device (IUD) for contraception. On physical examination, the patient looks ill. Her skin feels hot and dry. Her pulse is 110 beats/min and regular while sitting, 116 beats/min while standing; her respirations are 24 breaths/min and unlabored; and her BP is 122/74 mm Hg. The abdomen is very tender to palpation in all quadrants.
   a. This patient is most likely experiencing which of the following conditions?
      A. A threatened abortion
      B. An inevitable abortion
      C. A septic abortion
      D. An ectopic pregnancy
      E. Pelvic inflammatory disease (PID)

   b. List the steps you would take in managing this patient.

      (1)

      (2)

2. A 24-year-old woman calls for an ambulance because she says, "I think I have appendicitis." She has been having some crampy pain in the right lower quadrant for a couple of days, but today it got much worse. She cannot remember exactly when her last menstrual period was and says, "But I think I'm getting my period now because I had some spotting this morning." She is certain, in any case, that she could not possibly be pregnant. On physical examination, she appears anxious and in moderate distress. Her skin is cool and moist. Her pulse is 100 beats/min and regular while sitting, and 124 beats/min while standing; her respirations are 24 breaths/min and regular; and her BP is 110/70 mm Hg. Her abdomen is very tender to palpation.
   a. What is your field diagnosis of this patient?
      A. A threatened abortion
      B. An inevitable abortion
      C. A septic abortion
      D. An ectopic pregnancy
      E. Pelvic inflammatory disease (PID)

b. List the steps you would take in managing this patient.

(1)____________________

(2)____________________

(3)____________________

(4)____________________

(5)____________________

(6)____________________

(7)____________________

(8)____________________

True/False

If you believe the statement to be more true than false, write the letter "T" in the space provided. If you believe the statement to be more false than true, write the letter "F."

______ **1.** The paramedic should take a detailed history of a rape incident to enable the victim to vent her feelings about what happened.

______ **2.** An inflammation of the bladder that is caused by a yeast infection is called a Bartholin abscess.

______ **3.** The patient who has experienced a rape should be discouraged from cleaning up before being examined in the ED.

______ **4.** The rape victim's external genitalia should be routinely inspected for injury.

______ **5.** The insertion of an IUD can increase a woman's risk of developing PID.

______ **6.** Infection can cause the Bartholin glands to become cystic and abscessed.

______ **7.** Menarche is when a woman reaches menopause.

______ **8.** Endometritis is hereditary and runs in families.

______ **9.** The region of sexual stimulation is called the hymen.

______ **10.** The menstrual cycle is divided into the ovarian and the uterine cycles.

Short Answer

Complete this section with short written answers using the space provided.

1. You are summoned to a downtown apartment for a "sick woman." On arrival, you find a 24-year-old woman complaining of severe abdominal pain.

a. List 10 questions you would ask in taking this woman's history.

(1) ____________________

(2) ____________________

(3) ____________________

(4) ____________________

(5) ____________________

(6) ____________________

(7) ______________________________

(8) ______________________________

(9) ______________________________

(10) ______________________________

b. List two things you would look for in particular in performing the physical examination.

(1) ______________________________

(2) ______________________________

2. Ectopic pregnancy is more likely in some women than in others. List two factors that predispose a woman to ectopic pregnancy.

a. ______________________________

b. ______________________________

3. Three findings in the history make up the classic diagnostic triad for ectopic pregnancy, and a woman who has those three findings must be considered to be experiencing an ectopic pregnancy until proven otherwise. Which three findings make up the classic triad for ectopic pregnancy?

a. ______________________________

b. ______________________________

c. ______________________________

Fill in the Table

Fill in the missing parts of the table.

Elements of the Gynecologic History
Current symptoms: Vaginal bleeding? Amount? Any tissue passed?
Current symptoms: Vaginal discharge? Color, amount, odor, itching?
Current sexual activity? Birth control?
Prior pregnancies (gravidity)
Prior pregnancy complications or losses?
Other past medical history, medications, allergies

CHAPTER 23

Endocrine Emergencies

Prescription bottles can help pinpoint the patient's underlying medical problems and identify his or her physician.

Matching

Part I

Match each of the definitions in the left column to the appropriate terms in the right column.

______ **1.** A hormone produced by the pancreas that is vital to the control of the body's metabolism and blood glucose level. Glucagon stimulates the breakdown of glycogen to glucose.

______ **2.** Diabetes that develops during pregnancy in women who did not have diabetes before pregnancy.

______ **3.** Protrusion of the eyes from the normal position within the socket.

______ **4.** One of the three major female hormones at puberty; it brings about the secondary sex characteristics.

______ **5.** A hormone produced by the adrenal medulla that plays a vital role in the function of the sympathetic nervous system.

______ **6.** A hormone secreted by the thyroid gland that helps maintain normal calcium levels in the blood.

______ **7.** A hormone secreted by the posterior pituitary lobe of the pituitary gland, which constricts blood vessels and raises the blood pressure; also called vasopressin.

______ **8.** Male sex hormones that regulate body changes associated with sexual development (puberty), including growth spurts, deepening of the voice, growth of facial and pubic hair, and muscle growth and strength.

______ **9.** A hormone that stimulates the kidneys to reabsorb sodium from the uterine and excrete potassium by altering the osmotic gradient in the blood.

______ **10.** A hormone that targets the adrenal cortex to secrete cortisol (a glucocorticoid).

______ **11.** Abnormally high blood glucose level.

______ **12.** A type of hyperthyroidism in which the thyroid gland becomes enlarged as it is infiltrated by T lymphocytes and plasma cells.

______ **13.** An autoimmune disorder that causes thyroid gland hypertrophy and severe hyperthyroidism.

______ **14.** A visible mass in the anterior part of the neck caused by enlargement of the thyroid gland.

______ **15.** The passage of large quantities of urine containing glucose.

______ **16.** Acute adrenal insufficiency.

A. Addisonian crisis

B. Adrenocorticotrophic hormone (ACTH)

C. Aldosterone

D. Androgens

E. Antidiuretic hormone (ADH)

F. Calcitonin

G. Corticosteroids

H. Cortisol

I. Cushing syndrome

J. Diabetes

K. Diabetes insipidus (DI)

L. Diabetes mellitus

M. Diabetic ketoacidosis (DKA)

N. Diuresis

O. Dyslipidemia

P. Epinephrine

______	17. An excessive level of lipids (fats) circulating in the blood, which increases the risk of atherosclerosis and coronary artery disease.	Q. Estrogen
______	18. The production of large amounts of urine by the kidney.	R. Exophthalmos
______	19. A form of acidosis in uncontrolled diabetes in which certain acids accumulate when insulin is not available.	S. Gestational diabetes
______	20. Disease characterized by the body's inability to sufficiently metabolize glucose; it occurs either because the pancreas does not produce enough insulin or because the cells do not respond to the effects of the insulin that is produced.	T. Glucagon
______	21. A group of complex metabolic disorders with many causes, which include diabetes mellitus, gestational diabetes, hypoglycemia/hyperglycemia, diabetic ketoacidosis, and hyperosmolar hyperglycemic syndrome.	U. Glycosuria
______	22. A condition caused by an excess of cortisol production by the adrenal glands or by excessive use of cortisol or other similar corticosteroid (glucocorticoid) hormones.	V. Goiter
______	23. Hormones that stimulates most body cells to increase their energy production.	W. Graves disease
______	24. Hormones that regulate the body's metabolism, the balance of salt and water in the body, the immune system, and sexual function.	X. Hashimoto disease
______	25. A relatively uncommon disorder that has some of the same characteristics as diabetes, such as polyuria and polydipsia, in which the body is unable to regulate fluid owing to a lack of antidiuretic hormone or the kidneys are unable to respond appropriately.	Y. Hyperglycemia

Part II

Match each of the definitions in the left column to the appropriate terms in the right column.

______	1. An "orange peel" appearance and nonpitting edema of the skin on the anterior part of the leg below the knee.	A. Hyperosmolar hyperglycemic syndrome (HHS)
______	2. A condition identified in people who have certain risk factors associated with type 2 diabetes that exists when blood glucose levels or hemoglobin A1c levels are above normal levels, yet not high enough to be diagnosed as diabetes.	B. Hyperosmolar nonketotic coma (HONK)
______	3. Frequent and plentiful urination.	C. Hypoglycemia
______	4. Increased appetite.	D. Insulin
______	5. Significant thirst.	E. Insulin resistance
______	6. An endocrine disorder in which an excess of antidiuretic hormone results in a decrease in urinary output and, therefore, systemic fluid overload.	F. Islets of Langerhans
______	7. A hormone that inhibits insulin and glucagon secretion by the pancreas.	G. Ketonemia
______	8. A common condition characterized by a lack of adrenocorticotropic hormone (also called corticotrophin).	H. Lipolysis
______	9. Also known as Addison disease; a rare condition in which the adrenal glands produce an insufficient amount of adrenal hormones.	I. Luteinizing hormone
______	10. A hormone secreted by the parathyroid glands that acts as an antagonist to calcitonin; secreted when calcium blood levels are low.	J. Microangiopathy
______	11. The inadequate production or absence of the pituitary hormones, including adrenocorticotropic hormone (ACTH), cortisol, thyroxine, luteinizing hormone (LH), follicle-stimulating hormone (FSH), estrogen, testosterone, growth hormone, and antidiuretic hormone (ADH).	K. Myxedema coma
______	12. A hormone produced by the adrenal glands that is vital in the function of the sympathetic nervous system.	L. Testosterone

_____	**13.** The most important androgen in men.	**M.** Norepinephrine
_____	**14.** A rare condition that can occur in patients who have severe, untreated hypothyroidism.	**N.** Panhypopituitarism
_____	**15.** Microscopic deterioration of vessel walls caused primarily by adherence of blood lipids to vessel walls.	**O.** Parathyroid hormone
_____	**16.** A metabolic derangement that occurs principally in patients with type 2 diabetes; it is characterized by hyperglycemia and hyperosmolarity, in absence of significant ketosis; also known as hyperosmolar nonketotic coma.	**P.** Pheochromocytoma
_____	**17.** Another name for hyperosmolar hyperglycemic syndrome.	**Q.** Polydipsia
_____	**18.** Abnormally low blood glucose level.	**R.** Polyphagia
_____	**19.** A hormone produced by the pancreas that is vital to the control of the body's metabolism and blood glucose level; it causes sugar, fatty acids, and amino acids to be absorbed and metabolized by cells.	**S.** Polyuria
_____	**20.** Condition in which the pancreas produces enough insulin but the body cannot effectively use it.	**T.** Prediabetes
_____	**21.** A hormone that regulates the production of both eggs and sperm, as well as the production of reproductive hormones.	**U.** Pretibial myxedema
_____	**22.** The metabolism (breakdown or destruction) of stored fat that has been released into the circulation.	**V.** Primary adrenal insufficiency
_____	**23.** Excess amounts of ketone bodies in the blood.	**W.** Progesterone
_____	**24.** A specialized group of cells in the pancreas in which insulin and glucagon are produced.	**X.** Somatostatin
_____	**25.** A tumor of the adrenal gland, usually in the medulla, that causes excessive release of the hormones epinephrine and norepinephrine.	**Y.** Syndrome of inappropriate antidiuretic hormone secretion (SIADH)

Multiple Choice

Read each item carefully, and then select the best response.

_____ **1.** The endocrine system is made up of a network of glands that produce:

A. homeostasis.
B. glucose.
C. calcium.
D. hormones.

_____ **2.** The parathyroid glands assist in the regulation of:

A. sodium.
B. potassium.
C. calcium.
D. iron.

_____ **3.** Which part of the endocrine system has a role in hormone production as well as in digestion?

A. Hypothalamus
B. Pancreas
C. Thyroid
D. Parathyroid

_____ **4.** The pituitary gland stimulates other endocrine glands, including each of the following, EXCEPT:

A. calcitonin.
B. ACTH.
C. luteinizing hormone.
D. thyroid-stimulating hormone.

_____ **5.** The thyroid secretes:
A. iodine.
B. calcitonin.
C. cardiac enzymes.
D. norepinephrine.

_____ **6.** The adrenal glands consist of two parts: an outer part, called the adrenal cortex, and an inner part, called the:
A. adrenal cortex.
B. adrenal medulla.
C. posterior adrenal cortex.
D. inferior medulla.

_____ **7.** Epinephrine stimulates __________ nervous system receptors throughout the body.
A. parasympathetic
B. sympathetic
C. dopamine
D. neuron

_____ **8.** In the past, type 2 diabetes mellitus was called:
A. juvenile diabetes.
B. adult-onset diabetes.
C. diabetic hypoglycemia.
D. sweet diabetes.

_____ **9.** The most common form of diabetes is type 2 diabetes, also known as:
A. insulin intolerance.
B. insulin tolerance.
C. insulin resistance.
D. insulin opposition.

_____ **10.** Patients in diabetic ketoacidosis (DKA) are seldom:
A. comatose.
B. asymptomatic.
C. hyperglycemic.
D. hypoglycemic.

_____ **11.** Which of the following conditions is characterized by hyperglycemia, hyperosmolarity, and the absence of ketosis?
A. Hyperosmolar nonketotic coma (HONK)
B. Hyperosmolar hyperglycemic syndrome (HHS)
C. Cardiometabolic syndrome
D. Both A and B

_____ **12.** Signs and symptoms of acute adrenal insufficiency may appear suddenly and are commonly referred to as:
A. addisonian crisis.
B. adrenal insufficiency.
C. severe infection.
D. None of the above

_____ **13.** Cushing syndrome is caused by:
A. an excess of cortisol production.
B. an excess of glucocorticoid hormones.
C. tumors of the pituitary gland or adrenal cortex.
D. All of the above

_____ **14.** An extreme manifestation of untreated hypothyroidism that is accompanied by physiologic decompensation is called:

A. myxedema coma.
B. thyroid storm.
C. Cushing syndrome.
D. diabetic ketoacidosis.

_____ **15.** Thyrotoxicosis may be caused by all of the following, EXCEPT:

A. goiters.
B. Graves disease.
C. thyroid cancer.
D. ketoacidosis.

Labeling

Label the following diagrams with the correct terms.

1. Diabetic emergencies

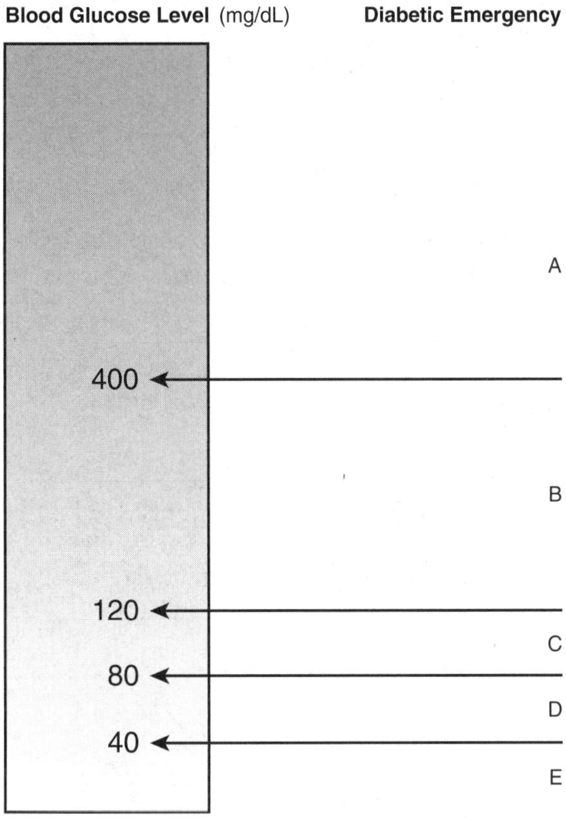

Blood Glucose Level (mg/dL) **Diabetic Emergency**

A

400

B

120

C

80

D

40

E

A. ______________________________

B. ______________________________

C. ______________________________

D. ______________________________

E. ______________________________

Fill in the Blank

Read each item carefully, and then complete the statement by filling in the missing word(s).

1. __________ coma is a metabolic and cardiovascular emergency. If not diagnosed and treated immediately, the mortality rate is approximately 40%.

2. The anterior pituitary gland secretes __________-__________ __________ in response to secretion of thyrotropin-releasing hormone by the hypothalamus.

3. Aldosterone regulates and maintains the __________ and __________ balance in the blood.

4. The goals of prehospital treatment for diabetic ketoacidosis are to begin __________ and to correct the patient's __________ and acid–base abnormalities.

5. Hyperglycemia usually progresses slowly, over a period of _____ to ______ hours, with the patient's level of consciousness ______ only gradually.

6. Symptoms of type 2 diabetes may include __________, __________, nausea, frequent urination, unexplained weight loss, blurred vision, unresponsiveness, and thirst

7. Two forms of diabetes exist: __________ __________ and __________ __________. Both types are serious conditions that affect many tissues and functions other than the glucose-regulating mechanism, and both require lifelong medical management.

8. The endocrine component of the pancreas is made up of the __________ __________ __________. These cell groups in the pancreas act like "an organ within an organ." The main hormones they secrete are __________, __________, and somatostatin, which are responsible for the regulation of blood glucose levels.

9. The pituitary gland secretions control, or regulate, the secretions of other __________ glands.

10. HHS, which stands for _______ hyperglycemic syndrome and is also called _________ nonketotic ______ (HONK), is a metabolic derangement that occurs principally in patients with type 2 diabetes.

Identify

Read the following case studies, and then list the chief complaint, vital signs, and pertinent negatives. Also identify the possible nature of the endocrine disorder.

1. It is a sunny but very cold and windy mid-February day. You and your partner would be content to remain inside the station practicing your advanced life support (ALS) skills. The silence is broken with a dispatch to a priority 1 call for an unconscious, unresponsive patient waiting for a prescription at the neighborhood pharmacy. On arrival, you find the 29-year-old woman being attended by the pharmacist, who states the patient was waiting for an insulin prescription. The patient is unresponsive. You note that respirations are shallow, and the patient is diaphoretic. Her radial pulse is 118 beats/min. Her blood pressure (BP) is 104/88 mm Hg. Her blood glucose is 48 mg/dL. As you prepare the electrocardiogram (ECG) monitor and intravenous (IV) equipment, the pharmacist pulls her history.

   a. Chief complaint:

   ____

   ____

   b. Vital signs:

   ____

   ____

   c. Pertinent negatives:

   ____

   ____

d. Nature of the endocrine disorder:

____

____

2. It is cold and flu season, and today is no exception. It seems these ailments are what everyone is calling in for. On arrival at the scene, you locate an elderly man sitting in his rocker, apparently short of breath. He states that he has had the flu for a number of days and cannot stop vomiting. He speaks in full, complete sentences, but he has an unusual breathing pattern and fruity breath odor. You quickly place the pulse oximeter probe on his finger. Surprisingly, his oxygen saturation is 95% on room air. You immediately follow up with high-flow supplemental oxygen as you begin your assessment. The patient states that he has a long history of diabetes. He further states that he has not been able to keep food down for several days but has been taking all of his medications. His blood glucose is 405 mg/dL. He is tachycardic, with a BP of 108/82 mm Hg. He has poor skin turgor, and skin tenting is present. The monitor is showing a sinus tachycardia. The patient complains of thirst.

a. Chief complaint:

____

____

b. Vital signs:

____

____

c. Pertinent negatives:

____

____

d. Nature of the endocrine disorder:

____

____

3. Once again today, you are requested to respond to a call to the local nursing home for a "routine" transport to the emergency department (ED). You are met by family members, who are concerned that Grandma's mental status has been rapidly deteriorating; she also appears to be cold. The family states that the patient has suddenly become confused and psychotic. The nursing home chart indicates a history of hypothyroidism. Her pulse rate is slightly bradycardic. She is also hypotensive. You cannot get an accurate pulse oximeter reading because of poor peripheral perfusion.

a. Chief complaint:

____

____

b. Vital signs:

____

____

c. Pertinent negatives:

d. Nature of the endocrine disorder:

Ambulance Calls

The following case scenarios provide an opportunity to explore the concerns associated with patient management and paramedic care. Read each scenario, and then answer each question.

1. A 22-year-old woman is found unconscious in her apartment. Her roommate, who is nearly hysterical, tells you between sobs, "I went away for the weekend, and when I got back tonight, I found her like this. She won't die, will she?" A neighbor arrives and helps calm the roommate while you and your partner carry out the primary assessment. That accomplished, you proceed to the secondary assessment. You find that the patient wakens to a painful stimulus but rapidly returns to sleep. Her skin is warm and flushed and tents when you pinch it. Her vital signs are as follows: Pulse is 110 beats/min and regular, respirations are 30 breaths/min and deep, and BP is 90/60 mm Hg. The patient's eyes look sunken, and her pupils are 5 mm and equal, round, and reactive to light and accommodation (PERRLA). The patient's breath smells like fruit-flavored gum (or nail polish remover). Her neck is not rigid, her chest is clear, and her abdomen is soft. There are multiple needle marks and skin changes over the anterior thighs. Completing your examination, you ask the patient's roommate, "Miss, does your friend by chance have diabetes?"

"Oh, didn't I mention that?" the roommate sniffles.

List the steps in treating this patient.

a.

b.

c.

d.

2. Over the course of a week of ambulance runs, four patients are found in a coma. You do not have any information about any of them except for the medications found at the scene or on the patient's person. Nonetheless, based on those medications, you can make an educated guess at least as to each patient's underlying illness(es). For each of the comatose patients whose medications are listed as follows, indicate the most probable underlying illness(es).

a. Patient 1 has glyburide (Micronase) on his bedside table.
Probable underlying illness(es):

b. A vial of insulin is found in patient 2's refrigerator.
Probable underlying illness(es):

c. Patient 3 has what appears to be an insulin pump. The patient's medical identification bracelet confirms your suspicion.
Probable underlying illness(es):

d. Patient 4, a 35-year-old insulin-dependent woman, had a sudden onset of a severe headache and blurred vision before she became unconscious and fell to the floor, striking her head on a concrete surface.
Probable underlying illness(es):

Complete the Patient Care Report (PCR)

Read the first incident scenario in the preceding Ambulance Calls section, and then complete the following patient care report (PCR).

EMS Patient Care Report (PCR)					
Date:	Incident No.:	Nature of Call:		Location:	
Dispatched:	En Route:	At Scene:	Transport:	At Hospital:	In Service:
Patient Information					
Age: Sex: Weight (in kg [lb]):			Allergies: Medications: Past Medical History: Chief Complaint:		
Vital Signs					
Time:	BP:	Pulse:	Respirations:	SpO_2:	
Time:	BP:	Pulse:	Respirations:	SpO_2:	
Time:	BP:	Pulse:	Respirations:	SpO_2:	
EMS Treatment (circle all that apply)					
Oxygen @ ______ L/min via (circle one): NC NRM Bag-mask device		Assisted Ventilation	Airway Adjunct	CPR	
Defibrillation	Bleeding Control	Bandaging	Splinting	Other:	
Narrative					

True/False

If you believe the statement to be more true than false, write the letter "T" in the space provided. If you believe the statement to be more false than true, write the letter "F."

_____ **1.** Cold, clammy skin is classically a sign of shock but may also signal severe hypoglycemia, as from an insulin reaction.

_____ **2.** Aldosterone stimulates the bladder to eliminate large quantities of potassium.

_____ **3.** Adult hypothyroidism is sometimes called myxedema.

_____ **4.** The anterior pituitary gland secretes thyroid-stimulating hormone (TSH) in response to the hypothalamus's secretion of thyrotropin-releasing hormone (TRH).

_____ **5.** The primary clinical manifestation of adrenal crisis is atrial fibrillation.

_____ **6.** The signs and symptoms of hypoglycemia and hyperglycemia can be quite similar.

_____ **7.** Normal blood glucose is approximately 70 to 120 mg/dL; hypoglycemia occurs when blood glucose drops to 35 mg/dL.

_____ **8.** Type 2 diabetes may be related to metabolic syndrome.

_____ **9.** Symptoms of type 2 diabetes may include fatigue; nausea; frequent urination; thirst; unexplained weight loss; blurred vision; frequent infections and slow healing of wounds; crankiness, confusion, or shakiness; unresponsiveness; and seizure.

_____ **10.** Most patients with diabetes do not live a normal life span, even if they adjust their lives to the demands of the disease, especially their eating habits and activities.

_____ **11.** Endocrine disorders can be caused by either hypersecretion or insufficient secretion of a gland.

_____ **12.** In addition to secreting somatostatin, the islets of Langerhans secrete glucagon and insulin, which are responsible for the regulation of blood glucose levels.

_____ **13.** When sodium is reabsorbed into the blood, water is secreted; this action decreases both blood volume and blood pressure.

_____ **14.** Iodine is an important component of thyroxine. Without the proper level of dietary iodine intake, thyroxine cannot be produced.

_____ **15.** Cushing syndrome is caused by an excess of testosterone.

Short Answer

Complete this section with short written answers using the space provided.

1. Define the following vocabulary words:

a. Hypoglycemia:

_____

_____

_____

b. Diabetic ketoacidosis (DKA):

_____

_____

_____

c. Thyrotoxicosis:

d. Insulin:

e. Cushing syndrome:

2. Explain the treatment for the following conditions:
   a. Myxedema coma:

   b. Adrenal insufficiency:

   c. Hyperosmolar nonketotic coma:

Fill in the Table

Fill in the missing parts of the table.

Oral Agents Used to Treat Type 2 Diabetes Mellitus		
Medication Class	**Function**	**Examples**
Sulfonylureas		Chlorpropamide (Diabinese) Glipizide (Glucotrol) Glyburide (Micronase, Glynase, DiaBeta) Glimepiride (Amaryl)
	Stimulate beta cells to produce more insulin	Repaglinide (Prandin) Nateglinide (Starlix)
Biguanides		Metformin (Glucophage)
	Increase insulin effectiveness in the muscle and decrease liver glucose production	Rosiglitazone (Avandia) Pioglitazone (ACTOS)
Alpha-glucosidase inhibitors		Acarbose (Precose) Miglitol (Glyset)
DPP-4 inhibitors	Inhibit the breakdown of GLP-1, a naturally occurring compound in the body that reduces blood glucose levels	Sitagliptin (Januvia) Saxagliptin (Onglyza)

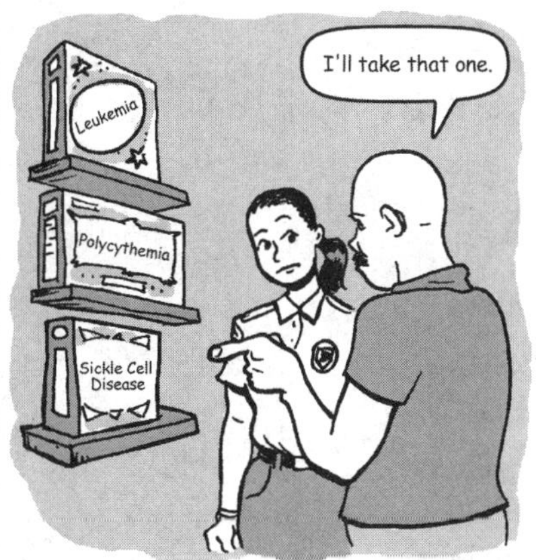

Your patient did not choose to have a disorder. Treat all of your patients with compassion.

CHAPTER 24

Hematologic Emergencies

Matching

Part I

Match each of the items in the left column to the appropriate definition in the right column.

______	**1.** The most common type of anemia.	**A.**	Acute chest syndrome
______	**2.** A bleeding and clotting abnormality.	**B.**	Acute splenic sequestration syndrome
______	**3.** The body's natural blood-clotting mechanism.	**C.**	Anemia
______	**4.** A bleeding disorder relating to the breakdown of red blood cells.	**D.**	Aplastic crisis
______	**5.** A disorder that is primarily hereditary, in which clotting does not occur or occurs insufficiently.	**E.**	Clotting cascade
______	**6.** Any disorder of the blood.	**F.**	Clotting factors
______	**7.** The proportion of red blood cells in the total blood volume.	**G.**	Coagulopathy
______	**8.** Red blood cells.	**H.**	Disseminated intravascular coagulation (DIC)
______	**9.** A condition that begins with widespread activation of the clotting cascade, which depletes the clotting factors and platelets and eventually results in uncontrolled hemorrhage.	**I.**	Erythrocytes
______	**10.** Any type of bleeding disorder that interferes with the activation or continuation of the clotting cascade or hemostasis.	**J.**	Hematocrit
______	**11.** A condition in which red blood cells break down quickly; it may occur as a result of sickle cell disease.	**K.**	Hematologic disorder
______	**12.** The iron-rich protein in the blood that carries oxygen.	**L.**	Hematology
______	**13.** The system that includes all blood components and the organs involved in their development and production.	**M.**	Hematopoietic system
______	**14.** The study of the physiology of blood.	**N.**	Hemoglobin
______	**15.** Substances in the blood that are necessary for clotting; also called coagulation factors.	**O.**	Hemolytic crisis
______	**16.** A vasoocclusive crisis that can be associated with pneumonia; common signs and symptoms include chest pain, fever, and cough; associated with sickle cell disease.	**P.**	Hemolytic disorder
______	**17.** A condition in which red blood cells become trapped in the spleen, causing a dramatic fall in hemoglobin available in the circulation; it usually occurs in infants or toddlers.	**Q.**	Hemophilia
______	**18.** A lower-than-normal hemoglobin or erythrocyte level.	**R.**	Hemostasis

______	**19.** A temporary halt in the production of red blood cells; it may occur as a result of sickle cell disease.	**S.** Hemostatic disorder
______	**20.** Lymphocytes that have been transformed because of stimulation by an antigen.	**T.** Iron-deficiency anemia
______	**21.** A reduction in the number of white blood cells.	**U.** Leukemia
______	**22.** An increase in the total number of white blood cells.	**V.** Leukocytes
______	**23.** White blood cells.	**W.** Leukocytosis
______	**24.** The process by which clotting factors work together to ultimately form fibrin.	**X.** Leukopenia
______	**25.** A cancer or malignancy of the blood-forming organs that particularly affects the white blood cells, which develop abnormally and/or excessively at the expense of normal blood cells.	**Y.** Lymphoblasts

Part II

Match each of the items in the left column to the appropriate definition in the right column.

______	**1.** Coagulation or clotting of blood in a blood vessel.	**A.** Lymphoid system
______	**2.** A condition in which the body produces too many platelets.	**B.** Lymphomas
______	**3.** The system in the body that is primarily used to defend against infection.	**C.** Multiple myeloma
______	**4.** Platelets.	**D.** Neutropenia
______	**5.** A type of anemia in which either not enough hemoglobin is produced or the hemoglobin is defective.	**E.** Plasma
______	**6.** Ischemia and pain caused by sickle-shaped red blood cells that obstruct blood flow to a portion of the body.	**F.** Polycythemia
______	**7.** A transfusion reaction characterized by increased pulmonary capillary permeability resulting in noncardiogenic pulmonary edema.	**G.** Reticuloendothelial system
______	**8.** A physiologic response that is similar to an anaphylactic reaction, in which the body reacts to the infusion of blood; it occurs rapidly and can cause severe circulatory collapse and death.	**H.** Sickle cell crisis
______	**9.** An overabundance or overproduction of red blood cells, white blood cells, and platelets.	**I.** Sickle cell disease
______	**10.** The system primarily made up of bone marrow, lymph nodes, and spleen, which participates in the formation of lymphocytes and immune responses.	**J.** Splenic sequestration crisis
______	**11.** Malignant diseases that arise within the lymphoid system; they include non-Hodgkin and Hodgkin lymphomas.	**K.** Stem cells
______	**12.** A disease in which the number of plasma cells in the bone marrow increases abnormally, causing tumors to form in the bones.	**L.** Thalassemia
______	**13.** Cells that can develop into other types of cells in the body.	**M.** Thrombocytes
______	**14.** An acute, painful enlargement of the spleen caused by sickle cell disease.	**N.** Thrombocytosis
______	**15.** A disease that causes the red blood cells to be misshapen, resulting in poor oxygen-carrying capability and potentially resulting in lodging of the red blood cells in blood vessels or the spleen.	**O.** Thrombosis
______	**16.** A component of blood, made of 92% water and 6% to 7% proteins, as well as electrolytes, clotting factors, and glucose; this component accounts for 55% of the total blood volume.	**P.** Transfusion reaction
______	**17.** An abnormally low number of neutrophils.	**Q.** Transfusion-related lung injury
______	**18.** A condition in which a patient with sickle cell disease experiences significant pain due to insufficient passage of oxygen and nutrients into tissues and joints because of vessel congestion.	**R.** Vasoocclusive crisis

Multiple Choice

Read each item carefully, and then select the best response.

_____ **1.** During the history taking and secondary assessment of a patient with a hematologic emergency, it is important to do all of the following, EXCEPT:

A. look for changes in level of consciousness.
B. obtain a SAMPLE history.
C. check for skin color changes and itching.
D. interview the family; confidentiality rules dictate that the family not be present.

_____ **2.** Common findings with patients with blood disorders include which of the following?

A. Bone fractures
B. Mental health disorders
C. "Clubbed" nails
D. Epistaxis

_____ **3.** Assessment and management of patients with hemophilia include which of the following procedures?

A. Controlling bleeding
B. Administering high-flow supplemental oxygen
C. Administering an analgesic
D. All of the above

_____ **4.** All of the following organs assist in the production of red blood cells (RBCs), EXCEPT the:

A. medulla.
B. liver.
C. spleen.
D. bone marrow.

_____ **5.** Sickle cell disease is associated with low readings of:

A. RBCs.
B. hematocrit.
C. thrombocytes.
D. hemoglobin.

_____ **6.** Which blood type is considered the universal donor?

A. AB
B. A
C. O
D. B

_____ **7.** Patients with leukemia may have which of the following signs and symptoms?

A. Frequent urinary tract infections
B. No symptoms
C. Unexplained bleeding
D. Spontaneous pneumothorax

_____ **8.** Disseminated intravascular coagulopathy (DIC):

A. has a mortality rate of 60% to 65%.
B. has a mortality rate of 10% to 15%.
C. is rarely fatal.
D. can be prevented with a large fluid bolus.

_____ **9.** Assessment and management of patients with multiple myeloma include which of the following procedures?

A. IV therapy using a Bone Injection Gun (BIG) device
B. Pain management
C. Supplemental oxygen via continuous positive airway pressure (CPAP)
D. Transport with multiple IV lines in place

______ **10.** Blood performs which of the following functions?

A. Transports oxygen from the lungs to the tissues
B. Ferries waste products of metabolism
C. Carries hormones from the endocrine glands to target tissues
D. All of the above

Labeling

Label the following diagrams with the correct terms.

1. Major organs for producing and regulating the blood

A. ______________________________

B. ______________________________

C. ______________________________

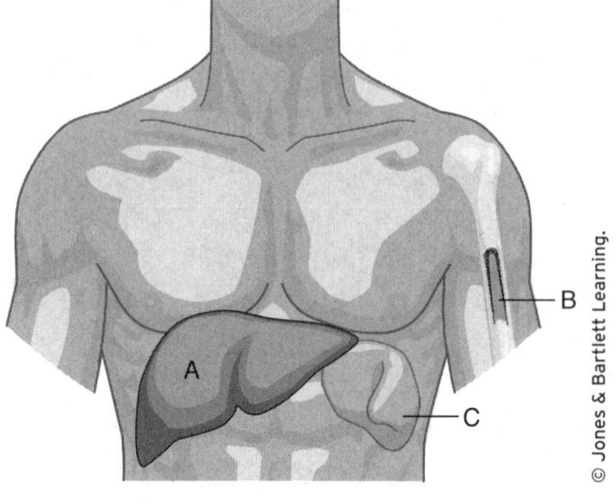

Fill in the Blank

Read each item carefully, and then complete the statement by filling in the missing word(s).

1. Blood is a(n) __________ tissue.

2. The __________ system includes blood components and the organs involved in their development and production.

3. The formed elements of blood include red __________ __________, white __________ __________, and __________.

4. Red blood cell production occurs within __________ __________.

5. __________ __________, __________ __________, and __________ are three common laboratory tests done on blood samples.

6. __________ are the smallest of the formed elements and are responsible for the clotting of blood.

7. __________ __________ is a painless, progressive enlargement of the lymphoid glands, most commonly affecting the spleen and the lymph nodes.

8. The most common inherited blood disorder is called __________ __________ __________.

9. Patients with leukemia frequently present with __________, __________, or __________.

10. Patients with lymphoma may require __________ management.

11. In __________, the body's ability to clot is decreased due to the absence of a key protein that is necessary for platelet adhesion.

12. The phenomenon in which oxygen-rich RBCs release oxygen as a result of being in an environment that contains higher concentrations of carbon dioxide is called the __________.

Identify

Read the following case studies, and then list the chief complaint, vital signs, and pertinent negatives.

1. You are called to the home of a 42-year-old woman with a history of metastatic cancer and bone marrow transplant. Her chief complaint is extreme weakness, fatigue, and exertional dyspnea. You find the patient lying in bed conscious and alert, although she appears very "withdrawn" and weighs about 90 lb. She denies chest pain or shortness of breath. She tells you that she does not have any energy, and the doctor's office wants her back in the hospital. Her vital signs are as follows: Pulse is 86 beats/min, slightly irregular, and difficult to palpate; blood pressure (BP) is also difficult to auscultate but appears to be 92/P mm Hg. The patient's skin is pale, warm, and dry. She has an oxygen saturation of 91% on ambient air. Her pupils are equal, round, and reactive to light and accommodation (PERRLA). She has a central IV port in place.
   a. Chief complaint:

   ____

   ____

   b. Vital signs:

   ____

   ____

   c. Pertinent negatives:

   ____

   ____

2. Your unit is dispatched to a high-priority "Charlie" response to Middle Road Elementary School. The dispatch information indicates the patient is a 10-year-old boy with near syncope. Once inside the nurse's office, you recognize your patient—you have transported him several times in the past. For years, he has been treated for leukemia. His mother is on the scene, and she appears comforted to see a familiar face. She explains that her son just returned to school full time after his latest round of treatments. As you speak to the patient, it is apparent that his mental status is slightly altered. However, when you ask him about his favorite topic, baseball, he becomes quite talkative. En route to the hospital, his vital signs indicate that he is now conscious and alert. He does not remember the near syncope. His radial pulses are equal bilaterally and regular at 86 beats/min. He currently denies any complaints as the baseball conversation continues. BP is 98/64 mm Hg. His skin is jaundiced but cool and dry. Pupils are PERRLA. The oxygen saturation is 98% on a nonrebreathing mask. The patient has central IV access. You contact medical control for direction and are told to continue transport while monitoring his ABCs. His IV will be activated in the emergency department (ED).
   a. Chief complaint:

   ____

   ____

   b. Vital signs:

   ____

   ____

   c. Pertinent negatives:

   ____

   ____

3. It has been a rather busy day, with mostly routine emergency calls. However, this call is a little different. A man with a history of sickle cell disease is having an acute crisis and is in extreme pain. He states that the pain is breaking through his oral morphine tablets and fentanyl transdermal patch. He reports his pain as a 9 on a scale of 1 to 10. According to the patient, this is the worst sickle cell pain that he has ever had. His vital signs are as follows: Pulse is 112 beats/min and regular; skin is pale, warm, and moist; and BP is 148/96 mm Hg. Pupils are PERRLA. His pulse oximetry reading is 91%. The patient is anxious and keeps telling you to "get the rubber on the road."
   a. Chief complaint:

   ____

   ____

   b. Vital signs:

   ____

   ____

   c. Pertinent negatives:

   ____

   ____

Ambulance Calls

The following case scenarios provide an opportunity to explore the concerns associated with patient management and paramedic care. Read each scenario, and then answer each question.

1. You are transporting a patient from the local community hospital to a regional trauma center. The patient's vital signs are stable when you start the transport. He has a unit of blood running. Shortly after you set out, the patient begins complaining of severe back pain. Soon thereafter he breaks out in a cold sweat, his lips take on a bluish tinge, and his neck veins seem to bulge out. You check his pulse, and it is 60 beats/min. A few minutes later, when you check it again, it is 110 beats/min.
   a. The patient is showing signs of a(n):
      (1) allergic reaction to the transfusion.
      (2) hemolytic reaction to the transfusion.
      (3) air embolism.
      (4) pyrogenic reaction to the transfusion.
      (5) thrombophlebitis.

   b. List the steps you will take to deal with the situation.

      (1)______________________________

      (2)______________________________

      (3)______________________________

      (4)______________________________

2. You and your partner receive a call for a 76-year-old man with a severe hemorrhage. On arrival, you find the patient's 49-year-old daughter hysterical on the front porch. She states that her father is "bleeding to death." She is too excited and emotional to provide any additional information. You enter the house and are directed to the bathroom. You are met by a rather pleasant but obviously frustrated 76-year-old man. There is a minimal amount of blood in the sink. He is holding a tissue to his carotid region and states that he cut himself shaving. He is very apologetic for and embarrassed about his daughter's behavior. He states that he has a history of a blood disorder called polycythemia, and he wears a medical identification bracelet.

a. What is polycythemia, and what are some of the symptoms?

____

____

____

b. How would you treat a patient who exhibits signs and symptoms of polycythemia?

____

____

____

True/False

If you believe the statement to be more true than false, write the letter "T" in the space provided. If you believe the statement to be more false than true, write the letter "F."

_____ **1.** White blood cells are responsible for transporting oxygenated blood.

_____ **2.** Red blood cell production occurs in the pancreas.

_____ **3.** "Clot busters" activate the fibrinolytic system, resulting in clot decomposition.

_____ **4.** The "universal donor" is a person with AB blood type.

_____ **5.** Malignant diseases that occur within the lymphoid system are called lymphomas.

_____ **6.** Phlebotomy is the treatment of choice for patients with disseminated intravascular coagulopathy.

_____ **7.** In multiple myeloma, abnormal plasma cells infiltrate the bone marrow.

_____ **8.** Patients with hematologic diseases might have symptoms that include vertigo, fatigue, or syncopal episodes.

_____ **9.** Oxygen is generally contraindicated for patients with red blood cell abnormalities.

_____ **10.** Paramedics should be supportive and communicate therapeutically with the patient with a suspected blood disorder.

Short Answer

Complete this section with short written answers using the space provided.

1. Blood disorders present differently from other typical injuries and diseases encountered by paramedics. Provide some of the common findings as they relate to the following:

a. Level of consciousness

____

____

____

b. Skin

____

____

____

c. Visual disturbances

____

____

____

d. Gastrointestinal system

____

____

____

e. Skeletal system

____

____

____

f. Cardiovascular system

____

____

____

g. Genitourinary system

____

____

____

2. Assessment and treatment of patients with blood disorders may differ slightly from assessment and treatment of patients with more typical diseases encountered by paramedics. Describe how the treatment and assessment of the following diseases differ.

a. Leukemia

(1) _______________

(2) _______________

(3) _______________

(4) _______________

(5) _______________

b. Hemophilia

(1) _______________

(2) _______________

(3) _______________

(4) _______________

c. Polycythemia
(1) ______
(2) ______
(3) ______
(4) ______
(5) ______
(6) ______

3. Define the following vocabulary words:
a. Leukopenia:
______
b. Polycythemia:
______
c. Reticuloendothelial system:
______
d. Pruritus:
______
e. Hematocrit:
______
f. Melena:
______

Fill in the Table

Fill in the missing parts of the table.

ABO Rh Type and Preferred and Alternative Donor Types		
Recipient Blood Type	**Preferred Donor Type**	**Additional Permissible Types**
A+	A+	A–, O+, O–
AB+	AB+	AB–, A+, A–, B+, B–, O+, O–
B+	B+	B–, O+, O–
O+	O+	O–

Data from: Applegate EJ. *The Anatomy and Physiology Learning System*. 4th ed. Philadelphia, PA: Saunders; 2011.

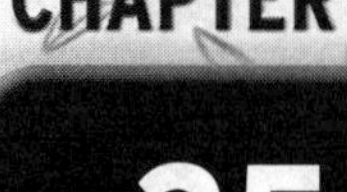

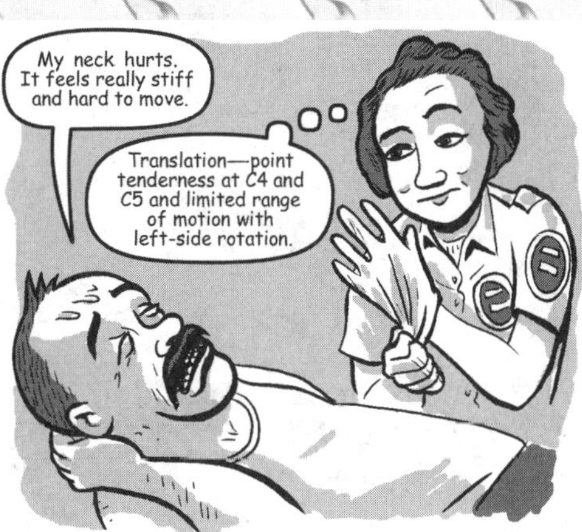

Immunologic Emergencies

Matching

Part I

Match each of the items in the left column to the appropriate definition in the right column.

_____	**1.** A group of autoimmune disorders that affect the collagen in tendons, bones, and connective tissues.	**A.** Absorption
_____	**2.** A chemical found in mast cells that, when released, causes vasodilation, capillary leaking, and bronchiole constriction.	**B.** Allergen
_____	**3.** Occurs when a patient reacts with exaggerated or inappropriate allergic symptoms after coming into contact with a substance the body perceives as harmful.	**C.** Allergic reaction
_____	**4.** White blood cells that work to produce chemical mediators during an immune response.	**D.** Anaphylactoid reaction
_____	**5.** A two-phase allergic reaction in which the patient's symptoms improve and then reappear without being exposed to the trigger (allergen) a second time; the symptoms can resurface up to 8 or more hours after the initial incident.	**E.** Anaphylaxis
_____	**6.** Chemicals that work to cause the immune or allergic response; for example, histamine.	**F.** Antibody
_____	**7.** Eating or drinking materials for absorption through the gastrointestinal tract.	**G.** Antigen
_____	**8.** In allergic reactions, foreign substances are breathed in through the respiratory system.	**H.** Basophils
_____	**9.** In allergic reactions, when foreign material is deposited on and moves into the skin.	**I.** Biphasic reaction
_____	**10.** A substance that produces allergic symptoms in a patient.	**J.** Chemical mediators
_____	**11.** An abnormal immune response the body develops when reexposed to a substance or allergen.	**K.** Collagen vascular diseases
_____	**12.** An agent that, when taken into the body, stimulates the formation of specific protective proteins called antibodies.	**L.** Histamine
_____	**13.** A protein the body produces ion response to an antigen; an immunoglobulin.	**M.** Hypersensitivity
_____	**14.** An extreme systemic form of an allergic reaction involving one, two, or more body systems.	**N.** Ingestion
_____	**15.** An extreme allergic response that does not involve IgE antibody mediation. The exact mechanism is unknown, but an event of this type may occur without the patient being previously exposed to the offending agent.	**O.** Inhalation

Part II

Match each of the items in the left column to the appropriate definition in the right column.

_____ 1. The ability to recognize a foreign substance the next time it is encountered.

_____ 2. The body's reaction when it is exposed to an antigen for which it already has antibodies, in which it responds by killing the invading substance.

_____ 3. An autoimmune connective tissue disease that causes fibrotic (scar tissue-like) changes to the skin, blood vessels, muscles, and internal organs.

_____ 4. Hives or reddened elevated patches on the skin.

_____ 5. A reaction that occurs throughout the body, possibly affecting multiple body systems.

_____ 6. A multisystem autoimmune disease.

_____ 7. Itching.

_____ 8. Anaphylaxis symptoms that continue over time, with time frames anywhere from 5 to 32 hours.

_____ 9. The first encounter with the foreign substance to begin the immune response.

_____ 10. In allergic reactions, when the skin is pierced, and foreign material is deposited into the skin.

_____ 11. When the body limits a response to a specific area after being exposed to a foreign substance.

_____ 12. Basophils that are located in the tissues.

A. Injection
B. Local reaction
C. Mast cells
D. Primary response
E. Prolonged (persistent) reaction
F. Pruritus
G. Scleroderma
H. Secondary response
I. Sensitivity
J. Systemic lupus erythematosus
K. Systemic reaction
L. Urticaria

Multiple Choice

For the following questions, select the best response based on the scenario provided.

It's been a slow shift, so you decide to grab a quick dinner at Bill's Steak 'n Lobster. You park your ambulance outside and find a table near the door, in case you have to leave in a hurry on a call. You've just had your medium-rare sirloin placed in front of you when you notice a woman at the next table who does not look well. You ask her if there is anything the matter. "I don't know," she says in a very squeaky voice. "I have this lump in my throat, and I feel like I'm going to die," whereupon she collapses to the floor.

_____ 1. This woman is MOST likely experiencing:
A. food poisoning.
B. choking.
C. strep throat.
D. anaphylaxis.

_____ 2. The treatment you need to give MOST urgently is:
A. pumping out her stomach.
B. administering 6 to 10 manual abdominal thrusts.
C. having her gargle with saltwater.
D. administering epinephrine.

_____ 3. Assuming the patient is having an acute anaphylactic reaction, what other medications might be helpful?
A. Nitroglycerin sublingual
B. Corticosteroids
C. Morphine sulfate
D. Narcan

_____ 4. You decide to administer diphenhydramine (Benadryl) to your patient as well. You determine that Benadryl may also be helpful at this time because it blocks:
A. beta receptor sites.
B. alpha receptor sites.
C. neurotransmitters that cause respiratory distress.
D. histamine receptors.

_____ **5.** While assessing and treating your patient, you discover a used EpiPen next to her collapsed body. The EpiPen auto-injector (if used properly) would have administered:

A. 1 mg of solution IM.
B. 1 mg of solution IV.
C. 0.5 mg of solution subcutaneously.
D. 0.3 mg of solution IM.

_____ **6.** The patient is responding slowly to the epinephrine. Which of the following medications may also be helpful if medical control concurs?

A. Glucagon
B. Albuterol
C. A corticosteroid
D. All of the above

The patient's mother explains that the baby had been up all night tugging at her ear and crying inconsolably. She has been running a low-grade fever that appears to respond well to pediatric Tylenol (acetaminophen). Today the baby went to the pediatrician, who prescribed liquid amoxicillin for an ear infection. After the first dose of the strawberry-flavored antibiotic, the baby began to vomit and appeared to stop breathing. Emergency Medical Services (EMS) was called. On your arrival, the child appeared conscious and alert and was acting appropriately for her age.

_____ **7.** The baby was MOST likely suffering from:

A. an anaphylactic reaction.
B. a localized reaction.
C. no reaction; sometimes sick children vomit and appear to hold their breath.
D. a systemic reaction.

_____ **8.** If the small child were having a reaction to the antibiotic, what would be the correct course of treatment?

A. Secure the ABCs, consider pharmacologic intervention in concert with medical control, and assess the need for rapid but safe transport to an appropriate facility.
B. Initiate rapid transport, and perform all assessment and treatment modalities en route.
C. After securing the patient's ABCs, administer IM Benadryl (diphenhydramine) immediately.
D. Contact medical control for further instructions.

_____ **9.** What was the "route" of exposure?

A. Exposure
B. Inhalation
C. Ingestion
D. Injection

_____ **10.** Of the following substances, which is NOT considered one of the body's chemical weapons designed to fight off the antigen?

A. Kinins
B. Serotonin
C. Norepinephrine
D. Prostaglandin

_____ **11.** What would be the prehospital implication for the paramedic caring for a lupus patient exhibiting symptoms of pneumonia?

A. You should assess for history of renal failure and electrolyte imbalance.
B. You should assess for a fever, tachypnea, cough, and/or worsening of chest pain.
C. You should monitor the patient for stroke and seizure precautions.
D. Be sure to collect a history that includes bloody stools and gastrointestinal (GI) distress.

_____ **12.** What is the MOST common type of transplant patient in the United States?

A. Liver
B. Heart
C. Skin
D. Kidney

Labeling

Use the following figure to answer the questions regarding anaphylaxis.

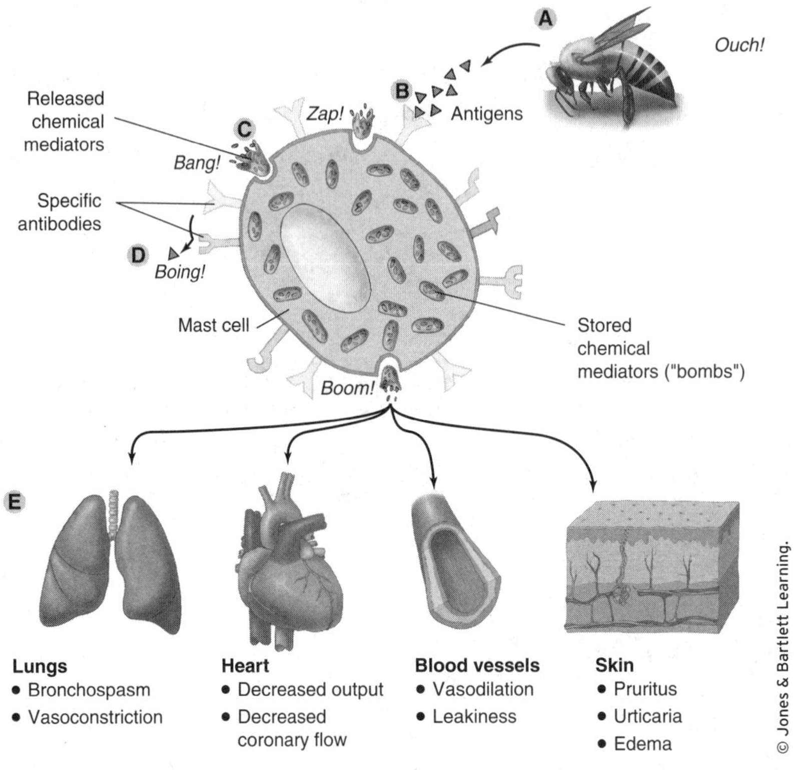

1. What is the first form of attack on the human body?

____

2. What types of cells are released?

____

3. What signs and symptoms may be present in the respiratory system?

____

4. What are the negative cardiovascular signs/symptoms that may be present?

____

5. Are there any effects to the circulatory system? If so, list them.

____

6. The skin is often the first place to show signs/symptoms; what are they?

____

Fill in the Blank

Read each item carefully, and then complete the statement by filling in the missing word(s).

1. Through the ________ response, the body develops ______, that is, the ability to recognize the antigen the next time it is encountered.

2. The _________ response occurs with ___________ to a foreign substance.

3. A protein the body produces in response to an antigen is a(n) __________.

4. __________ cells meet and greet invaders.

5. __________ is a chemical found in mast cells.

6. A(n) __________ __________ airway is an early sign of impending airway occlusion due to swelling.

7. A(n) _________ reaction occurs throughout the body, possibly affecting _______ body systems.

8. __________ occurs when a person's ________ system reacts with _______ or inappropriate symptoms after coming into contact with a substance perceived by the body to be harmful.

9. _________ vascular diseases are considered _________ diseases, which means that the body perceives its own tissues or cells as a dangerous invader.

10. High-flow __________ should be given to each anaphylactic patient.

Identify

In the following case studies, list the chief complaint, vital signs, and pertinent negatives.

1. You are treating a 16-year-old girl who was stung by a bee at her pool. She complains of hives and itching at the sting site. She denies respiratory distress or trouble swallowing. She states that she has never been stung before and doesn't carry an EpiPen. She is conscious and alert. Her skin color is normal, warm, and dry. Capillary refill is normal. Her oxygen saturation is 99%, blood pressure (BP) is 112/68 mm Hg, and pupils are equal, round, and reactive to light and accommodation (PERRLA).
   a. Chief complaint:

   ____

   ____

   b. Vital signs:

   ____

   ____

   c. Pertinent negatives:

   ____

   ____

2. You are called to a rural location for a 23-year-old man who states that he was bitten by a tick. He appears scared, but other than being "grossed-out," he has no complaint. The tick is still attached to his leg. After removing the tick, you assess his vital signs. He is conscious and alert. His pulse is 110 beats/min and regular, BP is 142/84 mm Hg, PERRLA, and skin is warm and moist. The patient has no previous medical history, no allergies, and no known drug allergies.
   a. Chief complaint:

   ____

   ____

   b. Vital signs:

   ____

   ____

c. Pertinent negatives:

______

______

3. A Priority One response directs you to Uptown Elementary School for an eighth grader complaining of trouble breathing and swallowing after ingesting brownies brought by a classmate. The student is in a class that has signs posted designating it as a "peanut-free" environment. The student has a medical identification bracelet indicating a severe allergy to peanuts and any by-products. The school nurse believes that the student accidentally ingested peanuts that were ingredients in the brownies. The student is conscious and alert, anxious, and speaking in a raspy voice. He has redness around his face and neck. Vital signs are pulse of 124 beats/min, oxygen saturation of 90%, and BP of 90/62 mm Hg.

a. Chief complaint:

______

______

b. Vital signs:

______

______

c. Pertinent negatives:

______

______

4. It's about 2200 hours. You respond to a call for an allergic reaction to seafood. On arrival, you are met by a 32-year-old woman who states that she's allergic to shellfish and iodine. She speaks in complete full sentences and complains of nausea and vomiting. While giving her medical history, she indicates that she has never had a reaction previously to eating fish. While assessing your patient, you note the following vital signs: Her pulse is 124 beats/min and regular, oxygen saturation is 90% on ambient air, and BP is easily auscultated at 112/62 mm Hg.

a. Chief complaint:

______

______

b. Vital signs:

______

______

c. Pertinent negatives:

______

______

5. It's late in the morning, and you are responding to a reported allergic reaction in a 10-month-old boy. Dispatch advises that the child was at the pediatrician today for a well-baby check. While there, the child received several immunizations. The child is now lethargic and gasping for breath. The child presents with urticaria all over. The baby has no other reported medical history or reported allergies. The apical pulse is 190 beats/min. The infant has delayed capillary refill and mottled skin.

a. Chief complaint:

______

______

b. Vital signs:

____

____

c. Pertinent negatives:

____

____

Ambulance Calls

The following case scenarios provide an opportunity to explore the concerns associated with patient management and paramedic care. Read each scenario, and then answer each question.

1. You are called to the suburban home of a 58-year-old man with "shortness of breath." You learn that while gardening, the patient was stung by numerous bees; within minutes, he noticed a tight feeling in his chest and started to wheeze. Now, 10 minutes after the sting, he looks flushed and very apprehensive and has a rash on the front of his chest. His vital signs are a pulse of 124 beats/min and slightly irregular, respirations of 36 breaths/min and shallow, and BP of 86/50 mm Hg. His SpO_2 is 93%.

a. List the steps in managing this patient.

(1)____

(2)____

(3)____

(4)____

(5)____

(6)____

(7)____

(8)____

b. One of the drugs that you will be giving is epinephrine. List the possible adverse effects or side effects of epinephrine.

(1)____

(2)____

(3)____

(4)____

(5)____

2. You are dining out on your night off at Fish Fare, a local restaurant. As you are just about to dig into your red snapper, you notice a woman at a nearby table looking distressed. "Aunt Gertrude, what's the matter?" asks another woman at the table.

"I don't know," squeaks the distressed woman. "I feel so peculiar. Like there's a lump in my throat. And my chest feels so tight."

Without waiting to hear another word, you bolt over to the telephone, dial 9-1-1, and ask for an ambulance posthaste. Then you go over to the woman in distress and introduce yourself as a paramedic. You notice that the woman's face is very flushed, and her eyes look puffy. Her pulse is weak and rapid.

"Oh, dear, I think I'm going to be sick," she says.
Just then, the ambulance pulls up. List the steps in treating this patient.

a. ____

b. ____

c. ____

d. ____

e. ____

3. Which of the following patients is most likely to be experiencing an anaphylactic reaction? (For those who are not, indicate what you think they are suffering from.)

a. A 45-year-old man is dining at a fast-food joint. Suddenly he grows very pale and lurches back from the table, clutching his throat, with his eyes popping. He staggers to his feet and then collapses to the floor—all in complete silence. His problem is most likely:

____

b. You are summoned for a 60-year-old man having a "bad reaction" to a medicine. Earlier in the day, the patient was prescribed erythromycin for a respiratory infection. Now he complains of severe abdominal distress and nausea. On physical examination, his skin is slightly pale and cool. His pulse is 72 beats/min and regular, his respirations are 22 breaths/min and unlabored, and his BP is 160/94 mm Hg. His problem is most likely:

____

c. A 22-year-old man is found sitting on the sidewalk in marked distress. He tells you hoarsely that he just got "a shot" at the venereal disease (VD) clinic down the street, and right after he was given the shot and sent home, he started to feel "real strange." He says he got hot and itchy all over, and now he feels like he's going to die. On physical examination, his face looks quite flushed and puffy. His pulse is 140 beats/min and thready, his respirations are 32 breaths/min and shallow, and his BP is 110/60 mm Hg. His problem is most likely:

____

4. List the steps you would take to manage the patient described in Question 3.

a. ____

b. ____

c. ____

d. ____

e. ____

5. After you report to medical control regarding the patient in Question 3, the physician instructs you to give diphenhydramine (Benadryl) as well. Per the Volume 1 Appendix, *Emergency Medications*, what are the contraindications to giving diphenhydramine?

a. ____

b. ____

c. ____

d. ____

e. ____

6. What are the correct dosage and route of administration in this case?

____

Complete the Patient Care Report (PCR)

Read the first incident scenario in the Ambulance Calls section, and then complete the following PCR.

EMS Patient Care Report (PCR)			
Date:	Incident No.:	Nature of Call:	Location:

Dispatched:	En Route:	At Scene:	Transport:	At Hospital:	In Service:

Patient Information	
Age: Sex: Weight (in kg [lb]):	Allergies: Medications: Past Medical History: Chief Complaint:

Vital Signs				
Time:	BP:	Pulse:	Respirations:	SpO_2:
Time:	BP:	Pulse:	Respirations:	SpO_2:
Time:	BP:	Pulse:	Respirations:	SpO_2:

EMS Treatment (circle all that apply)				
Oxygen @ ______ L/min via (circle one): NC NRM Bag-mask device		Assisted Ventilation	Airway Adjunct	CPR
Defibrillation	Bleeding Control	Bandaging	Splinting	Other:

Narrative

True/False

If you believe the statement to be more true than false, write the letter "T" in the space provided. If you believe the statement to be more false than true, write the letter "F."

_____ 1. All patients who exhibit signs and symptoms of allergic reaction should receive epinephrine.

_____ 2. Patients should be educated to wear medical identification tags and carry their prescribed anaphylaxis kit.

_____ 3. Corticosteroids can be used for anaphylaxis.

_____ 4. Epinephrine has beta-1 properties that cause the blood vessels to constrict, reducing vasodilation.

_____ 5. Bee stingers are best removed with sharp, pointy tweezers.

_____ 6. Millions of Americans are at risk for anaphylaxis.

_____ 7. Allergens can invade the body through the skin, respiratory tract, or GI tract.

_____ 8. The respiratory system usually protects the human body from substances and organisms that are considered foreign to the body.

_____ 9. An inhaled beta-adrenergic agent can be used for a patient with an allergic reaction with bronchospasm.

_____ 10. The time of onset after administration of corticosteroids is 4 to 6 hours.

Short Answer

Complete this section with short written answers using the space provided.

1. When an antigen combines with a specific antibody on the surface of a mast cell, the mast cell loses its chemical bombs ("degranulates," to use the technical term), releasing a variety of powerful mediators, such as histamine and serotonin. List seven effects produced by the mediator "histamine."

   a. ____________________

   b. ____________________

   c. ____________________

   d. ____________________

   e. ____________________

   f. ____________________

   g. ____________________

2. Besides bees, what other agents are commonly responsible for anaphylactic reactions? List at least four.

   a. ____________________

   b. ____________________

   c. ____________________

   d. ____________________

Fill in the Table

Fill in the missing parts of the table with examples of the common substances associated with anaphylaxis.

Causes of Anaphylactic Reactions	
Antigen, General Category	**Comments**
Foods	
Medications	
Insect stings	
Anti-cancer drugs	
Latex	
Animals	

Data from Mustafa S. Anaphylaxis. Medscape website. http://emedicine.medscape.com/article/135065-overview#a4. Updated February 22, 2017. Accessed March 31, 2017; and Peroni DG, Sansotta N, Bernardini R, et al. Muscle relaxants allergy. Int J Immunopathol Pharmacol. 2011;24(3 Suppl):S35-46. Pub Med Abstract. https://www.ncbi.nlm.nih.gov/pubmed/22014924. Accessed January 17, 2017.

CHAPTER 26

Infectious Diseases

The cycle of infection can often be easily broken by handwashing.

Matching

Part I

Match each of the items in the left column to the appropriate term in the right column.

_____ **1.** A sexually transmitted disease caused by the bacterium *Chlamydia trachomatis*; has the highest incidence in sexually transmitted diseases; signs and symptoms include inflammation of the urethra, epididymis, cervix, and fallopian tubes and discharge from the urethra.

_____ **2.** A pathogen is present but has produced no illness in the host; often progresses to active infection; a colonized host is often called a carrier because he or she can transmit the pathogen to others.

_____ **3.** An infectious disease that can be transmitted from one person to another by direct contact or by indirect contact through a vector or fomite; also called contagious disease.

_____ **4.** A virus that originated in Africa and is transmitted by the *Aedes aegypti* mosquito; signs and symptoms include fever that typically lasts from 5 to 7 days, and possibly incapacitating joint pain.

_____ **5.** A highly contagious sexually transmitted disease caused by the bacteria *Haemophilus ducreyi,* which causes painful sores (ulcers), usually of the genitals.

_____ **6.** Consistently present or prevalent in a population or geographic area.

_____ **7.** A virus formerly limited to West Africa, spread through direct contact through nonintact skin or mucous membranes, and whose initial symptoms include fever, intense weakness, muscle pain, headaches, and sore throat; both contact and droplet precautions are needed with this disease; approximately 10% of infected people experience internal or external bleeding.

_____ **8.** The transmission of an infectious agent by inhalation of relatively large particles generated when an infected person coughs or sneezes; these particles travel a short distance through the air before falling to the ground.

_____ **9.** Use of a surgical mask on the patient and airflow measures to prevent droplet transmission; used for patients with possible influenza, meningitis, pertussis (whooping cough), mumps, rubella (German measles), and Ebola.

_____ **10.** A person trained to ensure that proper postexposure medical treatment and counseling are provided to an exposure employee or volunteer.

_____ **11.** An overgrowth of bacteria in the vagina, characterized by itching, burning, or pain and possibly a fishy-smelling discharge.

A. Acquired immunodeficiency syndrome (AIDS)

B. Airborne precautions

C. Airborne transmission

D. Avian (bird) flu

E. Bacteria

F. Bacterial vaginosis

G. Bloodborne pathogens

H. Candidiasis

I. Carriers

J. Chancre

K. Chancroid

______	**12.** Small organisms that can grow and reproduce outside the human cell in the presence of the needed temperature and nutrients and cause disease by invading and multiplying in the tissues of the host.	**L.** Chikungunya
______	**13.** A disease caused by a virus that occurs naturally in the bird population; signs and symptoms include fever, sore throat, cough, and muscle aches.	**M.** Chlamydia
______	**14.** The transmission of an infectious agent by inhalation of small particles that become aerosolized when the infected person coughs, sneezes, talks, or exhales; particles remain suspended in this vapor and can be carried a short distance, usually 3 feet (1 m) to 6 feet (2 m).	**N.** Colonized
______	**15.** The use of a surgical mask on the patient and the use of airflow measures to prevent airborne transmission; apply to diseases that are large particle and can travel a distance of 6 feet (2 m), then drop to the floor.	**O.** Communicable disease
______	**16.** A virus transmitted by the mosquitos *Aedes aegypti* and *Aedes albopictus*, found throughout the world, in which the majority of people are asymptomatic; if the severe form develops, it is characterized by hypovolemic shock, hemorrhage, and potentially death.	**P.** Communicable period
______	**17.** The presence of blood or other potentially infectious materials on an item or surface.	**Q.** Contact precautions
______	**18.** The transmission of an infectious agent by means of direct or indirect contact with the infected persons, such as skin-to-skin contact or contact with the patient's environment and/or equipment.	**R.** Contact transmission
______	**19.** The use of precautions (gloves, gown, good handwashing, and cleaning of high-touch items) to prevent contact transmission; used for patients presenting with draining wounds, multidrug-resistant infection, lice, norovirus, and Ebola.	**S.** Contaminated
______	**20.** The period during which an infected person can transmit a communicable disease to someone else.	**T.** Dengue
______	**21.** The end-stage disease process caused by the human immunodeficiency virus; results in extreme vulnerability to numerous opportunistic bacterial, viral, and fungal infections that would not affect a person with an intact immune system.	**U.** Designated infection control officer (DICO)
______	**22.** The primary hard lesion or ulcer of syphilis that occurs at the entry site of the infection.	**V.** Droplet precautions
______	**23.** People who harbor an infectious agent and, although not personally ill, can transmit the infection to other people.	**W.** Droplet transmission
______	**24.** A vaginal infection that is not technically a sexually transmitted infection, and that can occur in a pregnant or nonpregnant female, but is more common in pregnancy; also called thrush or a yeast infection.	**X.** Ebola
______	**25.** Pathogenic microorganisms that are present in human blood and can cause disease in humans. These pathogens include, but are not limited to, hepatitis B virus, human immunodeficiency virus, hepatitis C virus, and syphilis.	**Y.** Endemic

Part II

Match each of the items in the left column to the appropriate term in the right column.

______	**1.** An infectious viral disease that occurs most often in late winter and spring; begins with a fever followed by a cough, running nose; and pinkeye; a rash spreads from the face and neck down the back and trunk.	**A.** Epidemic
______	**2.** A tick-borne disease that primarily affects the skin, heart, joints, and nervous system and is characterized by a round, red lesion or bull's-eye rash.	**B.** Enterococcus
______	**3.** Tiny, wingless, parasitic insects that feed on blood; an infestation is easily spread through close personal contact; types include head, body, and pubic lice.	**C.** Fomites

_____	**4.** The presence of excessive bile pigments in the bloodstream that give the skin, mucous membranes, and eyes a distinct yellow color; often associated with liver disease.	**D.** Fungi
_____	**5.** A disease originating from the Arabian peninsula, transmitted by close contact with camel urine or nasal secretions. Symptoms include fever, cough, and shortness of breath, and gastrointestinal disturbances; there is very low risk to health care providers and the general public in the United States.	**E.** Gastroenteritis
_____	**6.** A type of meningitis caused by the meningococcal bacterium, *Neisseria meningitidis*.	**F.** Genital warts
_____	**7.** An inflammation of the meningeal coverings of the brain and spinal cord; usually caused by a virus or bacterium; the viral type is not communicable and is less severe than the bacterial type, which can result in brain damage, hearing loss, learning disability, or death.	**G.** Gonorrhea
_____	**8.** The period between exposure to an organism and the first symptoms of illness, during which the organism multiplies within the body and starts to produce symptoms. This period is when the disease can be transmitted to another person.	**H.** Hantavirus
_____	**9.** The process of producing widespread immunity to a specific infectious disease among a targeted group by inoculating individual members of the population; can also refer to a set of vaccinations given together or on a recommended schedule.	**I.** Health care–associated infection
_____	**10.** The yellow appearance of the skin and other tissues caused by an accumulation of bile pigments.	**J.** Host resistance
_____	**11.** The most common sexually transmitted disease that can cause genital warts and some types of cancer.	**K.** Human immunodeficiency virus (HIV)
_____	**12.** The virus that may lead to acquired immunodeficiency syndrome; cells in the immune system are killed or damaged so that the body is unable to fight infections and certain cancers.	**L.** Human papilloma virus (HPV)
_____	**13.** A term that comprises many types of infections and irritations of the gastrointestinal tract; symptoms include nausea and vomiting, fever, abdominal cramps, and diarrhea; also called stomach flu.	**M.** Icterus jaundice
_____	**14.** Small organisms that can grow rapidly in the presence of the needed nutrients and organic material and can cause infection related to contact with decaying organic matter or from airborne spores in the environment such as molds.	**N.** Immunization
_____	**15.** Inanimate objects contaminated with microorganisms that serve as a means of transmitting an illness.	**O.** Incubation period
_____	**16.** A common, normal organism of the gastrointestinal tract, urinary tract, and genitourinary tract that can be pathogenic and become resistant to vancomycin.	**P.** Infectious disease
_____	**17.** An outbreak of disease that substantially exceeds what is expected based on recent experience.	**Q.** Infectious hepatitis
_____	**18.** A sexually transmitted disease that results in infection caused by the gonococcal bacteria *Neisseria gonorrhea*; signs and symptoms include pus-containing discharge from the urethra and painful urination in males and signs and symptoms of an acute abdomen in females.	**R.** Influenza
_____	**19.** Warts caused by the human papillomavirus, a sexually transmitted disease; also called condylomata acuminata or venereal warts.	**S.** Jaundice
_____	**20.** A type of virus found in wild rodents, which can also cause disease in humans, characterized by fever, headache, abdominal pain, loss of appetite, and vomiting; diseases caused are hemorrhagic fever with renal syndrome and hantavirus pulmonary syndrome.	**T.** Lice

_____	**21.** An infection acquired 2 days after admission to a health care setting or 30 days after discharge from one.	**U.** Lyme disease
_____	**22.** One's ability to fight off infection.	**V.** Measles
_____	**23.** The flu, a respiratory infection caused by a variety of viruses; differs from the common cold in that the flu involves a fever, headache, and extreme exhaustion.	**W.** Meningitis
_____	**24.** Another name for hepatitis A; an inflammation from a virus that causes mild fatigue, loss of appetite, fever, nausea, abdominal pain, and, eventually, jaundice, dark-colored urine, and pale, clay-colored stools.	**X.** Meningococcal meningitis
_____	**25.** A disease caused by pathogenic organisms.	**Y.** Middle East respiratory syndrome (MERS)

Multiple Choice

Read each item carefully, and then select the best response.

_____ **1.** Agencies responsible for protecting public health include the following, EXCEPT:

A. Occupational Safety and Health Administration (OSHA).
B. Centers for Disease Control and Prevention (CDC).
C. state health departments.
D. National Sanitary Foundation.

_____ **2.** Communicable diseases may be transmitted by:

A. droplets.
B. airborne particles.
C. vectors.
D. All of the above

_____ **3.** Host resistance refers to:

A. drug-resistant antibiotics.
B. the body's ability to fight off infection.
C. virulence of the invading microorganism.
D. the period of contagiousness.

_____ **4.** Which of the following best defines the key element of the Ryan White Comprehensive AIDS Resources Emergency Act?

A. A designated infection control officer (DICO) is required by federal law in each county.
B. The medical facility must release source patient tests to the DICO.
C. Emergency response personnel must be notified within 48 hours after a workplace exposure to tuberculosis.
D. Patients' health records are protected by federal law.

_____ **5.** Personal protective equipment (PPE) needs to be worn by a paramedic:

A. at all collision scenes.
B. at any multiple-casualty incident.
C. only while working in a contaminated environment.
D. according to your department's exposure control plan.

_____ **6.** No matter how high-tech PPE may be, it is only effective if:

A. proper removal techniques are employed.
B. it is used prior to the 36-month expiration.
C. the patient is in the incubation period.
D. the patient gives permission for you to use it.

______ **7.** An inflammation of the membranes that cover the brain and spinal cord is called:
- **A.** influenza.
- **B.** pertussis.
- **C.** meningitis.
- **D.** tuberculosis.

______ **8.** Most droplets and airborne disease exposures can be prevented by:
- **A.** placing a mask on patients with fevers and rashes.
- **B.** doing nothing; confining the patient's face may exacerbate secretions.
- **C.** the crew wearing level III biohazard suits.
- **D.** notifying the hospital in advance and having the patient decontaminated prior to admission.

______ **9.** All of the following are highly communicable viral diseases, EXCEPT:
- **A.** measles.
- **B.** mumps.
- **C.** pertussis.
- **D.** meningitis.

______ **10.** Lice and scabies infections may affect:
- **A.** patients.
- **B.** families.
- **C.** crews.
- **D.** All of the above

Fill in the Blank

Read each item carefully, and then complete the statement by filling in the missing word(s).

1. __________ __________ is the term used to describe infection control practices that reduce the opportunity of an exposure to occur in the daily care of patients.

2. A paramedic's major protective measure is __________.

3. Unfortunately, paramedics get exposed to communicable diseases. The third line of defense is considered __________ __________ __________-__________.

4. __________ __________ include bacteria, viruses, fungi, and parasites.

5. Mononucleosis is caused by the __________-__________ virus. Transmission occurs via direct contact with __________ secretions.

6. __________ __________ is caused when a deer tick's bite injects a bacterium into the bloodstream of the human host.

7. Gonorrhea, syphilis, and herpes are all considered __________ __________ __________.

8. An inflammation of the liver that may be produced by five distinct forms of virus is called __________ __________.

9. Methicillin-resistant *Staphylococcus aureus* (MRSA) is believed to be transmitted from __________ to __________ via __________ hands.

10. Severe acute respiratory syndrome (SARS) arose from the merger of viruses from __________ and __________.

Identify

Read the following case studies, and then list the chief complaint, vital signs, and pertinent negatives.

1. Your unit is called to the airport to meet an inbound flight. There is a patient reported to have flu-like symptoms that include fever, chills, and dry cough. The patient is conscious and alert but very weak. He is assisted from the aircraft when it arrives at the terminal gate. You note that the flight appears to be domestic in origin. While you are taking the patient's history, he denies any type of international travel but has been traveling extensively with very little sleep this past week. He denies other previous medical history. He denies medications and allergies to medications or prescription drugs. His skin is warm and dry. He feels febrile. After further discussion, you discover that his school-aged children were recently sick with a viral infection. His vital signs are as follows: Respiratory rate is 20 breaths/min, oxygen saturation on ambient air is 95%, pulse is 106 beats/min and regular, and blood pressure (BP) is 128/68 mm Hg.
   a. Chief complaint:

   ___

   ___

   b. Vital signs:

   ___

   ___

   c. Pertinent negatives:

   ___

   ___

2. It's a hot, humid day in the mid-90s and your advanced life support (ALS) unit is dispatched to assist the police department. You arrive on scene to discover several patrol vehicles located outside an unkempt house. You are met by one of the officers, who explains that the police department received a call from an out-of-town relative to check on the welfare of the elderly resident. Once inside the house, the police officers noticed a severe lice infestation. Many of the officers are exposed to the nasty critters. Although the exposure is not life threatening, the officers appear very annoyed. They describe the conditions as squalid. You request that the exposed officers assist the elderly patient out to his front yard so that you can properly decontaminate him and minimize the lice exposure to any additional providers and equipment. Once outside, the patient appears emaciated and is wearing soiled clothing, yet states he just put on the clean clothes the other morning. He has a bag of prescription medications that seem to indicate a mental health and cardiac history but says he rarely needs to take any pills. His vital signs are as follows: Pulse is 88 beats/min and irregular, BP is 98/72 mm Hg, and oxygen saturation is 88%. He is tachypneic, and there is obvious skin tenting and delayed capillary refill.
   a. Chief complaint:

   ___

   ___

   b. Vital signs:

   ___

   ___

   c. Pertinent negatives:

   ___

   ___

3. While preparing for an ALS interfacility transport, you are told by the nurse's station that the patient has MRSA. The patient has a number of drip medications, along with strict respiratory precautions. You are told that the patient is "stable" for transport. He is also on a nonrebreathing face mask and is conscious and alert. The patient is on a cardiac monitor and is in a sinus rhythm. His BP as noted on the noninvasive monitor is 98/54 mm Hg, and his heart rate is 62 beats/min. He has a lengthy medical history, including kidney transplant. He is on several immunosuppressants.
   a. Chief complaint:

   ____

   ____

   b. Vital signs:

   ____

   ____

   c. Pertinent negatives:

   ____

   ____

Ambulance Calls

The following case scenarios provide an opportunity to explore the concerns associated with patient management and paramedic care. Read each scenario, and then answer each question.

1. You are called to transport a 22-year-old college student from the college infirmary to the hospital. The nurse tells you that the student has a high fever. He complains of a severe headache and stiff neck, and he seems rather confused. He vomits twice en route to the hospital.
   a. What is the patient experiencing?

   ____

   ____

   b. How can the paramedic minimize the risk of catching the illness?

   ____

   ____

2. A 54-year-old man calls for an ambulance after he coughed up some blood. He says that over the past several weeks he has been waking up in the middle of the night with his pajamas and bedclothes soaked through with sweat. He has lost about 25 pounds in the last 2 or 3 months, and today he started noticing some blood in his sputum.
   a. What is the patient experiencing?

   ____

   ____

   b. How can the paramedic minimize the risk of catching the illness?

   ____

   ____

3. A 28-year-old man calls for an ambulance because he "feels lousy." He says that for a week or so, he hasn't had any energy at all. He doesn't feel like eating or doing anything; he just feels "done in." Even cigarettes "taste like cow dung." This morning, he noticed that his urine was very dark, and he got panicky. On examination, you observe that his eyes have a yellow tinge; he has a low-grade fever and aching joints. There are also needle tracks on both of his arms.
   a. What is the patient experiencing?

   ____

   ____

   b. How can the paramedic minimize the risk of catching the illness?

   ____

   ____

4. You are called to transport an 8-year-old boy who fell and sustained a laceration to his forehead. "I told him to stay in bed," his mother says, "but no, he has to go horsing around with his brother." According to the mother, both children have been sick for a week, with a fever, no appetite, and soreness under their ears. On examining the 8-year-old, you find a 2-inch laceration on the left side of the forehead, and you control the bleeding with pressure. He does seem a little warm to the touch and has a headache.
   a. Aside from the soft-tissue injury, what is the patient likely experiencing?

   ____

   ____

   b. How can the paramedic minimize the risk of catching the illness?

   ____

   ____

5. It's back to the college infirmary for another patient with a fever—this time a 19-year-old woman. She complains of headache and says the light bothers her a lot. Her eyes are reddened, and she is coughing. She has a blotchy, red rash over her face and neck, and when you examine her throat, you notice some little white spots on the mucous membranes in her mouth.
   a. What is the patient experiencing?

   ____

   ____

   b. How can the paramedic minimize the risk of catching the illness?

   ____

   ____

Complete the Patient Care Report (PCR)

Read the second scenario in the Ambulance Calls section, and then complete the following PCR.

EMS Patient Care Report (PCR)			
Date:	Incident No.:	Nature of Call:	Location:

Dispatched:	En Route:	At Scene:	Transport:	At Hospital:	In Service:

Patient Information	
Age: Sex: Weight (in kg [lb]):	Allergies: Medications: Past Medical History: Chief Complaint:

Vital Signs				
Time:	BP:	Pulse:	Respirations:	SpO_2:
Time:	BP:	Pulse:	Respirations:	SpO_2:
Time:	BP:	Pulse:	Respirations:	SpO_2:

EMS Treatment (circle all that apply)				
Oxygen @ ______ L/min via (circle one): NC NRM Bag-mask device		Assisted Ventilation	Airway Adjunct	CPR
Defibrillation	Bleeding Control	Bandaging	Splinting	Other:

Narrative

True/False

If you believe the statement to be more true than false, write the letter "T" in the space provided. If you believe the statement to be more false than true, write the letter "F."

_____ **1.** Ebola is a virus spread through direct contact with nonintact skin or mucous membranes.

_____ **2.** Patients with AIDS are abnormally susceptible to many opportunistic infections.

_____ **3.** AIDS can be acquired through casual contact, such as shaking hands with an HIV-positive patient.

_____ **4.** HIV is transmitted by airborne means.

_____ **5.** HIV type 1 was first identified in the late 1970s.

_____ **6.** Many health care workers have acquired HIV through contact with the blood or body fluids of patients.

_____ **7.** The majority of AIDS cases that have occurred in health care workers as a result of occupational exposure have been among emergency medical services (EMS) personnel.

_____ **8.** Complications of syphilis can include cardiac, ophthalmic, auditory, and central nervous system complications.

_____ **9.** Sexually transmitted diseases (STDs) require special standard precautions.

_____ **10.** The incubation period of genital herpes is 3 to 4 weeks.

Short Answer

Complete this section with short written answers using the space provided.

1. Carry out the following research project before you begin employment as a paramedic.

a. Check off the illnesses you had as a child or up to this point:

_____________ Measles

_____________ Mumps

_____________ Chickenpox

_____________ German measles (rubella)

_____________ Polio

_____________ Hepatitis B

b. Check off the immunizations you have had up to this point, and fill in the dates (obtain the records from your family doctor or the clinic where you received your immunizations):

_____________ Measles Date immunized: _____________

_____________ Mumps Date immunized: _____________

_____________ Rubella Date immunized: _____________

_____________ DPT (diphtheria/pertussis/tetanus)

#1 Date immunized: _____________

#2 Date immunized: _____________

#3 Date immunized: _____________

_____________ Most recent tetanus booster Date immunized: _____________

_____________ Oral polio #1 Date immunized: _____________

_____________ Oral polio #2 Date immunized: _____________

_____________ Oral polio #3 Date immunized: _____________

_____________ Hepatitis B Date immunized: _____________

c. Based on the preceding data you have compiled, what immunizations do you need to get before you start work?

____

____

a. List three ways that HIV can be transmitted from one person to another.

(1)____

(2)____

(3)____

b. List three things you can do to minimize the risk of acquiring HIV from a patient.

(1)____

(2)____

(3)____

Fill in the Table

Fill in the missing parts of the table.

1. Complete the following table, which outlines the PPE necessary in preventing transmission of HIV and HBV. Indicate "yes" or "no" for each task or activity.

Recommended Personal Protective Equipment for Preventing Transmission of Human Immunodeficiency Virus and Hepatitis B Virus in the Prehospital Setting				
Task or Activity	**Disposable Gloves**	**Gown**	**Mask**	**Protective Eyewear**
Bleeding control with spurting blood	Yes		Yes	
Bleeding control with minimal bleeding	Yes		No	
Emergency childbirth	Yes		Yes, if spatter	
Drawing blood samples	Yes		No	
Inserting an IV line	Yes		No	
Advanced airway insertion (eg, endotracheal intubation, laryngeal mask airway, Combitube)	Yes		No, unless spatter is likely[a]	
Oral/nasal suctioning, manually cleaning airway	Yes		No, unless spatter is likely[a]	
Handling and cleaning instruments with microbial contamination	Yes		No	
Measuring blood pressure	No		No	

Task or Activity	Disposable Gloves	Gown	Mask	Protective Eyewear
Measuring temperature	No		No	
Giving an injection	No		No	
[a]Spatter is often likely, so use personal protective equipment accordingly.				

Data from Centers for Disease Control and Prevention (CDC): Guidelines for prevention of transmission of human immunodeficiency virus and hepatitis B virus to health-care and public-safety workers: A response to P.L. 100-607 The Health Omnibus Programs Extention Act of 1988. MMWR. 1989;38(S-6):Table 4, (d)(3)(ix)(A)-(C). Available at: http://wonder.cdc.gov/wonder/prevguid/p0000114/p0000114.asp. Accessed November 10, 2011; and Ask the expert: gloves for injections. HCPro OSHA Heathcare Advisor website. http://blogs.hcpro.com/osha/2012/01/ask-the-expert-gloves-for-injections/; and Standard interpretations. United States Department of Labor, OSHA website. https://www.osha.gov/pls/oshaweb/owadisp.show_document?p_table=INTERPRETATIONS&p_id=20819

2. Indicate the mode(s) of transmission and recommended protective measures for each of the diseases in the following table.

Disease	Mode(s) of Transmission	Protective Measures
AIDS		
HAV		
HBV		
Meningitis		
Mumps		
Syphilis		
Tuberculosis		
MERS		
SARS		

CHAPTER 27

Toxicology

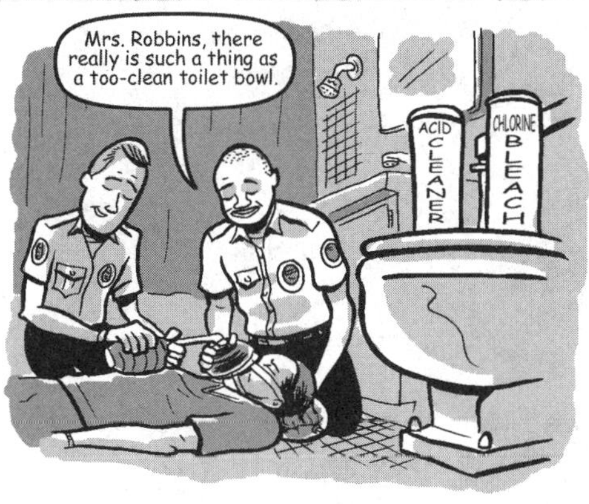

Matching

Part I

Match the definitions in the left column to the appropriate terms in the right column.

______	**1.** Any use of drugs that causes physical psychological, economic, legal, or social harm to the user or others affected by the user's behavior.	**A.** Alcoholism
______	**2.** Substance that has some therapeutic effect (such as reducing inflammation, fighting bacteria, or producing euphoria) when given in the appropriate circumstances and in the appropriate dose.	**B.** Amphetamines
______	**3.** A common houseplant that is also called dumb cane; ingestion leads to burns of the mouth and tongue and, possibly, paralysis of the vocal cords and nausea and vomiting; in severe cases, causes edema of the tongue and larynx, leading to airway compromise.	**C.** Antagonist
______	**4.** A severe withdrawal syndrome seen in people with alcoholism who are deprived of ethyl alcohol; characterized by restlessness, fever, sweating, disorientation, agitation, and seizures; can be fatal if untreated.	**D.** Antidote
______	**5.** The dried leaves and flower buds of the *Cannabis sativa* plant that are smoked to achieve a high.	**E.** Barbiturate
______	**6.** A common mood stabilizer used in the treatment of bipolar disorder.	**F.** Benzodiazepines
______	**7.** In relation to drugs, legalized drugs such as coffee, alcohol, and tobacco.	**G.** Caladium
______	**8.** A perennial flowering shrub with clusters of red berries that can lead to serious and even fatal poisoning. Also known as red sage or wild sage; ingestion causes stomach upset, muscle weakness, shock, and, sometimes, death.	**H.** Castor bean
______	**9.** A method of suicide that involves mixing certain household chemicals in an enclosed space to create toxic gases, such as hydrogen sulfide and hydrogen cyanide, as the chemicals combine; also called detergent suicide.	**I.** Caustics
______	**10.** Chemicals that are acids or alkalis; cause direct chemical injury to the tissues they contact.	**J.** Chemical suicide
______	**11.** A seed that contains the poison ricin; causes a variety of toxic effects; burning of the mouth and throat; nausea, vomiting, diarrhea, and severe stomach pains; prostration; failing vision; and kidney failure, which is the usual cause of death.	**K.** Cocaine
______	**12.** A common houseplant that contains calcium oxalate crystals; ingestion leads to nausea, vomiting, and diarrhea.	**L.** Delirium tremens (DTs)

______	**13.** In relation to drugs, illegal drugs such as marijuana, cocaine, and lysergic acid diethylamide.	**M.** Dieffenbachia
______	**14.** Compounds made up principally of hydrogen and carbon atoms mostly obtained from the distillation of petroleum.	**N.** Drug
______	**15.** An agent that produces false perceptions in any one of the five senses.	**O.** Drug abuse
______	**16.** A physical tolerance and psychological dependence on a drug or drugs.	**P.** Drug addiction
______	**17.** The family of sedative-hypnotics that provide muscle relaxation and mild sedation; most commonly used to treat anxiety, seizures, and alcohol withdrawal; include drugs such as diazepam (Valium) and midazolam (Versed).	**Q.** Foxglove
______	**18.** Potent sedative-hypnotics historically used as sleep aids, antianxiety drugs, and as part of the regimen for seizure control; include drugs such as thiopental (Pentothal, Trapanal) and methohexital (Brevital).	**R.** Habituation
______	**19.** Something to counteract the effect of a poison.	**S.** Hallucinogen
______	**20.** A molecule that blocks the ability of a given chemical to bind to its receptor, preventing a biologic response.	**T.** Hydrocarbons
______	**21.** A plant that contains cardiac glycosides used in making digitalis; ingestion of leaves causes nausea, vomiting, diarrhea, abdominal cramps, hyperkalemia, and a variety of dysrhythmias.	**U.** Illicit
______	**22.** A chronic disorder characterized by the compulsive use of a substance that results in physical, psychological, or social harm to the user, who continues to use the substance despite the harm.	**V.** Lantana
______	**23.** A stimulant; a naturally occurring alkaloid that is extracted from the *Erythroxylon coca* plant leaves found in South America.	**W.** Licit
______	**24.** A disorder characterized by a physical and psychological addiction to ethanol.	**X.** Lithium
______	**25.** A class of drugs that increase alertness and excitation (stimulants); including methamphetamine (crank or ice), methylenedioxyamphetamine (MDA, Adam), and methylenedioxymethamphetamine (MDMA, Eve, Ecstasy).	**Y.** Marijuana

Part II

Match the definitions in the left column to the appropriate terms in the right column.

______	**1.** A physiologic state of adaption to a drug, usually characterized by tolerance to the effects of the drug and a withdrawal syndrome if use of the drug is stopped, especially abruptly.	**A.** Methamphetamine
______	**2.** A substance whose chemical action could damage structures or impair function when introduced into the body.	**B.** Monoamine oxidase inhibitors (MAOIs)
______	**3.** Enhancement of the effect of one drug by another drug.	**C.** Narcotic
______	**4.** The emotional state of craving a drug to maintain a feeling of well-being.	**D.** Opiate
______	**5.** A predictable set of signs and symptoms, usually involving altered central nervous system activity that occurs after the abrupt cessation of a drug or after rapidly decreasing the usual dosage of a drug.	**E.** Opioid
______	**6.** A group of drugs used to treat severe depression and manage pain; minimal dosing errors can cause toxic results.	**F.** Organophosphates
______	**7.** A poison or harmful substance produced by bacteria, animals, or plants.	**G.** Overdose
______	**8.** The syndrome-like symptoms of any given class or group of poisonous agents.	**H.** Physical dependence
______	**9.** A highly addictive drug in the amphetamine family.	**I.** Poison
______	**10.** Psychiatric medication used primarily to treat atypical depression by increasing norepinephrine and serotonin levels in the central nervous system.	**J.** Potentiation

______	11. The generic term for opiates and opioids, drugs that act as a central nervous system depressant and produce insensibility or stupor.	K. Psychological dependence
______	12. Various alkaloids derived from the opium or poppy plant.	L. Rhabdomyolysis
______	13. The study of toxic or poisonous substances.	M. Salicylates
______	14. Medical emergencies caused by toxic agents such as poison; may be intentional or unintentional.	N. Sedative-hypnotic
______	15. Physiologic adaptation to the effects of a drug such that increasingly larger doses of the drug are required to achieve the same effect.	O. Selective serotonin reuptake inhibitors (SSRIs)
______	16. The action of two substances, such as drugs, in which the total effects are greater than the sum of the independent effects of the two substances.	P. Serotonin syndrome
______	17. A synthetic narcotic not derived from opium, with sedative properties; examples are fentanyl (Sublimaze) and alfentanil (Alfenta); also called narcotics.	Q. Spice
______	18. A class of chemical found in many insecticides used in agriculture and in the home.	R. Synergism
______	19. A condition that occurs when a drug (either licit or illicit) is taken in excess; can have toxic or lethal consequences.	S. Tolerance
______	20. The destruction of muscle tissue leading to a release of potassium and myoglobin.	T. Toxicologic emergencies
______	21. A primary ingredient in aspirin.	U. Toxicology
______	22. A drug used to reduce anxiety, calm agitated patients, and help produce drowsiness and sleep (central nervous system depressants).	V. Toxidrome
______	23. A class of antidepressants that inhibit the reuptake of serotonin.	W. Toxin
______	24. An idiosyncratic complication that occurs with antidepressant therapy in which patients have lower extremity muscle rigidity, confusion or disorientation, and/or agitation.	X. Tricyclic antidepressants (TCAs)
______	25. An illicit drug consisting of a blend of synthetic cannabinoids; it can produce delirium and short- and long-term psychotic effects.	Y. Withdrawal syndrome

Multiple Choice

Read each item carefully, and then select the best response.

______ 1. Poisoning by ingestion, in adults, is usually a result of:
- A. improperly labeled over-the-counter medications.
- B. improperly dispensed prescribed medications.
- C. suicide attempts or unintentional overdose.
- D. workplace mishaps involving chemicals and toxic exposures.

______ 2. All of the following are common routes of poisoning, EXCEPT:
- A. inhalation.
- B. ingestion.
- C. injection.
- D. excretion.

______ 3. Alcoholism is usually diagnosed when the patient has a demonstrated:
- A. problem handling his or her drinks in public.
- B. physical and psychological addiction to ethanol.
- C. medicinal need to relieve pain with alcohol.
- D. binge drinking at least two times in the last month.

______ 4. Alcohol abuse may cause a number of medical consequences, including:
- A. subdural hematoma.
- B. GI bleeding.
- C. a higher risk of burns.
- D. All of the above

_____ 5. Alcohol withdrawal may have life-threatening consequences, including delirium tremens. Delirium tremens, or the "DTs," are best characterized by:
A. tremors and diaphoresis.
B. confusion and fever.
C. restlessness and tachycardia.
D. All of the above

_____ 6. The general assessment approach for toxicologic emergencies includes all of the following tasks, EXCEPT:
A. primary survey.
B. scene size-up.
C. physical exam.
D. There is no "general assessment"; these patients should receive a secondary assessment.

_____ 7. You are called to the scene of a 4-year-old who ingested a common houseplant. The best source of information regarding the accidental ingestion is:
A. referring to the *Emergency Response Guidebook* (*ERG*).
B. contacting the Poison Center.
C. contacting CHEMTREC.
D. contacting medical control.

_____ 8. A chronic disorder characterized by the compulsive use of a substance resulting in physical, psychological, economic, legal, or social harm to the user who continues to use the substance despite the harm is considered:
A. tolerance.
B. drug addiction.
C. substance abuse.
D. antagonist.

_____ 9. The treatment for patients abusing cocaine, amphetamine, or methamphetamine is fundamentally the same. This treatment includes the following tasks, EXCEPT:
A. establishing and maintaining the airway; consider an advanced airway as needed.
B. establishing vascular access.
C. administering morphine for pain relief.
D. contacting medical control for sedation when behavior is violent.

_____ 10. Signs and symptoms of overdose with cardiac drugs may include:
A. hypotension.
B. weakness or confusion.
C. nausea and vomiting.
D. All of the above

_____ 11. Diarrhea, urination, miosis, muscle weakness, bradycardia, bronchospasm, bronchorrhea, emesis, lacrimation, seizures, salivation, and sweating are symptoms associated with a toxic exposure to:
A. psychedelics.
B. narcotics.
C. ketamine.
D. organophosphates.

_____ 12. Physical examination of a patient who has been poisoned with cyanide may reveal each of the following, EXCEPT:
A. an altered mental state.
B. respirations that are rapid and labored and that become slow and gasping.
C. a slow and thready pulse.
D. a bitter almond scent.

_____ **13.** The common symptoms of a tricyclic antidepressant overdose are:
- **A.** tachycardia, tachypnea, and hypotension.
- **B.** abdominal pain and nausea.
- **C.** internal bleeding and mottled skin.
- **D.** burning of the eyes, nose, and throat.

_____ **14.** An adult presenting with a potential salicylate overdose is likely to have:
- **A.** mistakenly taken too much Pepto-Bismol for a stomach ache.
- **B.** ingested a couple of extra Tylenol.
- **C.** a history of drug abuse or a psychiatric condition.
- **D.** a history of seizures or diabetes.

_____ **15.** Death from ingestion of large amounts of the plant foxglove usually occurs as a result of:
- **A.** acute respiratory distress.
- **B.** psychogenic shock.
- **C.** cardiac dysrhythmias.
- **D.** anaphylactic shock.

Fill in the Blank

Read each item carefully, and then complete the statement by filling in the missing word(s).

1. A(n) __________ is a substance that is toxic by nature, no matter how it gets into the body or in what quantities it is taken. By contrast, a(n) __________ is a substance that has some therapeutic effect when given in the appropriate dose.

2. __________ __________ usually fall under one of two general headings: __________ and __________.

3. Toxins cannot exert their effects until they enter the body. The four primary methods of entry are __________, __________, __________, and __________.

4. __________ are useful for remembering the assessment and management of different substances that fall under the same __________ __________.

5. The ________ effects of alcohol on the _______ produce a variety of _______, such as coagulopathies, hypoglycemia, and ____ bleeding.

6. _________, in both licit and illicit forms, can have devastating effects on those who _____ them. From smokable cocaine or _______ and methamphetamine to ________ diet aids and medications for attention deficit disorder (ADD), you will at some point care for a patient who is under the influence of __________.

7. Shortly after injecting __________, a user will appear to pass out. However, the user is typically quiet __________ and remains aware of what is being done or said.

8. Overdoses of cardiac medications are usually __________.

9. Treatment of carbon monoxide (CO) __________ in the field is aimed at providing the highest concentration of __________ possible to attempt to displace CO molecules from the __________.

10. Acids tend to be more __________-__________ than __________, and so they are often diluted relatively quickly. With __________, it is more important to keep water continually flowing because it usually takes much longer to rinse away the substance.

11. ______ is an analog of methamphetamine, and it may have similar toxic effects on the smaller scale.

12. Huffing ________ __________ can produce euphoria, anesthesia, weakness, ________, abdominal cramps, loss of coordination, neuropathy, blindness, and cardiac dysrhythmias.

13. Hydrocarbon products cause __________ __________, which results in severe abdominal __________, diarrhea, and belching. At the other end of the spectrum, just a single hydrocarbon substance exposure may cause life-threatening __________.

14. With a serious tricyclic antidepressant (TCA) overdose, be alert for electrocardiogram (ECG) changes, including a(n)_________ PR interval, _______, widening QRS, a terminal R wave greater than 3 mm in aVR, and a prolonged _____ interval.

15. Organic ______ is lipid soluble and quickly _______ in the ________.

Identify

In the following case studies, identify the appropriate toxidrome, and list two drugs associated with it.

1. You arrive on scene to find a 22-year-old woman who appears confused, has a blood pressure (BP) of 88/60 mm Hg, is slurring her speech, and is somewhat sleepy.
   a. Identify the appropriate toxidrome:

   ____

   b. Name two drugs that may fit this toxidrome.

   (1)______________________________

   (2)______________________________

2. Your advanced life support (ALS) ambulance arrives on scene at the request of law enforcement for a very agitated 42-year-old man. He won't stop talking and is paranoid.
   a. Identify the appropriate toxidrome:

   ____

   b. Name two drugs that may fit this toxidrome.

   (1)______________________________

   (2)______________________________

In the following case studies, identify the possible causative agent based on the presenting symptoms.

3. On arrival, you discover a 16-year-old boy with severe nausea and vomiting. You begin assessing the patient and immediately notice an odor that appears to be alcohol.

   ____

4. You are dispatched to a "delta" response (high priority) for a patient seizing. On arrival, you discover a 56-year-old man who is actively seizing and has snoring respirations. Family members state the patient has been recently depressed and withdrawn.

   ____

Ambulance Calls

The following case scenarios provide an opportunity to explore the concerns associated with patient management and paramedic care. Read each scenario, and then answer each question.

1. You are called to a somewhat rundown apartment building where the police have forcibly entered an apartment after neighbors reported that the occupant of the apartment has not been seen for a few days and has not answered his telephone. Inside, you find a man who looks to be about 30 years old lying unresponsive on a sofa in the living room. Some neighbors are milling around, giving information to the police officers.

a. List six questions you would ask the neighbors about the patient.

(1)____________________

(2)____________________

(3)____________________

(4)____________________

(5)____________________

(6)____________________

b. Besides the neighbors, what other sources of information might be present? What places in the apartment would you check? What would you be looking for?

(1)____________________

(2)____________________

(3)____________________

c. When you examine the patient, you detect the following findings. For each finding listed, indicate its possible diagnostic significance.

Finding	Possible Diagnostic Significance
Cold, dry skin	
Pulse = 110 beats/min, thready	
BP = 90/60 mm Hg	
Respirations = 12 breaths/min and shallow	
Pupils dilated and not reactive to light	
Breath smells of alcohol (ETOH)	

d. In assessing this patient's mental status, you find the following:

- He does not open his eyes.
- His arms flex when you pinch his leg.
- He does not make any sound in response to your calling his name or pinching him.

In view of those findings, he is best described as which of the following?

(1) Drowsy
(2) Lethargic
(3) Comatose
(4) Stuporous
(5) Obtunded

e. List steps in managing this patient.

(1)_____

(2)_____

(3)_____

(4)_____

(5)_____

(6)_____

(7)_____

(8)_____

(9)_____

(10)_____

2. You are called to the home of a frantic young couple who discovered their 3-year-old happily consuming the contents of a bottle from the cleaning cupboard. List five questions you would ask in taking the history of the incident.

a. _____

b. _____

c. _____

d. _____

e. _____

3. A middle-aged man is found unconscious in his garage. He has left a suicide note on the car windshield, but the hood of the car is cold, so you are reasonably sure the engine has not been run recently. List five things to which you would give particular attention in the physical examination of this patient.

a. _____

b. _____

c. _____

d. _____

e. _____

4. A 15-year-old boy swallowed about 20 of his father's tricyclic antidepressant pills in a suicide gesture after a family argument. You arrive at the scene, some 30 minutes distant from the nearest hospital, about 15 minutes after the ingestion. In a telephone consultation, Poison Control advises you to administer activated charcoal (if available) and monitor the airway and electrocardiogram (ECG) for dysrhythmias. The boy is alert, and vital signs are all within normal limits at this point.

a. What is the purpose of giving activated charcoal? That is, what is the therapeutic effect?

_____

b. List poisonings in which activated charcoal is contraindicated.

(1)_____

c. List the steps in treating this patient.

(1)______

(2)______

(3)______

(4)______

(5)______

(6)______

(7)______

(8)______

(9)______

(10)______

(11)______

(12)______

5. A 35-year-old man ingested "about a tablespoon" of drain buildup remover (Drano) crystals 10 to 15 minutes before your arrival. He is fully alert and complaining of severe pain in his throat and chest. His lips and mouth are very red, and there are still crystals sticking to the mucous membranes in his mouth.

a. From a management perspective, advanced life support care for a toxicologic emergency builds on the following basics:

(1)______

(2)______

(3)______

(4)______

(5)______

(6)______

(7)______

(8)______

(9)______

6. You are summoned to a location near the railway tracks where the local "down-and-outs" gather. A police officer at the scene gestures you toward two of the group members congregated there. "They looked in pretty bad shape," he says, "so I thought I'd better call EMS."

"Been drinking real bad stuff," one of the group chimes in. "Told 'em to stay away from that rotgut—you can go blind from drinkin' stuff like that."

The first patient is in severe respiratory distress. He says he hasn't had a drink since the previous day, when he drank "some stuff they left lying around the gas station—I don't know what it was—tasted pretty good." He says he threw up a few times about 6 hours after that. On physical examination, the patient is alert. There is no alcohol odor on his breath. His vital signs are a pulse of 120 beats/min and regular, respirations of 36 breaths/min and noisy, and BP of 180/105 mm Hg. The pupils are midposition, equal, and reactive to light. The gag reflex is present. The chest is full of crackles.

a. What do you think is this patient's problem?

______

b. List the steps you would take in managing this patient.

(1)________________________________

(2)________________________________

(3)________________________________

(4)________________________________

(5)________________________________

The second patient appears intoxicated. His speech is slurred, and he can scarcely walk. "Why ish it shnowing in Sheptember?" he mumbles. His breath smells of alcohol. His pulse is 108 beats/min and regular, his respirations are 30 breaths/min and deep, and his BP is 140/86 mm Hg. There is no evidence of head injury. The pupils are about 6 mm and equal and react sluggishly to light. The gag reflex is present. The chest is clear. The abdomen is very tender and nearly rigid to palpation.

c. What do you think is this patient's problem?

____

d. List the steps you would take in managing this patient.

(1)________________________________

(2)________________________________

(3)________________________________

(4)________________________________

(5)________________________________

7. You are staying with friends at their cabin in the mountains for a nice ski weekend. Your host takes considerable pride in the cabin, which he built himself. "Snug as a bug in a rug," he says. "Not a draft in the place." You have to admit that he did a good insulation job and that the place is nice and cozy with the Franklin stove in the corner.

When you get up the next morning, your friend's wife, asks, "Will you have a look at the baby? She's sick with something. She's been throwing up all morning." You don't know much about babies, and you don't feel so hot yourself, but you take a look at the baby. You find her pale and dehydrated, with a bounding pulse but no fever. As you are examining her, she has a grand mal seizure. "It must be the flu," says the baby's mother, "because I'm coming down with something, too. I feel really sick to my stomach." Meanwhile, your friend, just getting up, says, "Boy, do I have a headache; it's like Niagara Falls roaring through my skull."

a. What do you think is the baby's problem?

____

b. What steps should you take in this situation?

(1)________________________________

(2)________________________________

(3)________________________________

(4)________________________________

(5)________________________________

(6)________________________________

(7)________________________________

8. One fine Sunday afternoon, you are called to a suburban home for a "possible heart attack." On arrival, you find a middle-aged man, clad in shorts and a T-shirt, sprawled out on the sofa in the living room. "I don't know what happened," he says. "I was just sitting outside on the lawn, and I started to feel real dizzy and sick to my stomach, and real weak. And there's this tight feeling in my chest—"

"It's that stuff Mr. Greenthumb was spraying," his wife chimes in. "I'm sure of it. Why he has to spray his precious roses precisely when we're sitting in the garden is beyond me."

While you begin your assessment of the patient, your partner goes next door to talk with Mr. Greenthumb. You find the patient in considerable distress. His skin is pale and diaphoretic. His vital signs are a pulse of 42 beats/min and regular, respirations are 28 breaths/min and labored, and BP is 140/80 mm Hg. The pupils are very constricted. The patient is salivating profusely, and his breath smells like garlic. The neck veins are flat. The chest is full of wheezes. As you are completing the examination, your partner returns carrying a bottle labeled "parathion."

a. What do you think is this patient's problem?

____

b. What drug is used to treat this problem?

____

c. What is the correct dosage in this situation?

____

d. List the steps in treating this patient.

(1)____

(2)____

(3)____

(4)____

(5)____

(6)____

(7)____

(8)____

(9)____

9. You are called to a local junior high school where a 12-year-old boy had a grand mal seizure. The school nurse, who is kneeling on the floor of the boys' restroom beside the boy, tells you that the boy has no known seizure history. The boy is unconscious but can be roused by painful stimuli. You cannot find any abnormalities on physical examination save for signs that he indeed just had a seizure (slight bleeding of the tongue, incontinence). A search of his pockets, however, reveals a few small bottles of typewriter correction fluid. What steps will you take in managing this patient?

a. ____

b. ____

c. ____

d. ____

e. ____

f. ____

g. ____

Complete the Patient Care Report (PCR)

Read the ninth incident scenario in the Ambulance Calls section, and then complete the following PCR.

EMS Patient Care Report (PCR)					
Date:	Incident No.:	Nature of Call:		Location:	
Dispatched:	En Route:	At Scene:	Transport:	At Hospital:	In Service:

Patient Information	
Age: Sex: Weight (in kg [lb]):	Allergies: Medications: Past Medical History: Chief Complaint:

Vital Signs				
Time:	BP:	Pulse:	Respirations:	SpO_2:
Time:	BP:	Pulse:	Respirations:	SpO_2:
Time:	BP:	Pulse:	Respirations:	SpO_2:

EMS Treatment (circle all that apply)				
Oxygen @ ______ L/min via (circle one): NC NRM Bag-mask device		Assisted Ventilation	Airway Adjunct	CPR
Defibrillation	Bleeding Control	Bandaging	Splinting	Other:

Narrative

True/False

If you believe the statement to be more true than false, write the letter "T" in the space provided. If you believe the statement to be more false than true, write the letter "F."

_____ **1.** Your call to the Poison Control Center helps the center collect data on poisonings in your region. These data may be analyzed to help detect trends, spot developing public health problems, and evaluate current treatment protocols for different poisonings.

_____ **2.** Oxygen has a greater affinity than carbon monoxide (CO) to bind to hemoglobin on the red blood cells.

_____ **3.** There is an increasing trend of patients attempting suicide by mixing certain household chemicals while in a parked vehicle, which can be very dangerous to emergency response personnel.

_____ **4.** The major toxidromes are produced by stimulants, narcotics, cholinergics, anticholinergics, sympathomimetics, sedatives, and hypnotics.

_____ **5.** The more frequently consumption of alcohol takes place, the greater the irritation of the digestive system.

_____ **6.** The severity of alcohol withdrawal can vary according to the length and intensity of the patient's alcoholism. Minor withdrawal is characterized by restlessness, anxiousness, sleeping problems, agitation, and tremors.

_____ **7.** Prolonged heavy use of alcohol may cause ulcers, gastric esophageal reflux, and cancers of the mouth and throat.

_____ **8.** In a poisoning, the container and the remaining contents should never be taken with the patient to the hospital for fear of contaminating the emergency department.

_____ **9.** The trends in prevalence of cocaine use between 2013 and 2015 show that use is increasing.

_____ **10.** Patients who take lithium and nonsteroidal anti-inflammatory drugs (NSAIDs) have slowed renal clearance of the lithium, increasing the likelihood that they will inadvertently reach a toxic lithium level.

_____ **11.** Most patients who have swallowed caustic substances present with severe respiratory distress and pain in the mouth, throat, or chest.

_____ **12.** The primary goals when dealing with a patient who has inhaled hydrocarbons are to remove the patient from the noxious environment, give high-concentration supplemental oxygen, and promptly transport to the appropriate facility.

_____ **13.** Synthetic cathinones, also known as bath salts, refer to an emerging group of drugs similar to MDMA.

_____ **14.** Field treatment of a salicylate overdose should include the "universal antidote."

Short Answer

Complete this section with short written answers using the space provided.

1. List 10 medical problems to which alcoholics are particularly susceptible.

a. ______________________________

b. ______________________________

c. ______________________________

d. ______________________________

e. ______________________________

f. ______________________________

g. ______________________________

h. ______________________________

i. ______________________________

j. ______________________________

Fill in the Table

Fill in the missing parts of the table.

1. Although it is advisable to consult Poison Control for definitive identification of any ingested substance, it is nonetheless worthwhile to have a general knowledge of the categories of poisons and some of the more commonly encountered examples of each category. Fill in the following table with examples of each type of poison mentioned.

Common Poisons	
Type of Poison	**Examples**
Strong acid	
Strong alkali	
Hydrocarbons	
Toxic plants	

2. Fill in the amount of time it takes for the four stages of acetaminophen toxicity.

Signs and Symptoms of Acetaminophen Toxicity		
Stage	**Time Frame**	**Signs and Symptoms**
I		Nausea, vomiting, loss of appetite, pallor, malaise
II		Right upper quadrant abdominal pain; abdomen tender to palpation
III		Metabolic acidosis, renal failure, coagulopathies, recurring gastrointestinal (GI) symptoms
IV		Recovery slowly begins, or liver failure progresses, and the patient dies

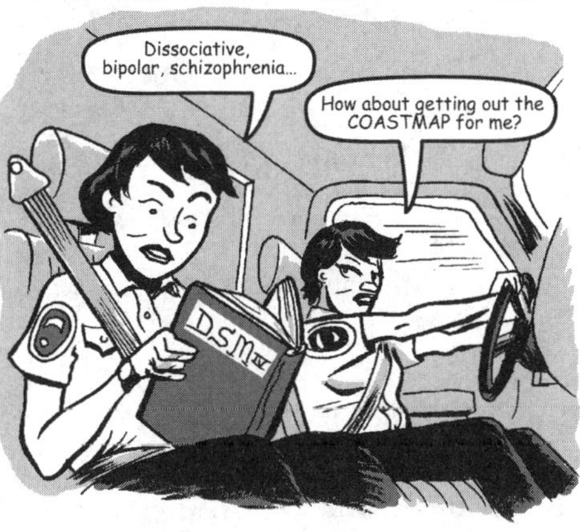

CHAPTER 28

Psychiatric Emergencies

Matching

Part I

Match each of the descriptions in the left column to the appropriate item in the right column.

______	**1.** A fixed belief that is not shared by others of a person's culture or background and that cannot be changed by reasonable argument; a false belief.	**A.** Activities of daily living (ADLs)
______	**2.** The slow onset of progressive disorientation, shortened attention span, and loss of cognitive function.	**B.** Acute dystonic reaction
______	**3.** A mental health disorder characterized by a persistent mood of sadness, despair, and discouragement; it may be a symptom of many different mental and physical disorders, or it may be a disorder on its own.	**C.** Affect
______	**4.** A condition in which a person is characterized by uncontrolled and disconnected thought, is usually incoherent or rambling in speech, and may or may not be oriented to person and place.	**D.** Agitated delirium
______	**5.** A condition in which a person may be confused about his or her identity, the location, and the time of day; one of the ways in which various conditions, such as schizophrenia or organic brain syndrome may present.	**E.** Agoraphobia
______	**6.** The basic activities a person usually accomplishes during a normal day, such as eating, dressing, and washing.	**F.** Anorexia nervosa
______	**7.** A syndrome that may occur in patients taking typical antipsychotic agents. The patient develops muscle spasms of the neck, face, and back within a few days of starting treatment with the medication.	**G.** Anxiety disorder
______	**8.** The outward expression of a person's inner feelings (eg, happy, sad, angry, fearful, withdrawn).	**H.** Atropine-like effects
______	**9.** An acute confrontational state characterized by global impairment of thinking, perception, judgment, and memory.	**I.** Behavior
______	**10.** Literally, "fear of the marketplace"; fear of entering a public place from which escape may be impeded.	**J.** Behavioral emergency
______	**11.** The use of medication to subdue a patient.	**K.** Bipolar mood disorder
______	**12.** Lacking expression or movement, or appearing rigid.	**L.** Borderline personality disorder
______	**13.** An eating disorder characterized by consumption of large amounts of food, for which the patient often compensates by using purging techniques.	**M.** Bulimia nervosa
______	**14.** A disorder characterized by disordered images of self, impulsive and unpredictable behavior, marked shifts in mood, and instability in relationships with others.	**N.** Catatonic

______	**15.** A disorder in which a person alternates between mania and depression.	**O.** Chemical restraint
______	**16.** Behavior that has a hidden meaning or intention that only the person understands.	**P.** Circumstantial thinking
______	**17.** Act of pointing out something of interest in the patient's conversation or behavior, thereby directing the patient's attention to something of which he or she may have been unaware.	**Q.** Compulsions
______	**18.** The invention of experiences to cover gaps in memory; seen in patients with certain organic brain syndromes.	**R.** Confabulation
______	**19.** Repetitive actions carried out to relieve the anxiety of obsessive thoughts.	**S.** Confrontation
______	**20.** Situation in which the patient includes many irrelevant details in his or her account of things.	**T.** Covert behavior
______	**21.** An eating disorder in which a person diets by exerting extraordinary control over his or her eating and loses weight to the point of jeopardizing his or her health and life.	**U.** Delusion
______	**22.** A mental disorder in which the dominant mood is fear and apprehension.	**V.** Dementia
______	**23.** Results of some antipsychotic medications that include adverse effects similar to atropine, resulting in dry mouth, blurred vision, urinary retention, and cardiac dysrhythmias.	**W.** Depression
______	**24.** How a person functions or acts in response to his or her environment.	**X.** Disorganization
______	**25.** The point at which a person's reactions to events interfere with activities of daily living; becomes a psychiatric emergency when it causes a major life interruption, such as attempted suicide.	**Y.** Disorientation

Part II

Match each of the descriptions in the left column to the appropriate item in the right column.

______	**1.** Temporary or permanent dysfunction of the brain, caused by a disturbance in the physical or physiologic functioning of brain tissue.	**A.** Echolalia
______	**2.** A collection of psychiatric disorders without psychotic symptoms and lacking the intense psychopathology or other mood disorders; includes anxiety disorders, phobias, and panic disorder.	**B.** Factitious disorder
______	**3.** A sense perception not founded on objective reality; a false perception.	**C.** Flat affect
______	**4.** The absence of speech.	**D.** Flight of ideas
______	**5.** A group of disorders in which the disturbance of mood is accompanied by full or partial manic or depressive syndrome.	**E.** Generalized anxiety disorder (GAD)
______	**6.** A severe form of anxiety that stems from a traumatic experience; characterized by the reliving of the stress and nightmares of the original situation.	**F.** Hallucination
______	**7.** Disorders involving an unreasonable fear, apprehension, or dread of a specific situation or thing.	**G.** Impulse control disorder
______	**8.** An abnormal and persistent dread of a specific object or situation.	**H.** Inappropriate affect
______	**9.** The condition in which a person behaves or thinks in a way that is dysfunctional or causes distress to other people.	**I.** Labile
______	**10.** Repeating the same idea over and over again.	**J.** Loosening of associations
______	**11.** Meaningless echoing of the interviewer's words by the patient.	**K.** Mania
______	**12.** A disorder in which a person wishes to be sick and intentionally produces or feigns physical or psychological signs or symptoms. Symptoms are under voluntary control, with no obvious physiologic reason.	**L.** Manic-depressive illness
______	**13.** The absence of emotion; appearing to feel no emotion at all.	**M.** Medication noncompliance
______	**14.** Accelerated thinking in which the mind skips very rapidly from one thought to the next.	**N.** Mental status exam (MSE)

_____	**15.** A disorder in which a person worries about everything for no particular reason, or in which the worrying is unproductive and the person cannot decide what to do about an upcoming situation.	**O.** Mood disorder
_____	**16.** Behavior that is open and generally understood by those around the person.	**P.** Mutism
_____	**17.** A disorder characterized by sudden, usually unexpected, and overwhelming feelings of fear and dread, accompanied by a variety of other symptoms produced by a massive activation of the autonomic nervous system.	**Q.** Neurotic disorders
_____	**18.** A bipolar disorder in which mood fluctuates between depression and mania. The alterations in mood are usually episodic and recurrent.	**R.** Organic brain syndrome
_____	**19.** A situation in which a patient chooses to not take his or her medications as prescribed, for reasons that may include undesirable adverse effects or prohibitive cost.	**S.** Overt behavior
_____	**20.** A tool for measuring the "mental vital signs" in a patient who is disturbed. The mnemonic COASTMAP can be used to conduct this exam, assessing consciousness, orientation, activity, speech, thought, memory, affect and mood, and perception.	**T.** Panic disorder
_____	**21.** A mental disorder characterized by abnormally exaggerated happiness, joy, or euphoria with hyperactivity, insomnia, and grandiose ideas.	**U.** Perseveration
_____	**22.** A situation in which the logical connection between one idea and the next becomes obscure, at least to the listener.	**V.** Personality disorder
_____	**23.** Rapidly shifting among different emotional states.	**W.** Phobia
_____	**24.** Emotion that is out of sync with the situation (eg, wearing a smile while discussing a parent's death).	**X.** Phobic disorders
_____	**25.** A condition in which a person lacks the ability to resist a temptation or cannot stop acting on a drive.	**Y.** Posttraumatic stress disorder (PTSD)

Part III

For each of the following signs and symptoms, indicate whether it is:

O: More typical of organic brain syndrome
P: More typical of psychiatric illness
B: Apt to be seen in both organic and psychiatric illnesses

_____ **1.** Obsessional thinking
_____ **2.** Flat affect
_____ **3.** Delirium
_____ **4.** Distractibility
_____ **5.** Compulsions
_____ **6.** Visual hallucinations
_____ **7.** Confabulation
_____ **8.** Anxiety
_____ **9.** Coma
_____ **10.** Circumstantial thinking

Part IV

For each of the psychiatric signs and symptoms listed, indicate whether it is a disturbance of:

A. Consciousness
B. Motor activity
C. Speech
D. Thinking
E. Affect or mood
F. Memory

G. Orientation
H. Perception

_____ 1. The patient cannot name three objects that you listed out loud 5 minutes earlier.
_____ 2. The patient is pacing back and forth.
_____ 3. The patient smiles pleasantly as he tells you that his daughter was run over by a truck.
_____ 4. The patient keeps shifting his attention from you to the television or to the window.
_____ 5. The patient seems to be having a conversation with an invisible friend.
_____ 6. The patient thinks the current year is 1931.
_____ 7. The patient thinks he is Albert Einstein.
_____ 8. The patient tells you, "All the world is my kingdumbell, and I'm the pellmellery scullop."
_____ 9. The patient is terrified of spiders.
_____ 10. The patient puts two fingers to his forehead in a salute every time he finishes speaking.
_____ 11. The patient complains of palpitations, nausea, tightness in his chest, and numbness around his lips.
_____ 12. The patient thinks that the sound of the wind is someone calling his name.

Multiple Choice

Read each item carefully, and then select the best response.

_____ 1. In an acute behavioral emergency, which of the following disease states may produce psychotic symptoms resulting from alcohol abuse, kidney failure, liver failure, and amphetamines?
- A. Toxic or deficiency states
- B. Infections
- C. Neurologic disease
- D. Endocrine disorders

_____ 2. Pressured speech, neologisms, echolalia, and mutism are examples of:
- A. disorders of thinking.
- B. disorders of mood and affect.
- C. disorders of motor activity.
- D. disorders of speech.

_____ 3. During the primary survey of patients with behavioral disorders, it is important for a paramedic to:
- A. hurry the call; you can't really assist the patient.
- B. assess the patient only en route to the hospital.
- C. convey that you have the time and concern.
- D. not gain consent because consent is never required.

_____ 4. The mental status exam includes:
- A. perception.
- B. affect and mood.
- C. memory.
- D. All of the above

_____ 5. Guilt, depressed appetite, sleep disturbances, lack of interest, low energy, and suicidal thoughts are diagnostic features of:
- A. depression.
- B. anxiety.
- C. mood disorders.
- D. manic-depressive illness.

_____ 6. Paramedics always need to take scene safety seriously. All of the following are risk factors for violence, EXCEPT:
- A. posture.
- B. speech.
- C. motor activity.
- D. prescription medication.

_____ **7.** Restraining a violent patient should include:
- **A.** a law enforcement presence.
- **B.** a Reeves stretcher.
- **C.** lots of duct tape.
- **D.** no more than two paramedics.

_____ **8.** A psychiatric emergency exists when a patient:
- **A.** threatens to harm himself or herself.
- **B.** threatens to harm other people.
- **C.** is delusional.
- **D.** All of the above

_____ **9.** All of the following drugs may sometimes cause a psychotic state, EXCEPT:
- **A.** steroids.
- **B.** Wellbutrin (bupropion).
- **C.** digitalis.
- **D.** LSD and PCP.

_____ **10.** Which of the following is considered a disturbance of behavior?
- **A.** Generalized anxiety disorder
- **B.** Organic brain syndrome
- **C.** Head injury
- **D.** Stroke

_____ **11.** The following are appropriate guidelines for the care of any patient with a psychiatric emergency, EXCEPT:
- **A.** being as calm and direct as possible.
- **B.** asking all the other disruptive family members to participate in the interview.
- **C.** maintaining a nonjudgmental attitude.
- **D.** developing a plan of action.

_____ **12.** A patient who has been diagnosed as having bipolar disorder, manic behavior, and depression is categorized as having what type of psychiatric disorder?
- **A.** Cognitive disorder
- **B.** Neurotic disorder
- **C.** Mood disorder
- **D.** Somatoform disorder

Fill in the Blank

Read each item carefully, and then complete the statement by filling in the missing word(s).

1. The causes of abnormal behavior can be classified into four broad categories: (1) causes that are __________ or __________ in nature, (2) causes resulting from a person's __________, (3) causes resulting from acute __________ or __________, and (4) causes that are __________-__________.

2. Identify yourself __________. Tell the patient who you are and what you are trying to do. If the patient is __________ or __________, you may have to explain yourself at __________ intervals.

3. Overwhelming feelings of __________ and __________, accompanied by a variety of other symptoms produced by a massive activation of the __________ nervous system, characterize panic disorder.

4. There are two major types of eating disorders: __________ __________ and __________ __________.

5. __________, __________, and __________ are common trade names for heterocyclic (tricyclic and tetracyclic) antidepressants.

6. One potential adverse effect of monoamine oxidase (MAO) inhibitors when taken by patients with a history of depression would be __________ __________, which although occasionally severe, usually responds to __________ therapy.

7. __________ is the second-leading cause of death among people aged 10 to 34 years and the fourth-leading cause of death among 35- to 54-year-olds.

8. One in __________ people will be affected by __________ in their lifetimes.

Identify

List the behavioral medications in the following scenarios.

1. You respond to a domestic dispute. When you arrive on scene, you are told by law enforcement that the scene is secure and safe. You and your partner proceed inside. The patient's wife is holding a bag of the patient's medications. The patient denies any complaint and simply states that he has a cardiac history and takes furosemide (Lasix) and digoxin. While you calm the patient, your partner reviews the bag of medications. He finds the furosemide and digoxin along with glyburide, fluoxetine (Prozac), and diazepam (Valium).

____

____

2. You are called to an outpatient mental health clinic for a patient requiring voluntary in-patient hospitalization. The patient has a history of hypercholesterolemia and depression. The patient is taking over-the-counter omega-3 and garlic. The patient is on the following prescription medications: phenelzine (Nardil), bupropion (Wellbutrin), simvastatin (Zocor), and atorvastatin (Lipitor).

____

____

3. You receive an emergency call for a "psychotic" patient. As you evaluate your patient, you review her medication list and discover the following prescriptions: tamoxifen, niacin (Niaspan), fluticasone/salmeterol inhaled (Advair), aripiprazole (Abilify), and famotidine (Pepcid).

____

____

Ambulance Calls

The following case scenarios provide an opportunity to explore the concerns associated with patient management and paramedic care. Read each scenario, and then answer each question.

1. The following is the transcript of an interview between an inexperienced paramedic and a disturbed patient. The interview illustrates several errors in approach. Read through the interview. Then, list the points in the interview that you think could have been handled or phrased in a better way.

   Paramedic (entering an apartment in which there is a lot of noise and confusion): Okay, which one of you is the patient?

   (Someone points to a young woman crouching in a corner, crying.)

   Paramedic (approaching the woman and standing in front of her): Now, dearie, what's the trouble?

   (Patient continues crying.)

   Paramedic: Now come on, get hold of yourself. Big girls don't cry.

   Patient (sobbing): Everything's just so hopeless.

   Paramedic: Things are never hopeless. You're probably just making a mountain out of a molehill, and by tomorrow, you'll wonder what you were making such a big fuss about.

   (Patient sits crying to herself.)

Paramedic: Well, if you don't want to tell me what's wrong, maybe one of your friends here can tell me. Is there anyone here who can tell me what's going on?

(Immediately the noise and confusion resume, as everyone starts talking at once. The patient huddles farther into the corner.)

List the things you think were done incorrectly in this interview, including errors of omission and errors of commission.

a. ____________________

b. ____________________

c. ____________________

d. ____________________

e. ____________________

f. ____________________

g. ____________________

h. ____________________

2. You are called to a downtown apartment building for a "sick man." Reaching the corridor outside the man's apartment, you are intercepted by a neighbor who had called for the ambulance. "I feel a little silly troubling you folks," she says, "but Mr. Crosby next door—he's just not himself lately—doesn't even poke his head out of that apartment. Doesn't want to see no one. He just says, 'Go away,' when I knock. So I got to worrying. I mean, I don't even think he's got himself anything to eat in there."

"Who's there?" someone finally says.

"We're paramedics, from the city ambulance service."

"Well, what do you want with me?"

"We just want to talk with you a bit," you say. "There are folks worried about you."

It takes some persuading, but finally, Mr. Crosby opens the door and admits you into his apartment. The place is in complete disarray, and it appears as if no one has washed a dish or tidied up in months. Here and there you note an empty liquor bottle lying on the floor.

So what do you want?" Mr. Crosby asks listlessly.

a. Where would you go from here? List some of the questions you would ask Mr. Crosby at this point.

____

____

____

____

b. In the course of your interview with Mr. Crosby, which seems to go very slowly, you learn that he is a 62-year-old widower. He has one son and says, "I never hear from him." He used to be a watchmaker, he says, "but I haven't been worth anything since I got this arthritis 10 years ago." In response to your query about why he has stopped going out of the apartment, he says, "What's there to go out for? Anyway, I don't have the energy to go rambling around the city."

"Don't you have to shop for food?" you ask.

"What for? I don't feel much like eating these days anyway."

This patient is showing clear symptoms of depression. List the symptoms of depression present in this case.

(1)____________________

(2)____________________

(3)____________________

(4)____________________

c. List four other symptoms or signs of depression.

(1)___

(2)___

(3)___

(4)___

d. List the risk factors for suicide present in this patient's history.

(1)___

(2)___

(3)___

(4)___

(5)___

e. List six other risk factors for suicide.

(1)___

(2)___

(3)___

(4)___

(5)___

(6)___

f. List three questions you would ask to try to evaluate the patient's risk of suicide.

(1)___

(2)___

(3)___

3. You are called to a downtown office building for a "possible heart attack." When you reach the building, you are escorted into an office by a harried-looking businessman. "It's my secretary," he says. "She's having some kind of cardiac attack." In the midst of a buzzing group of people, you see a woman who looks to be about 24 years old sitting wide-eyed and pale. People are fanning her with file folders and trying to get her to drink some water. You make your way through the crowd and ask the woman what her problem is.

"Can't breathe," she gasps. "Chest all tight (gasp). Feel like I'm going to pass out (gasp). Everything is unreal (gasp), like I'm dying (gasp)."

"Quick! Quick!" squeaks one of the bystanders. "Get her to the hospital!"

Ignoring the chorus demanding that you leave immediately for the hospital, you begin taking the woman's vital signs. Her pulse is 112 beats/min and regular, her respirations are 30 breaths/min and deep, and her blood pressure (BP) is 160/88 mm Hg. You notice that her skin is cold and sweaty and her hands are shaking.

a. What do you think is this patient's problem?

___

b. What signs and symptoms led you to that conclusion?

(1)____

(2)____

(3)____

(4)____

(5)____

(6)____

(7)____

c. Are there any other diagnoses you need to take into consideration? If so, what are they?

(1)____

(2)____

(3)____

(4)____

(5)____

d. How will you attempt to control the situation quickly?

(1)____

(2)____

(3)____

(4)____

(5)____

(6)____

4. You and your partner are called to a downtown bar to see a man who has apparently become disruptive there. A police officer meets you at the entrance to the bar. "Listen," he says, "the barkeeper called us to deal with an unruly customer, but personally, I think the guy's a psycho case—so I thought maybe you folks ought to take a look at him."

You enter the bar and find a well-dressed but disheveled man pacing rapidly up and down. "One week from today," he is announcing, "one week from today, I'll be one of the richest men in America. I'm putting together a business empire now that will rule Wall Street." He is talking a mile a minute, cracking jokes, and gesturing extravagantly. He catches sight of you and your partner and says, "Well, hello, fellas. Bartender, give these fine young people a drink, on me. They do a great public service. This country was built on public service—yes indeed, it was. So give them a public service drink."

"You haven't paid for the drinks you already ordered," says the bartender.

"Listen, fathead, I said give these nice people a drink."

"Uh, sir," you break in, "we're not allowed to drink while on duty. And we thought maybe you'd like to take a little ride with us to the hospital."

"Hospital? What do I need to go to the hospital for? Never felt better in my life. By next week, I'll be able to buy the hospital, buy this bar too, buy the whole damned town."

The police officer says, "Maybe you ought to go with them, sir, just to get a checkup."

"Any of you puts a hand on me," replies the man, "I'll sue the whole lot of you. Assault. Battery. False imprisonment. I'll sue you for the whole lot, and let me tell you, you don't want to tangle with my team of lawyers. Best legal talent in the country. You wouldn't stand a chance."

a. What do you think is this man's problem?

____

b. What symptoms and signs led you to that conclusion?

(1)______________________________

(2)______________________________

(3)______________________________

(4)______________________________

c. How will you manage this patient?

____

____

5. You are called to a downtown street corner where several police officers are standing around, apparently trying to talk to a somewhat wild-eyed man who could be anywhere from 55 to 75 years old. He is dressed in about six layers of tattered clothes and wearing a naval officer's cap. He clearly hasn't had a bath, shave, or haircut in weeks. "He was just walking down the middle of Main Street," says one of the police officers, "as if he didn't even notice the traffic—and all those horns blowing, people screeching on their brakes."

You introduce yourself to the man and ask whether you can be of help. He mumbles something that sounds like, "Dogs and cats."

"Sorry," you say, "I didn't quite catch what you said."

"Salt and pepper," he says. "Black and blue, I didn't, don't 'ya know, I didn't."

The police officer gives you a meaningful look.

How will you manage this case?

____

____

____

____

6. A middle-aged woman calls for an ambulance because "my son is acting real strange." When you arrive at the designated address, the woman greets you at the door. She tells you that her 20-year-old son won't come out of his room. He's been in there for 2 days now. Sometimes she hears him talking to someone, but there isn't anyone else there. "I'm sure it's all that karate stuff," she says. "It just went to his head, made him crazy, all that black-belt business."

You go up to the son's room and knock on the door.

"You're not going to get me," says a voice from the other side of the door. "You won't take me alive."

"Sir, we're paramedics. We've just come to talk with you."

"You can't fool me. I know you're from the FBI. Well, you'll have to shoot me to take me."

You try the door and find it's unlocked. Inside, a young man clothed in karate garb is sitting in an armchair, gripping the armrests.

You introduce yourselves again. The patient looks away.

"You won't take me alive," he says again in a monotone. He looks suddenly toward the wall. "I know, I know," he says to the wall.

"Who are you talking to?" you ask.

He looks startled. "The voices said you would come. They killed John Lennon, and the FBI is after me. The voices said not to let you take me alive."

a. This patient is showing signs of:

(1) a panic attack.

(2) psychosis.

(3) depression.

(4) mania.

(5) disorganization.

b. Are there any indications that he might become violent?

____

c. If so, what are four indications?

(1)______________________________

(2)______________________________

(3)______________________________

(4)______________________________

d. How will you attempt to manage this case?

____

____

____

____

____

____

True/False

If you believe the statement to be more true than false, write the letter "T" in the space provided. If you believe the statement to be more false than true, write the letter "F."

_____ **1.** The most important thing a paramedic can do to help a disturbed patient is to remain calm and steady.

_____ **2.** There should be a maximum sense of urgency in evacuating a disturbed patient to the hospital because there is nothing that can be done to help the patient in the field.

_____ **3.** It is essential to correct a patient's misinterpretations of reality.

_____ **4.** The disturbed patient should be reassured that everything will turn out all right.

_____ **5.** The paramedic should remain with the disturbed patient at all times until the emergency department (ED) staff takes over the patient's care.

_____ **6.** Police intervention is usually required to transport a disturbed patient against his or her will.

Short Answer

Complete this section with short written answers using the space provided.

1. Certain situations have a higher potential for violence than others do. List three scenarios that should activate the paramedic's "nose for danger."

   a. ______________________________

   b. ______________________________

   c. ______________________________

2. List four diagnostic groups that would activate the paramedic's "nose for danger."

   a. ______________________________

   b. ______________________________

   c. ______________________________

   d. ______________________________

Fill in the Table

Fill in the missing parts of the table with the conditions and substances that can produce psychotic symptoms.

Selected Disease States That May Produce Psychotic Symptoms	
Disease State	**Psychotic Symptoms**
	Drug-induced psychoses, especially from: • Digitalis • Steroids • Disulfiram • Amphetamines • LSD, PCP, and other psychedelics Nutrition disorders: • Alcohol abuse • Vitamin deficiencies Poisoning with bromide or other heavy metals • Kidney failure • Liver failure
	Syphilis Parasites Viral encephalitis (eg, after measles) Brain abscess
	Seizure disorders (especially temporal lobe seizures) Primary and metastatic tumors of the brain Dementia Stroke Closed head injury
	Low cardiac output (eg, in heart failure)
	Thyroid hyperfunction (thyrotoxicosis) Adrenal hyperfunction (Cushing syndrome)
	Electrolyte imbalances (eg, after severe diarrhea) Hypoglycemia Diabetic ketoacidosis

CHAPTER 29

Trauma Systems and Mechanism of Injury

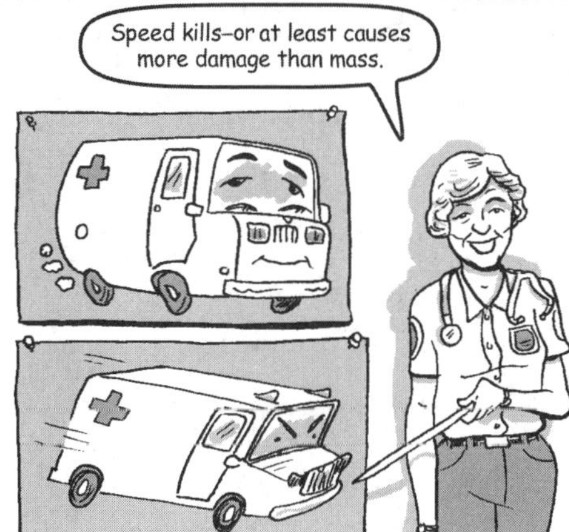

Matching

Part I

For each of the injuries listed in the left column, indicate which incident from the right column it is likely to be associated with. (Note: Some injuries may be associated with more than one type of mechanism.)

_____ 1. "Whiplash" injury
_____ 2. Multiple rib fractures
_____ 3. Fracture of the tibia/fibula
_____ 4. Fracture of the patella
_____ 5. Fracture of the humerus
_____ 6. Skull fracture
_____ 7. Laryngeal fracture
_____ 8. Flail chest
_____ 9. Pelvic fracture
_____ 10. Cervical spine injury

A. Head-on collision (unrestrained driver)
B. Lateral impact (unrestrained front-seat passenger)
C. Rear-impact collision (unrestrained driver)
D. Pedestrian struck by an oncoming car

Part II

Match each of the terms in the right column to the appropriate definition in the left column.

_____ 1. The shattering effect of a shock wave and its ability to cause disruption of tissues and structures.
_____ 2. An impact on the body by objects that cause injury without penetrating soft tissues or internal organs and cavities.
_____ 3. The leading edge of the shock wave.
_____ 4. The study of the physiology and mechanics of a living organism using the tools of mechanical engineering.
_____ 5. The energy that results from sudden changes in pressure as may occur in a diving accident or sudden decompression in an airplane.
_____ 6. A primary mechanism of tissue disruption from certain rifles in which pieces of the projectile break apart, allowing the pieces to create their own separate paths through tissues.
_____ 7. The way in which traumatic injuries occur; the forces that act on the body to cause damage.

A. Acceleration
B. Angle of impact
C. Arterial air embolism
D. Avulsing
E. Ballistics
F. Barometric energy
G. Biomechanics

______	**8.** The energy that results from motion (kinetic energy) or that is stored in an object (potential energy).	**H.** Blast front
______	**9.** The law of physics stating that energy can be neither created nor destroyed; it can only change form.	**I.** Blunt trauma
______	**10.** The study of the relationships among speed, mass, vector direction, and physical injury.	**J.** Brisance
______	**11.** The rate of change in velocity; speeding up.	**K.** Cavitation
______	**12.** The angle at which an object hits another; it characterizes the force vectors involved and has a bearing on patterns of energy dissipation.	**L.** Chemical energy
______	**13.** Air bubbles in the arterial blood vessels.	**M.** Deceleration
______	**14.** A tearing away or forcible separation.	**N.** Electrical energy
______	**15.** The study of nonpowered objects in flight; most often associated with rifle or handgun bullet travel.	**O.** Entrance wound
______	**16.** The energy delivered in the form of high voltage.	**P.** Exit wound
______	**17.** The point at which a penetrating object enters the body.	**Q.** Gravity
______	**18.** The point at which a penetrating object leaves the body, which may or may not be in a straight line from the entry wound.	**R.** Implosion
______	**19.** The acceleration of a body by the attraction of the earth's gravitational force, normally 32.2 ft/sec^2.	**S.** Index of suspicion
______	**20.** A bursting inward.	**T.** Kinetic energy (KE)
______	**21.** Cavity formation; shock waves that push tissues in front of and lateral to the projectile and may not necessarily increase the wound size or cause permanent injury but can result in cavitation.	**U.** Kinetics
______	**22.** The energy released as a result of a chemical reaction.	**V.** Law of conservation of energy
______	**23.** A negative acceleration; slowing down.	**W.** Mechanical energy
______	**24.** Anticipating the possibility of specific types of injury.	**X.** Mechanism of injury (MOI)
______	**25.** The energy associated with bodies in motion, expressed mathematically as half the mass times the square of the velocity.	**Y.** Missile fragmentation

Part III

Match each of the terms in the right column to the appropriate definition in the left column.

______	**1.** A score that relates to the likelihood of patient survival with the exception of a severe head injury. It is calculated on a scale from 1 to 16, with 16 being the best possible score. It takes into account the Glasgow Coma Scale (GCS) score, respiratory rate, respiratory expansion, systolic blood pressure, and capillary refill.	**A.** Multisystem trauma
______	**2.** A combination of hypothermia, coagulopathy (poor blood clotting), and acidosis that is a major contributor to death in patients with severe traumatic bleeding.	**B.** Negative wave pulse
______	**3.** Acute physiologic and structural change (injury) that occurs in a person's body as a result of the rapid dissipation of energy delivered by an external source.	**C.** Newton's first law of motion
______	**4.** Energy transferred from sources that are hotter than the body, such as a flame, hot water, and steam.	**D.** Newton's second law of motion

______	**5.** An applied force or pressure exerted against the surface and layers of the skin as tissues slide in opposite but parallel planes.	**E.** Pathway expansion
______	**6.** The path of crushed tissue produced by a missile traversing part of the body.	**F.** Penetrating trauma
______	**7.** Injury caused by objects that pierce the surface of the body, such as knives and bullets, and damage internal tissues and organs.	**G.** Permanent cavity
______	**8.** The tissue displacement that occurs as a result of low-displacement shock waves that travel at the speed of sound in tissue.	**H.** Positive wave pulse
______	**9.** The law of motion stating that the force that an object can exert is the product of its mass times its acceleration.	**I.** Potential energy
______	**10.** The law of motion stating that a body at rest will remain at rest unless acted on by an outside force.	**J.** Pulmonary blast injuries
______	**11.** An injury to the cervical vertebrae or its supporting ligaments and muscles, usually resulting from sudden acceleration or deceleration.	**K.** Revised Trauma Score (RTS)
______	**12.** A pattern of vehicle-versus-pedestrian injuries in children and people of short stature in which (1) the bumper hits pelvis and femur, (2) the chest and abdomen hit the grille or low hood, and (3) the head strikes the ground.	**L.** Shearing
______	**13.** The distance an object travels per unit time.	**M.** Thermal energy
______	**14.** The eardrum; a thin, semitransparent membrane in the middle ear that transmits sound vibrations to the internal ear by means of the auditory ossicles.	**N.** Trauma
______	**15.** The phase of an explosion in which pressure from the blast is less than atmospheric pressure.	**O.** Trauma lethal triad
______	**16.** Trauma caused by generalized mechanisms that affect numerous body systems.	**P.** Trauma score
______	**17.** A scoring system used for patients with head trauma.	**Q.** Tympanic membrane
______	**18.** Pulmonary trauma resulting from short-range exposure to the detonation of high explosives.	**R.** Velocity (V)
______	**19.** The amount of energy stored in an object, which is the product of mass, gravity, and height, and which is converted into kinetic energy and results in injury, such as from a fall.	**S.** Waddell triad
______	**20.** The phase of the explosion in which there is a pressure front with a pressure higher than atmospheric pressure.	**T.** Whiplash

Multiple Choice

Read each item carefully, and then select the best response.

______ **1.** Which of the following is NOT a criterion for referral to a regional trauma center?

- **A.** 45-year-old patient restrained in a low-speed auto crash
- **B.** Pelvic fracture
- **C.** Motorcycle crash at a speed greater than 20 mph
- **D.** A pregnant patient

______ **2.** The "platinum 10 minutes" refers to the:

- **A.** amount of time taken to extricate a patient from a motor vehicle crash.
- **B.** total response time to a traumatic incident.
- **C.** goal of the maximum time spent at a scene for a critical trauma patient.
- **D.** time deciding on your "transport decision."

_____ **3.** Which level of trauma center would be able to provide Advanced Trauma Life Support (ATLS) before transfer of patients to a higher-level trauma center?

A. Level I
B. Level II
C. Level III
D. Level IV

_____ **4.** Pediatric pedestrian injuries differ from adult pedestrian injuries because:

A. the skulls of children are not fused, which allows for energy absorption.
B. children are shorter, so they are more likely to be run over by the vehicle.
C. children are more likely to "fly over" the vehicle.
D. the bumper is more likely to strike children's femurs rather than their lower extremities.

_____ **5.** All of the following are important information to provide to the trauma team, EXCEPT the:

A. name of the street gang.
B. range at which the firearm was fired.
C. kind of bullet or projectile.
D. type of weapon used.

_____ **6.** Blast injuries may be seen in which of the following scenarios?

A. Mining mishaps
B. Chemical plants
C. Terrorist activities
D. All of the above

_____ **7.** All of the following are factors in the seriousness of firearms injuries, EXCEPT:

A. the type of tissue penetrated.
B. missile velocity.
C. fragmentation.
D. the firearm manufacturer.

_____ **8.** Which of the following is one type of mechanical energy?

A. Kinetic energy
B. Barometric energy
C. Electrical energy
D. Chemical energy

_____ **9.** Criteria for transport of an adult patient to a trauma center as defined by the American College of Surgeons Committee on Trauma (ACS-COT) and the Centers for Disease Control and Prevention (CDC) include all of the following, EXCEPT:

A. Glasgow Coma Scale score of 13 or less.
B. amputation proximal to the wrist or ankle.
C. ejection from an automobile.
D. falls from a height greater than 10 feet.

_____ **10.** A combination of facial injuries, pulmonary contusions, flail chest, ruptured aorta, and fractured sternum is an example of which of the following?

A. "Ring" of chest injuries
B. Typical injuries from lateral impacts
C. Typical injuries from head-on crashes
D. "Down and under pathway"

Labeling

Label the following diagram with the correct mechanisms of blast injuries.

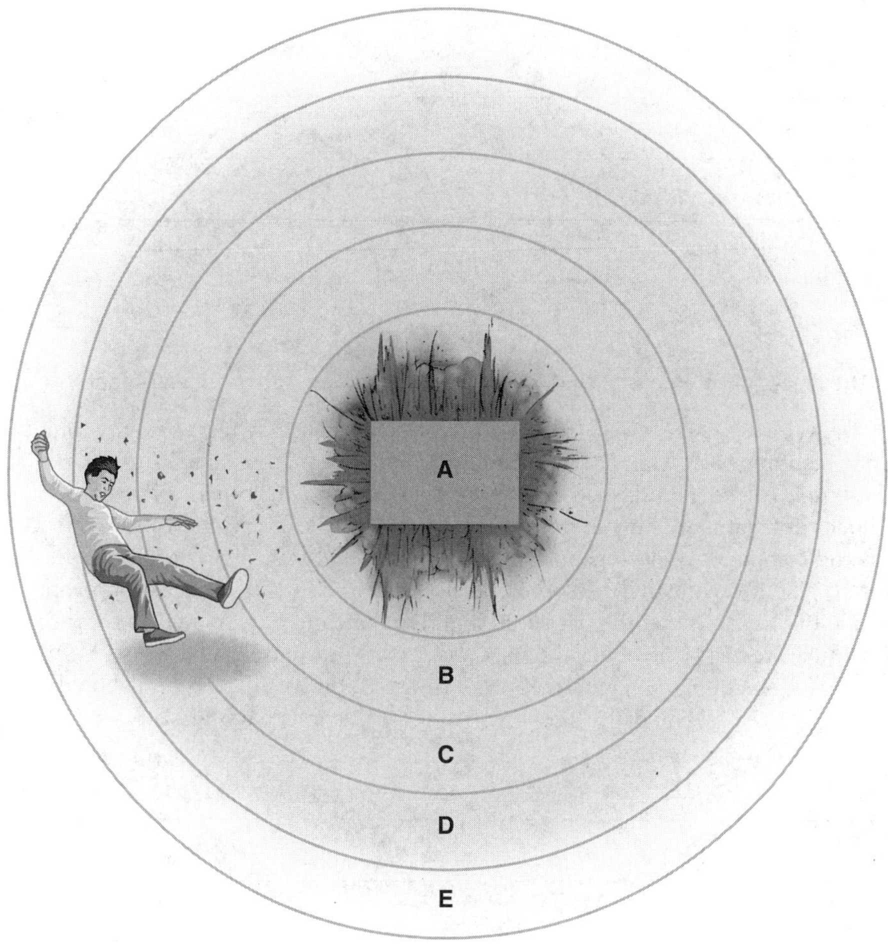

A. ______________________

B. ______________________

C. ______________________

D. ______________________

E. ______________________

Fill in the Blank

Read each item carefully, and then complete the statement by filling in the missing word(s).

1. The speed, duration, and pressure of the shock wave from an explosion are affected by the following factors:

a. ______________________

b. ______________________

c. ______________________

d. ______________________

2. The severity of a stab wound depends on the __________ area involved, depth of __________, blade length, and angle of penetration.

3. __________ __________ __________ is one of the most concerning of pulmonary blast injuries.

4. Severity of injuries in falls from heights depend on the following factors:

a. ______________________________

b. ______________________________

c. ______________________________

d. ______________________________

e. ______________________________

5. Specific injuries associated with seat belt use include __________ fractures due to flexion stresses and __________ sprains.

Identify

Read the following case studies, and then list the mechanism of injury, chief complaint, vital signs, and pertinent negatives.

1. While working in a paramedic first-response vehicle, you receive a call for a motor vehicle crash. On arrival, you find two patients who are out of the vehicle and standing along the roadside. You notice that the vehicle appears to have rolled over onto its side. No other patients are involved, and the scene is deemed safe for patient contact and treatment. One occupant denies any complaint and does not want anything to do with emergency medical services (EMS). The other patient is holding his right forearm and complains of neck pain. The injured occupant states that he had his seat belt on. You notice that the airbag deployed. The injured man denies loss of consciousness (LOC), shortness of breath, or other complaints. Your physical examination indicates that the patient is slightly ashen and has an obvious bruising and deformity to his right midshaft radius/ulna. He has positive distal pulses and motor and sensory function (PMS), along with the following findings: pulse is 110 beats/min and regular, respirations are 16 breaths/min and unlabored, blood pressure (BP) is 106/96 mm Hg, and Spo_2 is 98%. The patient denies significant previous medical history.

   a. Mechanism of injury:

   ____

   ____

   b. Chief complaint:

   ____

   ____

   c. Vital signs:

   ____

   ____

   d. Pertinent negatives:

   ____

   ____

2. Today you are assigned to work on an advanced life support (ALS) ambulance. Your response area includes many high-speed interstate highways. It is toward the end of your shift and, until now, the day has been uneventful. Medcom dispatches you, Priority 1 (a Charlie response), to a reported motorcycle crash with one critical injury. On arrival, you notice a long line of stopped traffic and concerned bystanders. They are frantically waving you toward the injured patient. You notice a one-vehicle, motorcycle-versus-guardrail collision. The patient appears to be talking, but you notice a pool of blood alongside him as well as a cracked helmet. He has a badly deformed lower leg that you quickly conclude is fractured or dislocated. The patient is in obvious pain and is able to communicate that he "hurts all over."

You quickly begin to assess the patient, and he appears agitated, ashen, diaphoretic, and slightly short of breath. He has delayed (more than 2 seconds) capillary refill, and he has diminished left-side breath sounds and no tracheal deviation. His pulse is 120 beats/min, respiratory rate is 28 breaths/min, BP is unobtainable, and Spo_2 is 92%. You note that the patient has a palpable femoral pulse but no radial or brachial pulse.

a. Mechanism of injury:

____

____

b. Chief complaint:

____

____

c. Vital signs:

____

____

d. Pertinent negatives:

____

____

3. You respond to a "routine" call at an adult care facility for a "fall." Your patient is an 82-year-old woman who is lying on a carpeted floor with a walker positioned beside her. She appears conscious but slightly confused. She does not really know why she fell or how she ended up on the ground. She asks you to help her up. You begin your primary survey of the patient, and she denies any knowledge of the incident. During the secondary assessment, she denies any chest discomfort, shortness of breath, or neck or back pain. You note some deformity and rotation of her right lower extremity. On palpation, it is tender to the touch. The patient is confused regarding her previous medical history. The staff tells you that she has a history of transient ischemic attacks (TIAs) and heart problems. She is on multiple medications and is allergic to morphine sulfate. Her abdomen is soft and nontender. Her vital signs are as follows: pulse 58 beats/min and irregular; BP 158/110 mm Hg; Spo_2 95%. Her skin is pale, cool, and dry.

a. Mechanism of injury:

____

____

b. Chief complaint:

____

____

c. Vital signs:

____

____

d. Pertinent negatives:

____

____

Complete the Patient Care Report

Reread the second case study in the preceding Identify exercise and then complete the following patient care report (PCR). Feel free to create the times and numbers as well as the date of the incident.

<table>
<tr><th colspan="6">EMS Patient Care Report (PCR)</th></tr>
<tr><td>Date:</td><td>Incident No.:</td><td colspan="2">Nature of Call:</td><td colspan="2">Location:</td></tr>
<tr><td>Dispatched:</td><td>En Route:</td><td>At Scene:</td><td>Transport:</td><td>At Hospital:</td><td>In Service:</td></tr>
<tr><th colspan="6">Patient Information</th></tr>
<tr><td colspan="3">Age:
Sex:
Weight (in kg [lb]):</td><td colspan="3">Allergies:
Medications:
Past Medical History:
Chief Complaint:</td></tr>
<tr><th colspan="6">Vital Signs</th></tr>
<tr><td>Time:</td><td>BP:</td><td>Pulse:</td><td>Respirations:</td><td colspan="2">SpO_2:</td></tr>
<tr><td>Time:</td><td>BP:</td><td>Pulse:</td><td>Respirations:</td><td colspan="2">SpO_2:</td></tr>
<tr><td>Time:</td><td>BP:</td><td>Pulse:</td><td>Respirations:</td><td colspan="2">SpO_2:</td></tr>
<tr><th colspan="6">EMS Treatment
(circle all that apply)</th></tr>
<tr><td colspan="2">Oxygen @ ______ L/min via (circle one):
NC NRM Bag-mask device</td><td>Assisted Ventilation</td><td>Airway Adjunct</td><td colspan="2">CPR</td></tr>
<tr><td>Defibrillation</td><td>Bleeding Control</td><td>Bandaging</td><td>Splinting</td><td colspan="2">Other:</td></tr>
<tr><th colspan="6">Narrative</th></tr>
<tr><td colspan="6"></td></tr>
</table>

Ambulance Calls

The following case scenarios provide an opportunity to explore the concerns associated with the mechanism of injury and trauma systems. Read each scenario, and then answer each question.

1. You are called to the scene of a backroad single-vehicle collision in which a car plowed into a utility pole. The driver of the car is sitting on the grass beside his wrecked vehicle, looking dazed and confused. Which parameters would you use to assess the mechanism of injury and suspected injuries and/or injury patterns?

   a. ______________________________

   b. ______________________________

   c. ______________________________

   d. ______________________________

   e. ______________________________

   f. ______________________________

2. You are summoned to the scene of a smoky apartment-house fire. When you arrive, one of the firefighters directs you to a casualty who has been carried to a spot just beyond the fire lines. The firefighter tells you that the man jumped from a window.

   a. Which further information do you need to obtain about this patient to evaluate the potential seriousness of the injuries he might have sustained in making that jump?

   ____

   ____

   ____

   ____

   ____

   ____

   b. Assuming the patient landed on his feet, which injuries might you expect him to have suffered?

   ____

   ____

3. On your next call, you are summoned to a housing project where a 2-year-old child managed to crawl over the edge of a second-story balcony and fall into the playground below. Which sort of injuries would this child most likely have sustained, and why?

   ____

   ____

4. You are called to a somewhat disreputable downtown area for a "man shot." You arrive on the scene to see the patient lying on the ground in the center of a small group of men, some of whom are apparently intoxicated and all of whom are talking at once.

a. What is the *first* action you will take before entering the scene?

____

b. Which information do you need to obtain regarding the shooting incident?

(1)______________________________

(2)______________________________

(3)______________________________

(4)______________________________

(5)______________________________

5. A fire at a warehouse of a large construction company ignites the stock of dynamite and produces an explosion that shatters windows for blocks around. As you respond to the scene, you review in your mind the different kinds of injuries you might soon have to deal with. List the four *mechanisms* of injury that can be produced by an explosion, and describe each one.

a. ______________________________

b. ______________________________

c. ______________________________

d. ______________________________

6. Among the patients whom you treat at the scene of the explosion is a young man who had been taking a walk about half a block from the construction company when the explosion occurred. The man states that the blast "knocked me clear off my feet." He complains of a "tight feeling in my chest" and blurry vision. On physical examination, he appears somewhat confused; he cannot tell you the date or what day of the week it is. His vital signs are as follows: pulse 100 beats/min, full and regular; respirations 30 breaths/min and somewhat shallow; BP 120/80 mm Hg. His skin is warm and dry. Aside from a little dried blood in the left ear canal, there are no other physical findings. Which tissues are at risk? What is the evidence for you thinking so?

Tissues at Risk	Evidence
1.	
2.	
3.	

True/False

If you believe the statement to be more true than false, write the letter "T" in the space provided. If you believe the statement to be more false than true, write the letter "F."

______ **1.** Solid organs are relatively protected from shock-wave injury but may be injured by secondary missiles or a hurled body.

______ **2.** A Level IV trauma center provides the most comprehensive trauma care possible.

______ **3.** Transport considerations are not necessary if the patient is seriously hurt.

______ **4.** Blunt trauma typically occurs in motor vehicle crashes.

______ **5.** The "paper-bag syndrome" can result in a pneumothorax.

_____ **6.** Small children should be seated in the front seats of motor vehicles so that they will benefit from the protection offered by airbags.

_____ **7.** Evaluation of the patient's GCS score is a component of step 1 in the 2011 CDC decision scheme for field trauma of injured patients.

_____ **8.** If a patient was riding a motorcycle and was involved in a crash at about 15 mph, he should automatically be taken to a trauma center based on the 2011 CDC decision scheme for field trauma of injured patients.

Short Answer

Complete this section with short written answers using the space provided.

1. A 2,000-lb automobile is traveling at 20 mph when it strikes a pedestrian.

a. What happens to the kinetic energy of the vehicle at the moment of impact?

____

____

____

b. If the vehicle weighed 6,000 lb instead of 2,000 lb, what difference would that make in terms of its kinetic energy?

____

____

____

c. If the vehicle were traveling at 60 mph rather than 20 mph, what difference would that make in terms of its kinetic energy?

____

____

____

2. A car traveling at 50 mph goes out of control and slams into a concrete wall. That sequence of events involves five phases of deceleration, each of which proceeds like a separate collision and each of which involves a transfer of kinetic energy (KE). Which objects are involved in each of the first three collisions, and what happens to the KE in each case?

a. Collision 1:

____

____

____

b. Collision 2:

____

____

____

c. Collision 3:

______

______

______

3. Careful inspection of a wrecked vehicle can enable the rescuer to detect injuries among the patients that might not otherwise be obvious. For each of the vehicular findings mentioned in the following list, list the injuries that are likely to be associated.

a. Deformed dashboard

(1)______

(2)______

(3)______

(4)______

(5)______

b. Deformed steering column

(1)______

(2)______

(3)______

(4)______

(5)______

(6)______

c. Cracked windshield

(1)______

(2)______

(3)______

(4)______

d. Door smashed in

(1)______

(2)______

(3)______

4. One of the most lethal objects in a motor vehicle is the steering wheel. Whenever you find structural damage to a steering wheel—indeed, whenever there is significant deformity to the front end of a car involved in a collision—you must be alert for the presence of the "ring of injuries" impact that the steering wheel may have produced in the driver of the car. List six injuries that may be associated with steering wheel trauma.

a. ______

b. ______________________________

c. ______________________________

d. ______________________________

e. ______________________________

f. ______________________________

Fill in the Table

Fill in the missing parts of the table.

1. Fill in the key elements for the corresponding definition.

Key Elements for Trauma Centers		
Level	**Definition**	**Key Elements**
Level I	A comprehensive regional resource that is a tertiary care facility. Capable of providing total care for every aspect of injury—from prevention through rehabilitation.	**1.** **2.** **3.** **4.** **5.**
Level II	Able to initiate definitive care for all injured patients.	**1.** **2.** **3.** **4.** **5.**
Level III	Able to provide prompt assessment, resuscitation, and stabilization of injured patients and emergency operations.	**1.** **2.** **3.** **4.** **5.**

Level IV	Able to provide ATLS before transfer of patients to a higher-level trauma center.	1. 2. 3. 4.

2. List the "ring" of chest injuries from impacting the steering wheel or dashboard.

"Ring" of Chest Injuries From Impact With the Steering Wheel or Dashboard
• _________________ • Soft-tissue neck trauma • Larynx and tracheal trauma • _________________ • _________________ • _________________ • Pulmonary contusion • Hemothorax, rib fractures • _________________ • _________________ • Intra-abdominal injuries

Problem Solving

Use the formula for kinetic energy to answer the following questions.

$$KE = M/2 \times V^2$$

You have responded to a motor vehicle crash. This was a collision involving a car and a stationary bridge abutment. There are two patients. Your patient appears to be a 6-feet man who weighs approximately 200 lb. The patient is conscious and alert. While talking to him, you discover that he was not wearing a seat belt, and his vehicle was traveling at 50 mph.

1. Use the formula for calculating kinetic energy (KE) to determine the KE units involved in this crash. The second passenger in the vehicle was also unbelted, and she weighs 120 lb.

2. How many KE units are involved for the second passenger?

CHAPTER 30

Bleeding

Left shoulder pain after a sports injury can signify a spleen injury.

Matching

Match each of the definitions in the left column to the appropriate term in the right column.

_____	**1.** A mass of blood in the soft tissues beneath the skin; it indicates bleeding into soft tissues and may be the result of a minor or a severe injury.	**A.** Afterload
_____	**2.** Blood in the urine.	**B.** Blood
_____	**3.** The proportion of red blood cells in the total blood volume.	**C.** Cardiac output
_____	**4.** Passage of stools containing bright red blood.	**D.** Compensated shock
_____	**5.** Vomited blood.	**E.** Decompensated (hypotensive) shock
_____	**6.** The body's natural blood-clotting mechanism.	**F.** Ejection fraction
_____	**7.** A condition in which volume is lost in the form of blood.	**G.** Exsanguination
_____	**8.** Bleeding.	**H.** Hematemesis
_____	**9.** Coughed-up blood.	**I.** Hematochezia
_____	**10.** A bleeding disorder that is primarily hereditary, in which clotting does not occur or occurs insufficiently.	**J.** Hematocrit
_____	**11.** An abnormal state associated with inadequate oxygen and nutrient delivery to the metabolic apparatus of the cell.	**K.** Hematoma
_____	**12.** The precontraction pressure in the heart, which increases as the volume of blood builds up.	**L.** Hematuria
_____	**13.** Small cells in the blood that are essential for clot formation.	**M.** Hemophilia
_____	**14.** A component of blood; made of 92% water, 6% to 7% proteins, and electrolytes, clotting factors, and glucose.	**N.** Hemoptysis
_____	**15.** The delivery of oxygen and nutrients to the cells, organs, and tissues of the body.	**O.** Hemorrhage
_____	**16.** The pressure in the aorta against which the left ventricle must pump blood; increasing this pressure can decrease cardiac output.	**P.** Hemorrhagic shock
_____	**17.** The fluid tissue that is pumped by the heart through the arteries, veins, and capillaries; it consists of plasma and formed elements or cells, such as red blood cells, white blood cells, and platelets.	**Q.** Hemostasis
_____	**18.** The amount of blood pumped by the heart per minute; calculated by multiplying the stroke volume by the pulse rate per minute.	**R.** Hypoperfusion

______	**19.** The early stage of shock, in which the body can still compensate for blood loss. The systolic blood pressure and brain perfusion are maintained.	**S.** Hypovolemic shock
______	**20.** The late stage of shock, when blood pressure is falling.	**T.** Melena
______	**21.** The loss of the total blood volume, resulting in death.	**U.** Perfusion
______	**22.** The percentage of blood that leaves the heart each time it contracts.	**V.** Plasma
______	**23.** Passage of dark, tarry stools.	**W.** Platelets
______	**24.** A condition that occurs when the circulating blood volume is inadequate to deliver adequate oxygen and nutrients to the body.	**X.** Preload
______	**25.** A condition that occurs when the level of tissue perfusion decreases below that needed to maintain normal cellular functions.	**Y.** Shock

Multiple Choice

Read each item carefully, and then select the best response.

______ **1.** __________ is a blood test that measures the portion of red blood cells (RBCs) in the whole blood.

- **A.** Plasma count
- **B.** Hematocrit
- **C.** Cardiac output
- **D.** Ejection fraction

______ **2.** Which of the following substances accounts for more than half of the body's blood volume?

- **A.** Erythrocytes
- **B.** Leukocytes
- **C.** Plasma
- **D.** Hemoglobin

______ **3.** A laceration or tear of a large artery can cause a patient to exsanguinate in as little as ________ minutes.

- **A.** 2
- **B.** 3
- **C.** 5
- **D.** 10

______ **4.** The body cannot tolerate an acute blood loss of __________. This loss will produce a significant change in vital signs of the adult patient, referred to as a Class III hemorrhage.

- **A.** less than 5%
- **B.** less than 15%
- **C.** 15% to 30%
- **D.** 30% to 40%

______ **5.** When you encounter a patient who is bleeding, the first thing you should do is:

- **A.** estimate the blood loss.
- **B.** apply direct pressure.
- **C.** check for breathing.
- **D.** don personal protective equipment.

______ **6.** A stool that contains bright red blood is called:

- **A.** hematochezia.
- **B.** melena.
- **C.** hematuria.
- **D.** epistaxis.

______ **7.** The coughing up of blood is referred to as:

- **A.** hematemesis.
- **B.** hematuria.
- **C.** hemoptysis.
- **D.** melena.

______ **8.** The initial stage of hemorrhagic shock is characterized by low circulating blood volume with:

A. a respiratory rate of 30 to 40 breaths/min.
B. minimal signs of hypoperfusion.
C. absent capillary refill.
D. a heart rate of more than 120 beats/min.

______ **9.** Which of the following statements about the use of an arterial tourniquet is correct?

A. It is rarely used in the field today.
B. It can be used only for arterial bleeding.
C. It should be placed proximal to the injury on the extremity.
D. It should be applied on and off every 20 minutes to save the limb.

______ **10.** A patient has the signs and symptoms of shock from a fracture or a burn. This is MOST likely due to which cause of shock?

A. Poor vessel function
B. Low fluid volume
C. Respiratory failure
D. Pump failure

Labeling

Label the following diagram with the correct terms.

1. The circulatory system

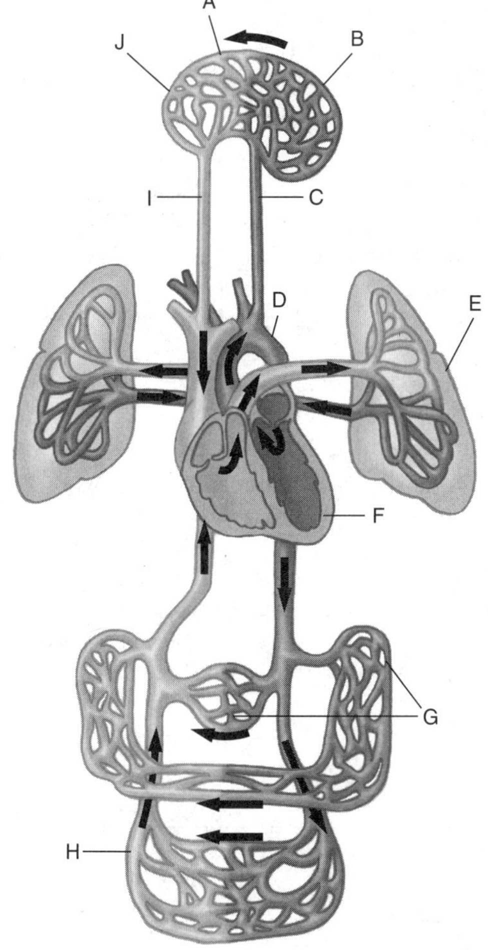

A. ______________________________

B. ______________________________

C. ______________________________

D. ______________________________

E. ______________________________

F. ______________________________

G. ______________________________

H. ______________________________

I. ______________________________

J. ______________________________

Fill in the Blank

Read each item carefully, and then complete the statement by filling in the missing word(s).

1. Red blood cells contain __________, a protein that gives blood its reddish color.
2. Blood circulation through an organ or tissue that meets the cells' current needs for oxygen, nutrients, and waste removal is known as __________.
3. __________ is the process in which platelets aggregate at the site, plugging the hole and sealing injured portions of the vessel.
4. A lower gastrointestinal (GI) bleed is indicated with the passing of __________, which is a dark, tarry-looking stool.
5. __________ is bleeding from the nose.
6. __________ happens when the level of tissue perfusion drops below normal limits.
7. When a patient is passing a bloody stool, this is referred to as __________ and can indicate hemorrhage near the external opening of the anus.
8. A small portion of the population lacks one or more of the blood's __________ factors. This condition is called __________.
9. As __________ increases and __________ drops, patients in shock develop cold, mottled, and pulseless extremities with __________ mental status.
10. The organs and organ systems with a high incidence of exsanguination from penetrating injuries include the __________, thoracic vascular system, abdominal vascular system, venous system, and __________.
11. The three phases of shock are __________, __________, and __________ shock.
12. The IV fluid of choice when replacing lost blood volume is either __________ __________ or __________ __________.
13. Do not give the patient with suspected hypovolemia anything by _______ because he or she is likely to ________.
14. Solutions that do not contain proteins or any other large molecules, and that are typically used in shock fluid resuscitation, are known as __________.

Identify

Read the following case study, and then list the chief complaint, vital signs, and pertinent negatives.

You are called to the scene of a local gas station where the 44-year-old man behind the counter was shot during a robbery. He is experiencing abdominal pain with a small bullet wound in the umbilical area. Upon arrival, the police determine that the perpetrator has fled the scene, so the scene is safe for you to proceed with your trauma assessment. John, the patient, is clutching his belly with a towel for bleeding control. You note there is no radial pulse, yet John is still alert and oriented. Your partner quickly places John on high-flow supplemental oxygen by a nonrebreathing mask and applies an occlusive dressing to the wound. You determine that John has no obvious injury to his chest, and his lung sounds are equal in both lungs. As he is being packaged to go to the trauma center, an electrocardiogram (ECG) monitor is applied, and you determine that John's heart is in a sinus tachycardia with a rate of 120 beats/min and no ectopy. He is breathing at 24 breaths/min, and his room air saturation is 92%. He is very anxious but comes around with the oxygen and is able to answer all your questions. His pupils are equal, round, and reactive to light and accommodation (PERRLA). His blood pressure (BP) is 80/56 mm Hg, and his skin is pale, cool, and diaphoretic. You determine that there are no other injuries, although you know that an abdominal gunshot wound (GSW) is significant, and it is difficult to tell how much internal bleeding he may have so far. En route to the trauma center, you start two large-bore IV lines of normal saline. You call ahead to prepare the emergency department (ED) for your arrival and then begin reassessment.

1. Chief complaint:

____

____

2. Vital signs:

____

____

3. Pertinent negatives:

____

____

Complete the Patient Care Report

Reread the case study in the preceding Identify exercise, and then complete the following patient care report (PCR) for the patient.

EMS Patient Care Report (PCR)					
Date:	Incident No.:	Nature of Call:		Location:	
Dispatched:	En Route:	At Scene:	Transport:	At Hospital:	In Service:

Patient Information	
Age: Sex: Weight (in kg [lb]):	Allergies: Medications: Past Medical History: Chief Complaint:

Vital Signs				
Time:	BP:	Pulse:	Respirations:	SpO_2:
Time:	BP:	Pulse:	Respirations:	SpO_2:
Time:	BP:	Pulse:	Respirations:	SpO_2:

EMS Treatment (circle all that apply)				
Oxygen @ ______ L/min via (circle one): NC NRM Bag-mask device		Assisted Ventilation	Airway Adjunct	CPR
Defibrillation	Bleeding Control	Bandaging	Splinting	Other:

Narrative

Ambulance Calls

The following case scenarios provide an opportunity to explore the concerns associated with patient management and paramedic care. Read each scenario, and then answer each question.

1. A middle-aged man was struck by a car as he was crossing the street. You find him lying by the side of the road, complaining of severe pain in his abdomen, where the car hit him. You would like to make an assessment of his state of perfusion. How will you assess the following?
   a. His *peripheral* perfusion:

   ____

   ____

   b. The perfusion to his *brain*:

   ____

   ____

2. You are called to a downtown bar where firearms were used to settle a difference of opinion. You find a man lying on the floor of the bar, unconscious, his trouser leg soaked in blood. In the correct sequence, list the steps you would take in treating this patient.

   a. ____

   b. ____

   c. ____

   d. ____

   e. ____

   f. ____

3. One rainy day, a car bomb was detonated in front of a foreign consulate. Some bystanders were injured by flying debris, including jagged pieces of metal torn from the car's body. The first patient you come upon is bleeding from multiple sites, including a deep gash on the right side of the neck and a laceration that has partially severed the right leg at the groin. The leg laceration is gushing blood; it is too proximal to benefit from a tourniquet. It is difficult to evaluate the patient's skin condition in the rain. Pulse is around 100 beats/min and somewhat weak; respirations are 30 breaths/min.
   a. Which steps would you take at the scene?

   (1)____

   (2)____

   (3)____

   (4)____

   b. Which steps would you take during transport?

   (1)____

   (2)____

   (3)____

4. A second patient from the car bombing, a young man, was sideswiped by a piece of flying debris, which made a clean 14-inch incision straight across his abdomen. He is conscious and in moderate distress. Pulse is 104 beats/min and regular, respirations are 28 breaths/min and slightly labored, and BP is 104/70 mm Hg. What looks to be a major portion of the patient's intestines is outside the abdomen.

a. Which steps would you take at the scene?

(1)__________

(2)__________

(3)__________

b. Which steps would you take during transport?

(1)__________

(2)__________

(3)__________

True/False

If you believe the statement to be more true than false, write the letter "T" in the space provided. If you believe the statement to be more false than true, write the letter "F."

______ **1.** One of the earliest signs of hypovolemic shock is a fall in the blood pressure.

______ **2.** Patients in hemorrhagic shock tend to have a normal pulse rate.

______ **3.** The IV fluid of choice to provide volume to a patient in hypovolemic shock is 5% dextrose in water (D_5W).

______ **4.** A patient may go into shock without losing any blood or fluid from the body.

______ **5.** The amount of blood pumped through the circulatory system in 1 minute is known as the cardiac output.

______ **6.** The function of plasma is to produce red blood cells (RBCs) and white blood cells (WBCs).

______ **7.** Nontraumatic internal bleeding usually happens in the gastrointestinal tract.

______ **8.** A 1-year-old child has a blood volume of approximately 800 mL.

______ **9.** You can use a wire, rope, or any narrow material as a tourniquet.

______ **10.** Definitive management for internal hemorrhage is in the hospital.

Short Answer

Complete this section with short written answers using the space provided.

1. Three components are required for a functioning circulatory system. If any one of those components is impaired, shock may result. List the three necessary components.

a. __________

b. __________

c. __________

2. The type of shock you will see most frequently in the prehospital setting is hemorrhagic shock. It is very important to detect hypovolemic shock early and to start treatment early. To do so, you must have a high index of suspicion in assessing patients at risk of hypovolemic shock, which means you must be aware of the situations in which hypovolemia is likely to occur. List four causes of hypovolemic shock.

a. __________

b. __________

c. __________

d. __________

3. Knowing the findings in hemorrhagic shock is important for you as a paramedic. For each of the following findings, note whether the value is increased, decreased, flat, or changed during suspected Class II fluid and blood loss.

Estimated Fluid and Blood Loss (for Class II)	
Heart rate (beats/min)	
Systolic blood pressure (mm Hg)	
Pulse pressure (mm Hg)	
Respiratory rate (breaths/min)	
Central nervous system/mental status	
Skin condition	
Urine output (mL/h)	

4. It is not necessary in the field to make a specific diagnosis of a patient's abdominal pain, but it is necessary to be able to recognize when a potentially life-threatening situation exists. Any patient with abdominal pain showing symptoms or signs of shock must be considered to be in danger. To recognize that danger, you must be able to spot the symptoms and signs of shock. List six symptoms and signs of shock.

a. ______

b. ______

c. ______

d. ______

e. ______

f. ______

5. List the four steps in managing external hemorrhage.

a. ______

b. ______

c. ______

d. ______

Fill in the Table

Fill in the missing parts of the table.

Compensated Versus Decompensated Shock	
Compensated	**Decompensated**
• ______	• Altered mental status (verbal to unresponsive)
• Sense of impending doom	• ______
• ______	• Labored or irregular breathing
• Clammy (cool, moist) skin	• ______
• ______	• Ashen, mottled, or cyanotic skin
• Shortness of breath	• ______
• ______	• Diminished urine output (oliguria)
• Delayed capillary refill in infants and children	• ______
• ______	
• Normal systolic blood pressure	

CHAPTER 31

Soft-Tissue Trauma

The paramedic is asked to be an island of calm and authority.

Matching

Part I

Match each of the terms in the right column to the appropriate definition in the left column.

	Definition		Term
______	**1.** Protein that gives tensile strength to the connective tissues of the body.	**A.**	Abrasion
______	**2.** A bruise; an injury that causes bleeding beneath the skin but does not break the skin.	**B.**	Amputation
______	**3.** A traumatic injury that results in the soft tissue of a part of the body being drawn downward like a glove being removed.	**C.**	Avulsion
______	**4.** The tendency toward constancy or stability in the body's internal environment.	**D.**	Bandage
______	**5.** A type of injury that occurs when a foreign material is forcefully injected into soft tissue.	**E.**	Chemotactic factors
______	**6.** A localized collection of blood in the soft tissues as a result of injury or a broken blood vessel.	**F.**	Closed wound
______	**7.** The continual shedding of the dead cells on the surface of the skin.	**G.**	Collagen
______	**8.** Material used to directly cover a wound.	**H.**	Contusion
______	**9.** Extravasation of blood under the skin, producing a "black-and-blue" mark.	**I.**	Degloving
______	**10.** The outermost layer of the skin.	**J.**	Dermis
______	**11.** Cells that contain granules.	**K.**	Desquamation
______	**12.** An infection commonly caused by *Clostridium perfringens*, which results in tissue destruction and gas production that may lead to death.	**L.**	Dressing
______	**13.** An injury in which a portion of the body is denuded of the epidermis by scraping or rubbing.	**M.**	Ecchymosis
______	**14.** An injury in which part of the body is completely or partially severed.	**N.**	High-pressure injection injury
______	**15.** An injury that leaves a piece of skin or other tissue partially or completely torn away from the body.	**O.**	Epidermis
______	**16.** The inner layer of skin, containing hair follicle roots, sweat glands, blood vessels, nerve endings, and sebaceous glands.	**P.**	Epithelialization
______	**17.** The formation of fresh epithelial tissue to heal a wound.	**Q.**	Erythema
______	**18.** Material used to secure a dressing in place.	**R.**	Fasciitis
______	**19.** The factors that cause cells to migrate into an area.	**S.**	Flexor tenosynovitis of the hand

_____ **20.** An injury in which damage occurs beneath the skin or mucous membrane but the surface remains intact. — **T.** Gangrene

_____ **21.** A closed-space infection of the hand. — **U.** Granulocytes

_____ **22.** Inflammation of the fascia. — **V.** Homeostasis

_____ **23.** Reddening of the skin. — **W.** Hematoma

Part II

Match each of the terms in the right column to the appropriate definition in the left column.

_____ **1.** Death of tissue from bacterial infection caused by more than one infecting organism—most commonly, *Staphylococcus aureus* and hemolytic streptococci; this condition has a high mortality rate. — **A.** Hypertrophic scar

_____ **2.** Inflammation of the muscle, usually caused by infection. — **B.** Incision

_____ **3.** A wound made by tearing or cutting tissues. — **C.** Integument

_____ **4.** Inflammation of a lymph channel. — **D.** Keloid scar

_____ **5.** The process by which the body maintains temperature through a combination of heat gain by metabolic processes and muscular movement and heat loss through breathing, evaporation, conduction, convection, and perspiration. — **E.** Laceration

_____ **6.** A disease caused by spores that enter the body through a puncture wound contaminated with animal feces, street dust, or soil or that enter through contaminated street drugs. — **F.** Lymphangitis

_____ **7.** The pattern of tautness of the skin, which is arranged over body structures and affects how well wounds heal. — **G.** Tetanus

_____ **8.** A surgical procedure to improve the appearance of a scar, reestablish function, or correct disfigurement from soft-tissue damage, surgical incision, or lesion. — **H.** Myositis

_____ **9.** Development of new blood vessels to aid in healing injured soft tissue. — **I.** Necrotizing fasciitis

_____ **10.** An injury in which there is a break in the surface of the skin or the mucous membrane, exposing deeper tissue to potential contamination. — **J.** Neovascularization

_____ **11.** Infection of the area around the fingernail bed. — **K.** Open wound

_____ **12.** A narrow strip of tissue by which an avulsed piece of tissue remains connected to the body. — **L.** Paronychia

_____ **13.** An abnormal scar with excess collagen that does not extend over the wound margins. — **M.** Pedicle

_____ **14.** A wound usually made deliberately, as in surgery; a clean cut, as opposed to a laceration. — **N.** Phagocytosis

_____ **15.** The skin. — **O.** Puncture wound

_____ **16.** An abnormal scar commonly found in people with darkly pigmented skin, which extends over a wound's margins. — **P.** Rabid

_____ **17.** Describes an animal that is infected with rabies. — **Q.** Scar revision

_____ **18.** An injury resulting from a piercing object, such as a nail or a knife; also referred to as a penetrating wound. — **R.** Thermoregulation

_____ **19.** The process in which one cell "eats" or engulfs a foreign substance to destroy it. — **S.** Tension lines

Multiple Choice

Read each item carefully, and then select the best response.

_____ **1.** The injury that occurs when high-pressure injected material enters the soft tissues can result in:
- **A.** no pain, initially.
- **B.** acute inflammation.
- **C.** chronic inflammation.
- **D.** All of the above

_____ **2.** Blood vessels, nerves, tendons, muscles, and internal organs can all be damaged by:
- **A.** compartment syndrome.
- **B.** improperly applied dressings.
- **C.** use of a wet dressing instead of a dry dressing.
- **D.** application of a tourniquet.

_____ **3.** When should the paramedic remove an impaled object in a patient's abdomen?
- **A.** When the object affects packaging and transport
- **B.** When the object does not stand up straight on its own
- **C.** When bleeding cannot be successfully controlled
- **D.** The paramedic should never remove an impaled object from that location.

_____ **4.** When a foreign material is forcefully injected into soft tissue, the resulting injury is called a(n):
- **A.** high-pressure injection injury.
- **B.** amputation.
- **C.** tympanic membrane rupture.
- **D.** blast injury.

_____ **5.** Patients with soft-tissue injuries:
- **A.** rarely have life-threatening injuries.
- **B.** should be "signed off" to save emergency medical services (EMS) system resources.
- **C.** should be treated with aggressive advanced life support (ALS) treatment in the event of unforeseen injury.
- **D.** have a high incidence of morbidity and mortality.

_____ **6.** The guidelines for the management of an amputation include each of the following, EXCEPT:
- **A.** do not place the amputated part in water.
- **B.** do not use dry ice to cool the part.
- **C.** keep the amputated part warm.
- **D.** wrap the part loosely in saline-moistened sterile gauze.

_____ **7.** There are numerous types of soft-tissue injuries. Many of them are relatively minor, but some have potentially serious outcomes. Which of the following injuries requires transportation?
- **A.** Abrasion
- **B.** Laceration
- **C.** Necrotizing fasciitis
- **D.** Incision

_____ **8.** Soft-tissue injuries often involve external hemorrhaging. All of the following measures would be considered appropriate bleeding management, EXCEPT:
- **A.** direct pressure with thick, bulky dressings.
- **B.** pressure with elastic bandages.
- **C.** "wet" dressings applied to the wound.
- **D.** tourniquet on a severely bleeding extremity.

_____ **9.** Soft-tissue injuries to the neck may lead to which of the following complications?
- **A.** Air embolism
- **B.** Spinal injury
- **C.** Airway disruption
- **D.** All of the above

_______ **10.** Which of the following can interfere with normal wound healing?

A. An underlying cardiac history
B. A seizure disorder
C. Carpal tunnel syndrome
D. A history of diabetes

Labeling

1. Label the components of the skin in the following diagram.

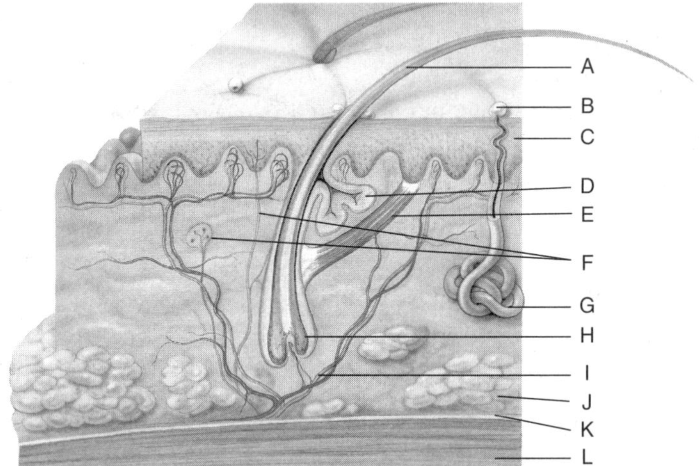

A. ______________________________ **G.** ______________________________

B. ______________________________ **H.** ______________________________

C. ______________________________ **I.** ______________________________

D. ______________________________ **J.** ______________________________

E. ______________________________ **K.** ______________________________

F. ______________________________ **L.** ______________________________

2. Determine which types of open wounds are shown in each of the following photos.

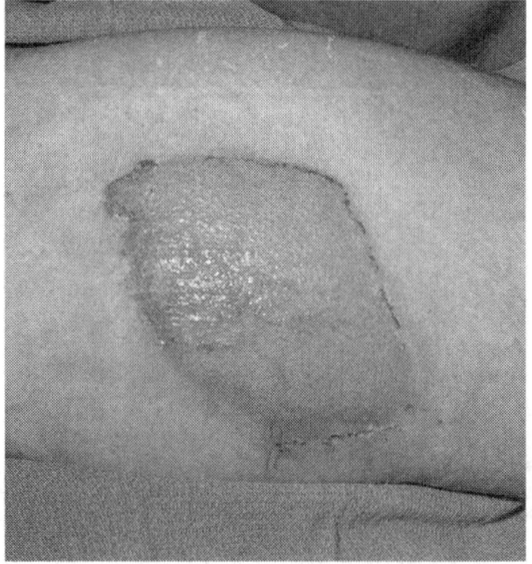

A. ______________________

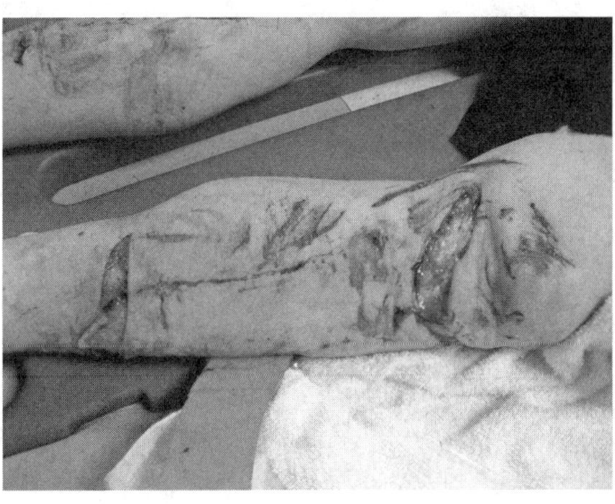

Courtesy of Rhonda Hunt.

B. ______________________________

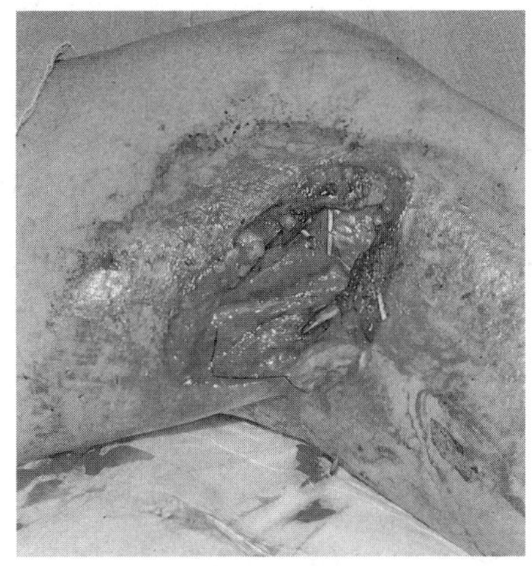

© Jones & Bartlett Learning.

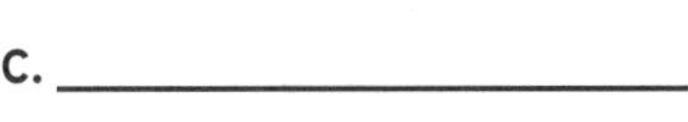

C. ______________________________

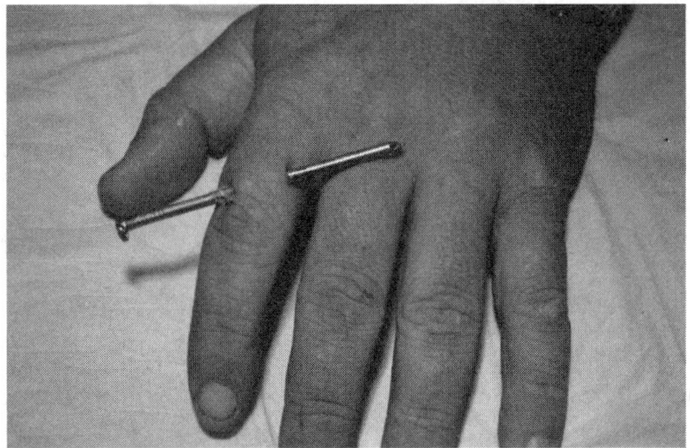

© Jones & Bartlett Learning.

D. ______________________________

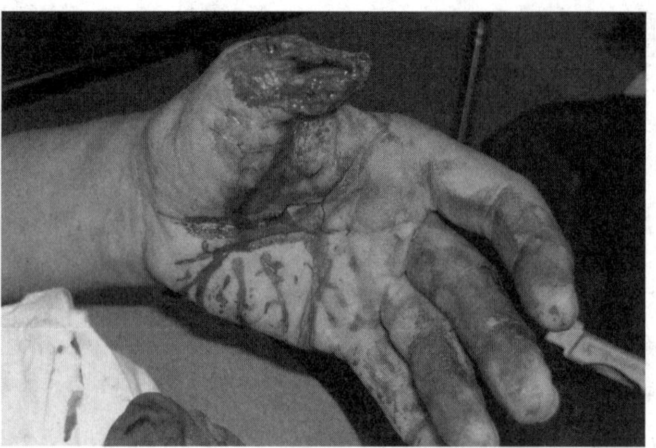

E. ____________________

Fill in the Blank

Read each item carefully, and then complete the statement by filling in the missing word(s).

1. __________ injuries require substantial irrigation and __________ before closing by an emergency practitioner.
2. Visible clues of infection include __________, __________, __________, __________, and __________ __________.
3. *Clostridium tetani* causes the body to produce a potent __________, which results in painful muscle __________ that are strong enough to fracture bones.
4. ____________ is dead tissue. It is caused when ________ supply delivery to tissue is interrupted or stopped.
5. ___________ is the most common infection of the hand in the United States.
6. Excessive _________ formation can occur if the healing process is not balanced between the building-up and breaking-down phases of healing.
7. Wet dressings have limited use in the field but are used in the care of _________ burns.

Identify

Read the following case studies, and then identify the type of soft-tissue injury and the care that you would provide.

1. You are called to the scene of a local campsite where a 10-year-old boy was playing with his pocket knife, whittling some wood, when he cut himself. The injury is a jagged incision to his right forearm. There is moderate darkish-red blood oozing from the site.

   ____

   ____

   ____

2. A patient was working in his home shop when he became distracted while using a circular saw. He inadvertently cut the fingers on his left hand. When you arrive, the patient is sitting in a chair, conscious and alert. He appears pale and sweaty. He has several blood-soaked towels covering his hand. You notice that his left middle and ring fingers are sitting on his wood-crafting bench.

____

____

____

3. It is a busy shift. On this call you are dispatched to a bar fight. On arrival, there is a crowd hovering around a woman who complains of pain in her right side and moderate shortness of breath. Her companion states that she was involved in a dispute and felt a sharp object impact her right side. The patient is somewhat angry and combative and wants to continue the dispute. As you examine the injury, you notice a minimal amount of bleeding that appears to have stopped. The patient has a quarter-inch circular opening to her chest. There appears to be a small amount of swelling and a rush of air when she breathes.

____

____

____

Ambulance Calls

The following case scenarios provide an opportunity to explore the concerns associated with patient management and paramedic care. Read each scenario, and then answer each question.

1. You are summoned to Bugsy's Butcher Shop to tend to the proprietor, Bugsy Butterfingers, who dropped a meat cleaver on his left leg. There is a large gash in the left calf, and it is bleeding profusely.
   a. List three methods you might use to try to control the bleeding, and put an asterisk next to the method likely to be the most effective. Please note that standard precautions are being done appropriately.

      (1)____

      (2)____

      (3)____

   b. Suppose Bugsy's wound had been on the forearm rather than on the leg. Which artery is most likely the cause of severe bleeding in the arm?

   ____

2. One of Bugsy's employees, Frank Fillet, becomes so distracted watching you care for his boss that he accidentally chops off two of his fingers while preparing an order of steaks.
   a. How will you treat Frank's injury?

   ____

   ____

   b. What will you do with the two fingers lying on the chopping board?

   ____

   ____

3. Yet another worker in the butcher shop, Hercules Hamburger, had been watching, slack-jawed and transfixed, as this drama was unfolding. So intent was he on the spectacle that he did not realize his right hand had entered the meat grinder—at least not until his hand became engaged in the grinding blades. Hearing his screams, a customer rushes

over to where Hercules is standing and manages to shut off the meat grinder, but not before Hercules's hand and forearm have been badly mangled. You already have your hands full with Bugsy and Frank, so you instruct the Good Samaritan who shut off the meat grinder, "Have him lie down, and try to control the bleeding—I'll be with him in just a minute." Obligingly, the customer grabs a piece of rope that he finds behind the counter, winds it around Hercules's upper arm, and slips a ballpoint pen into the knot to serve as a tourniquet. He twists the rope as tightly as he possibly can, secures the pen, and uses the butcher's apron to wrap the entire hand and arm.

Although the customer was trying to be helpful, in fact, he made several very serious mistakes. List the mistakes.

a. __________

b. __________

c. __________

d. __________

4. During deer-hunting season, two young backpackers were strolling through the woods when hunters, mistaking the pair for deer, discharged their crossbows at them. One arrow entered the eye of the first backpacker, while another arrow went straight through the cheek of the second backpacker.

a. Describe the steps you would take in treating the backpacker with the arrow in his eye. Please note that standard precautions are being done appropriately.

____

____

____

____

____

____

b. Describe the steps you would take in treating the backpacker who has an arrow impaled in his cheek.

____

____

____

____

____

____

5. You are folding up your deck chair when you happen to see a jogger running erratically down the beach toward you. His shorts are torn, and there is blood trickling down one leg. "What happened to you?" you ask.

"Some big Doberman tackled me as I was running. I figured the best thing to do was keep running to where I left my car." You note the tooth marks and a laceration on the runner's left leg.

How would you manage this patient? Please note that standard precautions are being done appropriately.

a. __________

b. __________

c. __________

d. __________

True/False

If you believe the statement to be more true than false, write the letter "T" in the space provided. If you believe the statement to be more false than true, write the letter "F."

_______ **1.** Amputation is a form of avulsion.

_______ **2.** Soft-tissue trauma is the leading form of injury.

_______ **3.** Sweating is regulated through the parasympathetic nervous system.

_______ **4.** Subcutaneous blood vessels have a crucial role in regulating body temperature.

_______ **5.** An incision is a clean (linear), intentional cut.

_______ **6.** Human bites carry a higher risk of infection than animal bites do.

_______ **7.** Keloid scars typically develop in areas of high tissue stress.

_______ **8.** Tetanus infection causes the body to produce a potent toxin that results in lockjaw.

_______ **9.** It is important to remove all other dressings before applying a hemostatic dressing.

_______ **10.** Bleeding control is a key principle in treating open wounds.

Short Answer

Complete this section with short written answers using the space provided.

1. You can appreciate the possible consequences of injury to the skin if you understand which functions healthy, intact skin performs. List four functions performed by the skin in a healthy person.

a. ______________________________

b. ______________________________

c. ______________________________

d. ______________________________

2. Healing of wounds is a natural process that involves several overlapping stages. List the five stages of wound healing.

a. ______________________________

b. ______________________________

c. ______________________________

d. ______________________________

e. ______________________________

3. Wounds are characterized as either closed or open. List the characteristics of closed wounds.

a. ______________________________

b. ______________________________

c. ______________________________

CHAPTER

Burns

32

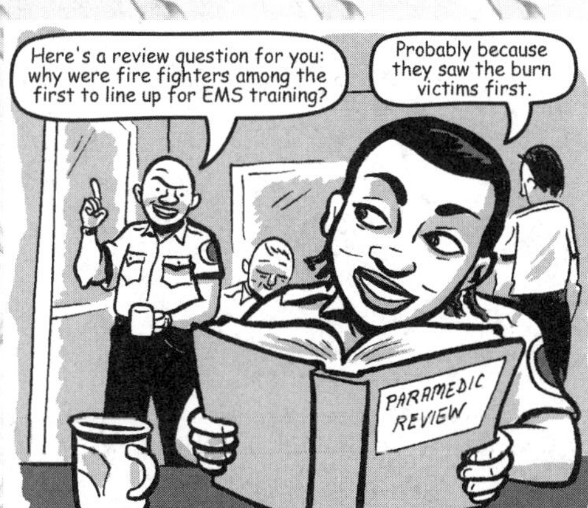

Matching

Part I

Match each of the patients with the appropriate treatment in question 1 and with the appropriate sequence in question 2.

1. In the course of a busy week, you are called on to treat eight burn victims in a variety of circumstances. In each case, you have to determine whether the patient has suffered a critical burn because, if so, he or she must be evacuated directly to the regional burn center, which is 24 miles away; noncritical burns, in contrast, can be managed by the community hospital right in town. A description of the patients you saw follows. Beside each description, indicate whether:

A. The patient has a critical burn and should be brought to a regional burn center.

B. The patient does not have a critical burn and can be managed in the community hospital.

_______ (1) A 2-year-old boy who overturned a pot of soup from the stovetop onto himself; both legs and the anterior trunk are burned.

_______ (2) A 57-year-old woman with diabetes and a scald burn of her left lower leg.

_______ (3) A 28-year-old woman with a scald burn of her entire right arm.

_______ (4) A lineman who suffered an electric shock. There is a small bull's-eye entrance wound on the left hand; you cannot find the exit wound. The lineman did not fall. His left leg feels rock hard.

_______ (5) A 22-year-old male short-order cook with partial-thickness (second-degree) burns over both anterior thighs, sustained when he spilled a pot of soup.

_______ (6) A 34-year-old woman rescued from a burning building, where she had been trapped in her smoke-filled bedroom. She has partial-thickness burns of the right forearm. She is coughing up sooty sputum.

_______ (7) A 25-year-old man who tripped and fell onto the hibachi on the back porch as he was preparing to grill some steaks. His hand went straight into the bed of red-hot charcoal, and his shirt caught fire. He has full-thickness (third-degree) burns of the left hand and forearm and partial-thickness burns of the anterior chest.

_______ (8) A plumber who spilled a bottle of industrial-strength liquid drain cleaner down the front of his pants.

2. You are called to treat a patient who was in a tenement fire. He is a middle-aged man who apparently fell asleep in an armchair while holding a lit cigarette. You arrive at the scene just as he is being carried, unresponsive, from the building and note that his clothes are still smoldering. Following, in random order, are the steps you will have to take in managing this patient. Arrange the steps in the correct sequence.

A. Administer supplemental oxygen.

B. Start an IV.

C. Open the airway manually.

D. Put out the fire.

E. Remove the patient's clothing.

F. Pass a nasogastric tube into his stomach.

G. Determine the extent and depth of the burn.

H. Intubate the trachea (if a basic life support [BLS] airway is not adequate).

I. Cover the burns with sterile dressings.

J. Obtain a set of baseline vital signs.

(1) ____________ (6) ____________
(2) ____________ (7) ____________
(3) ____________ (8) ____________
(4) ____________ (9) ____________
(5) ____________ (10) ____________

Part II

Match each of the terms in the right column to the appropriate definition in the left column.

	Definition	Term
_____	**1.** The skin.	**A.** Acute radiation syndrome
_____	**2.** Also referred to as burn shock; the shock or hypoperfusion caused by a burn injury and the tremendous loss of fluids; capillaries leak, resulting in intravascular fluid volume oozing out of the circulation and into the interstitial spaces, and cells take in increased amounts of salt and water.	**B.** Circumferential burn
_____	**3.** A tendency toward constancy or stability in the body's internal environment.	**C.** Coagulation necrosis
_____	**4.** A burn that extends through the epidermis and dermis into the subcutaneous tissues beneath; previously called a third-degree burn.	**D.** Collagen
_____	**5.** An electrothermal injury caused by arcing of electric current.	**E.** Consensus formula
_____	**6.** One of the complex materials found, along with collagen fibers and elastin fibers, in the dermis of the skin.	**F.** Contact burn
_____	**7.** A detailed version of the rule of nines chart that takes into consideration the changes in total body surface area that occur with growth.	**G.** Dermis
_____	**8.** A form of necrosis that results from the transformation of tissue into a liquid viscous mass (pus).	**H.** Elastin
_____	**9.** A description of the relationship between heat production, current, and resistance.	**I.** Epidermis
_____	**10.** The clinical course that usually begins within hours of exposure to a radiation source. Symptoms include nausea, vomiting, diarrhea, fatigue, fever, and headache. The long-term symptoms are dose related and are hematopoietic and gastrointestinal in nature.	**J.** Escharotomy
_____	**11.** A burn produced by touching a hot object.	**K.** Flame burn
_____	**12.** A formula that recommends giving 2 to 4 mL of normal saline for each kilogram of body weight, multiplied by the percentage of total body surface area burned; sometimes used to calculate fluid needs during lengthy transport times; formerly called the Parkland formula.	**L.** Flash burn
_____	**13.** A protein that gives tensile strength to the connective tissues of the body.	**M.** Full-thickness burn
_____	**14.** Cell death typically caused by ischemia or infarction.	**N.** Homeostasis
_____	**15.** A burn on the neck or chest, which may compress the airway, or on an extremity, which might act like a tourniquet.	**O.** Hypovolemic shock
_____	**16.** A thermal burn caused by flames touching the skin.	**P.** Integument
_____	**17.** A surgical cut through the eschar or leathery covering of a burn injury to allow for swelling and minimize the potential for development of compartment syndrome in a circumferentially burned limb or the thorax.	**Q.** Joule's law
_____	**18.** The outermost layer of the skin.	**R.** Liquefaction necrosis
_____	**19.** The inner layer of skin containing hair follicle roots, glands, blood vessels, and nerves.	**S.** Lund-Browder chart
_____	**20.** A protein that gives the skin its elasticity.	**T.** Mucopolysaccharide gel

Part III

Match each of the terms in the right column to the appropriate definition in the left column.

	Definition		Term
______	**1.** An injury caused by radiation or direct contact with a heat source on the skin.	**A.**	Ohm's law
______	**2.** Located above the glottis opening, as in the upper airway structures.	**B.**	Partial-thickness burn
______	**3.** A burn involving only the epidermis, which produces very red, painful skin; previously called a first-degree burn.	**C.**	Rule of nines
______	**4.** Located below the glottis opening, as in the lower airway structures.	**D.**	Rule of palms
______	**5.** A burn that has been caused by direct exposure to hot steam exhaust, as from a broken pipe.	**E.**	Scald burn
______	**6.** The peripheral area surrounding the zone of coagulation that has decreased blood flow and inflammation; it can undergo necrosis within 24 to 48 hours after the injury, particularly if perfusion is compromised due to burn shock.	**F.**	Steam burn
______	**7.** In a thermal burn, the area that is least affected by the burn injury; an area of increased blood flow where the body is attempting to repair injured but otherwise viable tissue.	**G.**	Subglottic
______	**8.** The reddened area surrounding the leathery and sometimes charred tissue that has sustained a full-thickness burn.	**H.**	Superficial burn
______	**9.** The formula that describes the relationship between voltage and resistance: Current (I) = Voltage (V) divided by Resistance (R).	**I.**	Supraglottic
______	**10.** A burn that involves the epidermis and part of the dermis, characterized by pain and blistering; previously called a second-degree burn.	**J.**	Thermal burn
______	**11.** A system that assigns percentages to sections of the body, allowing for calculation of the amount of total body surface area burned.	**K.**	Zone of coagulation
______	**12.** A system that estimates the total body surface area burned by comparing the affected area with the size of the patient's palm, which is roughly equal to 1% of the patient's total body surface area.	**L.**	Zone of hyperemia
______	**13.** A burn produced by hot liquids.	**M.**	Zone of stasis

Multiple Choice

Read each item carefully, and then select the best response.

______ **1.** What is the second "rule" when in a lightning storm?

- **A.** Take shelter in a structure.
- **B.** Avoid touching a conductor.
- **C.** Don't be the smallest conductor.
- **D.** Don't stand near the tallest conductor.

______ **2.** When dealing with acute radiation syndrome, which of the following is NOT likely to happen to the patient?

- **A.** Central nervous system changes
- **B.** Urinary changes
- **C.** Gastrointestinal changes
- **D.** Hematologic changes

______ **3.** There are three methods of calculating an area of burned skin. Which method is the fastest and most universally used?

- **A.** Rule of nines
- **B.** The Lund-Browder chart
- **C.** Rule of palms
- **D.** A Broselow tape

______ **4.** You have arrived on scene to find a 12-year-old girl who has been burned by chicken noodle soup from the stove. She has blisters and redness on her chest. How would you classify this burn?

A. Full-thickness burn
B. First-degree burn
C. Partial-thickness burn
D. Superficial burn

______ **5.** An adult man's entire back is worth what percentage when using the rule of nines?

A. 9%
B. 18%
C. 27%
D. 36%

______ **6.** What is the *immediate management* when dealing with a 45-year-old woman who fell asleep with a cigarette in her hand?

A. Managing the airway
B. Starting fluid resuscitation
C. Extinguishing the fire
D. Keeping the patient warm

______ **7.** The Consensus (Parkland) formula determines how much fluid a burn patient should receive:

A. during the first hour.
B. during transport to the hospital.
C. during the first 12 hours.
D. during the first 24 hours.

______ **8.** What is the BEST way to give pain medication to the burn patient?

A. IV route
B. Subcutaneous injection
C. By mouth
D. Intramuscular injection

______ **9.** What should you do first when treating a patient with a chemical burn?

A. Remove all the patient's clothing.
B. Begin flushing with copious amounts of water.
C. Brush the chemicals off the skin.
D. Wait for a hazardous materials team to arrive.

______ **10.** You arrive on the scene to find a child engaged in an electrical outlet. The child is "held" by the electricity. What should you do?

A. Use a wooden pole to push the child away from the source.
B. Throw a rope to the child and pull him away from the source.
C. Wait until someone shuts off the power to the source.
D. Cut the wires inside the electrical box.

Labeling

1. Label the layers of the skin in the following diagram.

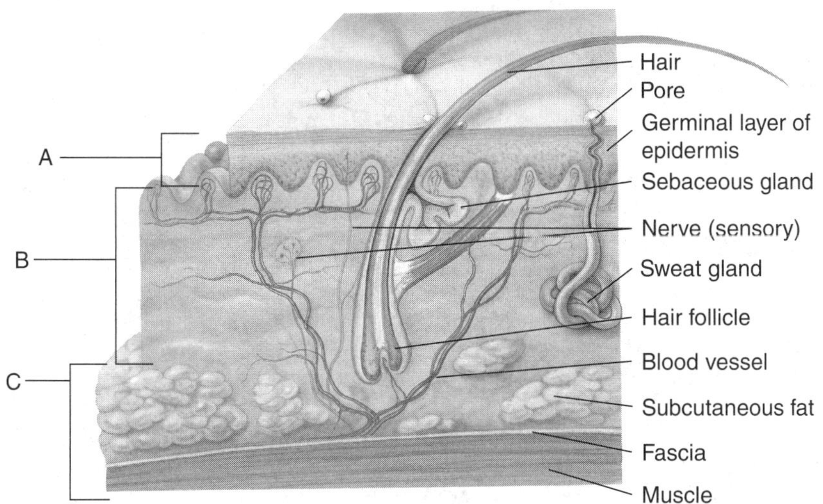

A. ______________________

B. ______________________

C. ______________________

2. Classify the following images as superficial, partial-thickness, or full-thickness burns.

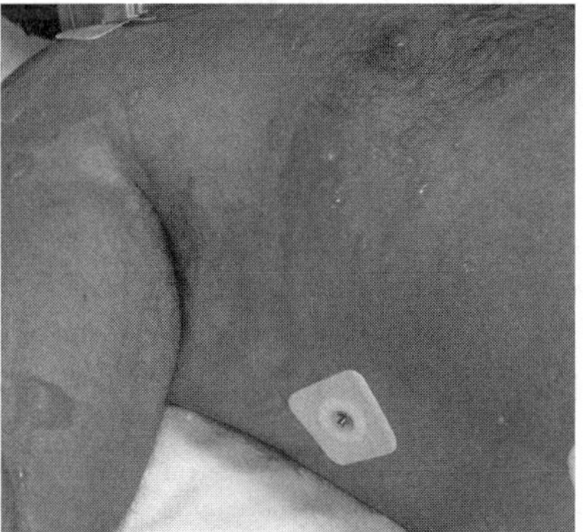

A. ______________________

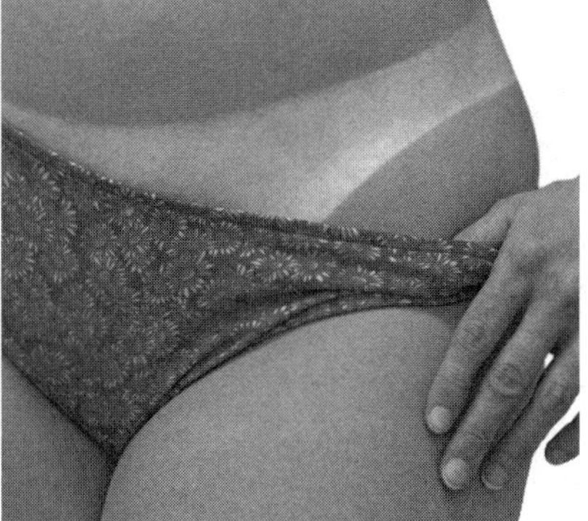

B. ______________________

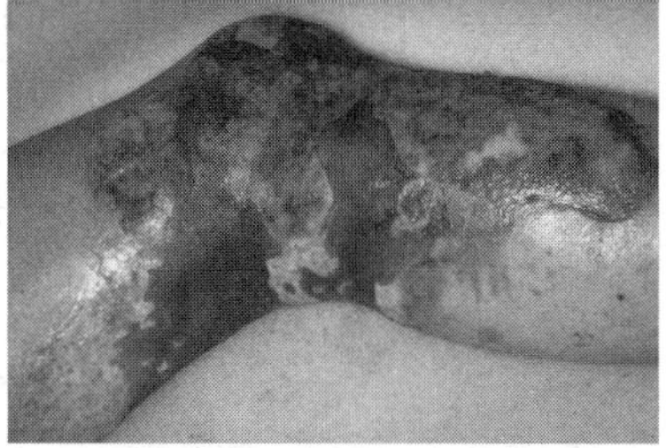

C. ______________________

Fill in the Blank

Read each item carefully, and then complete the statement by filling in the missing word(s).

1. The ________, or outermost layer, is the body's first line of defense, constituting the major barrier against water, dust, microorganisms, and mechanical stress.
2. Sweat glands are found in the __________.
3. A(n) __________ burn is most commonly seen in children and physically or developmentally challenged adults.
4. Chemical burns can occur when the skin comes in contact with __________, __________, or __________, or other corrosive materials.
5. __________ __________ cause exothermic reaction in addition to tissue destruction. They can also cause systemic poisoning.
6. You should always make sure the __________ __________ __________ before beginning any management of a patient struck by lightning.
7. There are three types of ionizing radiation: __________, __________, and __________.
8. The central area of a burn that has suffered the most damage is known as the __________ __________ __________.
9. When treating a full-thickness burn, you should apply a(n) __________ __________ to the area that has been burned.
10. A patient with a radiation burn must be __________ before being transported to the emergency department (ED).

Identify

Read the following case study, and then list the chief complaint, vital signs, and pertinent negatives.

Around noon, you are called to the local burger joint for a 56-year-old woman who has been burned by oil from a hot fryer. Upon arrival, you find her with holes in her jeans on the top of both thighs. She is crying and immediately rates her pain as unbearable. You cut the jeans away to find that there is an area covering most of the front of both thighs that is blistering and very red. The patient is breathing at 22 breaths/min, her oxygen saturation is 97%, and lung sounds are clear bilaterally. You apply supplemental oxygen via a nonrebreathing mask at 15 L/min. You have your partner take the rest of the vital signs as you apply a Water-Jel dressing to the burned areas. The patient's blood pressure is 150/100 mm Hg, her pulse is 114 beats/min, and her rhythm on the monitor is sinus tachycardia. You do catch a premature ventricular contraction on the monitor but do not see another after watching for a full minute. The patient's skin is cool to the touch, and you believe she might be going into shock. You cover her with a blanket and start an IV line of normal saline. The patient is able to answer all your questions, and she has no medical history or allergies. You find no other areas of burns as you do a secondary trauma assessment. The patient states she slipped on the floor when carrying the hot oil to the disposal. She splashed the oil on the front of her legs. She does rate her pain 10/10, so you give her 5 mg of morphine for the pain en route to the hospital. When you arrive at the hospital, which is only 10 minutes from the burger joint, her pain has dropped to a 3/10.

1. Chief complaint:

____

____

2. Vital signs:

____

____

3. Pertinent negatives:

____

____

Complete the Patient Care Report

Reread the case study in the preceding Identify exercise and then complete the following patient care report (PCR) for the patient.

<table>
<tr><th colspan="6">EMS Patient Care Report (PCR)</th></tr>
<tr><td>Date:</td><td>Incident No.:</td><td colspan="2">Nature of Call:</td><td colspan="2">Location:</td></tr>
<tr><td>Dispatched:</td><td>En Route:</td><td>At Scene:</td><td>Transport:</td><td>At Hospital:</td><td>In Service:</td></tr>
<tr><th colspan="6">Patient Information</th></tr>
<tr><td colspan="3">Age:
Sex:
Weight (in kg [lb]):</td><td colspan="3">Allergies:
Medications:
Past Medical History:
Chief Complaint:</td></tr>
<tr><th colspan="6">Vital Signs</th></tr>
<tr><td>Time:</td><td>BP:</td><td>Pulse:</td><td>Respirations:</td><td colspan="2">SpO_2:</td></tr>
<tr><td>Time:</td><td>BP:</td><td>Pulse:</td><td>Respirations:</td><td colspan="2">SpO_2:</td></tr>
<tr><td>Time:</td><td>BP:</td><td>Pulse:</td><td>Respirations:</td><td colspan="2">SpO_2:</td></tr>
<tr><th colspan="6">EMS Treatment
(circle all that apply)</th></tr>
<tr><td colspan="2">Oxygen @ ______ L/min via (circle one):
NC NRM Bag-mask device</td><td>Assisted Ventilation</td><td>Airway Adjunct</td><td colspan="2">CPR</td></tr>
<tr><td>Defibrillation</td><td>Bleeding Control</td><td>Bandaging</td><td>Splinting</td><td colspan="2">Other:</td></tr>
<tr><th colspan="6">Narrative</th></tr>
<tr><td colspan="6"></td></tr>
</table>

Ambulance Calls

The following case scenarios provide an opportunity to explore the concerns associated with patient management and paramedic care. Read each scenario, and then answer each question.

1. You are called to the scene of a smoky apartment-house fire to treat a man who jumped from his bedroom window approximately 15 feet above the ground. What you observe at first glance is the following: The patient is now lying unresponsive on the ground. His trousers are smoldering. His beard is partly burned off, and his lips are swollen. His left leg is splayed out at a peculiar angle. List, in the correct sequence, the steps you would take in managing this patient.

   a. ______________________________

   b. ______________________________

   c. ______________________________

   d. ______________________________

   e. ______________________________

   f. ______________________________

   g. ______________________________

   h. ______________________________

2. While you are securing the IV line on the patient described in question 1, firefighters lead the patient's wife over to you (they just rescued her from another room). A quick check does not reveal any injuries, but you give her supplemental oxygen by nasal cannula anyway because of her exposure to smoke. Meanwhile, you take advantage of the opportunity to get some information about her husband. List five questions you would ask this woman regarding her husband and what happened to him.

   a. ______________________________

   b. ______________________________

   c. ______________________________

   d. ______________________________

   e. ______________________________

3. Meanwhile, the firefighters bring you yet another victim of the fire, a college student who climbed down a fire escape in the back of the building. He has burns to the right side of his body and complains of severe pain in the right arm. On examination you find the following:
   - The *right arm* is mottled red and exquisitely sensitive to the lightest touch (even the breeze blowing past it causes pain).
   - The *right flank* is fiery red and very painful.
   - The *right lower leg* has a leathery appearance. In places, you can see thrombosed veins beneath the surface. When you touch the skin with a sterile needle, the patient does not feel the pinprick.

   a. The burn on the right arm is probably a(n) __________ burn.
   The appropriate treatment for that burn is:

   ____

   ____

   b. The burn on the flank is probably a(n) __________ burn.
   The appropriate treatment for that burn is:

   ____

   ____

c. The burn on the right leg is probably a(n) __________ burn.
The appropriate treatment for that burn is:

____

____

4. You are called to a construction site 20 miles out of town for a "man electrocuted." According to the person who telephoned your dispatcher, one of the construction workers apparently bulldozed through a buried electric cable. He dismounted his bulldozer and picked up the cable to toss it aside, not realizing that it was live, and his hand "froze" to the cable.

a. En route to the call, you review in your mind the types of injuries that may occur in connection with electrocution. You remember that there may be four different types of burns:

(1)____

(2)____

(3)____

(4)____

b. You also recall that high-voltage electricity may cause a variety of nonburn injuries. List six possible injuries or abnormal conditions that you need to be alert for in this patient.

(1)____

(2)____

(3)____

(4)____

(5)____

(6)____

c. When you reach the construction site, you see a knot of agitated people at one end of the site. One of them is holding a long two-by-four, with which he apparently jarred the victim loose from the cable. The victim is lying very still and appears to be unresponsive. The free end of the cable is now arcing along the ground like an angry snake. List the steps you will take in dealing with this situation in the sequence in which you will perform them.

(1)____

(2)____

(3)____

(4)____

(5)____

(6)____

(7)____

(8)____

(9)____

(10)____

5. You are summoned to a house fire where the firefighters have just rescued a young man from a particularly smoky part of the building. He is unresponsive, and you notice that his clothes are smoldering.

a. Whenever a person has been unresponsive in a smoky environment, you have to worry about the possibility of respiratory injury. List seven signs that should lead you to suspect the presence of respiratory injury in a burned patient.

(1)____

(2)____

(3)____

(4)____

(5)____

(6)____

(7)____

b. What is the *first* step you should take in dealing with this patient?

____

____

c. In due course, you remove the patient's clothing and examine him from head to toe to evaluate the depth and extent of the burn. You find the following:

- Full-thickness burns of the posterior surfaces of both legs, extending well into the buttocks and groin
- Partial-thickness burns of the entire left arm and a hand-sized patch of the left flank

(1) What percentage of the patient's body has been burned? __________%

(2) Does the patient have a critical burn? __________ If yes, according to which criteria?

(a) ____

(b) ____

(c) ____

d. Use the Consensus formula to calculate the rate at which you should run the patient's IV infusion. Assume that he weighs 70 kg and that your infusion set delivers 10 gtt/mL. (Show your calculations.)

The IV infusion should be run at __________ gtt/min.

e. After a few minutes of oxygen therapy, the patient regains consciousness and begins complaining of excruciating pain, especially in his groin and left arm. Medical control instructs you to administer morphine.

1. What is the correct dosage of morphine for this patient?

____

2. By which route should it be given?

____

3. List three possible adverse side effects that you should be ready to deal with.

(a) ______________________________

(b) ______________________________

(c) ______________________________

6. In examining a patient, you find that he has mixed partial- and full-thickness burns of his entire left leg and posterior right leg, extending into his groin. There are also partial-thickness burns over most of the left forearm.

a. What percentage of his body is burned? (Show your calculations.) __________%

b. Does he have a critical burn? __________ Explain the reason for your answer.

(1)______________________________

(2)______________________________

c. In doing the rapid trauma assessment, you are unable to detect either a dorsalis pedis pulse or an anterior tibial pulse in the left foot. What do you think is the most likely reason?

____

____

d. What are you going to do about it?

____

____

True/False

If you believe the statement to be more true than false, write the letter "T" in the space provided. If you believe the statement to be more false than true, write the letter "F."

______ 1. If you know the identity of the chemical that caused a burn, it is preferable to start treatment with a chemical antidote (eg, applying a weak acid to an alkali burn, and vice versa).

______ 2. When a person has been burned by a chemical agent, the skin should be flushed with copious amounts of water.

______ 3. It is important to use only sterile water to flush a chemical burn, lest you contaminate the burn wound.

______ 4. In burns caused by hot tar, it is crucial to remove the tar from contact with the skin as quickly as possible to prevent systemic tar poisoning.

______ 5. If chemicals have splashed into a patient's eyes, the eyes should be continuously irrigated with a steady stream of water.

______ 6. Burn shock occurs because of the fluid loss across the damaged skin and the volume shifts within the rest of the body.

______ 7. Although fire deaths continue to decrease, children younger than 5 years continue to be at a high risk of dying in a fire.

______ 8. Carbon monoxide binds to the hemoglobin 500 times faster than oxygen does.

______ 9. Currents as small as 0.1 A may cause ventricular fibrillation if the current passes through the heart.

______ 10. You should peel away clothing that has "melted" into the flesh of a burn patient.

Short Answer

Complete this section with short written answers using the space provided.

1. Discuss the four rules that can help you avoid being struck by lightning.

   a. ____

   b. ____

   c. ____

   d. ____

2. You would suspect that a patient with flame burns has a respiratory injury if any of the following signs are present:

   a. ____

   b. ____

   c. ____

   d. ____

   e. ____

   f. ____

   g. ____

3. Injury from a high-voltage electric source or from lightning may produce any of the following conditions:

   a. ____

   b. ____

   c. ____

   d. ____

   e. ____

   f. ____

Fill in the Table

Fill in the missing columns of the table.

Approximate the amount of fluid the burned patient will need by using the Consensus formula. During the first 24 hours, the burned patient will need:

$$2\text{–}4 \text{ mL} \times \text{body weight (in kg)} \times \text{percentage of body surface burned}$$

Consensus Formula Chart

% Burn	10 kg	20 kg	30 kg	40 kg	50 kg	60 kg	70 kg	80 kg	90 kg	100 kg
10	25			100	125	150	175		225	250
20	50			200	250	300	350		450	500
30	75			300	375	450	525		675	750
40	100			400	500	600	700		900	1,000
50	125			500	625	750	875		1,125	1,250
60	150			600	750	900	1,050		1,350	1,500
70	175			700	875	1,050	1,225		1,575	1,750
80	200			800	1,000	1,200	1,400		1,800	2,000
90	225			900	1,125	1,350	1,575		2,025	2,250
20 mL/kg	200			800	1,000	1,200	1,400		1,800	2,000

This table represents the fluid recommended in the *first hour* (one-eighth of the initial 8-hour dose) by the Consensus formula. The final row represents the amount of a 20-mL/kg bolus.

Note: Values in this table are based on the high end of the 2- to 4-mL range in the formula.

Problem Solving

Practice your calculation skills by solving the following math problems.

1. On examining the patient, you find burns covering the following areas:

- The whole right leg (front and back)
- The anterior left leg
- The anterior trunk
- The whole right arm

a. Use the rule of nines to calculate what percentage of the patient's body surface area is burned: __________ %. (Show your calculations.)

b. If the patient weighs 154 lb, at what rate should you run his IV infusion? Use the Consensus formula to calculate the rate (do not forget to convert the patient's weight to kilograms first!). (Show your calculations.)
IV infusion rate = __________ mL/h

c. If you have a standard infusion set that delivers 10 gtt/mL, at how many drops per minute do you have to run the IV infusion to deliver the volume you calculated?
IV infusion rate = __________ gtt/min

d. Which IV fluid will you use?

____

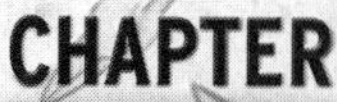

CHAPTER 33

Face and Neck Trauma

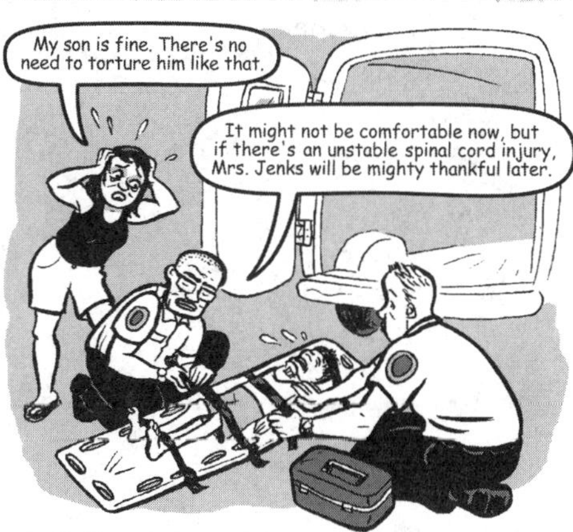

Matching

Part I

Match each of the terms in the right column to the appropriate definition in the left column.

______	**1.** An inflammation of the conjunctivae that usually is caused by bacteria, viruses, allergies, or foreign bodies; should be considered highly contagious if infectious in origin; also called pinkeye.	**A.**	Adnexa
______	**2.** A thin, transparent membrane that covers the sclera and internal surfaces of the eyelids.	**B.**	Alveoli
______	**3.** A fracture to the floor of the orbit, usually caused by a blow to the eye.	**C.**	Le Fort fractures
______	**4.** Nosebleed.	**D.**	Anterior chamber
______	**5.** Difficulty swallowing.	**E.**	Blowout fracture
______	**6.** Paralysis of gaze or lack of coordination between the movements of the two eyes.	**F.**	Conjunctiva
______	**7.** One of the three anatomic parts of the ear; the external portion of the tympanic membrane.	**G.**	Conjunctivitis
______	**8.** Small pits or cavities, such as the sockets for the teeth.	**H.**	Cornea
______	**9.** The surrounding structures and accessories of an organ; for the eye, these parts include the eyelids, lashes, and lacrimal structures.	**I.**	Craniofacial disjunction
______	**10.** The anterior area of the globe between the lens and the cornea, which is filled with aqueous humor.	**J.**	Crown
______	**11.** Maxillary fractures that are classified into three categories based on their anatomic location.	**K.**	Cusps
______	**12.** The colored portion of the eye.	**L.**	Dentin
______	**13.** One of the three anatomic parts of the ear; it consists of the cochlea and semicircular canals.	**M.**	Diplopia
______	**14.** The eyeball.	**N.**	Dysconjugate gaze
______	**15.** The bony anterior part of the palate that forms the roof of the mouth.	**O.**	Dysphagia
______	**16.** Coughing up blood.	**P.**	Epistaxis
______	**17.** Double vision.	**Q.**	External ear
______	**18.** The principal mass of the tooth.	**R.**	Globe
______	**19.** Points at the top of a tooth.	**S.**	Hard palate
______	**20.** A Le Fort III fracture that involves a fracture of all of the midface bones, which separates the entire midface from the cranium.	**T.**	Hemoptysis

______	**21.** The transparent anterior portion of the eye that overlies the iris and pupil.	**U.** Hyoid bone
______	**22.** Bleeding into the anterior chamber of the eye, resulting from direct ocular trauma.	**V.** Hyphema
______	**23.** A bone at the base of the tongue that supports the tongue and its muscles.	**W.** Inner ear
______	**24.** The part of the tooth that is external to the gum.	**X.** Iris

Part II

Match each of the terms in the right column to the appropriate definition in the left column.

______	**1.** Traumatic separation of the trachea from the layers.	**A.** Malocclusion
______	**2.** A thin membrane that separates the middle ear from the outer ear and sets up vibrations in the ossicles; also called the eardrum.	**B.** Mandible
______	**3.** A jellylike substance found in the posterior compartment of the eye between the lens and the retina.	**C.** Mediastinitis
______	**4.** An injury to the neck in which hyperextension occurs as a result of the head moving abruptly forward or backward; it can be difficult to differentiate from injuries that involve cervical bony structures and the spine.	**D.** Middle ear
______	**5.** The joint between the temporal bone and the posterior condyle that allows for movements of the mandible.	**E.** Oculomotor nerve
______	**6.** The movement of both eyes in unison.	**F.** Optic nerve
______	**7.** Stretching or tearing of a muscle or tendon.	**G.** Orbits
______	**8.** Stretching or tearing of ligaments.	**H.** Pinna
______	**9.** The act of declaring that a spinal injury is not present.	**I.** Pulp
______	**10.** The white part of the eye.	**J.** Pupil
______	**11.** Misalignment of the teeth.	**K.** Retina
______	**12.** The movable lower jaw bone.	**L.** Retinal detachment
______	**13.** Inflammation of the mediastinum, often a result of the gastric contents leaking into the thoracic cavity after esophageal perforation.	**M.** Sclera
______	**14.** A delicate, 10-layered structure of nervous tissue located in the rear of the interior of the globe; it receives light and generates nerve signals that are transmitted to the brain through the optic nerve.	**N.** Spinal clearance
______	**15.** The circular opening in the center of the eye through which light passes to the lens.	**O.** Sprain
______	**16.** Specialized connective tissue within the cavity of a tooth.	**P.** Strain
______	**17.** The third cranial nerve; it innervates the muscles that cause motion of the eyeballs and upper eyelid.	**Q.** Sympathetic eye movement
______	**18.** One of the three anatomic parts of the ear; it consists of the inner portion of the tympanic membrane and the ossicles.	**R.** Temporomandibular joint (TMJ)
______	**19.** The large outside portion of the ear through which sound waves enter the ear; also called the auricle.	**S.** Tracheal transection
______	**20.** Bony cavities in the frontal part of the skull that enclose and protect the eyes.	**T.** Tympanic membrane
______	**21.** Either of the secondary cranial nerves that enter the eyeball posteriorly, through the optic foramen.	**U.** Vitreous humor
______	**22.** Separation of the inner layers of the retina from the underlying choroid, the vascular membrane that nourishes the retina.	**V.** Whiplash

Multiple Choice

Read each item carefully, and then select the best response.

_____ 1. In addition to causing massive bleeding and shock, injury to the major arteries in the neck can cause:
- A. air embolism.
- B. cerebral infarct.
- C. cerebral hypoxia.
- D. All of the above

_____ 2. There are __________ facial bones that form the structure of the face.
- A. 6
- B. 14
- C. 9
- D. 21

_____ 3. How many adult teeth does the average adult have?
- A. 32
- B. 34
- C. 30
- D. 36

_____ 4. The large cartilaginous external portion of the ear is called the:
- A. organ of Corti.
- B. pinna.
- C. tympanic membrane.
- D. cochlea.

_____ 5. What is the name of the substance that forms the principal mass of the tooth?
- A. Alveolar ridge
- B. Cusp
- C. Pulp
- D. Dentin

_____ 6. What is the function of the oculomotor nerve?
- A. Causes motor function of the tongue
- B. Causes motion of eyeballs and upper eyelids
- C. Slows down the heart rate
- D. Causes the motor function of mastication

_____ 7. You are treating a patient who appears to have a fracture that has affected the upper jaw and the hard palate. What is the name for this fracture?
- A. Le Fort I
- B. Le Fort II
- C. Nasal fracture
- D. Mandibular fracture

_____ 8. Which of the following materials is NOT advisable for use when covering an injured eye?
- A. Aluminum eye shield
- B. Gauze
- C. Sterile dressing
- D. Cup

_____ **9.** A patient who has a maxillofacial fracture may have all of the following signs and symptoms, EXCEPT:

A. dental malocclusion.
B. swelling.
C. Battle sign.
D. blood or fluid running from the nose.

_____ **10.** What is the name of the fracture resulting from blunt trauma to the face that causes the face to appear flattened?

A. Hyoid bone fracture
B. Zygomatic bone fracture
C. Le Fort I fracture
D. Orbital bone injury

_____ **11.** You are treating a patient who sustained a blunt injury to his right eye from a fight. The patient reports that he is seeing flashing lights and specks. He MOST likely has the condition called:

A. diplopia.
B. hyphema.
C. retinal detachment.
D. conjunctivitis.

_____ **12.** The physical examination of the eyes involves evaluating the patient for all of the following, EXCEPT:

A. ecchymosis of the eyelids.
B. sympathetic eye movements.
C. redness of the globes.
D. foreign bodies in the cornea.

_____ **13.** When assessing a patient's eyes, you find visual field defects, which are also referred to as:

A. dysconjugate gaze.
B. hemianopsia.
C. conjunctivitis.
D. globe disruption.

_____ **14.** Which of the following is NOT a type of contact lens?

A. Rigid gas-permeable
B. Soft hydrophilic
C. Hard
D. Chemical

_____ **15.** You are treating a patient who has an injury to the anterior neck. She reports difficulty swallowing, hematemesis, and hemoptysis. What is her MOST likely injury?

A. Esophageal perforation
B. Neurologic impairment
C. Vascular injury
D. Laryngeal fracture

Labeling

Label the following diagrams with the correct terms.

1. Structures of the eye

Anterior compartment filled with aqueous humor
Anterior chamber
Posterior chamber
Posterior compartment filled with vitreous humor
Fovea
Vein
A
B
C
D
Suspensory ligaments
Ciliary muscle
Artery
G
F
Choroid
E

A. ______________________

B. ______________________

C. ______________________

D. ______________________

E. ______________________

F. ______________________

G. ______________________

2. Structures of the anterior neck

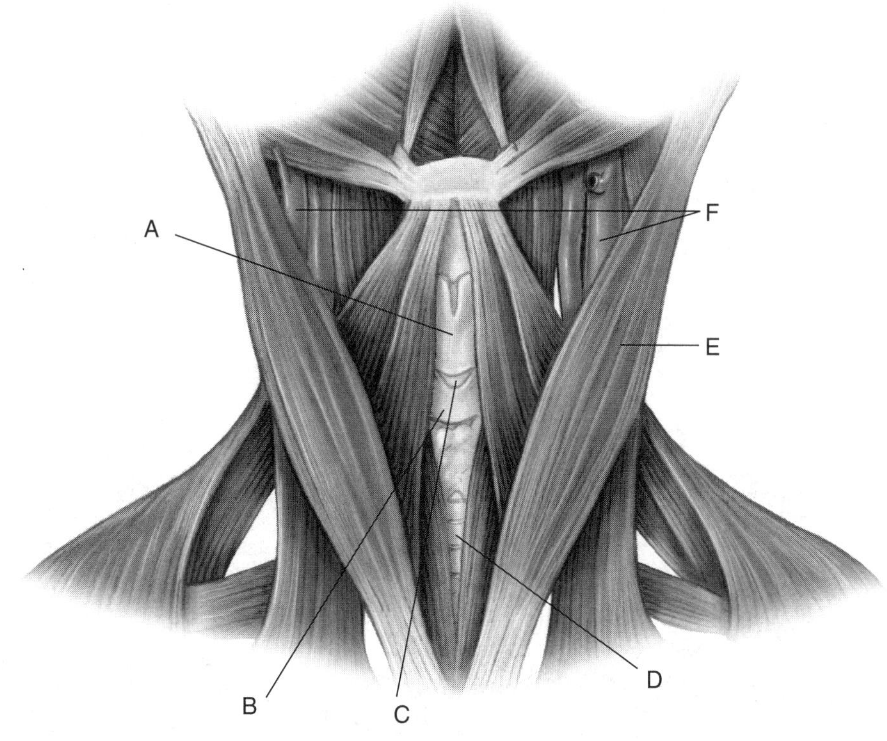

A. ______________________

B. ______________________

C. ______________________

D. ______________________

E. ______________________

F. ______________________

3. Arteries of the neck

A. ______________________________

B. ______________________________

C. ______________________________

D. ______________________________

E. ______________________________

F. ______________________________

G. ______________________________

H. ______________________________

I. ______________________________

Fill in the Blank

Read each item carefully, and then complete the statement by filling in the missing word(s).

1. The most common cervical strain is often called a(n) __________ injury.
2. A(n) __________ is a stretching or tearing of muscle or tendon.
3. The bones around the eye are thin, and with significant trauma to the face, the eye can be dislodged. This is called a(n) __________ fracture.
4. When assessing the ears, look for ______ from the ears and note if it is clear or _______.
5. Note the presence of enlarged ______ nodes on the neck on your assessment.
6. A(n) ________ fracture of the maxilla that involves the _____ ______ and the inferior maxilla, separating them from the rest of the skull, is called a Le Fort I fracture.
7. Massive ______ discharge of blood and possibly _____ may occur with an orbital fracture, and vision is often impaired.
8. The __________ __________ consists of the cochlea and semicircular canals.

9. When dealing with an impaled object in the face, the only time you should remove the object is when the patient has __________ complications.

10. Bleeding into the anterior chamber of the eye is called __________.

11. __________, __________, and __________ rays can burn the delicate tissues of the eyes.

12. If a patient has a burn to the eyes caused by a strong alkali or acid, you should irrigate the eye for __________ minutes.

13. The only indication for removing a contact lens in the field is a(n) __________ __________.

14. Reimplantation of a tooth may be successful for up to __________ hour(s) after it has been avulsed from the mouth.

15. Any open neck wounds should be covered with a(n) __________ dressing.

16. Chemicals, heat, and _____ rays can all burn the delicate tissues of the eye and _____ (the surrounding structures and accessories), often causing permanent damage.

17. When a patient has a facial injury, because __________ irritates the gastric lining, the risks of vomiting and aspiration are significant.

18. When a patient has a protruding eye, you should cover it with a moist, sterile dressing and stabilize it along with the uninjured eye to prevent further injury due to __________ __________ __________, the movement of both eyes in unison.

19. The paramedic should never exert __________ on or manipulate a patient's injured globe in any way.

20. A patient who has sustained a fracture of all midface bones, separating the entire midface from the cranium, has sustained a Le Fort III fracture, also called a(n) __________ __________.

Identify

Read the following case study, and then list the chief complaint, vital signs, and pertinent negatives; then answer the additional questions.

Tom and Dan arrive at the scene of a collision as additional help. It is 0030 hours, and a carload of teenagers has rolled into a cornfield. The corn is about shoulder high, and nobody can say for sure how many kids were in the car. Tom begins a search around the crash site as Dan helps with a patient. Tom hears something to his left and finds a 17-year-old girl on the ground.

The girl is lying face down, and when Tom carefully rolls her over, maintaining in-line manual stabilization with the assistance of two firefighters, he notices that she has severe facial injuries. The primary survey shows no life-threatening bleeding once her airway has been opened by positioning and the blood has been suctioned from her throat. The girl is a U on the AVPU scale, and Tom suspects that she may have gone through the windshield. Her respirations are 34 breaths/min and very deep, and oxygen saturation is 95%. Pupils are sluggish, blood pressure (BP) is 160/90 mm Hg, and pulse is 72 beats/min. The girl's skin is cool, but she has been lying on the ground for at least half an hour.

Help arrives, and they apply a cervical collar, secure the patient to a backboard, and get her in the unit.

The closest trauma center is half an hour away by helicopter, so Dan and Tom call for the life flight crew to meet them on the scene. Because the patient is unresponsive, Dan and Tom decide to insert an advanced airway and administer 100% supplemental oxygen to her. They place two large-bore IV lines and administer normal saline. They are careful not to overload this patient with fluid because of the potential for a head injury. The electrocardiogram (ECG) monitor now shows a sinus bradycardia, respiration is 56 breaths/min, and BP is now 168/88 mm Hg. Life flight then takes over and flies the patient to the regional trauma center.

Dan and Tom later find out that the patient survives. She had a Le Fort III fracture and has some neurologic defects from the closed head injury, from which it will take several months to years to recover.

1. Chief complaint:

____

____

2. Vital signs:

____

____

3. Pertinent negatives:

____

____

4. Why is it important to get this patient to the regional trauma center?

____

____

5. Why is it so important to keep this patient's airway clear of blood?

____

____

6. What are the patient's serial vital signs telling the paramedics?

____

____

Ambulance Calls

The following case scenarios provide an opportunity to explore the concerns associated with patient management and paramedic care. Read each scenario, and then answer each question.

1. While enjoying a weekend off at a ski resort, you happen to see a young woman trip over the steps at the lodge and fall. As you rush to her assistance, you see blood coming from her mouth, and closer inspection reveals that she has knocked out one of her lower teeth entirely. Which steps should you take?

   a. _______________

   b. _______________

   c. _______________

   d. _______________

   e. _______________

2. You volunteer to accompany the young lady to the nearest hospital, some 2 hours away by road. Just as you are pulling away from the ski resort in a friend's car, the resort manager comes running after you, waving for you to stop. "I have someone else here who needs to go to the hospital," he says. Behind him, two ski instructors are leading a young man along. The patient had been involved in a fistfight and now has two black eyes. A thorough examination of an injured eye includes assessment of which visible ocular structures and ocular functions?

a. ______________________________

b. ______________________________

c. ______________________________

d. ______________________________

e. ______________________________

f. ______________________________

g. ______________________________

h. ______________________________

3. A 12-year-old boy lost control of his bicycle as he was riding down a long, steep hill into town. At the base of the hill, his front wheel struck the curb, and he was catapulted from the bicycle straight through the show window of the local wedding dress shop. When you arrive, you find him bleeding from multiple lacerations. The most profuse bleeding seems to be coming from a large laceration on the left side of his neck.
a. What are the principal dangers associated with the laceration of the neck?

____

b. What should be done to the wound immediately?

____

True/False

If you believe the statement to be more true than false, write the letter "T" in the space provided. If you believe the statement to be more false than true, write the letter "F."

______ **1.** There are 22 facial bones that form the structure of the face without contributing to the cranial vault.

______ **2.** Floaters are specks the patient describes in his or her field of vision.

______ **3.** UV rays do not cause superficial burns to the eyes.

______ **4.** Double vision usually points to trauma involving the extraocular muscles, such as an orbit fracture.

______ **5.** Although painless to the patient, a ruptured tympanic membrane will not heal.

______ **6.** Nasal fractures are often complicated by the presence of epistaxis.

______ **7.** A Le Fort I fracture has a pyramidal shape and involves the nasal bone and inferior maxilla.

______ **8.** The patient who has sustained an orbital fracture may report symptoms of diplopia.

______ **9.** The avulsed tooth can be reimplanted successfully even if it has been out of the mouth for over a day.

______ **10.** Bruising and swelling are the first clues to a maxillofacial fracture.

______ **11.** To maintain an airway, it is acceptable to use blind nasotracheal intubation when there are signs of facial fractures.

______ **12.** Blunt eye trauma can lead to retinal detachment, which is common in sports injuries.

______ **13.** It is not necessary to cover both of the patient's eyes to prevent sympathetic eye movement.

______ **14.** The area above the angle of the mandible is referred to as zone III.

______ **15.** It may be difficult to determine the extent of bleeding in the mouth as a result of the patient swallowing the blood.

______ **16.** You should always apply an occlusive dressing to an open neck wound to prevent an air embolism.

______ **17.** Coughing up blood is known as dysphagia.

______ **18.** Hoarseness or voice changes may indicate laryngeal fracture.

______ **19.** A perforated tympanic membrane can occur from direct blows to the ear or pressure injuries.

______ **20.** If part of the patient's external ear has been avulsed in a fight, you should save the piece in a container of ice.

Short Answer

Complete this section with short written answers using the space provided.

1. Injuries to the face may be quite frightening to look at, but they do not by themselves ordinarily pose an immediate threat to life. However, facial injuries may be associated with other conditions or injuries that can threaten life or limb. List two potentially serious or life-threatening conditions that may be associated with maxillofacial trauma.

   a. ____________________

   b. ____________________

2. In examining a trauma patient, which findings would lead you to suspect maxillofacial fracture? List five signs of maxillofacial fracture.

   a. ____________________

   b. ____________________

   c. ____________________

   d. ____________________

   e. ____________________

Fill in the Table

Fill in the missing parts of the table.

1. Summary of maxillofacial fractures

Injury	Signs and Symptoms
Multiple facial bone fractures	• Massive facial swelling • ________________ • ________________ • Anterior or ________________ epistaxis
Zygomatic and orbital fractures	• Loss of sensation below the ________________ • Flattening of the ________________ • ________________ of upward gaze
Nasal fractures	• Crepitus and instability • Swelling, tenderness, ________________ • Anterior or ________________ epistaxis
Maxillary (Le Fort) fractures	• Mobility of the ________________ • Dental ________________ • Facial swelling
Mandibular fractures	• Dental malocclusion • ________________ instability

2. Signs and symptoms of injuries to the anterior part of the neck

Injury	Signs and Symptoms
Laryngeal fracture, tracheal transection	• Labored breathing or reduced ____________________ • Stridor • Hoarseness, voice changes • ____________________ (coughing up blood) • Subcutaneous emphysema • Swelling, edema • Structural irregularity
Vascular injury	• ____________________ bleeding • Signs of shock • Hematoma, swelling, edema • ____________________ deficits
Esophageal perforation	• ____________________ (difficulty swallowing) • ____________________ • ____________________ (suggests aspiration of blood)
Neurologic impairment	• Signs of a stroke (suggests air embolism or ____________________) • ____________________ or paresthesia • ____________________ nerve deficit • Signs of ____________________ shock

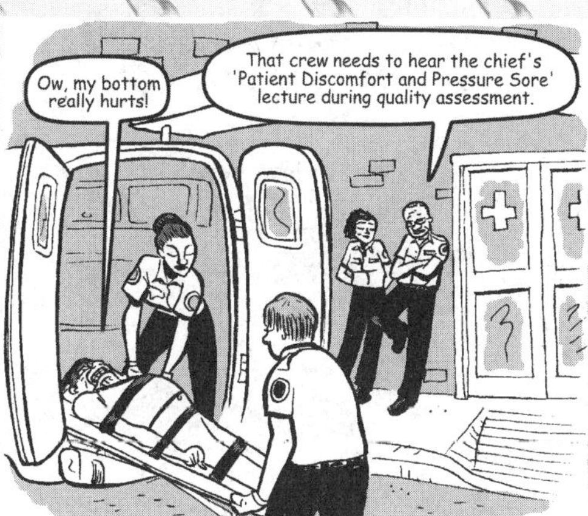

CHAPTER 34

Head and Spine Trauma

Matching

Part I

Match each of the terms in the right column to the appropriate definition in the left column.

_____ **1.** Fracture generally resulting from the extension of a linear fracture into the base of the skull; usually occurs after a diffuse impact to the head (as in a fall or motor vehicle crash) and can be difficult to diagnose, even with radiography.

_____ **2.** Upward movement of the toe(s) in response to stimulation to the sole of the foot. Under normal circumstances, the toe(s) move downward.

_____ **3.** A long, slender extension of a neuron (nerve cell) that conducts electrical impulses away from the neuronal soma.

_____ **4.** An increase in mean arterial pressure to compensate for decreased cerebral perfusion pressure; compensatory physiologic response that occurs in an effort to shunt blood to the brain; manifests clinically as hypertension.

_____ **5.** A late, life-threatening complication of spinal cord injury in which stimulation of the sympathetic nervous system below the level of injury generates a massive, uninhibited, uncompensated cardiovascular response; also known as autonomic hyperreflexia.

_____ **6.** A gradually increasing rate and depth of respirations followed by a gradual decrease with intermittent periods of apnea; associated with brainstem insult.

_____ **7.** The largest portion of the brain; responsible for higher functions, such as reasoning; divided into right and left hemispheres, or halves.

_____ **8.** Fluid produced in the ventricles of the brain that flows in the subarachnoid space and bathes the meninges.

_____ **9.** The pressure of blood flow through the brain; the difference between the mean arterial pressure and intracranial pressure.

_____ **10.** Excessive fluid in the brain; swelling of the brain.

_____ **11.** The middle membrane of the three meninges that enclose the brain and spinal cord.

_____ **12.** Loss of memory of events that occurred after an injury.

_____ **13.** A condition that occurs with flexion injuries or fractures, resulting in the displacement of bone fragments into the anterior portion of the spinal cord. Findings include paralysis below the level of the insult and loss of pain, temperature, and touch perception.

A. Anterior cord syndrome
B. Anterograde (posttraumatic) amnesia
C. Arachnoid
D. Autonomic dysreflexia
E. Autoregulation
F. Axon
G. Babinski reflex
H. Basilar skull fracture
I. Battle sign
J. Biot (ataxic) respirations
K. Brainstem
L. Brown-Séquard syndrome
M. Cauda equina

______	**14.** The midbrain, pons, and medulla, collectively.	**N.**	Cauda equina syndrome
______	**15.** Irregular pattern, rate, and depth of respirations with intermittent periods of apnea; results from increased intracranial pressure.	**O.**	Central cord syndrome
______	**16.** Bruising over the mastoid bone behind the ear often seen after a basilar skull fracture; also called retroauricular ecchymosis.	**P.**	Central neurogenic hyperventilation
______	**17.** The largest portion of the cerebrum; regulates voluntary skeletal movement and a person's level of awareness; a part of consciousness.	**Q.**	Cerebellum
______	**18.** A focal brain injury in which brain tissue is bruised and damaged in a defined area.	**R.**	Cerebral concussion
______	**19.** Injury that occurs when the brain is jarred around in the skull; a mild diffuse brain injury that does not result in structural damage or permanent neurologic impairment.	**S.**	Cerebral contusion
______	**20.** The brain region essential in coordinating muscle movements in the body; also called the athlete's brain.	**T.**	Cerebral cortex
______	**21.** A condition associated with penetrating trauma and characterized by hemisection of the spinal cord and complete damage to all spinal tracts on the involved side.	**U.**	Cerebral edema
______	**22.** The location where the spinal cord separates; composed of nerve roots.	**V.**	Cerebral perfusion pressure (CPP)
______	**23.** A neurologic condition caused by compression of the bundle of nerve roots located at the end of the spinal cord.	**W.**	cerebrospinal fluid (CSF)
______	**24.** A condition resulting from hyperextension injuries to the cervical area that damage the dorsal column of the spinal cord; characterized by hemorrhage or edema. Findings include greater loss of function in the upper extremities, with variable sensory loss of pain and temperature.	**X.**	Cerebrum
______	**25.** Deep, rapid respirations; similar to Kussmaul respirations, but without an acetone breath odor; commonly seen after brainstem injury.	**Y.**	Cheyne-Stokes respirations

Part II

Match each of the terms in the right column to the appropriate definition in the left column.

______	**1.** A specific, grossly observable brain injury.	**A.**	Complete spinal cord injury
______	**2.** A type of injury that results from forward movement of the head, typically as the result of rapid deceleration, such as in a car crash, or with a direct blow to the occiput.	**B.**	Coup-contrecoup injury
______	**3.** The joint on which each vertebra articulates with adjacent vertebrae.	**C.**	Cranial vault
______	**4.** An accumulation of blood between the skull and dura.	**D.**	Critical minimum threshold
______	**5.** The outermost layer of the three meninges that enclose the brain and spinal cord; the toughest meningeal layer.	**E.**	Cushing triad
______	**6.** Hypertension (with a widening pulse pressure), bradycardia, and irregular respirations; the classic findings associated with increased intracranial pressure.	**F.**	Decerebrate (extensor) posturing
______	**7.** Minimum cerebral perfusion pressure required to adequately perfuse the brain; 60 mm Hg in the adult.	**G.**	Decorticate (flexor) posturing
______	**8.** The bones that encase and protect the brain; the parietal, temporal, frontal, occipital, sphenoid, and ethmoid bones; also called the cranium or skull.	**H.**	Depressed skull fracture
______	**9.** Dual impacting of the brain into the skull, first at the point of impact and then on the opposite side of impact, as the brain rebounds.	**I.**	Dermatome
______	**10.** Total disruption of all spinal cord tracts, with permanent loss of all cord-mediated functions below the level of injury.	**J.**	Diffuse axonal injury (DAI)
______	**11.** Bleeding within the brain tissue (parenchyma) itself; also called an intraparenchymal hematoma.	**K.**	Diffuse brain injury

______	**12.** Spinal cord injury in which there is some degree of cord-mediated function; initial dysfunction may be temporary, and there may be potential for recovery.	**L.** Dura mater
______	**13.** A high body temperature.	**M.** Epidural hematoma
______	**14.** Extension of a limb or other body part beyond its usual range of motion.	**N.** Facet joint
______	**15.** Hyperacute pain to touch.	**O.** Flexion injury
______	**16.** Any injury that affects the entire brain.	**P.** Focal brain injury
______	**17.** Diffuse brain injury that is caused by stretching, shearing, or tearing of nerve fibers with consequent axonal damage.	**Q.** Frontal lobe
______	**18.** An area of the body innervated by sensor components of spinal nerves.	**R.** Hangman's fracture
______	**19.** Fracture caused by high-energy direct trauma applied to a small surface area of the skull with a blunt object (such as a baseball bat striking the head); commonly accompanied by bone fragments driven into the brain, causing further injury.	**S.** Head injury
______	**20.** Abnormal posture characterized by flexion of the arms and extension of the legs; indicates pressure on the brainstem.	**T.** Head trauma
______	**21.** A process in which tissue is forced out of its normal position, such as when the brain is forced from the cranial vault, either through the foramen magnum or over the tentorium.	**U.** Herniation
______	**22.** A general term that includes both head injuries and traumatic brain injuries.	**V.** Hyperesthesia
______	**23.** A traumatic insult to the head that may result in injury to soft tissues of the scalp and bony structures of the head and skull, not including the face.	**W.** Hyperextension
______	**24.** The most classic distraction injury, which occurs when a person is hanged by the neck. Bending and fractures occur at the C1 to C2 region, which quickly tear the spinal cord.	**X.** Hyperpyrexia
______	**25.** The portion of the brain that is important in voluntary motor actions and personality traits.	**Y.** Incomplete spinal cord injury
______	**26.** Abnormal posture characterized by extension of the arms and legs; indicates pressure on the brainstem.	**Z.** Intracerebral hematoma

Part III

Match each of the items in the left column to the appropriate injury in the right column. (Note: Some of the injury types can be applied more than once.)

______	**1.** A 15-year-old skateboarder has hit the side of his head after a fall. After an initial bout of unconsciousness, he regains consciousness, only to lapse again about an hour later. His mother cannot wake him up again.	**A.** Cerebral concussion
______	**2.** A football player comes off the field after a helmet-to-helmet hit. He is a little disoriented and cannot remember the play. The coach says he just "got his bell rung." The player shows no other signs later in the evening or the next day.	**B.** Cerebral contusion
______	**3.** The other football player also comes off the field. He is very confused. He loses consciousness in the locker room for about 3 minutes. He is confused for the next 2 days.	**C.** Epidural hematoma
______	**4.** A 40-year-old woman is scrubbing the floor. As she rises, she hits the back of her head on the sink. At the time, she gets a slight headache. Later in the evening, her speech becomes slightly slurred.	**D.** Subdural hematoma
______	**5.** A 12-year-old girl is hit on the head with a baseball bat by her brother. She is knocked out but wakes back up to tell her mother what happened. Her mother decides to have her checked out. On the way to the doctor's office, the girl appears to go to sleep. When they arrive, the mother cannot wake her.	**E.** Intracerebral hematoma

______ 6. The patient was the driver of a vehicle that was struck from the left side by another car. The door on the driver's side is dented. The patient is conscious, but witnesses say that he was "out cold" for a few minutes immediately after the collision. He complains of a headache and the feeling of pins and needles in his left hip and left leg. His skull is tender to palpation in the area just superior to the left ear. While he is under your care, his level of consciousness deteriorates until he is unconscious altogether, and his respirations become very slow.

F. Subarachnoid hemorrhage

______ 7. The patient was a participant in a barroom brawl. This patient was "knocked out cold" for a few minutes. Now he seems alert, but he cannot remember what happened. He complains of a little dizziness. His vital signs are normal.

______ 8. The patient was a front-seat passenger in a car that careened into a utility pole. He is confused and sleepy when you find him. His speech is slurred, and there is weakness of the right leg. He becomes increasingly more lethargic while under your care and vomits twice. The left pupil seems to be getting larger than the right.

______ 9. The patient was an unrestrained front-seat passenger in a car involved in a head-on collision with another car. He apparently struck his head on the windshield because the windshield in front of the patient is cracked. The patient is found unconscious. His left pupil is larger than the right. His pulse is 56 beats/min, and his blood pressure is 190/90 mm Hg. Respirations are irregular.

______ 10. You are called to a 70-year-old woman with a terrible headache. She hit her head on the cupboard about 2 hours ago. She initially had a severe headache at the site of the injury, but now it has moved to a larger area of her head. She is responsive only to questions and begins to vomit while you are taking care of her. She rapidly becomes unresponsive and begins to have a seizure.

Multiple Choice

Read each item carefully, and then select the best response.

______ 1. The majority of all skull fractures are:

- **A.** open skull fractures.
- **B.** basilar skull fractures.
- **C.** depressed skull fractures.
- **D.** linear skull fractures.

______ 2. The oculomotor nerve is the __________ cranial nerve.

- **A.** first
- **B.** second
- **C.** third
- **D.** fourth

______ 3. The brain consumes ________ of the body's total oxygen.

- **A.** 10%
- **B.** 20%
- **C.** 30%
- **D.** 40%

______ 4. Normally, the brain occupies about 80% of the space within the cranium. The remaining space is taken up by:

- **A.** muscle and fat.
- **B.** blood and CSF.
- **C.** water and glucose.
- **D.** lymph fluid.

_____ **5.** What is the reticular activating system (RAS) responsible for?
- **A.** Blood pressure
- **B.** Respiration
- **C.** Heart rate
- **D.** Consciousness

_____ **6.** When a patient has a basilar skull fracture, which of the following signs or symptoms would you LEAST expect to see?
- **A.** Raccoon eyes
- **B.** Battle sign
- **C.** Blowout fracture of the eye
- **D.** Draining of blood and CSF from the ear

_____ **7.** What is the minimum cerebral perfusion pressure in an adult that is required to perfuse the brain adequately?
- **A.** 15 mm Hg
- **B.** 30 mm Hg
- **C.** 45 mm Hg
- **D.** 60 mm Hg

_____ **8.** You are treating a patient who has starred the windshield in a car crash. The patient reports that he cannot remember what happened before the collision. This is called:
- **A.** anterograde amnesia.
- **B.** retrograde amnesia.
- **C.** amnesia.
- **D.** focal brain injury.

_____ **9.** After you drop off a patient whom you treated for a fall down the stairs, the doctor tells you she had bleeding into the brain tissue. What is the medical term for this condition?
- **A.** Epidural hematoma
- **B.** Intracerebral hematoma
- **C.** Subarachnoid hemorrhage
- **D.** Subdural hematoma

_____ **10.** What is the MOST important sign or symptom in evaluating a patient with a brain injury?
- **A.** Bleeding from the ears
- **B.** Pupil size and how the pupils react to light
- **C.** Level of consciousness
- **D.** Mechanism of injury

_____ **11.** Which of the following is NOT considered a sign or symptom of second-impact syndrome?
- **A.** Loss of eye movements
- **B.** A stunned appearance
- **C.** Coma
- **D.** Constricted pupils

_____ **12.** What is the MOST important step in managing any type of head injury?
- **A.** Maintaining airway and breathing
- **B.** Performing spinal immobilization
- **C.** Assessing where the bleeding is in the brain
- **D.** Establishing an IV line

_____ **13.** Which portion of the spine contains the most bones of the vertebral column?
- **A.** Cervical
- **B.** Thoracic
- **C.** Lumbar
- **D.** Sacral

_____ **14.** How many pairs of spinal nerves are there?
A. 12
B. 33
C. 31
D. 5

_____ **15.** The __________ plexus innervates the diaphragm.
A. cervical
B. sacral
C. lumbar
D. brachial

_____ **16.** Which of the following is NOT associated with high-risk mechanisms of injury (MOIs) for spinal injuries?
A. Penetrating trauma near the spine
B. Fall from two times the patient's height
C. Unrestrained in a rollover crash
D. Diving injury

_____ **17.** What is the initial step of assessment in a suspected spinal injury?
A. Ensuring scene safety
B. Clearing the airway
C. Checking for a pulse
D. Activating the trauma system

_____ **18.** What is the primary goal when immobilizing a patient with a spinal injury?
A. Determining whether the patient will be paralyzed
B. Determining where the exact injury is
C. Preventing further injuries to the patient
D. Securing the airway of the patient

_____ **19.** Which of the following is NOT done prior to applying a cervical collar to a patient?
A. Determine the need for the collar.
B. Perform manual stabilization of the head.
C. Assess the extremities for distal pulse, motor, and sensory (PMS) functions.
D. Check the patient's ability to move the neck.

_____ **20.** In which of the following situations should you NOT perform a rapid extrication?
A. The patient's legs are tingling.
B. The patient's condition requires immediate transport.
C. The vehicle or scene is unsafe.
D. You are unable to manage the airway.

_____ **21.** How many rescuers does it take to properly remove a helmet from a patient?
A. One
B. Two
C. Three
D. Never remove the helmet.

_____ **22.** The nerve root located at T4 is responsible for which dermatome area?
A. Umbilicus
B. Back of the leg
C. Apex of axilla
D. Nipple line

Labeling

Label the following diagrams with the correct terms.

1. Sections of the cervical, thoracic, and lumbar spine

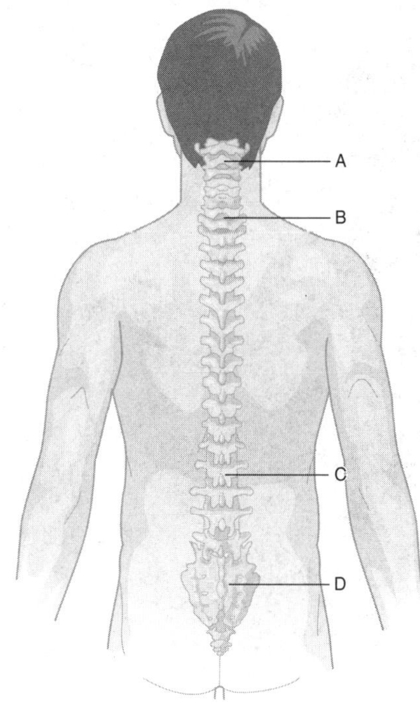

A. ______________________________

B. ______________________________

C. ______________________________

D. ______________________________

2. The meninges

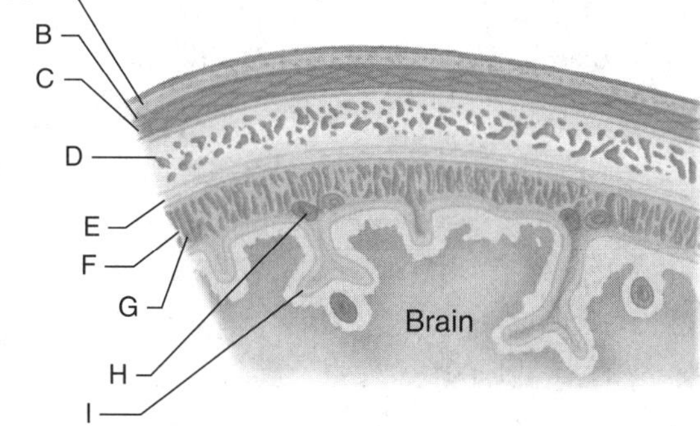

A. ______________________________

B. ______________________________

C. ______________________________

D. ______________________________

E. ______________________________

F. ______________________________

G. ______________________________

H. ______________________________

I. ______________________________

3. Major regions of the brain

DIENCEPHALON
A
B
CEREBRUM
C
D
E
I
BRAIN STEM
CEREBELLUM
H
G
F

A. ______________________

B. ______________________

C. ______________________

D. ______________________

E. ______________________

F. ______________________

G. ______________________

H. ______________________

I. ______________________

Fill in the Blank

Read each item carefully, and then complete the statement by filling in the missing word(s).

1. The ______ body, the anterior weight-bearing structure, is made of bone that supports and stabilizes the body.
2. The vertebral components include the _____, ______, and spinous processes.
3. The __________ is responsible for higher functions and is the largest portion of the brain.
4. The brainstem contains the midbrain, __________, and the __________.
5. The second layer of the meninges, which is a delicate, transparent membrane, is called the __________.
6. A(n) __________-__________ injury happens when the brain sloshes forward and hits the front of the skull and then recoils and hits the back part of the skull.
7. Increased intracranial pressure (ICP) can produce signs of __________, bradycardia, and irregular respirations. This set of findings is known as __________ __________.
8. A(n) __________ hematoma is the collection of blood between the dura mater and the skull.
9. Because of clenched teeth, the paramedic may have to perform __________ __________ __________ to intubate the patient with head injury safely.
10. Unlike patients who experience shock, the patient with a head injury can develop a very high __________ __________.
11. The components of the vertebral body are the spinous process, __________, and the __________.

12. The two vertebrae in the cervical area that allow for the rotational movement of the skull are __________ and __________.

13. The two components of the central nervous system are the __________ and the __________ __________.

14. The three components of the brainstem are the __________, __________, and __________.

15. The spinal cord attaches to the brain through the __________ __________, which is a hole in the base of the skull.

16. The nerves can also be injured at the _______ level, which is outside the spinal cord.

17. __________ spinal cord injury is total disruption of all tracts of the spinal cord, with all cord-mediated functions below the level of transaction being lost permanently.

18. The signs and symptoms of __________ __________ are hypotension and bradycardia, accompanied by warm, dry, flushed skin.

19. In most adults, the ______ cord extends from the base of the skull to L2; here it separates into the ________ equina.

20. During an assessment of the feet of a patient, when you stimulate the bottom of the feet, normally the toes move __________; with a positive Babinski reflex, the toes move __________.

Identify

Read the following case studies, and then list the chief complaint, vital signs, and pertinent negatives.

Part I

Tom and Janet, two off-duty paramedics, are leaving the midnight show at the local movie theater when they witness a collision between a car with two occupants and an 18-wheel tractor trailer flying down the highway. It is 0230 hours, and it looked like the car misjudged the speed of the truck when making a right-hand turn onto the main boulevard. The small car was struck on the left-side driver's door, spinning the vehicle and rolling it a couple times before it stopped by a telephone pole in the upright position. Tom begins a search around the crash site as he calls on his cell phone for the police, EMS, and the fire department for an engine and rescue. Janet begins to deal with traffic and then starts to check out the patients in the car.

Janet quickly recognizes the male driver is pinned behind the wheel and will require extrication. The female front-seat occupant probably did not have her seatbelt on as she struck the windshield and was thrown out the side door to the ground.

The woman is on her back with her arms drawn up to her chest, and her feet seem to be rigid and slightly turned in. A primary survey shows minor bleeding from the scalp but no life-threatening bleeding. The girl is a U on the AVPU scale, and Tom determines she is a 7 on the Glasgow Coma Scale (GCS). Her respirations are 34 breaths/min and very deep, and oxygen saturation is 98%. Pupils are sluggish, blood pressure (BP) is 160/90 mm Hg, and her pulse is 64 beats/min. The woman's skin is cool.

Help arrives. Fire personnel take over extrication of the male patient, while paramedics begin care for the female patient. The paramedics apply a cervical collar to the female patient, secure her to scoop stretcher, and load her into their ambulance.

The closest trauma center is 15 minutes away by helicopter, so the paramedics call for the life flight crew to meet them in a landing zone near the scene. Because the patient is unresponsive (and the paramedics know they should consider intubating a patient with a GCS score of less than 8), they decide to insert an advanced airway and administer 100% supplemental oxygen to the patient. They place two large-bore IV lines and administer normal saline. The paramedics are careful not to overload this patient with fluid because of the rising intracranial pressure (ICP). The ECG monitor now shows a sinus bradycardia. Respirations are 56 breaths/min, and the BP is now 168/88 mm Hg. An air ambulance then takes over and flies the patient to the regional trauma center. Ultimately, the patient makes it but has some neurologic defects, from which it will take several months to years to recover.

Answer the following questions regarding the female patient.

1. Chief complaint:

____

____

2. Vital signs:

3. Pertinent negatives:

4. Why is it important to get this patient to the regional trauma center?

5. What does the patient's position on the ground tell the paramedics?

6. What do the patient's serial vital signs tell the paramedics?

Part II

Your unit is called to a two-vehicle collision. It is a dark morning, and it is misting outside. The patient is a young woman with long hair who is trapped in a vehicle that has landed on its wheels after rolling two or three times. Her hair is trapped between the roof of the car and the headrest, and you are unable to get inside because of the damage of the collision. You find that the patient responds to a few of your questions, but the only thing she can remember is her first name. You need the Jaws of Life to get her out. After the car is cut apart, you can finally get in the car to perform manual stabilization. A cervical collar is applied, and you and your partners—with some help from a firefighter—do a rapid extrication, being very careful to move the patient in straight lines onto the backboard.

En route to the hospital, you perform a rapid trauma assessment, which reveals no bleeding from anywhere. The patient is very cold, and you learn that the crash happened about an hour before anyone found the two cars. She has a BP of 100/62 mm Hg and a pulse of 124 beats/min. Her oxygen saturation is 96% before applying supplemental oxygen via nonrebreathing mask at 15 L/min. Her rate of breathing is 26 breaths/min and somewhat shallow. Lungs are clear. You are unable to find a pulse in either of the feet. She is unable to move her legs, and she does not respond to you when you touch or pinch her feet, knees, or hips. The monitor shows sinus tachycardia with no ectopy. You start two large-bore IV lines with warm normal saline and use active rewarming, turning the heat on high in the unit to help bring the patient's body temperature back up. Her serial vital signs remain largely unchanged except for the oxygen saturation, which has increased to 98%. After a 500-mL bolus of fluid, her BP has come up slightly to 108/64 mm Hg. The next day, you learn the patient had a broken L2 vertebra and is paralyzed from there down.

1. Chief complaint:

2. Vital signs:

3. Pertinent negatives:

Complete the Patient Care Report (PCR)

Read the incident scenario in the preceding Identify, Part II, exercise, and then complete the following PCR for the patient.

<table>
<tr><th colspan="6">EMS Patient Care Report (PCR)</th></tr>
<tr><td>Date:</td><td>Incident No.:</td><td colspan="2">Nature of Call:</td><td colspan="2">Location:</td></tr>
<tr><td>Dispatched:</td><td>En Route:</td><td>At Scene:</td><td>Transport:</td><td>At Hospital:</td><td>In Service:</td></tr>
<tr><th colspan="6">Patient Information</th></tr>
<tr><td colspan="3">Age:
Sex:
Weight (in kg [lb]):</td><td colspan="3">Allergies:
Medications:
Past Medical History:
Chief Complaint:</td></tr>
<tr><th colspan="6">Vital Signs</th></tr>
<tr><td>Time:</td><td>BP:</td><td>Pulse:</td><td>Respirations:</td><td colspan="2">SpO_2:</td></tr>
<tr><td>Time:</td><td>BP:</td><td>Pulse:</td><td>Respirations:</td><td colspan="2">SpO_2:</td></tr>
<tr><td>Time:</td><td>BP:</td><td>Pulse:</td><td>Respirations:</td><td colspan="2">SpO_2:</td></tr>
<tr><th colspan="6">EMS Treatment
(circle all that apply)</th></tr>
<tr><td colspan="2">Oxygen @ ______ L/min via (circle one):
NC NRM Bag-mask device</td><td>Assisted Ventilation</td><td>Airway Adjunct</td><td colspan="2">CPR</td></tr>
<tr><td>Defibrillation</td><td>Bleeding Control</td><td>Bandaging</td><td>Splinting</td><td colspan="2">Other:</td></tr>
<tr><th colspan="6">Narrative</th></tr>
<tr><td colspan="6"></td></tr>
</table>

Ambulance Calls

The following case scenarios provide an opportunity to explore the concerns associated with patient management and paramedic care. Read each scenario, and then answer each question.

1. In the old cowboy movies, one of the standard ways of preventing the bad guys from making their getaway was to tie a rope securely between two trees on either side of the road, at a height about 8 or 9 feet off the ground. When the bad guys came galloping down the road, the rope would catch them across the chest or neck and throw them from their horses.

Imagine, then, that you are the Dodge City paramedic, called to attend a bad guy who has just been thrown from his horse after riding precipitously into a rope stretched across the road. You find the bad guy lying on the road and moaning. His voice is quite hoarse as he replies to your questions about what happened, and he seems very short of breath. On examination, you find a prominent bruise over the anterior neck. The patient's face and neck appear bloated, and the skin there has a crinkly feel to it.

a. Which serious injury or injuries do you have to consider in this patient, given the mechanism of injury and the findings on examination?

____

____

b. List the steps you would take in treating this patient.

(1)____

(2)____

(3)____

2. A 15-year-old boy was shot in the abdomen during a gang dispute. You find him lying supine on the sidewalk. He is conscious, alert, and crying out, "I can't move my legs! I can't move my legs!" You find an entrance wound just to the left of the umbilicus. You cannot find an exit wound. On examination, sensation is absent from the toes up to the bottom of the ribs. The patient cannot move either leg, but he has normal strength in both hands.

a. At approximately which level of the spinal cord has this patient probably been injured?

____

b. Suppose that your examination also revealed a systolic blood pressure of 80 mm Hg. What could you conclude from that finding?

____

3. A 34-year-old man has been injured in a road incident in which his head apparently struck the windshield with some force. When you first reach the scene, the patient is unconscious. He is breathing 8 breaths/min, inhaling approximately 500 mL of air with each breath.

a. What is his minute volume? __________

b. Is that volume greater or less than normal? __________

c. Therefore, you can conclude that the patient's arterial P_{CO_2} will tend to __________ (increase or decrease?), so his pH will __________ (increase or decrease?). The net effect will be an acid–base disorder called a __________ (respiratory or metabolic?) __________ (acidosis or alkalosis?). The way you can help correct that abnormality is to __________.

d. One reason to try to correct hypoventilation in a patient with a head injury is that hypoventilation may, through its effects on acid–base balance, worsen cerebral edema and thereby accelerate the increase in ICP. How would you know if this patient is developing an increase in ICP? List five signs of increasing ICP.

(1)____

(2)____

(3)__________

(4)__________

(5)__________

e. Here are the findings of your initial neurologic assessment of the patient:
- He opens his eyes only when pinched, not when spoken to.
- He pulls his whole arm and shoulder away when you pinch his hand.
- He makes garbled sounds that you cannot understand.

(1) What is his AVPU? __________

(2) What is his score on the GCS? __________

4. Score each of the patients described in the following scenarios according to the AVPU scale and the GCS.

a. The patient is found unconscious. He opens his eyes in response to a loud voice. He does not follow commands, but he pulls his hand away when pinched and makes a few garbled noises that you cannot understand.

AVPU scale __________ GCS score __________

b. The patient is found apparently unconscious, but he opens his eyes at the sound of your voice. He can follow simple commands, but he is a bit confused and cannot tell you what month it is or what day of the week it is.

AVPU scale __________ GCS score __________

c. The patient is found unconscious. He does not open his eyes when pinched or try to pull away from the painful stimulus; instead, his arms flex spasmodically across his chest while his legs go into hyperextension. He makes no sound.

AVPU scale __________ GCS score __________

d. The patient is found conscious. He gives you a coherent account of what happened to him, his name, and the day of the week, and he can follow simple commands.

AVPU scale __________ GCS score __________

5. You are called to attend to a patient who was injured in an altercation that took place in a downtown drinking establishment. In the course of the dispute, someone broke a whiskey bottle over the patient's head. You find the patient conscious, bleeding profusely from his scalp, and in a distinctly unfriendly frame of mind, which he manifests by hurling tables and chairs in all directions while screaming uncomplimentary names at his assailants. List the steps you would take in treating this patient.

a. __________

b. __________

c. __________

d. __________

True/False

If you believe the statement to be more true than false, write the letter "T" in the space provided. If you believe the statement to be more false than true, write the letter "F."

______ **1.** The cranial vault consists of 10 bones.

______ **2.** The cerebral perfusion pressure (CPP) is the pressure of blood flow through the brain.

______ **3.** The reticular activating system is responsible for maintenance of hearing and reading skills.

______ **4.** According to the "90-90-9 rule" a single drop of the Spo_2 below 90% increases the chance of a brain injured patient's death.

______ **5.** The frontal lobe of the brain is responsible for personality traits.

_____ **6.** The vagus nerve originates from the pons.

_____ **7.** CSF is manufactured in the ventricles of the brain.

_____ **8.** Motor vehicle crashes are among the most common causes of head injury.

_____ **9.** The body's response to a decrease of cerebral perfusion pressure is to increase mean arterial pressure.

_____ **10.** Decerebrate posturing is seen when the patient pulls the arms into the core of the body.

_____ **11.** Subarachnoid hematoma will usually present with a sudden and severe headache.

_____ **12.** The outermost of the meninges is the dura mater.

_____ **13.** There are 32 pairs of spinal nerves that emerge from the spinal cord.

_____ **14.** The vagus nerve is part of the parasympathetic nervous system.

_____ **15.** A flexion injury is usually caused by a rapid deceleration or a direct blow to the occipital region.

_____ **16.** Most fractures sustained in a vertical compression are classified as unstable.

_____ **17.** In central cord syndrome, the patient will demonstrate a greater loss of function in the lower extremities than in the upper extremities.

_____ **18.** The diaphragm is innervated by the phrenic nerve between C3 and C5.

_____ **19.** When there is an absent pulse in a patient with a spinal cord injury, it is acceptable not to start cardiopulmonary resuscitation (CPR) because of the region of the injury.

_____ **20.** A normal neurologic exam can immediately rule out a spinal cord injury.

_____ **21.** The preferred method of immobilizing a person to a long backboard is the two-person log-roll method.

_____ **22.** You should assess the pulse, motor, and sensory (PMS) functions in each extremity before and after placing the patient on a long backboard.

_____ **23.** A rapid extrication technique should be used for every patient who is in a seated position in a car crash.

_____ **24.** It is acceptable to release manual stabilization of the neck while you are measuring for a cervical collar. Make sure, however, to let your patient know not to move the head.

Short Answer

Complete this section with short written answers using the space provided.

1. When a patient has sustained a potential injury to the spinal cord, it does not pay to wait until there are symptoms and signs of spinal cord damage. By then, it may be too late to prevent permanent disability. The only sure way to prevent such disability is to anticipate spinal injury under the appropriate circumstances and handle the patient in a way that will protect his or her spinal cord from damage. List eight high-risk MOIs that strongly suggest spine injury.

a. ______________________________

b. ______________________________

c. ______________________________

d. ______________________________

e. ______________________________

f. ______________________________

g. ______________________________

h. ______________________________

Fill in the Table

Fill in the missing parts of the tables.

1. Signs and symptoms of head trauma

____________, contusions, or ____________ to the scalp
Soft area or ____________ noted on palpation of the scalp
Visible skull ____________ or ____________
____________ sign or ____________ eyes
CSF rhinorrhea or ____________
Traumatic Brain Injury
Pupillary abnormalities
• ____________ pupil size
• Sluggish or ____________ pupils
A period of unresponsiveness
Confusion or disorientation
Repeatedly asks the same questions (perseveration)
Amnesia (____________ and/or ____________)
Combativeness or other abnormal behavior
Numbness or tingling in the ____________
Loss of sensation and/or motor function
Focal ____________ deficits
Seizures
____________ triad: hypertension, ____________, and irregular or erratic respirations
Dizziness
Visual disturbances, blurred vision, or double vision (____________)
Seeing "stars" (flashes of light)
Nausea or vomiting
Posturing (____________ and/or ____________)

2. Dermatomes

Nerve Root	Anatomic Location	Nerve Root	Anatomic Location
C2	____________________	T10	Umbilicus
C3	____________________	L1	____________________ line
C5	Lateral side of ____________________	L2	Mid-anterior thigh
C6	Thumb and medial index finger (6-shooter)	L3	Medial aspect of the ____________________
C7	____________________ finger	L5	____________________
C8	____________________ finger	S1–S3	Back of ____________________
T2	____________________	S4–S5	____________________ area
T4	____________________ line		

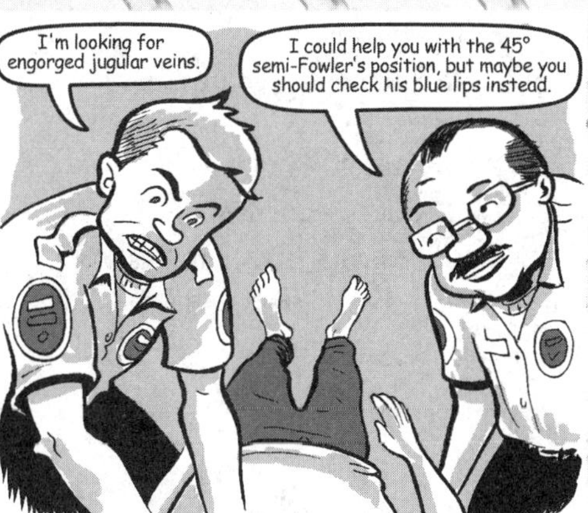

CHAPTER 35

Chest Trauma

Matching

Part I

Match each of the items in the right column to the appropriate description in the left column.

______	**1.** Blunt force injury to the heart that results in capillary damage, interstitial bleeding, and cellular damage in the area.	**A.** Atelectasis
______	**2.** A prominence of the jugular veins due to increased volume or increased pressure within the central venous system or the thoracic cavity.	**B.** Cardiac tamponade
______	**3.** The collection of blood within the normally closed pleural space.	**C.** Clavicle
______	**4.** A collection of blood and air in the pleural cavity.	**D.** Commotio cordis
______	**5.** An injury that involves two or more adjacent ribs fractured in two or more places, allowing the segment between the fractures to move independently of the rest of the thoracic cage.	**E.** Crepitus
______	**6.** Alveolar collapse that prevents use of that portion of the lungs for ventilation and oxygenation.	**F.** Exophthalmos
______	**7.** A condition in which the atria and right ventricle are collapsed by a collection of blood or other fluid within the pericardial sac, resulting in diminished cardiac output.	**G.** Flail chest
______	**8.** An S-shaped bone, also called the collarbone, that articulates medially with the sternum and laterally with the shoulder.	**H.** Hemopneumothorax
______	**9.** An event in which an often-fatal cardiac dysrhythmia is produced by a sudden blow to the thoracic cavity.	**I.** Hemothorax
______	**10.** A grating sensation made when two pieces of broken bone rub together or subcutaneous emphysema is palpated.	**J.** Jugular venous distention (JVD)
______	**11.** A pattern of injuries seen after a severe force is applied to the thorax, forcing blood from the great vessels and back into the head and neck.	**K.** Myocardial contusion
______	**12.** Dissection or rupture of the aorta.	**L.** Myocardial rupture
______	**13.** The collection of blood within the sclera of the eye, presenting as a bright red patch of blood over the sclera but not involving the cornea.	**M.** Needle decompression
______	**14.** The superior aspect of the thoracic cavity; this ring-like opening is created by the first vertebral vertebra, the first rib, the clavicles, and the manubrium.	**N.** Open pneumothorax
______	**15.** A life-threatening collection of air within the pleural space; the volume and pressure both collapse the involved lung and cause a shift of the mediastinal structures to the opposite side.	**O.** Pericardial sac
______	**16.** A procedure in which a needle or angiocatheter is introduced into the pericardial sac to relieve cardiac tamponade.	**P.** Pericardiocentesis

______	**17.** The collection of air within the normally closed pleural space.	**Q.** Pneumothorax
______	**18.** Injury to the lung parenchyma that results in capillary hemorrhage into the tissue.	**R.** Pulmonary contusion
______	**19.** Protrusion of the eyes from the normal position within the socket.	**S.** Pulsus paradoxus
______	**20.** A physical finding of air within the subcutaneous tissue.	**T.** Subconjunctival hematoma
______	**21.** The potential space between the layers of the pericardium.	**U.** Subcutaneous emphysema
______	**22.** The result of a defect in the chest wall that allows air to enter the thoracic space.	**V.** Tension pneumothorax
______	**23.** A procedure in which a needle or angiocatheter is introduced into the pleural space in an attempt to relieve a tension pneumothorax; also referred to as needle thoracentesis.	**W.** Thoracic inlet
______	**24.** An acute traumatic perforation of the ventricles, atria, intraventricular septum, intra-atrial septum, chordae, papillary muscles, or valves.	**X.** Traumatic asphyxia
______	**25.** A drop in the systolic blood pressure of 10 mm Hg more than during inspiration; commonly seen in patients with cardiac tamponade or severe asthma.	**Y.** Traumatic aortic disruption

Part II

Certain signs identify specific lung injuries. Match the types of lung injuries to the signs.

______	**1.** Hemoptysis, lack of tracheal deviation, and dullness noted on the side affected during percussion.	**A.** Simple pneumothorax
______	**2.** Jugular vein distention, and tracheal deviation and absence of breath sounds on affected side.	**B.** Open pneumothorax
______	**3.** Diminished breath sounds heard on auscultation, a finding that is best heard anteriorly if the patient is in the supine position or in the apices if the patient is upright.	**C.** Tension pneumothorax
______	**4.** A sucking chest wound or bubbling wound may be noted.	**D.** Massive hemothorax
______	**5.** Evidence of underlying injury may include contusions, tenderness, crepitus, or paradoxical motion. Auscultation may reveal wheezes or crackles (formerly known as rales).	**E.** Pulmonary contusion

Multiple Choice

Read each item carefully, and then select the best response.

______ **1.** While riding his bicycle fast down a hill, a 16-year-old boy falls and sustains an injury to the chest. While palpating the chest, you feel what you believe to be the fracture of a number of adjacent ribs and observe that the patient is having paradoxical respirations. What you are feeling and observing is likely which type of injury?

A. Flail chest
B. Subcutaneous emphysema
C. Commotio cordis
D. Pulmonary contusion

______ **2.** When a knife wound to the chest wall allows air to enter the thoracic space, what is the condition called?

A. Pulmonary contusion
B. Tension pneumothorax
C. Open pneumothorax
D. Myocardial contusion

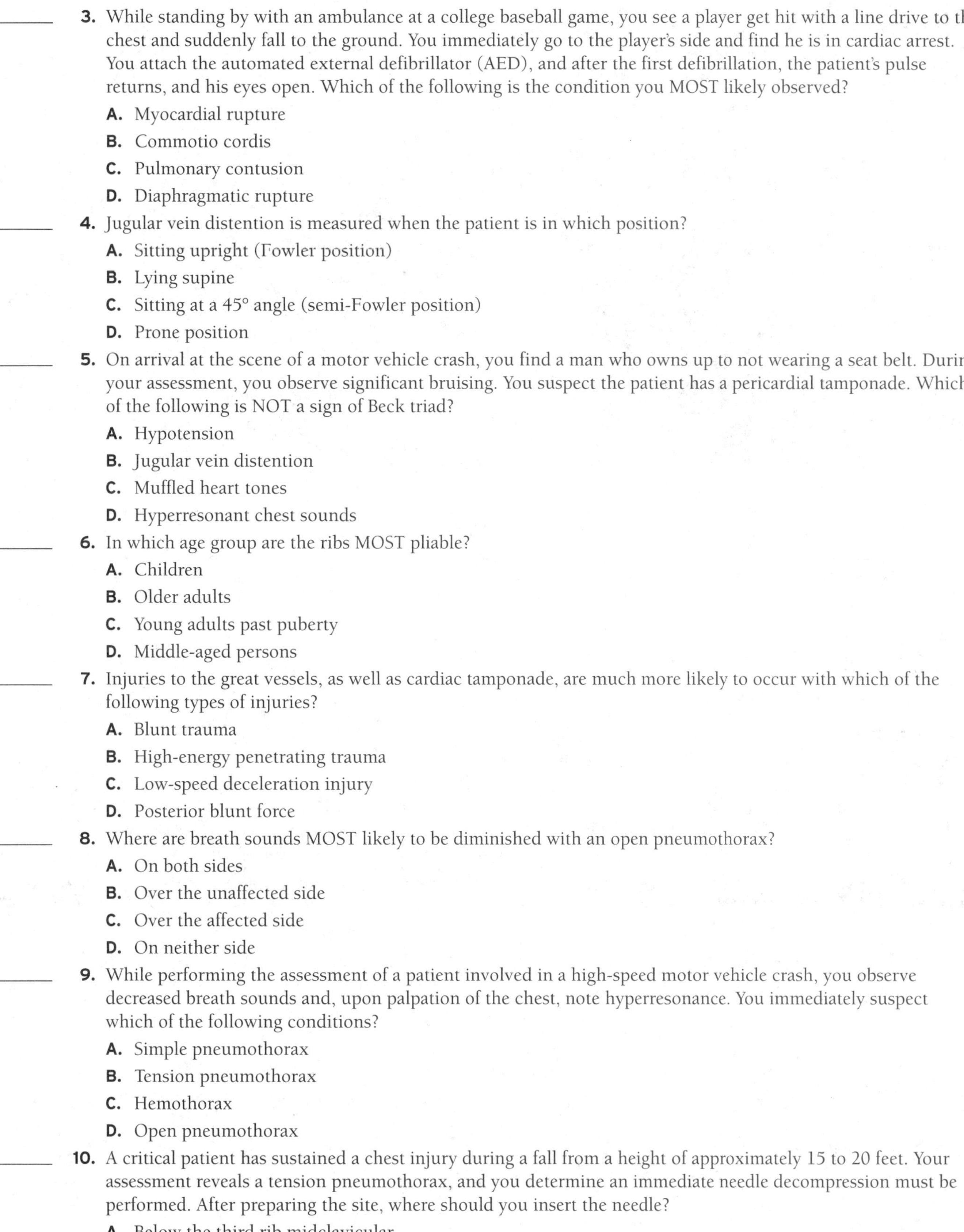

_____ **3.** While standing by with an ambulance at a college baseball game, you see a player get hit with a line drive to the chest and suddenly fall to the ground. You immediately go to the player's side and find he is in cardiac arrest. You attach the automated external defibrillator (AED), and after the first defibrillation, the patient's pulse returns, and his eyes open. Which of the following is the condition you MOST likely observed?

A. Myocardial rupture
B. Commotio cordis
C. Pulmonary contusion
D. Diaphragmatic rupture

_____ **4.** Jugular vein distention is measured when the patient is in which position?

A. Sitting upright (Fowler position)
B. Lying supine
C. Sitting at a 45° angle (semi-Fowler position)
D. Prone position

_____ **5.** On arrival at the scene of a motor vehicle crash, you find a man who owns up to not wearing a seat belt. During your assessment, you observe significant bruising. You suspect the patient has a pericardial tamponade. Which of the following is NOT a sign of Beck triad?

A. Hypotension
B. Jugular vein distention
C. Muffled heart tones
D. Hyperresonant chest sounds

_____ **6.** In which age group are the ribs MOST pliable?

A. Children
B. Older adults
C. Young adults past puberty
D. Middle-aged persons

_____ **7.** Injuries to the great vessels, as well as cardiac tamponade, are much more likely to occur with which of the following types of injuries?

A. Blunt trauma
B. High-energy penetrating trauma
C. Low-speed deceleration injury
D. Posterior blunt force

_____ **8.** Where are breath sounds MOST likely to be diminished with an open pneumothorax?

A. On both sides
B. Over the unaffected side
C. Over the affected side
D. On neither side

_____ **9.** While performing the assessment of a patient involved in a high-speed motor vehicle crash, you observe decreased breath sounds and, upon palpation of the chest, note hyperresonance. You immediately suspect which of the following conditions?

A. Simple pneumothorax
B. Tension pneumothorax
C. Hemothorax
D. Open pneumothorax

_____ **10.** A critical patient has sustained a chest injury during a fall from a height of approximately 15 to 20 feet. Your assessment reveals a tension pneumothorax, and you determine an immediate needle decompression must be performed. After preparing the site, where should you insert the needle?

A. Below the third rib midclavicular
B. Below the third rib midaxillary
C. Above the third rib midaxillary
D. Above the third rib midclavicular

Labeling

Label the following diagram with the correct terms.

1. The thorax

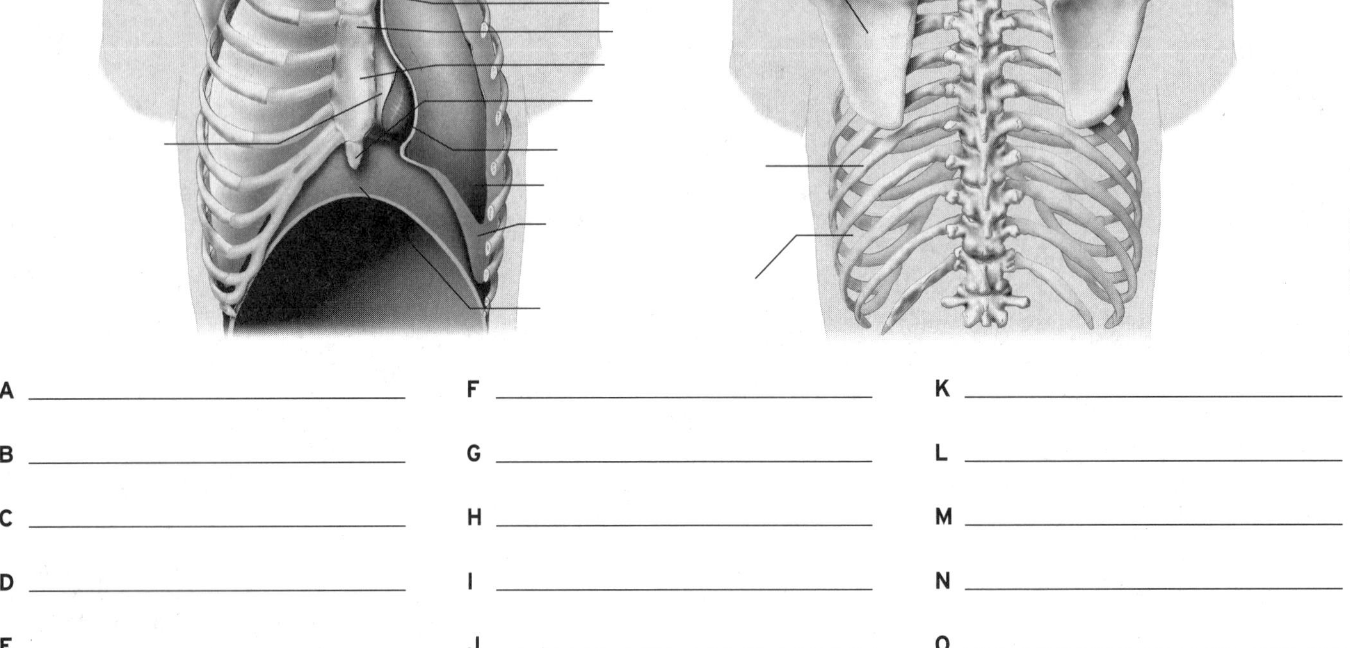

A ______________________ F ______________________ K ______________________

B ______________________ G ______________________ L ______________________

C ______________________ H ______________________ M ______________________

D ______________________ I ______________________ N ______________________

E ______________________ J ______________________ O ______________________

Fill in the Table

Fill in the possible injuries for each of the following situations.

Many, if not most, serious chest injuries cannot be specifically identified in the field. An understanding of the mechanism of injury (MOI), however, should enable you to anticipate the injuries that might be present in any given case and thereby to assess the potential urgency of the situation. For each of the following MOIs or associated injuries, indicate the serious chest injury or injuries that are likely to be present. The MOI, or easily detected injuries, may give clues to the presence of injuries that are harder to find.

If you find:	The patient may have:
1. Steering wheel imprint on anterior chest	
2. Caved-in door on driver's side	
3. Fall from a height	
4. Bullet entrance wound in fifth left intercostal space	
5. Fracture of ribs 5–7 in a young man	
6. Fracture of first and second ribs	

Identify

Read the following case study, and then list the chief complaint, physical findings, and signs of Beck triad.

1. A 35-year-old man was involved in a motor vehicle crash. The patient is quickly extricated from the vehicle. You are the first paramedic to evaluate the patient. He is verbal, and when asked about pain and other symptoms, he states, "My chest hurts." During your assessment, you observe bruising on the lower chest, diaphoresis, cyanosis, dyspnea, and jugular vein distention. While assessing the vital signs, you identify equal bilateral breath sounds, tachycardia, weak peripheral pulses, hypotension, and muffled heart tones. An electrocardiogram (ECG) displays electrical alternans.
   a. Chief complaint:
   b. Physical findings:
   c. Signs of Beck triad:
   d. Do you suspect this patient has a pericardial tamponade or a tension pneumothorax?

Read the following trauma scenario, and then list the physical findings that indicate pulmonary contusion. Also describe the Spalding effect, inertial effects, and implosion in this scenario.

2. You respond to an assault of a 16-year-old boy. The patient has been struck in the chest with a baseball bat. Upon your arrival, he is conscious. You immediately perform a primary survey. The airway is open, and the patient is breathing with only mild distress. Crackles are heard upon auscultation. The pulse identifies a sinus tachycardia, and other vital signs are within normal limits. An ECG shows ischemic changes. There are no other signs of hypovolemia. You apply supplemental oxygen and initiate an IV line while en route to the hospital.

   You suspect this patient has sustained a pulmonary contusion. You believe that the pressure waves generated by the blunt trauma disrupted the capillary-alveolar membrane. The pressure created by the trauma compressed the gases within the lung. The tissues accelerated and decelerated at different rates, causing a tear.
   a. Physical findings:
   b. Spalding effect:
   c. Inertial effects:

d. Implosion:

____

____

e. Would you run the IV infusion wide open for this patient?

____

____

Ambulance Calls

The following case scenarios provide an opportunity to explore the concerns associated with patient management and paramedic care. Read each scenario, and then answer each question.

1. A 26-year-old woman was an unrestrained front-seat passenger in a car that was involved in a head-on collision. You find her lying unresponsive on the front seat, her face covered with blood. The dashboard on her side is dented in, and the windshield in front of her is smashed.

a. List four things that might jeopardize the airway in this patient.

(1)______________________________

(2)______________________________

(3)______________________________

(4)______________________________

b. Specify precisely what you would check in assessing the patient's breathing in the primary survey.

(1) LOOK for:

(a) ______________________________

(b) ______________________________

(c) ______________________________

(d) ______________________________

(2) LISTEN for:

(a) ______________________________

(b) ______________________________

(c) ______________________________

(3) FEEL for:

(a) ______________________________

(b) ______________________________

(c) ______________________________

c. Which steps would you take at this point to ensure adequate breathing?

(1)____

(2)____

d. Specify precisely what you would check in assessing the patient's circulation in the primary survey.

(1)____

(2)____

(3)____

(4)____

(5)____

2. A 22-year-old man was shot at close range by a "friend" wielding a shotgun. You find the patient slumped in a chair and in considerable respiratory distress. There is a ragged 2-inch hole in his left anterior chest, and the left chest does not seem to move with respirations.

a. This patient has a(n):

(1) simple pneumothorax.

(2) tension pneumothorax.

(3) open pneumothorax.

(4) spontaneous pneumothorax.

b. Which steps would you take to manage this situation?

(1)____

(2)____

(3)____

(4)____

(5)____

3. A 71-year-old woman was crossing the street when she was struck by a car and thrown to the ground. She is complaining of severe pain in her right chest (she points to the exact spot, over the fifth right rib in the anterior axillary line). She says the pain is much worse when she coughs or takes a deep breath. On examination, she is conscious and alert and leaning toward her right side. Her skin is warm and moist. There is no cyanosis. Her pulse is 88 beats/min and regular; respirations are 24 breaths/min and shallow. Blood pressure is 160/90 mm Hg. The neck veins are flat. There is no tracheal deviation. There is extreme tenderness over the right fifth rib in the anterior axillary line. Breath sounds are diminished over the right chest, which sounds somewhat hollow to percussion. The rest of the exam seems to be within normal limits.

a. This patient probably has:

____

b. What is the principal danger associated with the type of injury or injuries the patient has suffered?

____

c. Which treatment is necessary in the field?

(1)____________________

(2)____________________

(3)____________________

d. As you are transporting this patient to the hospital (a 20-minute drive from the collision scene), she suddenly becomes very restless and agitated and complains that she cannot breathe. Her skin becomes cold and sweaty, and her pulse gets very weak. Her neck veins seem to bulge out.

(1) What do you think has happened?

____

____

____

(2) Which measures will you take?

____

____

____

4. You are called to the scene of a two-car collision. A convertible going south on the interstate apparently jumped the median divider and plowed head-on into a station wagon traveling in the northbound lane. The driver of the convertible is lying unresponsive in the road. Your primary survey reveals gurgling respirations; broken teeth; flat neck veins; asymmetric chest movement; cold, sweaty skin; weak, rapid pulse; poor capillary refill; and brisk bleeding from wounds on the scalp and neck. You are 10 minutes from a regional trauma center. List in order the steps you would take in this case.

a. ____________________

b. ____________________

c. ____________________

d. ____________________

e. ____________________

f. ____________________

g. ____________________

5. A passenger was in a car that was struck from the right side by a truck running a red light. The right-hand front door of the car is rammed in, deforming the passenger compartment of the car. The patient, a middle-aged woman, is conscious and in considerable distress. Her skin is cold and moist. Her neck veins are distended. Her chest moves only minimally on respiration, and you have difficulty hearing breath sounds on the right. You cannot really assess the percussion note because of all the noise at the scene. The patient's pulse is 120 beats/min and weak, and her respirations are 36 breaths/min and shallow.

a. Which steps would you take at the scene?

(1)____________________

(2)____________________

(3)__________

(4)__________

b. Which steps would you take during transport?

(1)__________

(2)__________

(3)__________

6. A passenger car has been involved in a head on collision with a pickup truck. When you arrive at the scene, you find the driver of the passenger car propped up against a tree, where he had been placed by bystanders who pulled him from the wreckage. The patient has numerous cuts on his face and arms and is in severe respiratory distress. He seems confused. His skin is cold, cyanotic, and sweaty, and his pulse is rapid and very weak. He can barely talk, but he manages to gasp, "Can't breathe..." You notice that the veins of his neck are bulging out. List in order the steps you would take in assessing and managing this patient.
Assessment:

a. __________

b. __________

(1)__________

c. __________

(1)__________

(2)__________

(3)__________

(4)__________

(5)__________

(6)__________

d. __________

(1)__________

(2)__________

(3)__________

e. __________

(1)__________

f. __________

(1)__________

g. __________

Management:

a. ______________________________

b. ______________________________

c. ______________________________

d. ______________________________

e. ______________________________

f. ______________________________

g. ______________________________

h. ______________________________

7. For each of the following patients, indicate what the MOST likely diagnosis is, and list the steps of prehospital management.

A. Tension pneumothorax
B. Massive hemothorax
C. Flail chest
D. Cardiac tamponade
E. Traumatic asphyxia

______ **a.** A 20-year-old driver of a car that rammed a utility pole at high speed. He is in severe distress. His pulse is rapid and feeble, and every so often, you can hardly palpate a pulse at all. His neck veins are distended. There is a steering wheel imprint on his chest. The rib cage is stable. Breath sounds are equal bilaterally. It is too noisy to hear heart sounds. You are 30 minutes from the nearest hospital. Steps of management:

(1) ______________________________

(2) ______________________________

(3) ______________________________

(4) ______________________________

______ **b.** A 23-year-old driver of a car that rammed a utility pole at high speed. His face, neck, and chest are cyanotic and look very bloated. His eyes are bloodshot and bulging. He is vomiting blood. Breathing is labored. His pulse is rapid and very weak. The chest looks caved-in. You are 5 minutes from a regional trauma center. Steps of management:

(1) ______________________________

(2) ______________________________

(3) ______________________________

(4) ______________________________

(5) ______________________________

_____ **c.** A 70-year-old driver of a car that rammed a utility pole at high speed. He is conscious but in severe respiratory distress. The pulse is 92 beats/min, strong, and slightly irregular. Neck veins are flat. There are bruises on the anterior chest and point tenderness along the left sternal border and over the left fifth, sixth, seventh, and eighth ribs in the anterior axillary line. The chest seems to move asymmetrically on respiration. Breath sounds seem equal. It is too noisy to hear heart sounds. You are 10 minutes from the hospital. Steps of management:

(1) ____________________

(2) ____________________

(3) ____________________

(4) ____________________

(5) ____________________

(6) ____________________

_____ **d.** A 42-year-old front-seat passenger in a car that was struck from the right side by an ambulance that ran a red light. The patient is in severe respiratory distress. Her pulse is rapid and very weak. Her skin is cold and sweaty. The neck veins are distended. Breath sounds are decreased on the right side of the chest, which is hyperresonant to palpation. It is too noisy to hear heart sounds. You are 15 minutes from the nearest hospital. Steps of management:

(1) ____________________

(2) ____________________

(3) ____________________

(4) ____________________

(5) ____________________

(6) ____________________

(7) ____________________

(8) ____________________

_____ **e.** A 22-year-old man who was stabbed in the left chest. The patient is in severe distress. His pulse is rapid and very weak. His skin is cold and sweaty. His neck veins are flat. Breath sounds are decreased in the left chest, which is dull to percussion. It is too noisy to hear heart sounds. You are 15 minutes from the nearest hospital. Steps of management:

(1) ____________________

(2) ____________________

(3) ____________________

True/False

If you believe the statement to be more true than false, write the letter "T" in the space provided. If you believe the statement to be more false than true, write the letter "F."

_____ **1.** Children's ribs are pliable, so underlying structures may be injured even if the ribs are not fractured.

_____ **2.** In a traumatic asphyxia, the sudden compression of the chest causes pressure to be translated into the major veins of the head, neck, and kidneys.

_____ **3.** Cardiac tamponade is defined as fluid in the myocardium causing compression of the heart and decreasing cardiac output.

_____ **4.** Commotio cordis occurs when the thorax receives a direct blow during the critical portion of the heart's repolarization period, resulting in cardiac arrest.

_____ **5.** Atelectasis is alveolar collapse that prevents the use of a portion of the lung.

_____ **6.** Blunt disruptions of the diaphragm are usually associated with herniation of all or part of the liver into the right side of the chest.

_____ **7.** Esophageal injuries are not usually serious injuries.

_____ **8.** Jugular vein distention is usually an early sign of tension pneumothorax.

_____ **9.** Hypotension, as a late finding, should not be considered to either confirm or exclude the possibility of a tension pneumothorax.

_____ **10.** One physical finding of tension pneumothorax is distended neck veins.

Short Answer

Complete this section with short written answers using the space provided.

A 22-year-old man was shot in the right chest with a handgun at a range of 10 feet. There is an entrance wound in the right midclavicular line about 2 fingerbreadths below the right nipple. A slightly larger exit wound is visible 3 inches (7.5 cm) to the right of the vertebral column just below the lowest rib. Which organs are most likely to have been in the path of the bullet?

____

____

____

CHAPTER

36

Abdominal and Genitourinary Trauma

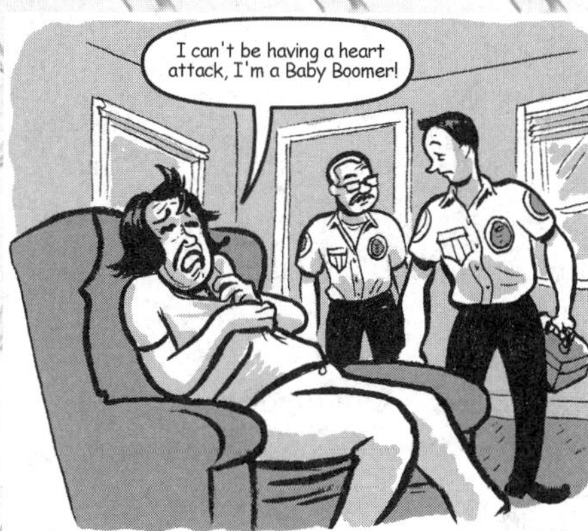

Matching

Part I

Match each of the items in the right column with the appropriate definition in the left column.

______	**1.** Crampy, aching pain deep within the body, the source of which is usually difficult to pinpoint; common with genitourinary problems.	**A.**	Evisceration
______	**2.** The area in the abdomen containing the aorta, vena cava, pancreas, kidneys, ureters, and portions of the duodenum and large intestine.	**B.**	Hematuria
______	**3.** Localized pain, usually felt deeply, that represents irritation or injury to tissue, causing activation of peripheral nerve tracts.	**C.**	Hemoperitoneum
______	**4.** Displacement of an organ outside the body.	**D.**	Kehr sign
______	**5.** The presence of blood in the urine.	**E.**	Mesentery
______	**6.** The presence of extravasated blood in the peritoneal cavity.	**F.**	Peritoneal cavity
______	**7.** Left shoulder pain that may indicate a ruptured spleen.	**G.**	Peritoneum
______	**8.** A membranous double fold of tissue in the abdomen that attaches various organs to the body wall.	**H.**	Peritonitis
______	**9.** Pertaining to the area around the umbilicus.	**I.**	Periumbilical
______	**10.** Inflammation of the peritoneum, the protective membrane that lines the abdominal and pelvic cavities.	**J.**	Retroperitoneal space
______	**11.** The area in the abdomen encased in the peritoneum. It consists of an upper and a lower part. The upper portion contains the diaphragm, liver, spleen, stomach, gallbladder, and transverse colon. The lower portion contains the small bowel, sigmoid colon, parts of the descending and ascending colon, and, in women, the internal reproductive organs.	**K.**	Somatic pain
______	**12.** A membrane in the abdomen encasing the liver, spleen, diaphragm, stomach, and transverse colon.	**L.**	Visceral pain

Part II

Match each of the items in the left column to the appropriate injuries in the right column.

For each of the patients described here, given the mechanism of injury (MOI) and the clinical findings, indicate which injury from the right-hand column he or she is most likely to have experienced. (Note: A patient may have sustained more than one of the injuries listed.)

_____ **1.** A 15-year-old girl was kicked in the left side by a horse. She is conscious and alert. Her pulse is rapid. She has a bruise over the left 10th rib in the anterior axillary line and has severe tenderness at that point.

_____ **2.** A 50-year-old man was a passenger in a car that slammed into a wall. He was wearing a lap seat belt. He complains of shortness of breath and abdominal pain. He winces when he coughs. His vital signs are as follows: pulse, 92 beats/min and regular; respirations, 36 breaths/min and shallow; and blood pressure, 120/80 mm Hg.

_____ **3.** An 18-year-old man was shot in the right upper quadrant by his girlfriend, who wielded a .38 special at a distance of about 10 feet. The patient is conscious. He has cold, sweaty skin and a weak, rapid pulse. There is an entrance wound in the right upper quadrant, about 2 fingerbreadths below the costal margin in the midclavicular line. The exit wound is near the left buttock.

_____ **4.** A 60-year-old man was struck by a car as he was crossing the street. The patient presents with gross hematuria; suprapubic pain and tenderness; difficulty voiding; and abdominal distention, guarding, and rebound tenderness.

_____ **5.** A 42-year-old construction worker is extricated from underneath a pile of concrete blocks that caved in on top of him. He is unresponsive, with cold and clammy skin. His pulse is very weak. There are no bruises on the chest, which moves symmetrically with respiration. The abdomen is not rigid, but there seems to be a fullness in the center of the lower quadrant. The pelvis is unstable.

_____ **6.** Your team is assessing a conscious, alert 18-year-old man who was involved in a high-speed car crash against a bridge abutment. The patient was unrestrained. The patient has an odor of ethyl alcohol; he is currently complaint-free. While you are evaluating the patient, you note ecchymosis of the flanks.

_____ **7.** It's another weekend night and another stabbing. On arrival, you have a conscious, alert male patient. He is lying on the ground with what appears to be exposed abdominal contents.

_____ **8.** A patient is struck by falling debris. He was struck on the lower left quadrant and is found to be in profound shock. His lower left quadrant has point tenderness and is rigid.

_____ **9.** A patient is a victim of blunt trauma; he is anxious and short of breath. He appears to have associated thoracic, abdominal, head, and extremity injuries.

_____ **10.** A woman fell from a height while hiking. You are assessing the patient and recognize that she has Kehr sign.

A. Diaphragm injury

B. Ruptured spleen

C. Liver laceration

D. Torn or ruptured bladder

E. Retroperitoneal injuries

F. Cullen sign

G. Evisceration

Multiple Choice

Read each item carefully, and then select the best response.

_____ **1.** The physical examination conducted as a part of the secondary assessment of abdominal injuries includes all of the following, EXCEPT:

A. inspection.

B. palpation.

C. percussion.

D. determination of baseline vital signs.

_____ **2.** A ruptured kidney will usually present with:
A. flank pain.
B. pain on inspiration in abdomen.
C. gross hematuria.
D. All of the above

_____ **3.** All of the following are considered hollow organs or structures of the abdomen, EXCEPT the __________, which is considered part of the genitourinary system.
A. esophagus
B. stomach
C. bladder
D. gallbladder

_____ **4.** Hollow organs are less likely to be injured, unless:
A. they are empty.
B. the MOI is a motor vehicle crash.
C. they are full.
D. the patient is a pregnant woman.

_____ **5.** The largest organ in the abdominal cavity and the most vascular is the:
A. large intestine.
B. pancreas.
C. spleen.
D. liver.

_____ **6.** Because of the nature of abdominal trauma in patients, which of the following should be required in your management plan?
A. Obtaining a 12-lead ECG
B. Securing the cervical spine
C. Consulting with medical control on analgesia
D. Establishing IV access for administration of fluids

_____ **7.** Injuries to the retroperitoneal space may include injuries to all of the following, EXCEPT the:
A. pancreas.
B. kidneys.
C. vascular structures.
D. liver.

_____ **8.** Crushing injuries may be caused by:
A. crushing of abdominal contents by the abdominal wall and the spinal column.
B. the dashboard of a car.
C. the hood of the car.
D. All of the above

_____ **9.** In penetrating trauma, it is helpful to:
A. identify the type of weapon used.
B. explore the wound to detect the path of destruction.
C. cleanse the wound site to prevent life-threatening infection.
D. remove all exposed foreign bodies.

_____ **10.** The primary survey for abdominal injuries should include all of the following, EXCEPT:
A. road rash.
B. bruising.
C. swelling.
D. epistaxis.

Labeling

Label the following diagrams with the correct terms.

1. Organs in the peritoneum

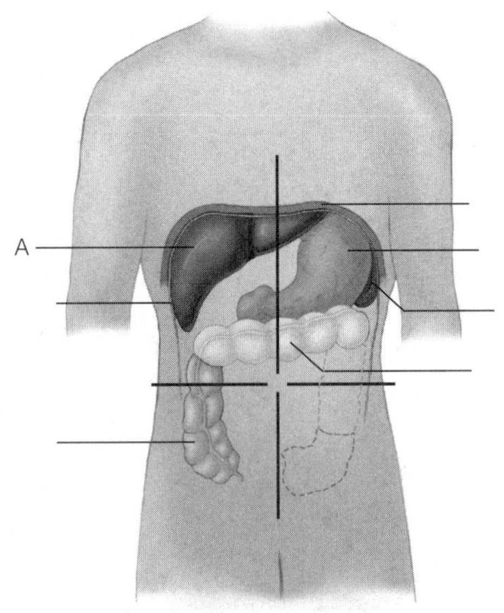

A. ______________________

B. ______________________

C. ______________________

D. ______________________

E. ______________________

F. ______________________

G. ______________________

2. Organs in the retroperitoneal space

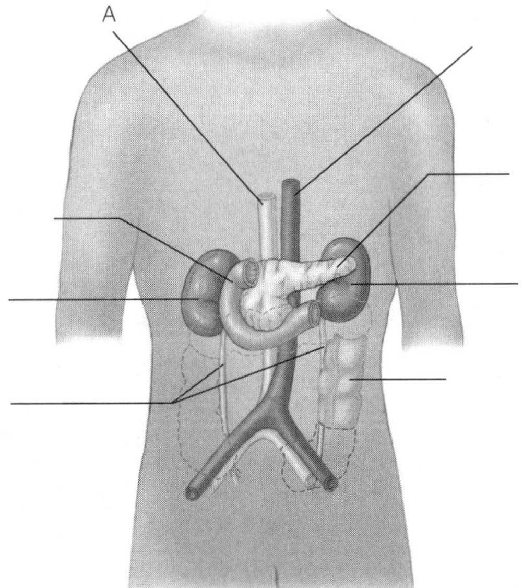

A. ______________________

B. ______________________

C. ______________________

D. ______________________

E. ______________________

F. ______________________

G. ______________________

H. ______________________

3. Organs in the pelvis

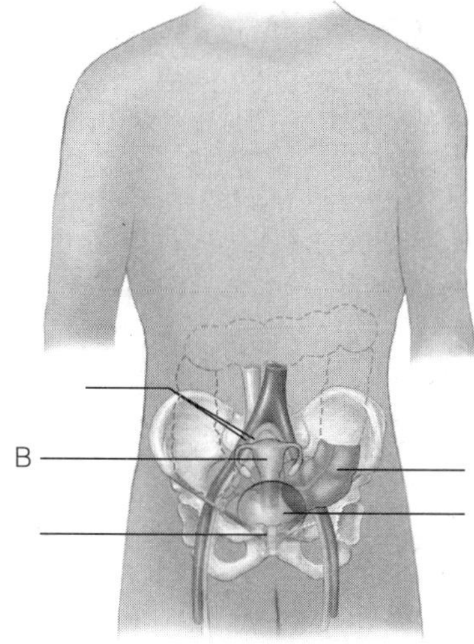

A. ____________________

B. ____________________

C. ____________________

D. ____________________

E. ____________________

Fill in the Blank

Read each item carefully, and then complete the statement by filling in the missing word(s).

1. A(n) __________ is externalization of ______ organs through a wound in the abdominal wall.
2. Retroperitoneal bleeding can lead to ecchymosis of the flanks, commonly referred to as __________ __________ __________.
3. Retroperitoneal bleeding can lead to ecchymosis around the umbilicus, commonly referred to as __________ __________.
4. An injury to the ______ can cause signs and symptoms of ventilatory ________..
5. The __________ is relatively well protected due to its location in the __________.
6. The stomach is an intraperitoneal __________ organ that lies in the left upper quadrant and epigastric region.
7. The intestines are most commonly injured from ______ trauma, although they can be injured from severe ____ trauma as well.
8. The spillage of toxins into the abdominal cavity due to trauma is called __________ and can be a potentially life-threatening infection.

Identify

Read the following case studies, and then list the chief complaint, vital signs, and pertinent negatives.

1. You receive a Priority 1 response for a conscious and alert 54-year-old man involved in a domestic violence incident. When you arrive, you are advised that the scene is safe and secured by law enforcement. The patient denies any complaint. You notice that the patient's shirt is soaked with blood, and the police have placed a kitchen knife in an evidence bag. The patient is not very cooperative, and he appears ashen, diaphoretic, and slightly short of breath. After several minutes of prodding, the patient agrees to remove his shirt. The patient denies any previous medical history. You observe a half-inch laceration above his umbilicus. The wound is not actively bleeding. The patient denies chest pain or other injuries. His vital signs are as follows: pulse is 120 beats/min and regular; skin is ashen, cool, and diaphoretic; oxygen saturation is 90%; blood pressure (BP) is 86/60 mm Hg; and sinus tachycardia is found on the electrocardiogram (ECG).
   a. Chief complaint:

   ____

   ____

   b. Vital signs:

   ____

   ____

   c. Pertinent negatives:

   ____

   ____

2. Your unit is standing by at the local arena for an indoor motocross event. This high-speed motorcycle race features numerous elevated jumps and turns. The riders are well protected by helmets and specialized outerwear. While you are watching, you observe a rider crash into a retaining wall. He initially appears unresponsive. As you approach, the patient is alert and speaking clearly. He attempts to stand and get back on his motorcycle. You quickly notice that bystanders are pointing to the patient's abdomen; when you follow their signals, you see what appears to be a small protrusion of abdominal contents from the patient's left upper quadrant. It's obvious that the patient has an evisceration. You quickly assess the ABCs and immobilize the patient. He has the following vital signs: pulse is 100 beats/min and irregular; skin is pale, warm, and dry; oxygen saturation is 97% on room air; and BP is 160/90 mm Hg. After quickly treating the patient and initiating rapid transport, you become suspicious because of the patient's vital signs. The patient states he has a history of atrial fibrillation and hypertension. He currently denies chest pain.
   a. Chief complaint:

   ____

   ____

   b. Vital signs:

   ____

   ____

   c. Pertinent negatives:

   ____

   ____

Ambulance Calls

The following case scenarios provide an opportunity to explore the concerns associated with patient management and paramedic care. Read each scenario, and then answer each question.

1. You are called to the scene of an interstate collision in which an apparently intoxicated 25-year-old driver plowed his car into a bridge abutment at high speed. The front end of his vehicle is accordioned against the bridge. As you approach the disabled vehicle, your keen powers of observation enable you to perceive that the patient is conscious (he is screaming obscenities at a police officer). Describe the steps in evaluating this patient for possible abdominal injuries. In particular, which issues will you be looking for?

a. ______________________________

b. ______________________________

c. ______________________________

d. ______________________________

2. A 20-year-old man was the unrestrained driver of a car that was struck on the passenger side by another vehicle. The crash caused the empty bucket seat beside the driver to be jammed into his right side. On your arrival at the collision, you find the patient conscious but anxious and restless. His skin is ashen, cool, and diaphoretic. The patient has a delayed capillary refill greater than 2 seconds. His vital signs are a pulse of 140 beats/min and thready, respirations of 40 breaths/min and shallow, and BP of 72/40 mm Hg. There is a bruise over the right lower ribs. A large portion of the small bowel is eviscerated through an avulsion in the right side of the abdomen. The right elbow appears to be fractured. List the injuries and your priorities in managing this case.

Injuries:

a. ______________________________

b. ______________________________

c. ______________________________

d. ______________________________

Priorities:

a. ______________________________

b. ______________________________

c. ______________________________

d. ______________________________

e. ______________________________

f. ______________________________

g. ______________________________

3. During the usual Saturday night festivities at the local Knife & Gun Club, a 16-year-old boy is stabbed with a hunting knife in the left lower quadrant of the abdomen. When you arrive, you find him lying on the ground moaning. The knife is still embedded up to its hilt in the patient's abdomen. The patient's skin is pale, warm, and moist. Vital signs are a pulse of 100 beats/min, respirations of 32 breaths/min, and BP of 100/80 mm Hg. List the steps in managing this case.

a. ______

b. ______

c. ______

d. ______

e. ______

True/False

If you believe the statement to be more true than false, write the letter "T" in the space provided. If you believe the statement to be more false than true, write the letter "F."

______ 1. Hollow organs are less likely to cause life-threatening injuries.

______ 2. Contusions of the testicles or scrotal sac result in painful hematomas.

______ 3. Cullen sign is best described as ecchymosis around the umbilicus.

______ 4. Treatment of impaled abdominal objects includes removal of the object to allow for proper immobilization and transport of the patient.

______ 5. Delay in recognizing intra-abdominal or pelvic injury leads to early death from hemorrhage.

______ 6. The diaphragm plays a large role in the mechanical process of breathing.

______ 7. Visceral pain comes from organs inside the body that are affected by injury or illness.

______ 8. Severe injuries to the testicles are rare.

______ 9. Bladder injury should be suspected in any patient with trauma to the lower abdomen or pelvis.

______ 10. A saddle-type injury is likely to cause damage to the kidneys in a female patient.

Fill in the Table

Fill in the missing parts of the table.

1. Organs of the abdomen and their location.

Organ	Location: Peritoneal Cavity, Retroperitoneal Space, Pelvis (Fill in One of the Three Locations Below)
1. Liver	1.
2. Spleen	2.
3. Stomach	3.
4. Duodenum	4.
5. Kidney	5.
6. Aorta	6.
7. Uterus	7.
8. Rectum	8.
9. Bladder	9.

Short Answer

Complete this section with short written answers using the space provided.

1. Which of the abdominal organs is most likely to be injured in association with each of the following injuries?

   a. Rapid deceleration in a motor vehicle crash or a fall from a height: liver, __________, intestines, and spleen

   b. Right-sided chest trauma as well as abdominal trauma: __________

   c. Fracture of the pelvis: __________

   d. Stab wound to the right upper quadrant: __________

CHAPTER 37

Orthopaedic Trauma

Some ranges of motion are pretty clear without your checking them.

Matching

Part I

Match the orthopaedic trauma term on the right with its best definition on the left.

_____ **1.** Compression of the ulnar nerve at the tunnel along the outer edge of the elbow, causing numbness, tingling, and possible partial loss of function of the little finger and medial aspect of the ring finger.

_____ **2.** A condition that arises after a body part that has been compressed for a significant period is released, leading to the entry of potassium and other metabolic toxins into the systemic circulation.

_____ **3.** A grating sensation felt when moving the ends of a broken bone.

_____ **4.** A fracture in which the bone is broken into two or more completely separate pieces.

_____ **5.** An increase in tissue pressure in a closed fascial space or compartment that compromises the circulation to the nerves and muscles within the involved compartment.

_____ **6.** Musculoskeletal injuries that commonly occur together.

_____ **7.** Inflammation of the joints.

_____ **8.** The part of the skeleton comprising the upper and lower extremities.

_____ **9.** The presence of an abnormal angle or bend in an extremity.

_____ **10.** Pain, paralysis, paresthesias, pulselessness, pallor, and pressure.

_____ **11.** The displacement of a bone from its normal position within a joint.

_____ **12.** An increase in the distance between the two sides of a joint.

_____ **13.** The loss of blood to a part of the body.

_____ **14.** A fracture in which the broken region of the bone is pushed deeper into the body than the remaining intact bone.

_____ **15.** The formation of a blood clot within the larger veins of an extremity, typically following a period of prolonged stabilization.

_____ **16.** A common incomplete fracture in children in which the cortex of the bone fractures from an excessive compression force; also called a torus fracture.

_____ **17.** A fracture of the head of the fifth metacarpal that usually results from striking an object with a clenched fist.

_____ **18.** The part of the skeleton comprising the skull, spinal column, and rib cage.

A. Six Ps of musculoskeletal assessment
B. Angulation
C. Appendicular skeleton
D. Arthritis
E. Associated fractures
F. Avascular necrosis
G. Avulsion fracture
H. Axial skeleton
I. Boxer's fracture
J. Buckle fracture
K. Buddy splinting
L. Bursitis
M. Cancellous bone
N. Carpal tunnel syndrome
O. Closed fracture
P. Comminuted fracture
Q. Compartment syndrome
R. Complete fracture

______	**19.** A fracture that occurs when a piece of bone is torn free at the site of attachment of a tendon or ligament.	**S.**	Crepitus
______	**20.** Tissue death resulting from the loss of blood supply.	**T.**	Crush syndrome
______	**21.** A fracture in which the bone is broken into three or more pieces.	**U.**	Cubital tunnel syndrome
______	**22.** A fracture in which the skin is not broken.	**V.**	Deep vein thrombosis
______	**23.** Compression of the median nerve at the wrist where it passes through the carpal canal, causing numbness and tingling in the hand and possible pain.	**W.**	Depression fracture
______	**24.** Trabecular or spongy bone.	**X.**	Devascularization
______	**25.** Inflammation of a bursa.	**Y.**	Diastasis
______	**26.** Securing an injured digit to an adjacent uninjured one to allow the intact digit to act as a splint.	**Z.**	Dislocation

Part II

Match the orthopaedic trauma term on the right with its best definition on the left.

______	**1.** A fracture that runs parallel to the long axis of a bone.	**A.**	Displaced fracture
______	**2.** A force that is directed from the side toward the midline of the body.	**B.**	Distraction injury
______	**3.** A fracture that occurs in the region between the lesser and greater trochanters.	**C.**	Dorsiflex
______	**4.** An injury that results from a force that is applied to one region of the body but leads to an injury in another area.	**D.**	Fascia
______	**5.** A fracture in which the bone does not fully break.	**E.**	Fatigue fracture
______	**6.** A painful disorder characterized by the crystallization of uric acid within a joint.	**F.**	Femoral shaft fracture
______	**7.** The process by which the kidneys filter the blood, removing excess wastes and fluids.	**G.**	Fracture
______	**8.** The socket in the scapula in which the head of the humerus rotates.	**H.**	Glenoid fossa
______	**9.** A break or rupture in the bone.	**I.**	Glomerular filtration
______	**10.** A break in the diaphysis of the femur.	**J.**	Gout
______	**11.** A fracture that results from multiple compressive loads.	**K.**	Greenstick fracture
______	**12.** A strong, fibrous membrane that covers, supports, and separates muscles.	**L.**	Hyperkalemia
______	**13.** To bend the foot or hand backward.	**M.**	Hyperphosphatemia
______	**14.** An injury that results from a force that tries to increase the length of a body part or separate one body part from another.	**N.**	Hyperuricemia
______	**15.** A break in which the ends of the fractured bone move out of their normal positions.	**O.**	Impacted fracture
______	**16.** The subluxation of the radial head that often results from pulling on an outstretched arm.	**P.**	Incomplete fracture
______	**17.** A break in which the bone remains aligned in its normal position.	**Q.**	Indirect injury
______	**18.** The loss of the nerve supply, blood supply, or both to a region of the body, typically distal to a site of injury; characterized by alterations in sensation.	**R.**	Intertrochanteric fracture
______	**19.** Muscle pain.	**S.**	Lateral compression
______	**20.** An avulsion fracture of the extensor tendon of the distal phalanx caused by jamming a finger into an object.	**T.**	Linear fracture
______	**21.** A broken bone in which the cortices of one bone become wedged into another bone, as could be the case in a fall from a significant height.	**U.**	Luxation
______	**22.** High levels of uric acid in the blood.	**V.**	Mallet finger
______	**23.** An abnormally elevated serum phosphate; often associated with decreased calcium. Normal phosphate levels are between 0.81 and 1.45 mmol/L.	**W.**	Myalgia
______	**24.** An abnormally elevated level of potassium in the blood.	**X.**	Neurovascular compromise
______	**25.** A type of fracture occurring most frequently in children in which there is incomplete breakage of the bone.	**Y.**	Nondisplaced fracture
______	**26.** A complete dislocation.	**Z.**	Nursemaid's elbow

Part III

Match the orthopaedic trauma term on the right with its best definition on the left.

______	**1.** The wrist bone that is found just beyond the most distal portion of the radius.	**A.**	Oblique fracture
______	**2.** An inflammatory disorder that affects the entire body and leads to degeneration and deformation of joints.	**B.**	Olecranon
______	**3.** The destruction of muscle tissue leading to a release of potassium and myoglobin.	**C.**	Open-book pelvic fracture
______	**4.** The arc of movement of an extremity at a joint in a particular direction.	**D.**	Open fracture
______	**5.** Obstruction of a pulmonary artery or arteries by solid, liquid, or gaseous material swept through the right side of the heart into the lungs.	**E.**	Osteoarthritis (OA)
______	**6.** A type of disorder in which multiple nerves become dysfunctional.	**F.**	Osteoporosis
______	**7.** The tenderness that is sharply localized at the site of the injury, found by gently palpating along the bone with the tip of one finger.	**G.**	Overriding
______	**8.** The large bone that arises in the area of the last nine vertebrae and sweeps around to form a complete ring.	**H.**	Paresthesia
______	**9.** Stretching or tearing of a muscle by excessive stretching or overuse.	**I.**	Pathologic fracture
______	**10.** A fracture of the pelvis that results from landing on the peroneal region.	**J.**	Pectoral girdle
______	**11.** An injury, including a stretch or a tear, to the ligaments of a joint that commonly leads to pain and swelling.	**K.**	Pelvic girdle
______	**12.** A break in a bone that appears like a spring on a radiograph.	**L.**	Point tenderness
______	**13.** Any break in a bone in which the overlying skin has been damaged.	**M.**	Polyneuropathy
______	**14.** A life-threatening fracture of the pelvis caused by a force that displaces one or both sides of the pelvis laterally and posteriorly.	**N.**	Pulmonary embolism
______	**15.** The proximal bony projection of the ulna at the elbow; the part of the ulna that constitutes the “funny bone.”	**O.**	Range of motion
______	**16.** A fracture that travels diagonally from one side of the bone to the other.	**P.**	Rhabdomyolysis
______	**17.** The region at the base of the thumb where the scaphoid may be palpated.	**Q.**	Rheumatoid arthritis (RA)
______	**18.** The dorsal deformity of the forearm that results from a Colles fracture.	**R.**	Scaphoid
______	**19.** Inflammation of a joint based on a bacterial or fungal infection.	**S.**	Segmental fracture
______	**20.** A bone that is broken in more than one place.	**T.**	Septic arthritis
______	**21.** The shoulder girdle.	**U.**	Silver fork deformity
______	**22.** A fracture that occurs in an area of abnormally weakened bone.	**V.**	Anatomic snuffbox
______	**23.** An abnormal sensation such as burning, numbness, or tingling.	**W.**	Spiral fracture
______	**24.** The overlap of a bone that occurs from the muscle spasm that follows a fracture, leading to a decrease in the length of the bone.	**X.**	Sprain
______	**25.** A condition characterized by decreased bone density and increased susceptibility to fractures.	**Y.**	Straddle fracture
______	**26.** The degeneration of a joint surface caused by wear and tear that lead to pain and stiffness.	**Z.**	Strain

Part IV

Match the musculoskeletal injury on the left with the complication or other injury that is most likely to be associated with it on the right.

______	**1.** Pelvic fracture	**A.**	Fracture of the lumbar spine
______	**2.** Calcaneal fracture	**B.**	Volkmann ischemic contracture
______	**3.** Humeral shaft fracture	**C.**	Fracture dislocation of the ipsilateral hip
______	**4.** Posterior dislocation of the clavicle	**D.**	Compartment syndrome
______	**5.** Elbow fracture	**E.**	Deceleration injuries
______	**6.** Posterior dislocation of the hip	**F.**	Possible damage to underlying structures (eg, subclavian artery)
______	**7.** Open fracture	**G.**	Infection
______	**8.** Patellar fracture	**H.**	Ruptured bladder

Multiple Choice

Read each item carefully, and then select the best response.

_____ 1. Which of the following is considered one of the most common reasons that patients seek medical attention?
- A. Trauma
- B. Musculoskeletal injuries
- C. Dislocations
- D. Fractures

_____ 2. Which of the following is considered one of the functions of the musculoskeletal system?
- A. Providing support to the soft tissues
- B. Allowing the body to maintain an erect position
- C. Protecting internal organs
- D. All of the above

_____ 3. A fall on an outstretched hand is a mechanism that produces a characteristic ____________ deformity.
- A. twisting.
- B. silver fork.
- C. crushing.
- D. glove.

_____ 4. Stress fractures are often referred to as ____________ fractures.
- A. fatigue
- B. greenstick
- C. comminuted
- D. oblique

_____ 5. Crepitus is BEST described as a:
- A. loss of distal sensation.
- B. sure sign of dislocation.
- C. sign that occurs with fractures.
- D. grating sensation with fractures.

_____ 6. Which of the following statements MOST accurately describes an Achilles tendon rupture?
- A. It is rarely seen in adults.
- B. It often accompanies arthritis.
- C. It occurs with tendonitis.
- D. It can be identified with the Thompson test.

_____ 7. Assessing extremity injuries should include all of the following, EXCEPT:
- A. scene size-up.
- B. auscultation.
- C. inspection.
- D. examination.

_____ 8. Which of the following is the MOST common result of splinting fractured extremities?
- A. Increased pain
- B. Delay in transport
- C. Increased bleeding and nerve damage
- D. Reduced risk of further injury and less discomfort

_____ 9. Which of the following statements MOST accurately describes compartment syndrome?
- A. It can be one of the most devastating consequences of a musculoskeletal injury.
- B. It occurs as a result of loosely applied bandages.
- C. It does not occur with open fractures.
- D. It generally is not a painful injury.

_____ **10.** Pelvic fractures occur infrequently; however, they are:
A. never fatal.
B. responsible for a relatively high percentage of deaths.
C. not to be splinted in the prehospital setting.
D. rarely painful, and as a result, they are often misdiagnosed.

Labeling

Label the following diagram with the correct terms.

1. Types of fractures

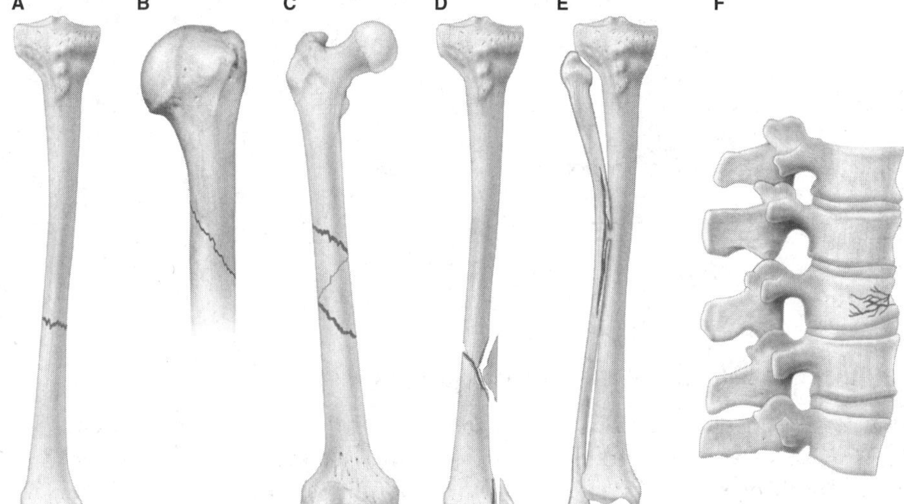

A. ______________________
B. ______________________
C. ______________________
D. ______________________
E. ______________________
F. ______________________

Fill in the Blank

Read each item carefully, and then complete the statement by filling in the missing word(s).

1. Vocabulary

a. Within a limb, groups of muscles are surrounded by an inelastic membrane called _______.

b. Inflammation of the joints is called __________.

c. The process by which toxins and waste products are removed from circulating blood is called __________________.

d. The _________, also called the carpal navicular, is located just distal to the radius.

e. A(n) _________ fracture is a fracture of the neck of the fifth metacarpal.

f. A(n) _________ finger occurs when a finger is jammed into an object, such as a basketball.

g. The kneecap is also called the __________.

h. The ____________ test can be performed in the field to identify an Achilles tendon rupture.

i. The shoulder girdle is also called the __________ __________.

2. To detect a fracture, you have to know what a fractured extremity looks and feels like. Fill in the following signs and symptoms of fractures. (Some letters in the words have been provided as hints.)

a. Unnatural shape: ______ ______ F ______ ______ ______ ______ ______ ______

b. Reduced length: ______ ______ ______ R ______ ______ ______ ______ ______ ______

c. Fracture of the small finger: ______ ______ ______ E ______ ______ F ______ ______ ______ ______ ______ ______ ______

d. Numbness or tingling: ______ ______ R ______ ______ T ______ ______ ______ ______ ______ ______

e. Grating: ______ ______ ______ ______ ______ T ______ ______

f. Devastating consequence of musculoskeletal injuries: D ______ ______ ______ ______ ______ ______ ______ ______ ______

g. Protecting from movement: ______ ______ ______ R ______ ______ ______ ______

h. Hurts to touch it: ______ ______ ______ ______ ______ ______ ______ ______ ______ ______ ______ ______ E ______ ______

i. Patient with a fracture may report this: Heard a S ______ ______ ______

j. Seen in open fracture: ______ X ______ ______ ______ ______ ______ ______ O ______ ______ ______ N ______ ______

Identify

Read the following case studies, and then list the chief complaint, vital signs, and pertinent negatives.

1. It is a snowy night in the Big Apple, and most people have decided to stay indoors. You are dispatched to the scene where a 48-year-old man slipped on the ice and snow while working late on Wall Street. As you turn the corner to the scene, you notice that law enforcement is already on scene. You mentally note to yourself that the scene is safe.

   Your patient states that he slipped and fell on the icy sidewalk. He complains of right ankle pain. The patient further states that he tried to catch himself and landed on his left wrist. He complains of severe wrist pain. You notice that the wrist is deformed, and the patient appears to be supporting it against his chest with his right arm.

   By questioning the patient, you discover that he has a previous medical history of angina, atrial fibrillation, and hypertension. He also takes one 81-mg aspirin tablet per day and an antihypertensive medication. He denies loss of consciousness and any head or neck pain. The patient denies any respiratory distress and any current chest discomfort. He denies any medical condition that may have caused him to fall. He adamantly states that he simply slipped on ice and fell. After quickly assessing the patient, you decide to move him into the warm ambulance for further treatment and evaluation.

   The patient's baseline vital signs reveal a pulse of 116 beats/min and irregular, respirations of 16 breaths/min and nonlabored, oxygen saturation on room air at 98%, and blood pressure (BP) of 150/90 mm Hg. His electrocardiogram (ECG) shows a rapid atrial fibrillation. Pupils are equal, round, and reactive to light and accommodation (PERRLA). Normal capillary refill of < 2 seconds. Skin is, warm, dry, and a normal color.

   a. Chief complaint:

   ____

   ____

   b. Vital signs:

   ____

   ____

   c. Pertinent negatives:

   ____

   ____

2. A 48-year-old woman was injured while waiting in line for a popular clothing store to open during the annual President's Day sale. This is the one day of the year when all the designer handbags are on sale. Unfortunately, at "crunch" time, the woman tripped on the curb in the parking lot and fell to the ground. Luckily, she wasn't trampled by the hordes of bargain shoppers as the doors opened. She did catch herself with her two outstretched arms. Besides her injured pride, she complains of bilateral wrist injuries and is found in extreme pain.

When you approach this patient, she is sitting in a chair with ice packs already applied and mall security providing first aid. You notice that both her wrists appear bruised and deformed. Her initial mental status is conscious and alert. Her skin is slightly ashen and diaphoretic, and she has positive distal motor and neurologic sensations in both hands. She denies other injuries. Her capillary refill is > 2 seconds, and she has bilateral radial pulses that appear to be equal.

Her blood pressure is obtainable only by palpation at 86 mm Hg. Her oxygen saturation is 96% on ambient air. She denies taking any medications or having allergies.

a. Chief complaint:

____

____

b. Vital signs:

____

____

c. Pertinent negatives:

____

____

3. You believe that this is just another medical evacuation. As you take off from the hospital's rooftop pad and head toward the scene, you pay attention to the radio as the patient information, landing zone description, coordinates, and weather are relayed through your headset. You have a 25-minute estimate time of arrival (ETA) and request any vital signs and relevant patient information. After several minutes, you begin to realize that this call is anything but routine. The flight dispatcher describes a farm mishap in which a tractor rolled on top of and is now pinning a 64-year-old man. The flight dispatcher advises that the ground crew is requesting medicated facilitated intubation immediately on your arrival. Once again, you request vital signs as you prepare the medications. Prior to your arrival, the patient is unresponsive, with a Glasgow Coma Scale (GCS) score < 8, severe respiratory distress, bilateral open femoral fractures, and a possible dislocated or fractured hip or pelvis. Further transmissions indicate a delayed capillary refill, sinus tachycardia, pulse of 128 beats/min, and BP of 64 mm Hg by palpation. The ground medics are attempting IV access while rescue crews are attempting to extricate the patient.

a. Chief complaint:

____

____

b. Vital signs:

____

____

c. Pertinent negatives:

____

____

Complete the Patient Care Report (PCR)

Reread the first incident scenario in the preceding Identify exercise, and then complete the following PCR for the patient.

EMS Patient Care Report (PCR)					
Date:	Incident No.:	Nature of Call:		Location:	
Dispatched:	En Route:	At Scene:	Transport:	At Hospital:	In Service:
Patient Information					
Age: Sex: Weight (in kg [lb]):			Allergies: Medications: Past Medical History: Chief Complaint:		
Vital Signs					
Time:	BP:	Pulse:	Respirations:	SpO_2:	
Time:	BP:	Pulse:	Respirations:	SpO_2:	
Time:	BP:	Pulse:	Respirations:	SpO_2:	
EMS Treatment (circle all that apply)					
Oxygen @ ______ L/min via (circle one): NC NRM Bag-mask device		Assisted Ventilation	Airway Adjunct	CPR	
Defibrillation	Bleeding Control	Bandaging	Splinting	Other:	
Narrative					

Ambulance Calls

The following case scenarios provide an opportunity to explore the concerns associated with patient management and paramedic care. Read each scenario, and then answer each question.

1. Some injuries frequently come in pairs because they share a common mechanism of injury. When you find one of such a pair, you should be alert for the presence of the other. For each of the following cases, indicate which other injury or injuries you would look for in particular, given the injury already detected.
   a. A young man jumped from a second-story window to escape a fire. He complains of severe pain in the left heel, which is quite bruised and swollen. Which other injury or injuries might you expect to find in this patient?

   ____

   ____

   b. A 50-year-old woman was the front-seat passenger in a car that was hit head-on by an oncoming vehicle. Her right knee is bruised and swollen. Which other injury or injuries might you expect to find in this patient?

   ____

   ____

   c. A 60-year-old man fell sideways onto his outstretched hand. There is ecchymosis and tenderness at the base of his thumb. Which other injury or injuries might you expect to find in this patient?

   ____

   ____

   d. A construction worker has been extricated from under a pile of concrete blocks that fell on top of him, pinning him in a prone position, when part of a building collapsed. He has bruising over the left shoulder blade, and he cannot move the shoulder on that side. Which other injury or injuries might you expect to find in this patient?

   ____

   ____

2. For each of the following patients, list the most likely field diagnosis, answer any questions asked about the patient, and describe how you would manage the case.
   a. A 14-year-old boy fell from his skateboard onto his extended right elbow. The elbow is massively swollen and ecchymotic. The right hand is cool and pale, and the patient cannot feel a pinprick over the dorsum of the hand in the web space between the thumb and index finger.

   (1) What is the most likely field diagnosis?

   ____

   ____

   (2) Is there any particular danger in this case? If so, what is the danger?

   ____

   ____

   (3) How would you manage this case?

   ____

   ____

b. The mother of the boy just described fell over her son's skateboard as she was rushing to his assistance, and her outstretched left hand took the brunt of the impact as she hit the ground. As she walks toward the ambulance, she is gripping the dorsum of her left wrist with her right hand and holding the left wrist against her abdomen. When you inspect the left wrist from the side, it has a peculiar curve, rather like that of a dinner fork.

(1) What is the most likely field diagnosis?

____

____

(2) Is there any particular danger in this case? If so, what is the danger?

____

____

(3) How would you manage this case?

____

____

c. A front-seat passenger in a car that hit a tree is found with his right hip flexed, adducted, and internally rotated. The right leg looks shorter than the left leg. There are no other obvious injuries, and baseline vital signs are normal.

(1) What is the most likely field diagnosis?

____

____

(2) Is there any particular danger in this case? If so, what is the danger?

____

____

(3) How would you manage this case?

____

____

d. The driver of the vehicle in the preceding crash is unresponsive behind the wheel. His skin is cold and sweaty. When you are extricating him from the vehicle, you notice that his hips are unstable.

(1) What is the most likely field diagnosis?

____

____

(2) Is there any particular danger in this case? If so, what is the danger?

____

____

(3) What would your primary survey of this patient involve? How would you manage this case?

______

______

______

______

______

______

e. As your 250-lb partner leaps from the ambulance to attend to the patients of a car crash, his ankle buckles underneath him. "Ow," he says, "that is rather painful." He manages to complete his work at the scene by hopping around on one foot, but by the time he gets back to the station, his ankle is quite swollen and hurts a lot. Aside from the swelling, there is no obvious deformity and no ecchymosis.

(1) What is the most likely field diagnosis?

______

______

(2) Is there any particular danger in this case? If so, what is the danger?

______

______

(3) How would you manage this case?

______

______

f. You are watching the championship football game pitting your local high school team against last year's regional champions. Your team's quarterback, who is about 5 feet 6 inches tall and weighs perhaps 150 pounds, is looking to pass when he gets sacked and buried under a horde of 225-pound defensive linemen from the other team. When the linemen unpile, your quarterback is very slow in getting up. Of course, you race over to offer your assistance. After peeling off the boy's shirt, shoulder pads, and other gear, you notice that his chest is not symmetric. There seems to be a hollow area just to the left of the sternum, at the base of the neck, and that spot is very tender. The boy, meanwhile, is quite pale, and he gasps, "I'm choking."

(1) What is the most likely field diagnosis?

______

______

(2) Is there any particular danger in this case? If so, what is the danger?

______

______

(3) How would you manage this case?

____

____

g. A 25-year-old man was struck by a car while crossing the street. The bumper caught him in the middle of his shin. His lower leg is severely angulated and bleeding from an open wound. He complains of severe pain in his leg and of "pins and needles" in his foot.

(1) What is the most likely field diagnosis?

____

____

(2) Is there any particular danger in this case? If so, what is the danger?

____

____

(3) How would you manage this case?

____

____

h. Another 25-year-old man was shot in the thigh at close range. The left thigh is swollen compared to the right, and the left leg as a whole looks shorter than the right leg. The left dorsalis pedis pulse seems weaker than that on the right side.

(1) What is the most likely field diagnosis?

____

____

(2) Is there any particular danger in this case? If so, what is the danger?

____

____

(3) How would you manage this case?

____

____

(4) If your management of this case included a splint, why did you use a splint? List three reasons for splinting an injured extremity.

(a) ______________________________

(b) ______________________________

(c) ______________________________

i. You are spending a weekend on the ski slopes. While you are sailing down a particularly challenging hill, you see a skier stopped in the middle of the slope, admiring the view. Seconds later, about five other skiers come careening down the slope and, one after another, pile into the stationary skier. When the pile is unraveled, the skier at the bottom is found to have a severely deformed right knee, which seems to be swelling before your eyes.

(1) What is the most likely field diagnosis?

____

____

(2) Is there any particular danger in this case? If so, what is the danger?

____

____

(3) How would you manage this case?

____

____

3. You are called to the scene of a hit-and-run collision. A 45-year-old man is lying unresponsive in the street, surrounded by a crowd of highly agitated people. No one actually saw how the crash happened. At first glance, you can see that the man's right thigh is angulated, and the trouser leg on that side is soaked in blood.

a. Arrange the following steps in his management in the correct sequence. One step will be performed twice.

______ Start an IV line.

______ Take the vital signs.

______ Cut away the trouser leg.

______ Determine whether the patient is breathing (he is).

______ Secure the patient to a backboard or scoop stretcher.

______ Put manual pressure on the bleeding site.

______ Open the airway.

______ Start transport.

______ Move the patient to a backboard or scoop stretcher.

______ Check for a carotid pulse (pulse is present).

______ Check for a dorsalis pedis pulse on the right side.

______ Do the AVPU "mental status" check.

______ Check for an open or tension pneumothorax.

______ Put a pressure dressing over the open wound on the leg.

b. Have any steps been omitted? If so, which step(s)?

____

4. A 56-year-old woman was struck by a car as she was crossing the street. You find her lying in the street, near the curb; her left leg is severely angulated and bleeding. She is conscious. There is no tenderness to palpation over the chest or spine (you don't want to remove her shirt in the middle of the street to inspect the chest). Her skin is warm. Pulse is 108 beats/min and regular, respirations are 28 breaths/min, and BP is 132/90 mm Hg. There is an open fracture of the left tibia. The dorsalis pedis pulses are equal, and sensation to pinprick is intact in both feet.

a. Which steps would you take at the scene?

(1)____________________

(2)____________________

(3)____________________

(4)____________________

b. Which steps would you take during transport?

(1)____________________

(2)____________________

(3)____________________

True/False

If you believe the statement to be more true than false, write the letter "T" in the space provided. If you believe the statement to be more false than true, write the letter "F."

______ **1.** Severely angulated fractures should be straightened before they are splinted.

______ **2.** An air splint is also known as a pneumatic splint.

______ **3.** There is no need to straighten or manipulate a fracture involving joints unless there is no distal pulse.

______ **4.** A femoral shaft fracture places the patient at risk for fat emboli.

______ **5.** Fingers or toes should be left out of the splint so that distal circulation can be monitored.

______ **6.** A patient who sustained multitrauma is in unstable condition. One should splint the whole axial skeleton as a unit, on a long backboard or scoop stretcher, rather than take time to splint individual fractures.

______ **7.** Vacuum splints consist of a sealed mattress that is filled with air and small plastic beads.

Fill in the Table

Fill in the missing parts of the table.

Potential Blood Loss From Fracture Sites

Fracture Site	Potential Blood Loss (mL)
Pelvis	
Femur	
Humerus	
Tibia or fibula	
Ankle	
Elbow	
Radius or ulna	

Short Answer

Complete this section with short written answers using the space provided.

1. Fractures of the forearm or lower leg may be complicated by compartment syndrome when significant bleeding and swelling occur within one of the tight muscular compartments of the injured limb. Compartment syndrome, by cutting off the blood supply, can jeopardize the whole limb, so it is important to recognize the symptoms and signs that suggest that this condition may be developing. List six symptoms and signs of compartment syndrome.
   a. ______
   b. ______
   c. ______
   d. ______
   e. ______
   f. ______

2. Review the case of the man injured on the ski slope, which is repeated here. List the steps you would take in examining him. Looking for the signs of compartment syndrome is, in fact, only part of the assessment of an injured extremity.

   You are spending a weekend on the ski slopes. While you are sailing down a particularly challenging hill, you see a skier stopped in the middle of the slope, admiring the view. Seconds later, about five other skiers come careening down the slope and, one after another, pile into the stationary skier. When the pile is unraveled, the skier at the bottom is found to have a severely deformed right knee, which seems to be swelling before your eyes.
   a.
   ______
   ______
   b.
   ______
   ______
   c.
   ______
   ______

3. The equipment you should grab and take with you when you rush to the side of a severely injured patient should include the following items:
   a. ______
   b. ______
   c. ______
   d. ______
   e. ______
   f. ______
   g. ______

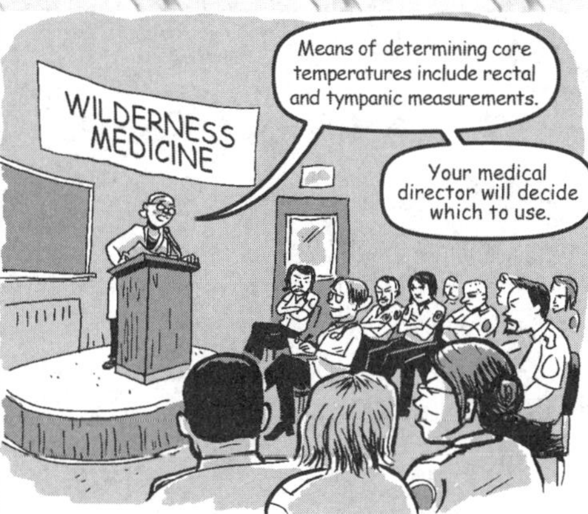

CHAPTER 38

Environmental Emergencies

Matching

Part I

Match each of the terms in the right column to the appropriate definition in the left column.

_____ **1.** A condition due to prolonged exertion in hot environments coupled with excessive hypotonic fluid intake that leads to nausea, vomiting, and, in severe cases, mental status changes and seizures.

_____ **2.** The conversion of a liquid to a gas.

_____ **3.** Medical conditions caused or exacerbated by the weather, terrain, or unique atmospheric conditions, such as high altitude or underwater.

_____ **4.** The injecting of venom via a bite or sting.

_____ **5.** Mechanism by which body heat is picked up and carried away by moving air currents.

_____ **6.** Transfer of heat to a solid object or a liquid by direct contact.

_____ **7.** Secretion of large amounts of urine in response to cold exposure and the consequent shunting of blood volume to the body core.

_____ **8.** A serious heat illness that usually occurs during heat waves and is most likely to strike very old, very young, or bedridden people.

_____ **9.** The heat energy produced at rest from normal body metabolic reactions, determined mostly by the liver and skeletal muscles.

_____ **10.** Injury resulting from pressure disequilibrium across body surfaces.

_____ **11.** A measurement of ambient pressure; the weight of air at sea level, equivalent in pressure to 33 feet of seawater (fsw).

_____ **12.** Inability to coordinate the muscles; often used to describe a staggering gait.

_____ **13.** A condition in which lung tissue is damaged, characterized by hypoxemia, low lung volume, and pulmonary edema.

_____ **14.** An altitude illness characterized by headache plus at least one of the following: fatigue or weakness, gastrointestinal symptoms (nausea, vomiting or anorexia), dizziness or light-headedness, or difficulty sleeping.

_____ **15.** Continued fall in core temperature after a victim of hypothermia has been removed from a cold environment, due at least in part to the return of cold blood from the body surface to the body core.

_____ **16.** Conditions caused by the effects from hypobaric (low atmospheric pressure) hypoxia on the central nervous system and pulmonary systems as a result of nonacclimated people ascending to altitude; range from acute mountain sickness to high-altitude cerebral edema and high-altitude pulmonary edema.

A. Acute lung injury
B. Acute mountain sickness (AMS)
C. Afterdrop
D. Altitude illness
E. Arterial gas embolism (AGE)
F. Ataxia
G. Atmosphere absolute (ATA)
H. Barotrauma
I. Basal metabolic rate (BMR)
J. Boyle's law
K. Breath-hold diving
L. Chilblains
M. Classic heatstroke
N. Cold diuresis
O. Conduction
P. Convection

_____ **17.** A type of frostbite in which the affected part looks white, yellow-white, or mottled blue-white and is hard, cold, and without sensation.

_____ **18.** A broad range of signs and symptoms caused by nitrogen bubbles in blood and tissues coming out of solution on ascent.

_____ **19.** A term for decompression sickness (DCS) and air gas embolism (AGE).

_____ **20.** Each gas in a mixture exerts the same partial pressure that it would exert if it were alone in the same volume, and the total pressure of a mixture of gases is the sum of the partial pressures of all the gases in a mixture.

_____ **21.** The resultant gaseous emboli from the forcing of gas into the vasculature from barotrauma.

_____ **22.** Itchy, red and purple, swollen lesions that occur primarily on the extremities, due to longer exposure to temperatures just above freezing or sudden rewarming after exposure to cold.

_____ **23.** Also called free diving; a type of diving that does not require any equipment, except sometimes a snorkel.

_____ **24.** At a constant temperature, the volume of a gas is inversely proportional to its pressure (if you double the pressure on a gas, you halve its volume); written as $PV = K$, where P = pressure, V = volume, and K = a constant.

_____ **25.** The temperature in the part of the body comprising the heart, lungs, brain, and abdominal viscera.

_____ **26.** The process of experiencing respiratory impairment from submersion or immersion in liquid.

Q. Core body temperature (CBT)
R. Dalton's law
S. Decompression illness (DCI)
T. Decompression sickness (DCS)
U. Deep frostbite
V. Drowning
W. Envenomation
X. Environmental emergencies
Y. Evaporation
Z. Exercise-associated hyponatremia (EAH)

Part II

Match each of the terms in the right column to the appropriate definition in the left column.

_____ **1.** A condition that can result from common anesthesia medications (notably succinylcholine) and that presents with hyperthermia, muscular rigidity, altered mental status, and a hyperdynamic state.

_____ **2.** A potentially fatal condition resulting from a brown recluse spider bite that begins with a painful, inflamed vesicle that may progress to a gangrenous sloughing of the skin.

_____ **3.** Severe constriction of the larynx in response to allergy, noxious stimuli, or illness.

_____ **4.** Low oxygen levels in the arterial blood.

_____ **5.** Condition in which the core body temperature is significantly below normal.

_____ **6.** The amount of gas dissolved in a liquid is directly proportional to the partial pressure of the gas above the liquid.

_____ **7.** An orthostatic or near-syncopal episode that typically occurs in nonacclimated people who may be under heat stress.

_____ **8.** The least common and most deadly heat illness, caused by a severe disturbance in thermoregulation, usually characterized by a core temperature of more than 104°F (40°C) and altered mental status.

_____ **9.** The increase in core body temperature due to inadequate thermolysis.

_____ **10.** A clinical syndrome characterized by volume depletion and heat stress that is thought to be a milder form of heat illness and on a continuum leading to heatstroke.

_____ **11.** Acute and involuntary muscle pains, usually in the lower extremities, the abdomen, or both that occur because of profuse sweating and subsequent sodium losses in sweat.

_____ **12.** Permanent cell death.

A. Exertional heatstroke
B. Feet of seawater (fsw)
C. Frostbite
D. Frostnip
E. Gangrene
F. Heat cramps
G. Heat exhaustion
H. Heat illness
I. Heatstroke
J. Heat syncope
K. Henry's law
L. High-altitude cerebral edema (HACE)

_____	**13.** Early frostbite, characterized by numbness and pallor without significant tissue damage.	**M.**	High-altitude pulmonary edema (HAPE)
_____	**14.** Localized damage to tissues resulting from prolonged exposure to extreme cold.	**N.**	Homeostasis
_____	**15.** An indirect measure of pressure under water, equal to one atmosphere absolute (ATA).	**O.**	Hypercapnia
_____	**16.** A serious type of heatstroke usually affecting young and fit people exercising in hot and humid conditions.	**P.**	Hyperthermia
_____	**17.** A fall in blood pressure that occurs when moving from a recumbent to a sitting or standing position.	**Q.**	Hypothalamus
_____	**18.** Painful swallowing.	**R.**	Hypothermia
_____	**19.** A state resembling alcohol intoxication produced by nitrogen gas dissolved in the blood at high ambient pressure; also called rapture of the deep.	**S.**	Hypoxemia
_____	**20.** A condition caused by antipsychotic and even common antiemetic medications that presents with hyperthermia, muscular rigidity, altered mental status, and a hyperdynamic state.	**T.**	Laryngospasm
_____	**21.** Portion of the brain that regulates a multitude of body functions, including core temperature.	**U.**	Loxoscelism
_____	**22.** Unusually elevated body temperature.	**V.**	Malignant hyperthermia
_____	**23.** Carbon dioxide in the blood.	**W.**	Neuroleptic malignant syndrome (NMS)
_____	**24.** Processes that balance the supply and demand of the body's needs.	**X.**	Nitrogen narcosis
_____	**25.** An altitude illness characterized by at least two of the following: dyspnea at rest, cough, weakness or decreased exercise performance, or chest tightness or congestion. Also, at least two of the following signs: central cyanosis, audible crackles or wheezing in at least one lung field, tachypnea, or tachycardia.	**Y.**	Odynophagia
_____	**26.** An altitude illness in which there is a change in mental status and/or ataxia in a person with acute mountain sickness or the presence of mental status changes and ataxia in a person without acute mountain sickness.	**Z.**	Orthostatic hypotension

Part III

Place the letters HP next to the factors that increase heat production and the letters HL next to the factors that interfere with heat loss (dissipation).

_____ **1.** High ambient temperature
_____ **2.** Physical exertion
_____ **3.** Heavy or tight clothing
_____ **4.** Diabetic peripheral neuropathies
_____ **5.** Hyperthyroidism
_____ **6.** Response to infection
_____ **7.** Alcoholism
_____ **8.** Overdosing on such drugs as cocaine, caffeine, or Ecstasy
_____ **9.** Impaired vasodilation
_____ **10.** Agitated and tremulous state (such as from Parkinson disease or drug withdrawal)

Multiple Choice

Read each item carefully, and then select the best response.

_____ **1.** Heat syncope is seen in nonacclimated people who may be under heat stress and typically occurs in all of the following situations, EXCEPT:

A. after standing suddenly.
B. at mass outdoor gatherings.
C. after prolonged standing.
D. after swimming on a very hot day.

_____ **2.** The major contributors to the basal metabolic rate (BMR), the heat energy produced at rest from normal body metabolic reactions, are the:

A. spleen and lungs.
B. kidneys and heart.
C. liver and skeletal muscles.
D. kidneys and gallbladder.

_____ **3.** The loss of heat that takes place when moving air picks up heat and carries it away is:

A. evaporation.
B. convection.
C. radiation.
D. conduction.

_____ **4.** A call to the scene of an outdoor high school track meet is for a 15-year-old student who was running the mile race. It is a humid day with the temperature in the 90s. The patient presents with muscle pain in the lower extremities and abdomen. Based on these symptoms, what is the MOST likely problem?

A. Heat cramps
B. Heat exhaustion
C. Heatstroke
D. Heat syncope

_____ **5.** You are called to an apartment building on a hot July afternoon for a bedridden 78-year-old woman. Upon entering the apartment, you notice that it is extremely hot, and the patient is very warm with dry skin. The SAMPLE history identifies that the patient has heart failure and is taking beta-blockers and diuretics. Her blood glucose is normal. You should suspect:

A. exertional heatstroke.
B. malignant hyperthermia.
C. neuroleptic malignant syndrome.
D. classic heatstroke.

_____ **6.** All of the following factors increase heat loss, EXCEPT:

A. vasoconstriction.
B. wet clothes.
C. alcohol.
D. diabetic neuropathies.

_____ **7.** Which unique finding might be observed on an electrocardiogram (ECG) of a patient with a low core body temperature?

A. Alternans
B. Osborn waves
C. Spiked waves
D. Inverted T waves

_____ **8.** You are called to a local boat dock for a patient returning from a scuba dive. His dive computer shows the maximum depth was 120 feet. The patient is reported by his buddy to have demonstrated inappropriate behavior while getting ready to ascend. The ascent was controlled with a safety stop for a few minutes at around 20 feet. Back in the dive boat, the patient complains of tingling in his lips and legs. He has no other reported symptoms. You most likely suspect that the patient may have a mild case of:

A. arterial gas embolism.
B. nitrogen narcosis.
C. pulmonary overpressurization syndrome.
D. barotitis externa.

______ **9.** You are dispatched to the pool at a private residence for an unresponsive teenager. Upon arrival, you are told that the patient was competing with a friend to see who could hold his breath underwater for the longest amount of time. He was swimming underwater, and while coming to the surface, he went limp and was pulled from the water. You find the patient is breathing, and you administer supplemental oxygen and continue with an assessment. What do you expect is the patient's problem?

A. Decompression sickness

B. Barotrauma

C. Shallow-water blackout

D. Bends

______ **10.** Deep frostbite usually involves the hands or feet, and the extremity may initially exhibit all of the following colors, EXCEPT:

A. white.

B. yellow-white.

C. mottled blue-white.

D. red.

Labeling

Label the following diagrams with the correct terms.

1. Dangerous snakes

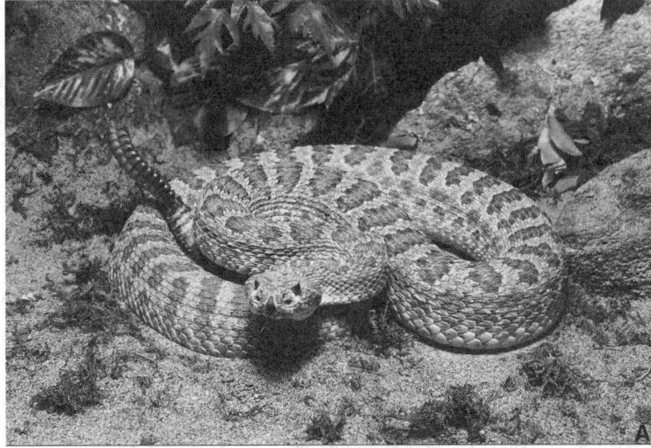

© Photos.com/Getty.

A. 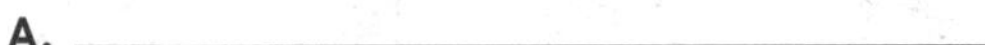

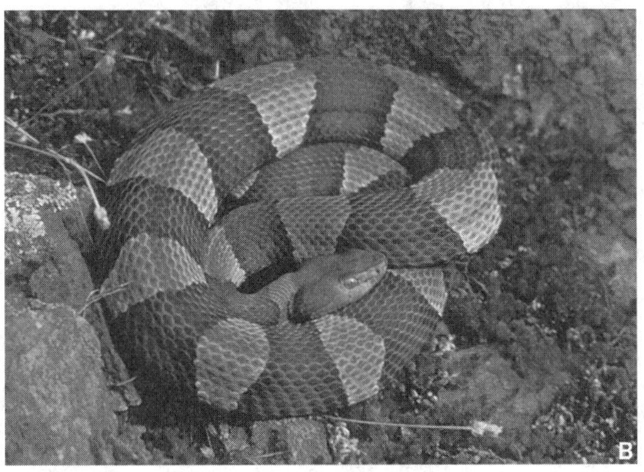

Courtesy of Ray Rauch/U.S. Fish & Wildlife Service.

B. 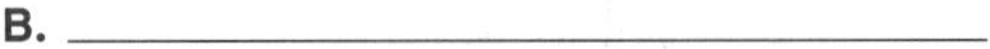

C. ____________________________________

© SuperStock/Alamy.

D. ____________________________________

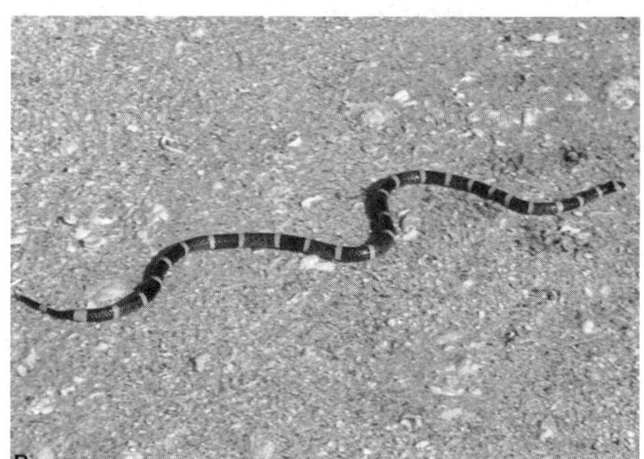

Courtesy of Luther C. Goldman/U.S. Fish & Wildlife Service.

Fill in the Blank

Read each item carefully, and then complete the statement by filling in the missing word(s).

1. The core temperature of the human body at any given moment represents a balance between the heat produced by the body and the heat shed by the body.
   a. List the potential sources of body heat and the mechanisms by which body heat can be dissipated.

Sources of Body Heat	Ways of Shedding Heat
1.	1.
2.	2.
3.	3.
4.	

   b. The body's mechanisms for dissipating excess heat have certain limitations. First, all of the mechanisms depend on __________ __________ to shunt blood from the core to the body surface. Furthermore, to be effective, three of the body's cooling mechanisms require a temperature gradient between the body and the outside. None of these three mechanisms—__________, __________, or __________—can work if the outside temperature is not at least a few degrees cooler than the body core. Finally, one of the body's cooling mechanisms is dependent on the ambient humidity. When the humidity is high, that mechanism—namely, __________ __________ __________—is ineffective in lowering the core temperature.
   c. A hatless hiker standing still on a mountaintop on a windless day loses heat from his head by __________. A breeze picks up. Now the hiker loses heat by __________ as well.
   d. A white-water enthusiast who capsizes his canoe in a swift-running river loses body heat by __________.
   e. A soldier on maneuvers in the desert in ambient temperatures of more than 37.7°C (100°F) can shed heat only by __________ __________ __________.

Identify

Read the following case study, and then list the chief complaint, vital signs, and pertinent negatives.

1. You are riding on Squad 5 and are dispatched to an incident in which a person fell through the ice at a local pond. Upon arrival, you find an 18-year-old man who is shivering with a blanket wrapped around him. It is reported that a Good Samaritan threw a rope and helped the patient get to shore. When you question the patient, he says that he was trying to walk home and didn't realize he had gotten lost. There is a smell of alcohol on the patient's breath. You immediately place the patient in your squad and turn the heat on high. The patient's wet clothes are removed, and he is wrapped in a number of blankets. He is placed on supplemental oxygen and a cardiac monitor. The ECG rhythm is regular, with no ectopy, but you do observe Osborn waves. You establish an IV line using warm crystalloid solution. The patient is transferred to the regional trauma center, which is located 15 minutes away. You continue to monitor the patient and perform a reassessment en route. You take serial vital signs every 5 minutes.

a. Chief complaint:

____

____

b. Vital signs:

____

____

c. Pertinent negatives:

____

____

d. Which three pieces of information not included in this scenario would be helpful to know?

(1)____

(2)____

(3)____

e. Based on this scenario, which of the following four methods of heat loss is most responsible for the greatest amount of heat lost by this patient?

A. Radiation
B. Conduction
C. Convection
D. Evaporation

f. You determine the patient is moderately hypothermic. How much IV fluid should you infuse initially?

____

Complete the Patient Care Report (PCR)

Reread the incident scenario in the preceding Identify exercise, and then complete the following PCR for the patient.

<table>
<tr><th colspan="6">EMS Patient Care Report (PCR)</th></tr>
<tr><td>Date:</td><td>Incident No.:</td><td colspan="2">Nature of Call:</td><td colspan="2">Location:</td></tr>
<tr><td>Dispatched:</td><td>En Route:</td><td>At Scene:</td><td>Transport:</td><td>At Hospital:</td><td>In Service:</td></tr>
<tr><th colspan="6">Patient Information</th></tr>
<tr><td colspan="3">Age:
Sex:
Weight (in kg [lb]):</td><td colspan="3">Allergies:
Medications:
Past Medical History:
Chief Complaint:</td></tr>
<tr><th colspan="6">Vital Signs</th></tr>
<tr><td>Time:</td><td>BP:</td><td>Pulse:</td><td>Respirations:</td><td colspan="2">SpO₂:</td></tr>
<tr><td>Time:</td><td>BP:</td><td>Pulse:</td><td>Respirations:</td><td colspan="2">SpO₂:</td></tr>
<tr><td>Time:</td><td>BP:</td><td>Pulse:</td><td>Respirations:</td><td colspan="2">SpO₂:</td></tr>
<tr><th colspan="6">EMS Treatment
(circle all that apply)</th></tr>
<tr><td colspan="2">Oxygen @ ______ L/min via (circle one):
NC NRM Bag-mask device</td><td>Assisted Ventilation</td><td>Airway Adjunct</td><td colspan="2">CPR</td></tr>
<tr><td>Defibrillation</td><td>Bleeding Control</td><td>Bandaging</td><td>Splinting</td><td colspan="2">Other:</td></tr>
<tr><th colspan="6">Narrative</th></tr>
<tr><td colspan="6"></td></tr>
</table>

Ambulance Calls

The following case scenarios provide an opportunity to explore the concerns associated with patient management and paramedic care. Read each scenario, and then answer each question.

1. At the morning briefing, you are told that you will be doing a standby at an outdoor festival at a local college campus. These assignments are usually boring, but you will make the best of it. It is a very hot and humid day in late spring, and except for a few scrapes and blisters, you have few requests for service. The concert has been going for about an hour when you are called to a person who has passed out. When you arrive, you find an unresponsive man approximately 20 years old. His friends tell you that he had been standing listening to the concert and suddenly fell. As you are assessing the patient, he starts to regain consciousness. You can tell he has been drinking. You ask how many beers he had, and he tells you he drank two. In your mind, you at least double that number. You load the patient into the ambulance and turn up the air conditioner. The assessment indicates dehydration.

a. What is the probable cause of the syncopal episode, and what may be some contributing underlying causes?

____

____

____

b. How would you manage this patient?

____

____

____

c. If the patient does not recover and stabilize quickly, what may be another presenting problem to consider?

____

____

2. You are called to the local high school playing field on a hot, sticky August afternoon to deal with a "casualty" of preseason football training—a 16-year-old fullback who "became crazy" during practice. You see him over near the goalposts, where several of his teammates are trying to restrain him. "None of my boys ever messed around with drugs before," the coach tells you, "and I sure never would have pegged Chuck as a junkie. But I don't know how else to explain his behavior. He's been touchy all afternoon, and he just started acting crazy."

You find the fullback to be agitated and combative. He seems completely disoriented. His skin is warm and sweaty. His vital signs are as follows: Pulse is 120 beats/min and bounding, respirations are 30 breaths/min and shallow, blood pressure (BP) is 150/90 mm Hg, and oral temperature is 41.7°C (107°F). His pupils are widely dilated and react only sluggishly to light.

a. This patient most likely has:

____

____

b. List the steps in managing this case.

(1)______________________________

(2)______________________________

(3)______________________________

(4)______________________________

(5)______________________________

(6)______________________________

(7)______________________________

3. The following day, it is even hotter, but mercifully, the humidity has dropped considerably. You are called to the very same playing field for another casualty of preseason football training—this time, a 14-year-old running back. You find him lying at midfield, writhing in pain. "I swear I didn't clip him," one of the other players is insisting. "I didn't even get near him. He just fell down by himself."

"Sure, sure," says the coach, who is trying to massage the cramps out of the boy's legs. When you ask the boy what his problem is, he just moans and says, "My legs, my legs."

On examination, the patient's skin is cool and sweaty. His pulse is 100 beats/min and regular, respirations are 30 breaths/min and shallow, BP is 110/70 mm Hg, and oral temperature is 37°C (98.6°F). There are no signs of injury to the extremities.

a. This patient most likely has:

____

____

b. List the steps in managing this case.

(1)____

(2)____

(3)____

(4)____

4. "As long as you folks are already here," says the coach, "maybe you could take a look at our quarterback. I think he's coming down with something, and I have to decide whether to send him home."

You find the quarterback sitting on the bench looking quite miserable. He says that his girlfriend has mononucleosis, and he thinks he may be coming down with it as well because he feels very tired and achy. On examination, he is sweating profusely, and his skin feels clammy. His pulse is 110 beats/min and somewhat weak, respirations are 28 breaths/min and shallow, BP is 100/60 mm Hg, and oral temperature is 39.4°C (103°F).

a. This patient most likely has:

____

____

b. List the steps in managing this case.

(1)____

(2)____

(3)____

(4)____

(5)____

c. Which advice should you give the football coach?

____

____

5. On the very same day, you are called to a local supermarket for a "sick baby." You arrive to find a nearly hysterical woman who looks scarcely out of her teens holding a comatose baby. "I just left her in the car for a minute while I ran in to buy a couple of things," she says, although you note three full shopping bags in the woman's cart. The baby, a 6-month-old, is unresponsive (AVPU = U). The pulse is 180 beats/min, respirations are 60 breaths/min, and BP is 100/80 mm Hg. The baby's rectal temperature is 43.3°C (110°F).

a. This patient most likely has:

____

____

b. List the steps in managing this case.

(1)____

(2)____

(3)____

(4)____

(5)____

(6)____

(7)____

6. You are enjoying a week off at a mountain ski resort. On your first morning there, the manager of the resort asks for volunteers to join a search-and-rescue party that is going out to look for three skiers who failed to return to the lodge the previous night. You, of course, volunteer, and you set off with a team on skis to comb the slopes. You are all carrying two-way radios so that you can summon a snowmobile to help transport the lost skiers if you find them. Eventually, you locate two of the skiers, about 15 miles from the ski lodge, dug into a makeshift shelter in the snow (and unaware that only about 50 m away, beyond a stand of trees, is an empty cabin). Both skiers are alert.

a. The first skier tells you that he lost all sensation in his left leg sometime during the night. On examination, the leg is white, cold, and very hard. This patient most likely has:

____

____

b. Describe how you would manage this patient.

(1)____

(2)____

(3)____

(4)____

(5)____

c. The second skier says, "I think I've got the same problem in my left foot." On examination, the foot has a waxy, white appearance. The skin feels very stiff, but there is "give" underneath when you press down hard on the skin. This patient most likely has:

____

____

d. How would you manage this patient?

(1)____

(2)____

(3)____

(4)____

(5)____

e. Not long after those two skiers have been evacuated on stretchers by snowmobile, you find the third skier. He is sitting up against a tree, unresponsive. Apparently, he did not realize that he had come within 100 m of the main road. His skin is very cold. You cannot detect any pulse. The patient's pupils are dilated and unreactive. He does seem to be breathing, although only about once or twice a minute. You radio for a paramedic-staffed ambulance to meet you at the road. This patient most likely has:

____

____

f. Describe the management of this patient both until the ambulance comes and en route to the hospital.

(1)____

(2)____

(3)____

(4)____

(5)____

(6)____

(7)____

(8)____

7. You and your crew are at the local lake on a chilly November afternoon, covering an annual speedboat race that invariably produces a few minor casualties (mostly from indigestion among the picnicking spectators). While making a hairpin turn at high speed, one of the speedboats capsizes. After what seems like a very long time, you see the boat's driver bob to the surface of the water (he is wearing a life jacket) and begin swimming for shore. Describe the actions you should take in this situation.

a. ____

b. ____

c. ____

d. ____

e. ____

f. ____

g. ____

h. ____

8. During the first spell of bitterly cold weather of the season, you are called to the downtown bus terminal for a "man down." When you reach the scene, a police officer waves you over. "Sorry to bother you folks with this," he says. "He's just a vagrant who's been sleeping in the place for a few days, and probably all he needs is a night in the lockup to sober up." You find the patient, being restrained by another police officer, over in a corner. His speech is slurred, and he staggers when he tries to walk. His breath smells of wine. His skin is pale and cold.

a. List at least three diagnoses you must consider in this case.

(1)___

(2)___

(3)___

b. In view of the diagnostic possibilities, describe how you would manage this case.

(1)___

(2)___

(3)___

(4)___

(5)___

(6)___

(7)___

9. You decide to take a week's vacation to do some climbing in the Canadian Rockies. Of course, you are carrying a medical kit because it's hard for you to accept the idea that you are really on vacation. On your first day out, one of your buddies starts complaining of a headache—"probably because I didn't sleep really well last night," he says. You're a little concerned that he might be suffering from the altitude, but he shrugs it off and insists that you all keep going.

a. At that point, how could you check whether your friend has a serious case of acute altitude sickness?

___

___

b. As things turn out, you decide to continue climbing. About an hour later, you feel a tug on the rope and look back to see your friend really dragging. He seems out of breath. Now you're really concerned. List four signs or symptoms that would suggest your friend may have high-altitude pulmonary edema.

(1)___

(2)___

(3)___

(4)___

c. Assuming that you do find signs of high-altitude pulmonary edema (HAPE), which steps should you take to treat your friend?

(1)___

(2)___

(3)___

10. When your next vacation comes up, you decide you won't make the same mistake twice: no more mountains where emergencies will spoil your relaxation. Instead, you sign up for a cruise to the West Indies—a week of sun and sand and steel drum bands. On the ship with you is a group of scuba enthusiasts who don't miss any opportunity to explore the local coral reefs each time you anchor.

One fine afternoon, as you are sunning yourself on deck with a rum swizzle in hand, you hear a commotion off to the starboard side of the ship. You leap from your chair and peer over the rail to see some of the diving crowd in a state of agitation in the rubber raft from which they've been diving. One of their number is lying motionless in the raft, and another two are just emerging from the water and climbing into the raft to join them. The captain, having spotted the situation, has already lowered a winch to bring up the raft and everyone in it.

As soon as the divers are back aboard the ship, you race to the side of the diver who is unresponsive. His friends tell you that he was the least experienced of their group. He had surfaced first, and a minute or so after being pulled onto the raft, he complained of chest pain, and his voice had sounded funny. Then, he just blacked out.

a. What do you think has happened to this diver?

____

____

b. Which steps should you take to manage this situation?

(1)____

(2)____

(3)____

(4)____

(5)____

(6)____

c. About an hour later, while you are monitoring the condition of the diver pending more definitive treatment, you hear one of his friends who was in the water with him saying to another member of the group, "Gee, my back is sure killing me. I must have pulled a muscle when I did my backflip off the raft. The hell of it is that I can't pee, either." You perk up your ears when you hear that because this bit of information makes you suspect that the speaker has:

____

____

True/False

If you believe the statement to be more true than false, write the letter "T" in the space provided. If you believe the statement to be more false than true, write the letter "F."

_____ **1.** A superficial frostbitten extremity is best warmed in front of a campfire or heater.

_____ **2.** With deep frostbite, the extremity feels cold and rock hard.

_____ **3.** If rescue circumstances require it, a patient with deep frostbite may walk on a frostbitten leg as long as the leg is not rewarmed in the field.

_____ **4.** Elapidae is the same family of snakes that includes mambas, cobras, and sea snakes.

_____ **5.** A frostbitten extremity will be excruciatingly painful until it is rewarmed.

_____ **6.** Injuries from the cold most often affects the tips of the ears, nose, fingers, and toes.

_____ **7.** Heat exhaustion is a clinical syndrome thought to represent a milder form of heat illness on a continuum leading to heatstroke.

_____ **8.** Classic heatstroke is less apt to affect older patients with chronic illnesses.

_____ **9.** Patients with heatstroke usually have dilated pupils.

_____ **10.** Radiation accounts for more than 65% of heat loss in a cooler setting.

Short Answer

Complete this section with short written answers using the space provided.

1. The body's normal response to entering a hot environment can place considerable stress on a person who has a limited cardiovascular reserve. Explain why.

____

____

____

2. Anyone can succumb to a heat wave, but some people are more vulnerable than others. List five factors that increase a person's risk of experiencing significant heat illness in response to heat stress.

a. ______________________________

b. ______________________________

c. ______________________________

d. ______________________________

e. ______________________________

3. Paramedics, like other public safety personnel, do not have the luxury of postponing heavy exertion until weather conditions are favorable. Instead, they must do their job whatever the weather, which means they may be exposed to a significant risk of heat illness during periods of high temperature.

a. List five measures you can take to reduce your risk of becoming ill from the heat.

(1)______________________________

(2)______________________________

(3)______________________________

(4)______________________________

(5)______________________________

b. If you do start to experience early symptoms of heat illness, you must stop your activities immediately. To do so, you must be able to recognize the warning symptoms of heat illness when they occur. List four warning symptoms of heat illness.

(1)______________________________

(2)______________________________

(3)______________________________

(4)______________________________

4. People wouldn't experience cold injury if they simply heeded the advice of their mothers. Mothers always know, even without taking a paramedic course, how to keep warm on cold days. Following are several statements you have probably heard at least once from your mother. Each statement reflects an intuitive knowledge of the ways in which the body generates and loses heat. For each statement, explain why your mother was right.

a. "Don't go out without a hat and scarf; it's freezing out there." Mother was right because:

____

____

b. "Stop rolling around in the snow. You'll get a death of a chill." Mother was right because:

____

____

c. "Get out of those wet clothes this minute." Mother was right because:

____

____

d. "Those skates are much too tight. Your toes will fall off." Mother was right because:

____

____

e. "Make sure you wear your windbreaker. It's blowing a gale out there." Mother was right because:

____

____

f. "Eat. Eat. You have to have something to keep you going in this weather." Mother was right because:

____

____

5. The body has only a limited repertoire of defenses against the cold. List three ways the body can defend itself against a drop in core temperature.

a. ____

b. ____

c. ____

6. Although anyone can experience cold injury, certain factors predispose a person to experience ill effects from the cold.

a. List five factors that predispose a person to experience frostbite when exposed to freezing conditions.

(1) ____

(2) ____

(3) ____

(4) ____

(5) ____

b. List four factors that predispose a person to experience hypothermia.

(1) ____

(2) ____

(3) ____

(4) ____

7. The stories that many of us learned as children contain many cautionary tales about cold exposure.

a. When the three little kittens lost their mittens, they became most vulnerable to:

____

b. Sitting on an ice-cold tuffet on a winter day, Little Miss Muffet was losing heat from her body by:

____

c. Who is at greater risk of experiencing hypothermia—Jack Sprat (who ate no fat) or his wife (who ate no lean)?

____

d. Before venturing outside to try out his new ice skates, little Jack Horner retreated to a corner and ate his Christmas pie. Was that a good idea? Why or why not?

____

e. Swinging about in the treetop is Baby in his cradle. When the wind blows, the cradle will rock. Furthermore, when the wind blows, Baby will lose heat from his body by the process called:

____

Fill in the Table

Fill in the missing parts of the table.

1. Factors that predispose to cold illness

Increase Heat Loss	Impair Thermoregulatory Mechanism	Decrease Heat Production
______________	Dehydration	______________
Wet clothes	Parkinson disease or dementia	Age (very young or very old)
______________	______________	______________
Impaired judgment from drugs/alcohol	Anorexia nervosa	______________
	Central nervous system (CNS) bleeding or ischemia, spinal cord injury with neurogenic shock	Inability to shiver and immobility
______________		
Diabetic peripheral neuropathies	______________	
	Drugs interfering with vasoconstriction	

SHOCK AND RESUSCITATION

CHAPTER 39

Responding to the Field Code

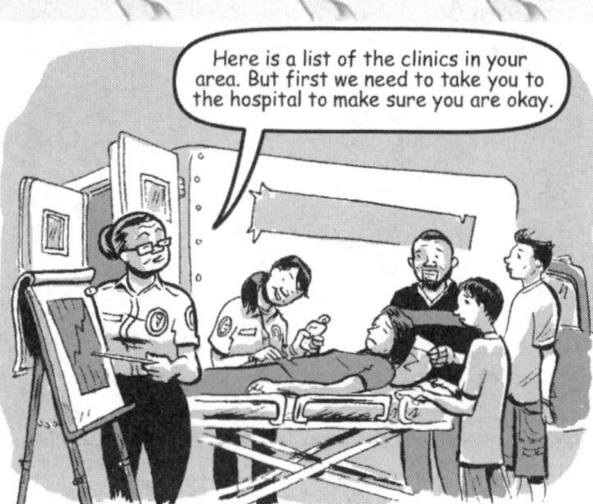

Paramedics should take every opportunity to educate their patients.

Matching

Match each of the terms in the right column to the appropriate definition in the left column.

______	**1.** In cardiopulmonary resuscitation (CPR), when two rescuers perform ventilations and compressions individually; ventilations are not timed and do not require waiting for the other rescuer to pause.	**A.**	Active compression-decompression CPR
______	**2.** A defibrillator that can analyze the patient's heart rhythm and determine whether a defibrillating shock is needed to terminate ventricular fibrillation (VF) or ventricular tachycardia (VT).	**B.**	Asynchronous
______	**3.** The code team member who has the responsibility for managing the rescuers or team members during a cardiac arrest, as well as choreographing the effort of the group.	**C.**	Automated external defibrillator (AED)
______	**4.** A member of the resuscitation team trying to revive the patient.	**D.**	Automatic transport ventilator (ATV)
______	**5.** The use of an unsynchronized direct current electric shock to terminate VF or VT.	**E.**	Code team leader
______	**6.** A mode available on automated external defibrillators, allowing the paramedic to interpret the cardiac rhythm and determine whether defibrillation is indicated (rather than the monitor making the determination).	**F.**	Code team member
______	**7.** The return of spontaneous heartbeat and blood pressure during the resuscitation of a patient in cardiac arrest.	**G.**	Compression fraction
______	**8.** A mnemonic used to describe the objectives of a community-based program to improve the survival of patients in out-of-hospital cardiac arrest: Specific, Measurable, Attainable and Achievable, Realistic and Relevant, and Timely.	**H.**	Defibrillation
______	**9.** An indication of how well the team is minimizing pauses in CPR; it is calculated by dividing the amount of time compressions are delivered by the amount of time compressions are indicated.	**I.**	Manual defibrillation
______	**10.** A portable mechanical ventilator attached to a control box that allows the variables of ventilation (such as rate and tidal volume) to be set.	**J.**	Return of spontaneous circulation (ROSC)
______	**11.** A procedure intended to lower body temperature in patients who are in a coma after return of spontaneous circulation; ideally performed in the hospital setting; formerly called therapeutic hypothermia.	**K.**	SMART
______	**12.** A manual technique that involves compressing the chest and then actively pulling it back up to its neutral position or beyond (decompression); may increase the amount of blood that returns to the heart and, thus, the amount of blood ejected from the heart during the compression phase.	**L.**	Targeted temperature management (TTM)

Multiple Choice

Read each item carefully, and then select the best response.

_____ **1.** Which of the following is NOT considered a link in the chain of survival?
- **A.** Recognition and activation of the emergency response system
- **B.** Immediate high-quality CPR
- **C.** Early clotbuster therapy in the field
- **D.** Rapid defibrillation

_____ **2.** For which types of incidents does simulation training provide valuable preparation?
- **A.** High-frequency, low-risk incidents
- **B.** Low-frequency, high-risk incidents
- **C.** Low-frequency, low-risk incidents
- **D.** High-frequency, high-risk incidents

_____ **3.** With the issuance of the 2005, 2010, and 2015 ECC Guidelines, there was a strong emphasis on:
- **A.** advanced airway procedures.
- **B.** choices of cardiac medications.
- **C.** increasing the ventilation rates.
- **D.** high-quality compressions.

_____ **4.** When placing an advanced airway during resuscitation, the MOST important consideration would be:
- **A.** not to take any longer than 30 seconds.
- **B.** not to interrupt chest compressions for more than 10 seconds.
- **C.** to hyperventilate the patient as soon as possible.
- **D.** to insert the largest tube that will fit the patient.

_____ **5.** High-quality CPR, in the adult patient, consists of each of the following, EXCEPT:
- **A.** compressions at a rate of 100 to 120 per minute.
- **B.** allowing complete chest recoil after each compression.
- **C.** avoiding excessive ventilations.
- **D.** compression depth of 1½ inches on the adult patient.

_____ **6.** For the purposes of the ECC Guidelines, an infant is:
- **A.** age 1 year to adolescence.
- **B.** age 1 month to 1 year.
- **C.** within the first few hours after birth.
- **D.** within the first month after birth.

_____ **7.** When there are two health care providers doing CPR, the infant compression-to-ventilation ratio should be:
- **A.** 30:2.
- **B.** 15:1.
- **C.** 15:2.
- **D.** 30:1.

_____ **8.** When a pediatric patient needs to be defibrillated with an AED, it is acceptable to:
- **A.** use the pediatric dose-attenuator system.
- **B.** use a manual defibrillator.
- **C.** use the standard adult pads if that is all that is available.
- **D.** All of the above

_____ **9.** You are treating an adult patient who has overdosed from a narcotic. The patient is in respiratory arrest, and your partner is obtaining the naloxone (Narcan). What is the rate of ventilations that should be given to the patient prior to inserting an advanced airway?
- **A.** 1 breath every 5 to 6 seconds
- **B.** 2 breaths every 30 compressions
- **C.** 1 breath every 3 seconds
- **D.** 2 breaths every 3 seconds

_____ **10.** Of the following treatments for the patient with ROSC, which would NOT be appropriate?

A. Normalize the blood pressure (BP) with dopamine (Intropin) or norepinephrine infusion to at least 100 mm Hg systolic.

B. Elevate the patient's head to 30° if the BP allows.

C. Stabilize the cardiac rhythm with an antidysrhythmic.

D. Begin TTM if the patient is alert.

Labeling

Label the following diagrams with the correct terms.

1. CPR devices

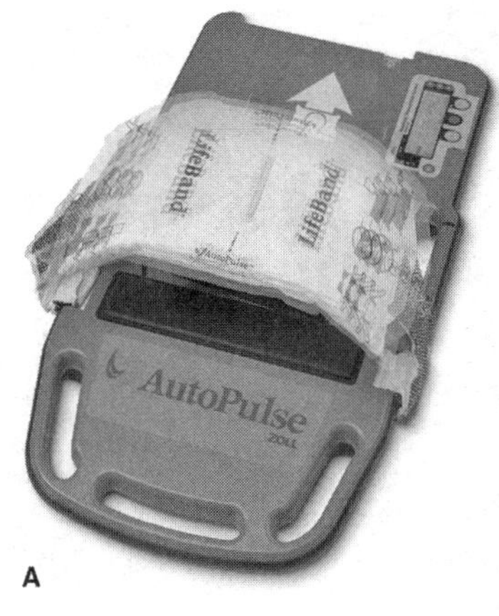

A

Courtesy of ZOLL.

A. 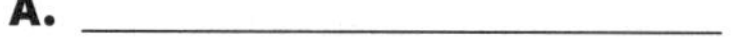

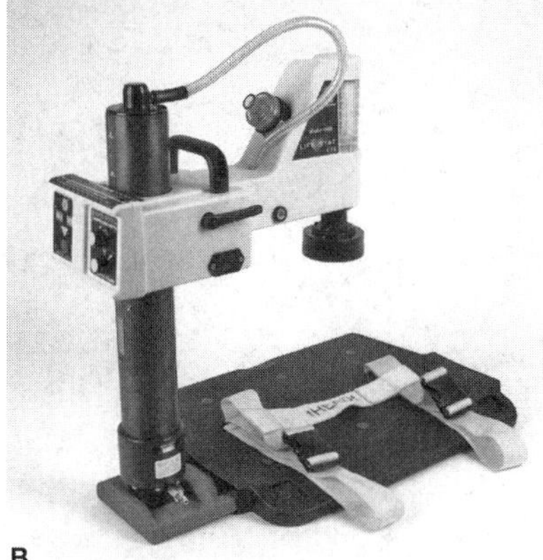

B

Courtesy of Michigan Instruments, Inc.

B. ______________________

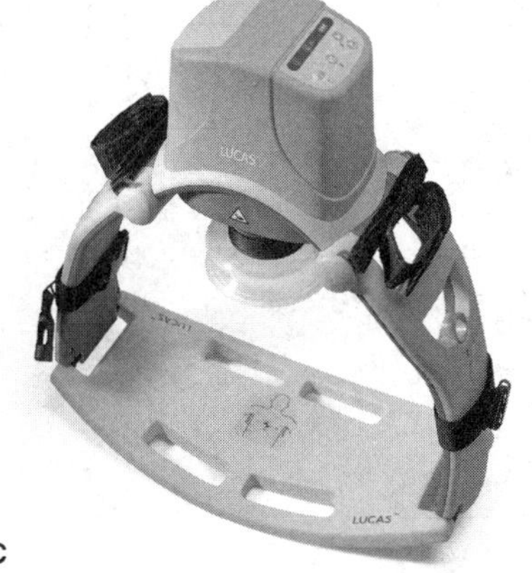

C

Courtesy of Physio-Control, Inc.

C. ______________________

2. Resuscitation pyramid

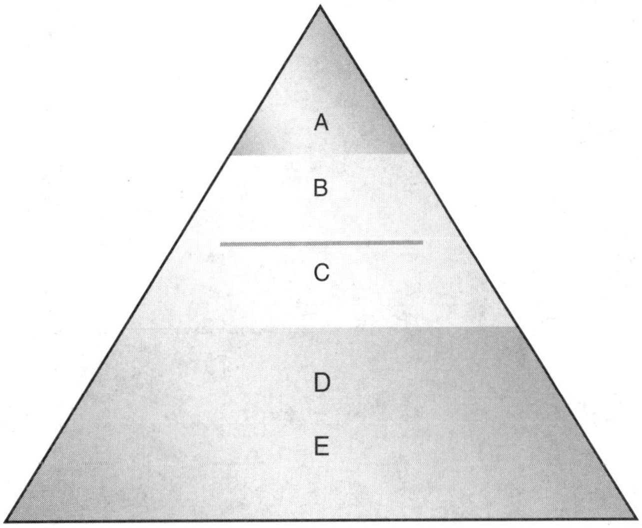

A
B
C
D
E

A. ______________________

B. ______________________

C. ______________________

D. ______________________

E. ______________________

Fill in the Blank

Read each item carefully, and then complete the statement by filling in the missing word(s).

1. The __________ is an adjunct to adult CPR that provides both continuous chest compressions and ventilations.

2. If a(n) __________ __________ is in place, then the compressions and ventilations become asynchronous.

3. The __________ __________ __________ is marketed as the ResQPOD in the United States.

4. If an advanced airway is inserted, you should switch to __________ compressions of 100 to 120 per minute and ventilate every __________ seconds.

5. For __________ or __________, do not deliver shocks.

6. Drug therapy for pulseless electrical activity (PEA) or asystole includes the __________ (epinephrine).

Identify

Read the following case study, and then list the chief complaint, vital signs, and pertinent negatives.

1. You are riding on Medic 480 and are dispatched along with a basic life support (BLS) unit to a person who is unresponsive in the shopping mall restroom. Upon arrival, you find a bystander and a security guard doing CPR on a 58-year-old man. When you question the patient's spouse, she says that he was complaining of pressure in his chest and indigestion before he went into the bathroom. She stated that he was only in there for a couple of moments when the bystander who started chest compressions had his son come out to get her and call 9-1-1. The security guard arrived soon thereafter with the AED. You immediately rotate the compressor, who is starting to get tired, and determine that the initial rhythm is not a shockable rhythm. As the other unit arrives, you begin to choreograph the resuscitation, making sure the patient is receiving high-quality chest compressions with as few interruptions as possible. Your partner is placing an intraosseous (IO) line in the leg so that the first epinephrine can be administered. At this point, the emergency medical technician (EMT) doing the ventilations reports that bag-valve mask ventilation is working just fine. After 2 minutes (of five cycles of compressions and ventilations), you note a rhythm change to VF, so the defibrillator is charged, and a shock is administered. After the shock is administered, the chest compressions are started immediately. Within moments, you note that the monitor is now showing a "normal"-looking electrocardiogram (ECG), so you stop the compressions and note that the patient has a strong carotid pulse. Because the patient is not yet breathing on his own, you decide to intubate and start your region's ROSC protocol. The wife, who has been observing all of the care, is very happy when the pulse returns. Further history reveals that the patient has been having these periods of chest discomfort for the past few weeks. He has no allergies and takes only vitamins each day. He has never had previous problems with his heart, head, or lungs, although his father did die from heart problems at a young age. En route to the hospital, a 12-lead ECG is taken, and the patient's BP is 108 mm Hg systolic, and his pulse rate is 96 beats/min and regular.

After delivering the patient right to the coronary catheterization lab for post–successful resuscitative measures, you note that the success of this resuscitation was definitely due to the bystander's immediate actions!

a. Chief complaint:

____

____

b. Vital signs:

____

____

c. Pertinent negatives:

____

____

d. What medication would most likely be administered to this patient?

____

____

e. Based on this scenario, what are the links in the chain of survival for this patient and all victims of sudden cardiac arrest?

(1)______________________________

(2)______________________________

(3)______________________________

(4)______________________________

(5)______________________________

Complete the Patient Care Report (PCR)

Reread the incident scenario in the preceding Identify exercise, and then complete the following PCR for the patient.

<table>
<tr><th colspan="6">EMS Patient Care Report (PCR)</th></tr>
<tr><td>Date:</td><td>Incident No.:</td><td colspan="2">Nature of Call:</td><td colspan="2">Location:</td></tr>
<tr><td>Dispatched:</td><td>En Route:</td><td>At Scene:</td><td>Transport:</td><td>At Hospital:</td><td>In Service:</td></tr>
<tr><th colspan="6">Patient Information</th></tr>
<tr><td colspan="3">Age:
Sex:
Weight (in kg [lb]):</td><td colspan="3">Allergies:
Medications:
Past Medical History:
Chief Complaint:</td></tr>
<tr><th colspan="6">Vital Signs</th></tr>
<tr><td>Time:</td><td>BP:</td><td>Pulse:</td><td>Respirations:</td><td colspan="2">SpO$_2$:</td></tr>
<tr><td>Time:</td><td>BP:</td><td>Pulse:</td><td>Respirations:</td><td colspan="2">SpO$_2$:</td></tr>
<tr><td>Time:</td><td>BP:</td><td>Pulse:</td><td>Respirations:</td><td colspan="2">SpO$_2$:</td></tr>
<tr><th colspan="6">EMS Treatment
(circle all that apply)</th></tr>
<tr><td colspan="2">Oxygen @ ______ L/min via (circle one):
NC NRM Bag-mask device</td><td>Assisted Ventilation</td><td>Airway Adjunct</td><td colspan="2">CPR</td></tr>
<tr><td>Defibrillation</td><td>Bleeding Control</td><td>Bandaging</td><td>Splinting</td><td colspan="2">Other:</td></tr>
<tr><th colspan="6">Narrative</th></tr>
<tr><td colspan="6"></td></tr>
</table>

Ambulance Calls

The following case scenarios provide an opportunity to explore the concerns associated with patient management and paramedic care. Read each scenario, and then answer each question.

1. At morning briefing, you are interrupted by a call for a possible cardiac arrest. The police have just arrived on the scene, and the supervisor is also en route to the call. As you arrive, you are met by a neighbor who states, "Mr. Jones was out shoveling snow when he suddenly collapsed. He was told by his heart doctor to leave the heavy work for his grandson!" Apparently, the grandson found him, carried him into the garage, called 9-1-1, and began hands-only CPR. As you and your partner are bringing in your equipment, you think to yourself, *The good news is CPR was started . . . The bad news is that he has a cardiac history.* Just then, a backup unit pulls up, as does the supervisor's truck. That means there are two medics (including you), two EMTs, a supervisor, and a police officer, and you will need to assign tasks so that this code runs with the speed and precision of a NASCAR pit stop.

a. What is the highest priority during the entire code?

____

____

____

b. If your role is that of the code team leader, what are your responsibilities?

(1)____

(2)____

(3)____

(4)____

(5)____

(6)____

(7)____

(8)____

(9)____

c. If you need to assign roles to the code team members, what do they include?

(1)____

(2)____

(3)____

(4)____

2. Based on the scenario just described, if the grandson had come home to find his grandfather on the floor in the kitchen in cardiac arrest, and there was an unknown downtime before calling 9-1-1, the results could be entirely different. On your arrival at the scene this time, the grandson was not doing hands-only CPR because he missed that day when it was taught in high school.

a. What are the criteria for NOT starting resuscitation?

____

____

____

b. With regard to the success of this resuscitation, what is the significance of chest compressions not being started prior to your arrival on the scene?

____

____

____

3. Later that day, you and your partner respond to a private home where, on entering the living room, you note there is a hospital bed set up in the corner of the room. The daughter has called 9-1-1 because she thinks her father, who has been suffering for a long time, has passed away. She leads you to the bathroom, where you can hear the son counting "19 and 20 and 21 and ..." as he provides chest compressions to his father on the floor of the small bathroom. The daughter states, "We just didn't know what to do. Dad wouldn't have wanted all this." You and your partner quickly move the patient, who weighs about 100 pounds, out into the living room, where there is more room.

a. List the conditions (termination rules) when it would be appropriate to stop the resuscitation in consult with medical control.

(1)______________________________

(2)______________________________

(3)______________________________

(4)______________________________

b. From the scenario described, what might lead you to ask if the patient was in a hospice program or has a do not resuscitate (DNR) order?

(1)______________________________

(2)______________________________

(3)______________________________

(4)______________________________

True/False

If you believe the statement to be more true than false, write the letter "T" in the space provided. If you believe the statement to be more false than true, write the letter "F."

_____ **1.** A possible cause of PEA is hypovolemia.

_____ **2.** A clue to the patient in cardiac arrest due to cardiac tamponade may be jugular venous distention.

_____ **3.** Beyond managing a cardiac arrest, if you suspect a tension pneumothorax, you should do a needle decompression on the affected side.

_____ **4.** Putrefaction is a discoloration of the skin caused by pooling of blood.

_____ **5.** If the patient has torsades de pointes, the paramedic should consider administering magnesium.

_____ **6.** Once you start CPR in the field, you should not stop until 15 minutes have gone by.

_____ **7.** An impedance threshold device (ITD) selectively prevents excess air from rushing into the chest during resuscitation.

_____ **8.** Once ROSC occurs, the ITD can be used to assist in the patient's ventilations.

_____ **9.** The two-hands encircling method should be used by a single rescuer doing infant CPR.

_____ **10.** In an adult who is unresponsive, where you suspect a foreign body airway obstruction, CPR chest compressions are used to attempt to clear the obstruction.

Short Answer

Complete this section with short written answers using the space provided.

1. The 2015 Institute of Medicine (Health and Medicine Division of the National Academies of Science, Engineering, and Medicine) report entitled *Strategies to Improve Cardiac Arrest Survival: A Time to Act* included key recommendations. List five of the recommendations:

a. ______________________________

b. ______________________________

c. ______________________________

d. ______________________________

e. ______________________________

2. The chapter describes a plan for prehospital response to a cardiac arrest with a five-person team. This is just an example of a "best practice" that could be practiced in your community, but it certainly is not the only way to manage a cardiac arrest; each community has different responders and resources. List the roles of the five-person team, and describe what they are responsible for.

a. ______________________________

____

____

____

____

b. ______________________________

____

____

____

____

c. ______________________________

____

____

____

____

d. ______________________________

____

____

____

____

e. ______________________________

____

____

____

____

Fill in the Table

Fill in the missing parts of the table.

Key Elements of CPR for Adults, Children, and Infants			
Procedure	**Age 9 to Adult**	**Age 1–8 Years**	**Younger Than 1 Year**[a]
Circulation			
Recognition	Unresponsive with no breathing or only agonal (gasping) respirations		
Pulse check	______________	______________	Brachial artery
Compression location	In the center of the chest (lower half of the sternum)	In the center of the chest (lower half of the sternum)	______________
Hand placement	Heel of both hands	______________	Two-fingers or two-thumb encircling-hands technique
Compression depth	At least 2 in. (5 cm); not to exceed 2.4 in. (6 cm)	At least one-third of anterior-posterior diameter of chest; approximately 2 in. (5 cm)	______________
Compression rate	______________		
Chest wall recoil	Allow full chest recoil in between compressions. No ______________!		
	Rotate rescuers delivering compressions every 2 min		
Interruptions	Limit interruptions in delivery of chest compressions to less than 10 s		
Compression-to-ventilation ratio (until an advanced airway is inserted)	______________	______________ (one rescuer); ______________ (two professional rescuers)	
Airway			
Airway positioning	Head tilt-chin lift maneuver; jaw-thrust maneuver if ______________ is suspected		
Breathing			
Untrained rescuer	Compressions only		
Ventilations without advanced airway	2 breaths with a duration of ______________ each, with enough volume to produce ______________[b]		

Key Elements of CPR for Adults, Children, and Infants			
Procedure	**Age 9 to Adult**	**Age 1-8 Years**	**Younger Than 1 Year**[a]
Ventilations with advanced airway	1 breath every 6 s (10/min) ___________ with chest compressions; duration of 1 s each, with enough volume to produce chest rise	*Age 1 month to the onset of puberty:* 1 breath every 6-8 s (8-10 breaths/min); chest compressions delivered continuously at a rate of at least 100/min with no pauses for ventilations; duration of 1 s each, with enough volume to produce visible chest rise	
Rescue breathing	1 breath every ___________ (10-12 breaths/min)	1 breath every ___________ (12-20 breaths/min)	1 breath every ___________ (12-20 breaths/min)
Defibrillation			
Device	Adult AED	Use ___________ unit if available; if unavailable, then use adult unit	Use ___________ if available; if unavailable, use unit with pediatric dose-attenuator; if neither is available, then use adult unit
Procedure	Attach AED as soon as it is available. If two rescuers are available, then one should immediately begin CPR while the second retrieves and applies the AED. Minimize CPR interruptions. Resume CPR immediately after shock, beginning with ___________.		
Airway Obstruction			
Foreign body obstruction	Responsive: ___________	Responsive: ___________	Responsive: ___________
	Unresponsive: ___________[c]		

Abbreviations: AED, automated external defibrillator; CPR, cardiopulmonary resuscitation.

[a]Excluding newborns, in whom arrest is usually the result of asphyxiation and requires the rescue ventilations.

[b]Pause compressions to deliver ventilations.

[c]Look in the mouth for objects before delivering breaths in a patient with a known airway obstruction.

Data from: Kleinman ME, Brennan EE, Goldberger ZD, et al. Part 5: Adult basic life support and cardiopulmonary resuscitation quality: 2015 American Heart Association Guidelines Update for Cardiopulmonary Resuscitation and Emergency Cardiovascular Care. Circulation. 2015;132(suppl 2):S414-S435; Atkins DL, Berger S, Duff JP, et al. Part 11: Pediatric basic life support and cardiopulmonary resuscitation quality: 2015 American Heart Association Guidelines Update for Cardiopulmonary Resuscitation and Emergency Cardiovascular Care. *Circulation*. 2015;132(suppl 2):S519-S525.

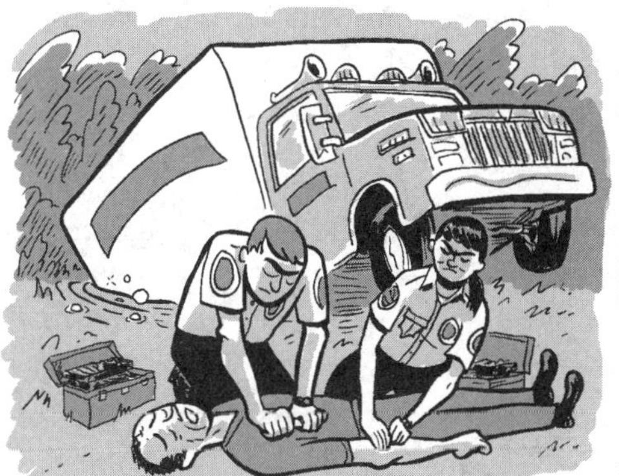
Some people, when they think they're up to their ears in alligators, forget to look out for a swamp.

CHAPTER 40

Management and Resuscitation of the Critical Patient

Matching

Part I

Match each of the terms in the right column to the appropriate definition in the left column.

	Definition	Term
______	**1.** Sense organs that monitor the levels of oxygen and carbon dioxide and the pH of cerebrospinal fluid and blood and provide feedback to the respiratory centers to modify the rate and depth of breathing based on the body's needs at any given time.	**A.** Aerobic metabolism
______	**2.** A condition that consists of cardiogenic shock and obstructive shock (Weil–Shubin classification).	**B.** Afterload
______	**3.** Failure of the heart and blood vessels; shock.	**C.** Anaerobic metabolism
______	**4.** A condition caused by loss of 40% or more of the functioning myocardium; the heart is no longer able to circulate sufficient blood to maintain adequate oxygen delivery.	**D.** Anaphylactic shock
______	**5.** The volume of blood pumped through the circulatory system in 1 minute.	**E.** Anchoring bias
______	**6.** The blood pressure required to sustain organ perfusion; roughly 60 mm Hg in the average person.	**F.** Angioedema
______	**7.** The point at which shock has progressed to a terminal stage, resulting in death.	**G.** Baroreceptors
______	**8.** Pattern recognition and pattern matching, based on your own past experiences.	**H.** Capacitance vessels
______	**9.** A condition that occurs when the circulating blood volume is inadequate to deliver adequate oxygen and nutrients to the body.	**I.** Cardiac output
______	**10.** A condition that occurs when the level of tissue perfusion decreases below that needed to maintain normal cellular functions; also called shock.	**J.** Cardiogenic shock
______	**11.** A patient who is in premorbid condition, has experienced major trauma, or is in the peri-arrest period.	**K.** Cardiovascular collapse
______	**12.** A type of bias that occurs with the tendency to gather and rely on information that confirms your existing views and to avoid or downplay information that does not conform to your preexisting hypothesis or field diagnosis.	**L.** Central shock
______	**13.** The early stage of shock, in which the body can still compensate for blood loss. The systolic blood pressure and brain perfusion are maintained.	**M.** Chemoreceptors
______	**14.** The smallest venules.	**N.** Compensated shock
______	**15.** Receptors in the blood vessels, kidneys, brain, and heart that respond to changes in pressure in the heart or main arteries to help maintain homeostasis.	**O.** Confirmation bias

	Definition	Term
______	**16.** Recurrent large areas of subcutaneous edema of sudden onset, usually disappearing within 24 hours, which is seen mainly in young women, frequently as a result of an allergy to food or drugs.	**P.** Critical patient
______	**17.** A type of bias in which an initial reference point distorts your estimates.	**Q.** Decompensated shock
______	**18.** A principle that states the movement and use of oxygen in the body are dependent on an adequate concentration of inspired oxygen, appropriate movement of oxygen across the alveolar–capillary membrane into the arterial bloodstream, adequate number of red blood cells to carry the oxygen, proper tissue perfusion, and efficient offloading of oxygen at the tissue level.	**R.** Differential diagnosis
______	**19.** A condition that occurs when there is widespread dilation of the resistance vessels, the capacitance vessels, or both.	**S.** Diffusion
______	**20.** A process in which molecules move from an area of higher concentration to an area of lower concentration.	**T.** Distributive shock
______	**21.** The process of weighing the probability of one disease versus other diseases by comparing clinical findings that could account for a patient's illness; also refers to the list of possible conditions considered based on the patient's signs and symptoms.	**U.** Fick principle
______	**22.** The late stage of shock, when blood pressure is falling.	**V.** Hypoperfusion
______	**23.** A severe hypersensitivity reaction that involves bronchoconstriction and cardiovascular collapse.	**W.** Hypovolemic shock
______	**24.** Metabolism that takes place in the absence of oxygen.	**X.** Intuition
______	**25.** The pressure in the aorta against which the left ventricle must pump blood.	**Y.** Irreversible shock
______	**26.** Metabolism that can proceed only in the presence of oxygen.	**Z.** Mean arterial pressure (MAP)

Part II

Match each of the terms in the right column to the appropriate definition in the left column.

	Definition	Term
______	**1.** The initial stretching of the cardiac muscle prior to contraction. It is related to the chamber volume of blood just prior to the contraction.	**A.** Multiple-organ dysfunction syndrome (MODS)
______	**2.** A condition that consists of hypovolemic shock and distributive shock (Weil–Shubin classification).	**B.** Myocardial contractility
______	**3.** The period either just before or just after cardiac arrest when the patient is critical and care must be taken to prevent progression or regression into cardiac arrest.	**C.** Neurogenic shock
______	**4.** The delivery of oxygen and nutrients to the cells, organs, and tissues of the body.	**D.** Nonhemorrhagic shock
______	**5.** A drop in systolic blood pressure when moving a patient from a sitting to a standing position.	**E.** Obstructive shock
______	**6.** The one diagnosis from a differential list used to base the patient's treatment plan.	**F.** Orthostatic hypotension
______	**7.** The amount of time that specific tissues of the body are deprived of oxygen, typically as a result of an injury or arterial occlusion.	**G.** Perfusion
______	**8.** The resistance to blood flow within all of the blood vessels except the pulmonary vessels.	**H.** Peri-arrest period
______	**9.** The amount of blood that the left ventricle ejects into the aorta per contraction.	**I.** Peripheral shock
______	**10.** The local neurologic condition that occurs after a spinal injury produces motor and sensory losses (which may not be permanent).	**J.** Preload
______	**11.** Shock that occurs when there is a block to blood flow in the heart or great vessels, causing an insufficient blood supply to the body's tissues.	**K.** Premorbid condition
______	**12.** Shock that occurs as a result of fluid loss contained within the body, such as in dehydration, burn injury, crush injury, and anaphylaxis.	**L.** Psychogenic shock

_____	**13.** Circulatory failure caused by paralysis of the nerves that control the size of the blood vessels, leading to widespread dilation; seen in patients with spinal cord injuries.	**M.** Pulse pressure
_____	**14.** The ability of the heart to contract.	**N.** Resistance vessels
_____	**15.** A circular muscular wall of capillaries that constricts and dilates, acting as a gate to increase or decrease blood flow.	**O.** Sensitization
_____	**16.** A progressive condition usually characterized by combined failure of several organs, such as the lungs, liver, and kidneys, along with some clotting mechanisms, which occurs after severe illness or injury.	**P.** Septic shock
_____	**17.** An abnormal state associated with inadequate oxygen and nutrient delivery to the metabolic apparatus of the cell; also called hypoperfusion.	**Q.** Shock
_____	**18.** Shock caused by severe infection, usually a bacterial infection.	**R.** Sphincter
_____	**19.** Developing a sensitivity to a substance that initially caused no allergic reaction.	**S.** Spinal shock
_____	**20.** The smallest arterioles.	**T.** Stroke volume
_____	**21.** The difference between the systolic blood pressure and the diastolic blood pressure.	**U.** Systemic vascular resistance
_____	**22.** A sudden reaction of the nervous system that produces a temporary, generalized vascular dilation, resulting in syncope (vasovagal syncope).	**V.** Warm ischemic time
_____	**23.** A condition preceding the onset of disease.	**W.** Working diagnosis

Multiple Choice

Read each item carefully, and then select the best response.

_____ **1.** The short list of potential causes of the patient's presenting condition is called the:
- **A.** definitive diagnosis.
- **B.** presenting problem.
- **C.** differential diagnosis.
- **D.** disposition.

_____ **2.** Conditions that come before the onset of disease are called:
- **A.** peri-arrest conditions.
- **B.** premorbid conditions.
- **C.** risk factors.
- **D.** congenital defects.

_____ **3.** With a patient who has a chief complaint of altered mental status, a starting point for the differential diagnosis can be remembered using the acronym:
- **A.** SAMPLE.
- **B.** M-T-SHIP.
- **C.** OPQRST.
- **D.** AVPU.

_____ **4.** Intuition has a definite role in the assessment of critical patients by experienced providers. Intuition can:
- **A.** forewarn you of what may happen next.
- **B.** lead you to make treatment errors.
- **C.** be difficult to teach.
- **D.** All of the above

_____ **5.** A tendency to gather and rely on information that confirms your existing assessment views is called a(n):
- **A.** personal bias.
- **B.** confirmation bias.
- **C.** relieved decision.
- **D.** anchoring bias.

_____ **6.** The amount of circulation of blood within an organ or tissue in adequate amounts to meet the cells' current needs for oxygen, nutrients, and waste removal is referred to as:
- **A.** stroke volume.
- **B.** contractility.
- **C.** preload.
- **D.** perfusion.

_____ **7.** The initial stretching of the cardiac muscle prior to contraction is called the:
- **A.** cardiac output.
- **B.** preload.
- **C.** afterload.
- **D.** stroke volume.

_____ **8.** Your patient has a blood pressure of 110/70 mm Hg. What is his mean arterial pressure?
- **A.** 40
- **B.** 56
- **C.** 83
- **D.** 92

_____ **9.** Stimulation of the sympathetic nervous system can cause the pupils to __________ and the heart rate to __________.
- **A.** dilate; increase
- **B.** dilate; decrease
- **C.** constrict; increase
- **D.** constrict; decrease

_____ **10.** Stimulation of the parasympathetic nervous system can cause the gastrointestinal tract to:
- **A.** decrease motility.
- **B.** shut down.
- **C.** increase salivation.
- **D.** All of the above

_____ **11.** Of the following, which is NOT considered an essential element of the Fick principle?
- **A.** Proper tissue perfusion
- **B.** Adequate number of white blood cells to carry oxygen
- **C.** Adequate concentration of inspired oxygen
- **D.** Efficient offloading of oxygen at the tissue level

_____ **12.** The perfusion triangle includes each of the following, EXCEPT:
- **A.** the blood volume.
- **B.** the heart.
- **C.** insulin release by the pancreas.
- **D.** the blood vessels.

_____ **13.** A progressive condition characterized by the combined failure of two or more organs or organ systems that were initially unharmed by the patient's initial illness is called:
- **A.** cardiovascular collapse.
- **B.** compensated shock.
- **C.** decompensated shock.
- **D.** multiple-organ dysfunction syndrome.

_____ **14.** Your patient has sustained a serious internal injury. He is agitated, anxious, and restless. He complains of nausea and thirst and has a normal blood pressure. What phase of shock is he MOST likely in?
- **A.** Irreversible shock
- **B.** Compensated shock
- **C.** Decompensated shock
- **D.** Terminal shock

_____ 15. Pediatric patients are unique, as compared to adults, in that they can often compensate even when they have lost up to __________ of their blood volume.

A. 15%

B. 25%

C. 35%

D. 45%

Labeling

Label the following diagram with the correct terms.

1. Relationship between the organism and the cells

A
B
C
D
E

A. ______________________

B. ______________________

C. ______________________

D. ______________________

E. ______________________

Fill in the Blank

Read each item carefully, and then complete the statement by filling in the missing word(s).

1. When the paramedic allows his or her initial reference point to distort an estimate while conducting the assessment, this is known as a(n) __________ bias.

2. To protect vital organs, the body attempts to __________ by __________ blood flow from organs that are more tolerant of low flow to vital organs that cannot tolerate hypoperfusion.

3. Blood flow through capillary beds is regulated by the capillary __________, circular muscular walls that constrict and dilate to increase or decrease flow.

4. Along with the baroreceptors are __________, which measure subtle shifts in the amount of carbon dioxide in the arterial blood.

5. The switch from __________ metabolism to __________ metabolism is a critical point that begins to produce lactic acidosis from this inefficient form of metabolism.

6. Effects of norepinephrine are primarily __________ and __________ in nature and center on vasoconstriction and __________ (increasing/decreasing) peripheral vascular resistance.

7. A reduction in __________ blood flow produces acute tubular __________, which in turn leads to __________ (urine output of less than 20 mL/h).

8. The last phase of shock, when this condition has progressed to a terminal stage, is __________ shock.

9. In cases of suspected __________ __________, you must recognize the need for expeditious transport for pericardiocentesis at the emergency department (ED).

10. __________ shock occurs when the heart is unable to circulate sufficient blood to maintain adequate peripheral oxygen delivery.

Identify

In the following case study, list the chief complaint, vital signs, and pertinent negatives.

You are called to the home of a 74-year-old man who is experiencing chest pain. Upon arrival, you begin your chest pain protocol. John, the patient, is experiencing tightness in his chest and left arm. You place John on high-flow supplemental oxygen and obtain a 12-lead electrocardiogram (ECG). You determine that John's heart is in a sinus bradycardia with a rate of 52 beats/min. Both his lungs have some crackles at their bases, he is breathing 24 breaths/min, and his room air saturation is Spo_2 92%. He is slightly confused, but he comes around with the oxygen and is able to answer all your questions. His pupils are equal, round, and reactive to light and accommodation (PERRLA). You are unable to feel a pulse in his wrist. His blood pressure (BP) is 80/56 mm Hg, and he is diaphoretic. You determine that the rate and strength of John's heart are causing the problem. You realize that John could be in cardiogenic shock. You start an IV line and a low-dose dopamine (Intropin) drip. You feel that John is a top priority and head to the most appropriate hospital as quickly as possible.

1. Chief complaint:

____

____

2. Vital signs:

____

____

3. Pertinent negatives:

____

____

Complete the Patient Care Report (PCR)

Reread the case study in the preceding Identify exercise, and then complete the following PCR for the patient.

EMS Patient Care Report (PCR)			
Date:	Incident No.:	Nature of Call:	Location:

Dispatched:	En Route:	At Scene:	Transport:	At Hospital:	In Service:

Patient Information	
Age: Sex: Weight (in kg [lb]):	Allergies: Medications: Past Medical History: Chief Complaint:

Vital Signs				
Time:	BP:	Pulse:	Respirations:	SpO_2:
Time:	BP:	Pulse:	Respirations:	SpO_2:
Time:	BP:	Pulse:	Respirations:	SpO_2:

EMS Treatment (circle all that apply)				
Oxygen @ ______ L/min via (circle one): NC NRM Bag-mask device		Assisted Ventilation	Airway Adjunct	CPR
Defibrillation	Bleeding Control	Bandaging	Splinting	Other:

Narrative

Ambulance Calls

The following case scenarios provide an opportunity to explore the concerns associated with patient management and paramedic care. Read each scenario, and then answer each question.

1. A 45-year old woman was struck by a motorcycle as she attempted to cross the street. You find her lying by the side of the road, reporting severe pain in her abdomen where the motorcycle hit her. To assess her state of perfusion, how will you assess the following?
   a. Her peripheral perfusion:

   ____

   b. The perfusion to her vital organs:

   ____

2. You are called to a downtown concert venue in which firearms may have been deployed. You find a man lying on the floor, unresponsive, with obvious bleeding on his leg. In the correct sequence, list the steps you will take in treating this patient who you suspect may be in shock.

   a. ______________________________

   b. ______________________________

   c. ______________________________

   d. ______________________________

   e. ______________________________

   f. ______________________________

3. A bomb exploded at a bus stop, injuring a number of bystanders. There was flying debris, including pieces of metal torn from the "backpack bomb." The first patient you come upon has multiple wounds, including a deep gash on the right side of the neck and a laceration that has partially severed the left leg near the groin. The leg laceration is gushing blood; it is too proximal to benefit from a tourniquet. Pulse is around 100 beats/min and somewhat weak; respirations are 30 breaths/min, and you suspect that the patient is already in shock.
   a. What steps would you take at the scene?

   (1)______________________________

   (2)______________________________

   (3)______________________________

   (4)______________________________

   b. What steps would you take during transport?

   (1)______________________________

   (2)______________________________

   (3)______________________________

4. A second patient from the bombing incident, an 18-year-old male, was injured by flying debris, which made a clean 10-inch incision straight across his abdomen. He is responsive and in moderate distress. This patient is a picture of shock. His pulse is 104 beats/min and regular, respirations are 28 breaths/min and slightly labored, and BP is 104/70 mm Hg. You see the patient's intestines outside his abdomen.

a. What steps would you take at the scene?

(1)________________________________

(2)________________________________

(3)________________________________

b. What steps would you take during transport?

(1)________________________________

(2)________________________________

(3)________________________________

5. A third patient from the car bombing incident is a 20-year-old female in considerable respiratory distress. There is a 2-inch-wide hole in her right chest through which you can hear air being sucked on inhalation. Her skin is warm. Her pulse is 108 beats/min and regular, respirations are 30 breaths/min and gasping, and BP is 112/64 mm Hg.

a. What steps would you take at the scene?

(1)________________________________

(2)________________________________

(3)________________________________

b. What steps would you take during transport?

(1)________________________________

(2)________________________________

(3)________________________________

6. A 55-year-old female was the driver of a car that crashed into a bridge abutment in the early hours of the morning. The patient is responsive but very restless. She is sweating profusely. Her chest is stable (it's too dark to see whether there are bruises). She can move all her extremities. Her pulse is 88 beats/min, respirations are 28 breaths/min, and BP is 100/68 mm Hg.

a. What steps would you take at the scene?

(1)________________________________

(2)________________________________

(3)________________________________

(4)________________________________

(5)________________________________

b. What steps would you take during transport?

(1)______________________________

(2)______________________________

(3)______________________________

(4)______________________________

True/False

If you believe the statement to be more true than false, write the letter "T" in the space provided. If you believe the statement to be more false than true, write the letter "F."

______ **1.** The patient with obstructive shock may have jugular vein distention.

______ **2.** Cardiogenic shock can lead to warm skin and hypertension.

______ **3.** Severe bacterial infection can lead to septic shock.

______ **4.** Simple fainting is also called psychogenic shock.

______ **5.** The capacitance vessels are the small arterioles.

______ **6.** When a patient is in "cold shock," he or she may benefit from epinephrine.

______ **7.** Neurogenic shock usually results from spinal cord injury.

______ **8.** Sensitization means developing a heightened reaction to a substance.

______ **9.** A recurrent large area of subcutaneous edema of sudden onset, usually disappearing within 24 hours and mainly seen in young women, is called angioedema.

______ **10.** Poor vessel function, a cause of shock, can be caused by infection and/or drug abuse.

Short Answer

Complete this section with short written answers using the space provided.

1. List what each of the following could indicate using the acronym M-T-SHIP:

M.______________________________

T.______________________________

S.______________________________

H.______________________________

I.______________________________

P.______________________________

2. Karl Weick's "five-step process" for communicating intuitive decisions and obtaining feedback from team members includes:

a. ______________________________

b. ______________________________

c. ______________________________

d. ______________________________

e. ______________________________

Fill in the Table

Fill in the missing parts of the tables.

1. The "H and T" questions of cardiac arrest

Reversible Causes of Cardiac Arrest	Questions to Ask Your Team
Hypovolemia	Does this patient have any evidence of internal or external bleeding or fluid loss?
________________	How well is the patient oxygenating? Could there have been a respiratory event that led to this cardiac arrest?
Hydrogen ion (acidosis)	Is there any reason for metabolic or respiratory acidosis in this patient?
________________	Does this patient undergo renal dialysis? Might the electrolytes be altered (ie, is the patient on a liquid diet)?
Hypothermia	Does the patient feel cold to touch? If so, obtain the core body temperature.
________________	Does the patient have diabetes? What is the blood glucose level?
Tension pneumothorax	Does the patient have bilateral breath sounds? Is the patient becoming difficult to ventilate? Consider the need for chest decompression.
________________	Is there penetrating trauma to the patient's heart? Consider the need for pericardiocentesis or ultrasound (in the emergency department).
Toxins	Consider substance abuse (ie, narcotics or opiates). Consider naloxone (Narcan) intravenously/intramuscularly/intranasally.
________________	Does the patient have a history of blood clots? Does the patient smoke and/or take birth control? Has the patient had a recent long-bone immobilization?
Thrombosis (coronary)	Does the patient have a large acute myocardial infarction developing? Is this patient a candidate for percutaneous coronary intervention (PCI)?
________________	Is there a mechanism of injury for life-threatening trauma?

2. Compensated versus decompensated shock

Compensated Shock	Decompensated Shock
• Agitation, anxiety, restlessness • ________________ • Weak, rapid (thready) pulse • Clammy (cool, moist) skin • ________________ • ________________ • Nausea, vomiting • Delayed capillary refill in infants and children • ________________ • ________________	• Altered mental status (verbal to unresponsive)[a] • ________________ • ________________ • Thready or absent peripheral pulses • Ashen, mottled, or cyanotic skin • ________________ • Diminished urine output (oliguria) • ________________

[a]Mental status changes are late indicators.

3. Types of shock

Types of Shock	Examples of Potential Causes	Signs and Symptoms	Assessment and Treatment
________	Inadequate heart function Disease of muscle tissue Impaired electrical system Disease or injury	Chest pain Irregular pulse Weak pulse Low BP Cyanosis (lips, under nails) Cool, clammy, mottled, or flushed skin Anxiety Rales Pulmonary edema Hepatomegaly	________ ________
________	Mechanical obstruction of the cardiac muscle causing a decrease in cardiac output **1.** Tension pneumothorax **2.** Cardiac tamponade	Dependent on cause: • Dyspnea • Rapid, weak pulse • Rapid, shallow breaths • Decreased lung compliance • Unilateral, decreased, or absent breath sounds • Decreased BP • JVD • Subcutaneous emphysema • Cyanosis • Tracheal deviation toward affected side • Beck triad (cardiac tamponade): – JVD – Narrowing pulse pressure – Muffled heart tones	________ ________ ________ ________
________	Severe bacterial infection	Warm, unstable skin temperatures Tachycardia Low blood pressure	________ ________ ________
________	Cervical or thoracic spinal cord injury, which causes widespread blood vessel dilation	Bradycardia (slow pulse) or normal pulse Low BP Signs of neck injury	________ ________
________	Extreme life-threatening allergic reaction	Develop within seconds Mild itching or rash Burning skin Vascular dilation Generalized edema Coma Rapid death	________ ________ ________ ________

______________	Temporary, generalized vascular dilation Anxiety, bad news, sight of injury or blood, prospect of medical treatment, severe pain, illness, tiredness	Rapid pulse Normal or low BP	______________ ______________
______________	Blood or fluid loss	Rapid, weak pulse Low BP Change in mental status Cyanosis (lips, nail beds) Cool, clammy skin Increased respiratory rate	______________ ______________ ______________
______________	Severe chest injury, airway obstruction	Rapid, weak pulse Low BP Change in mental status Cyanosis (lips, nail beds) Cool, clammy skin Increased respiratory rate	______________ ______________ ______________

Abbreviations: BP, blood pressure; CPAP/BPAP, continuous positive airway pressure/bilevel positive airway pressure; IM, intramuscularly; JVD, jugular venous distention; KVO, keep vein open.

CHAPTER 41

Obstetrics

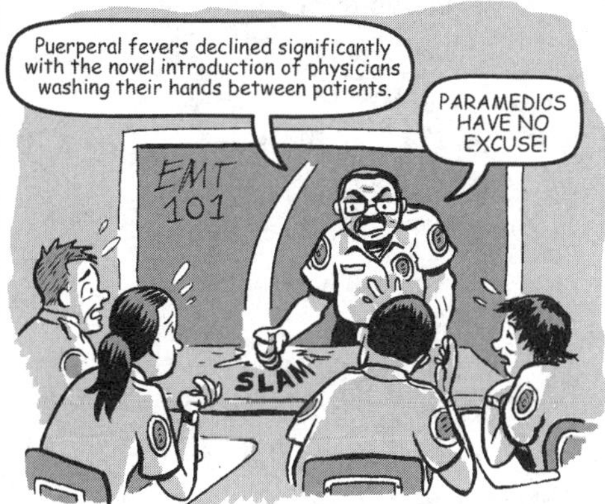

Matching

Part I

Match each of the items in the left column to the appropriate term in the right column.

_____ 1. The developing, unborn infant inside the uterus.

_____ 2. A situation in which a fetus is large, usually defined as weighing more than 4,500 g (almost 9 pounds); also known as "large for gestational age."

_____ 3. An incision in the perineal skin made to prevent tearing during childbirth.

_____ 4. Intentional expulsion of the fetus.

_____ 5. Thinning and shortening of the cervix; a normal process that occurs as the uterus contracts.

_____ 6. A disease of the liver that occurs only during pregnancy, in which hormones affect the gallbladder by slowing down or blocking the normal bile flow from the liver; the most common symptom is profuse, painful itching, particularly of the hands and feet.

_____ 7. The interior of the cervix.

_____ 8. A situation in which the head of the fetus is larger than the woman's pelvis; in most cases, cesarean section is required for such a delivery.

_____ 9. A delivery in which the buttocks come out first.

_____ 10. A plug of mucus, sometimes mixed with blood, that is expelled from the dilating cervix and discharged from the vagina.

_____ 11. The fluid-filled, baglike membrane in which the fetus develops.

_____ 12. An extremely rare, life-threatening condition that occurs when amniotic fluid and fetal cells enter the pregnant woman's pulmonary and circulatory system through the placenta via the umbilical veins, causing an exaggerated allergic response from the woman's body.

_____ 13. A watery fluid that provides the fetus with a weightless environment in which to develop.

_____ 14. A premature separation of the placenta from the wall of the uterus.

_____ 15. Expulsion of the fetus, from any cause, before 20 weeks' gestation.

_____ 16. A scoring system for assessing the status of a newborn that assigns a number value to each of five areas of assessment.

_____ 17. The term for an oocyte once it has been fertilized and multiplies into cells.

_____ 18. A hormone produced by the anterior pituitary gland that is important in the menstrual cycle.

A. Abortion
B. Abruptio placenta
C. Amniotic fluid
D. Amniotic fluid embolism
E. Amniotic sac
F. Apgar scoring system
G. Blastocyst
H. Bloody show
I. Breech presentation
J. Cephalopelvic disproportion
K. Cervical canal
L. Cholestasis
M. Chronic hypertension
N. Complete abortion
O. Corpus luteum
P. Crowning
Q. Cytomegalovirus (CMV)
R. Eclampsia

______	**19.** The stage of labor that begins with the onset of regular labor pains (crampy abdominal pains) during which the uterus contracts and the cervix effaces.	**S.** Ectopic pregnancy
______	**20.** An egg that attaches outside the uterus, typically in a fallopian tube.	**T.** Effacement
______	**21.** Seizures that result from severe hypertension in a pregnant woman.	**U.** Elective abortion
______	**22.** A herpesvirus that can produce symptoms of prolonged high fever, chills, headache, malaise, extreme fatigue, and an enlarged spleen.	**V.** Episiotomy
______	**23.** The appearance of the newborn's body part (usually the head) at the vaginal opening at the beginning of labor.	**W.** Fetal macrosomia
______	**24.** The remains of a follicle after an oocyte has been released; secretes progesterone.	**X.** Fetus
______	**25.** Expulsion of all products of conception from the uterus.	**Y.** First stage of labor
______	**26.** A blood pressure that is equal to or greater than 140/90 mm Hg and exists prior to pregnancy, occurs before the 20th week of pregnancy, or persists postpartum.	**Z.** Follicle-stimulating hormone (FSH)

Part II

Match each of the items in the left column to the appropriate term in the right column.

______	**1.** A dark green-black material in the amniotic fluid that indicates fetal distress, and that can be aspirated into the fetus's lungs during delivery; the fetus's first bowel movement.	**A.** Gestational hypertension
______	**2.** The vaginal discharge of blood and mucus that occurs following delivery of a newborn; it usually lasts several days and then gradually decreases over the weeks following delivery.	**B.** Gestational period
______	**3.** In pregnancy, a feeling of relief of pressure in the upper abdomen; a premonitory sign of labor.	**C.** Gravidity
______	**4.** The mechanism by which the fetus and the placenta are expelled from the uterus.	**D.** Habitual abortion
______	**5.** A protein that plays a key role in the menstrual cycle by triggering release of follicle-stimulating hormone.	**E.** Human immunodeficiency virus (HIV)
______	**6.** The outer protective layer of tissue in the uterus.	**F.** Hydramnios
______	**7.** The number of live births a woman has had.	**G.** Hyperemesis gravidarum
______	**8.** A mature oocyte.	**H.** Imminent abortion
______	**9.** A situation in which the umbilical cord is wrapped around the fetus's neck; cord compression may occur during labor, causing the fetal heart rate to slow and resulting in fetal distress.	**I.** Incomplete abortion
______	**10.** The middle layer of tissue in the uterus.	**J.** Inhibin
______	**11.** A situation in which the umbilical cord comes out of the vagina before the newborn.	**K.** Labor
______	**12.** The state of the pregnant woman before birth.	**L.** Lightening
______	**13.** A condition of late pregnancy that involves gradual onset of hypertension, headache, visual changes, and swelling of the hands and feet; also called pregnancy-induced hypertension or toxemia of pregnancy.	**M.** Lochia
______	**14.** The period of time after a woman has given birth.	**N.** Meconium
______	**15.** A condition in which the placenta develops over and covers the cervix.	**O.** Missed abortion
______	**16.** A situation in which a fetus has died during the first 20 weeks of gestation, but has remained in utero.	**P.** Myometrium
______	**17.** The tissue attached to the uterine wall that nourishes the fetus through the umbilical cord.	**Q.** Nuchal cord
______	**18.** Expulsion of the fetus that results in some products of conception remaining in the uterus.	**R.** Ovum

______	**19.** A spontaneous abortion that cannot be prevented.	**S.** Parity
______	**20.** A condition of persistent nausea and vomiting during pregnancy.	**T.** Perimetrium
______	**21.** A condition in which there is too much amniotic fluid; also known as polyhydramnios.	**U.** Placenta
______	**22.** The time that it takes for the fetus to develop in utero, normally 38 weeks.	**V.** Placenta previa
______	**23.** The total number of times a woman has been pregnant, including the current pregnancy.	**W.** Postpartum
______	**24.** Three or more consecutive pregnancies that end in miscarriage.	**X.** Preeclampsia
______	**25.** An infection that causes acquired immune deficiency syndrome (AIDS).	**Y.** Prenatal
______	**26.** High blood pressure that develops after 20th week of pregnancy in women with previously normal blood pressures, and that resolves spontaneously in the postpartum period; formerly known as pregnancy-induced hypertension.	**Z.** Prolapsed umbilical cord

Part III

Match each of the items in the left column to the appropriate term in the right column.

______	**1.** A potentially fatal complication of childbirth in which the placenta fails to detach properly and results in the uterus turning inside out.	**A.** Rh factor
______	**2.** The interior of the body of the uterus.	**B.** Second stage of labor
______	**3.** The conduit connecting the pregnant woman to the fetus via the placenta; it contains two arteries and one vein.	**C.** Septic abortion
______	**4.** A delivery in which the fetus lies crosswise in the uterus; one hand may protrude through the vagina.	**D.** Shoulder dystocia
______	**5.** Expulsion of the fetus that occurs naturally; also called miscarriage.	**E.** Spontaneous abortion
______	**6.** A complication of delivery in where there is difficulty delivering the shoulders of a newborn; the shoulder cannot get past the woman's symphysis pubis.	**F.** Supine hypotensive syndrome
______	**7.** A life-threatening emergency in which the uterus becomes infected following any type of abortion.	**G.** Third stage of labor
______	**8.** The stage of labor in which the newborn's head enters the birth canal, during which contractions become more intense and more frequent.	**H.** Threatened abortion
______	**9.** Expulsion of the fetus that is attempting to take place but has not occurred yet; usually occurs in the first trimester.	**I.** TORCH syndrome
______	**10.** The stage of labor in which the placenta is expelled.	**J.** Toxoplasmosis
______	**11.** Low blood pressure resulting from compression of the inferior vena cava by the weight of the pregnant uterus when the woman is supine.	**K.** Transverse presentation
______	**12.** A protein found on the red blood cells of most people; when a woman without this protein is impregnated by a man with this protein, the woman's body can create antibodies against the protein that attack future pregnancies.	**L.** Umbilical cord
______	**13.** An infection caused by a parasite that pregnant women may get from handling or eating contaminated food or exposure from handling cat litter; the fetus can become infected.	**M.** Uterine cavity
______	**14.** An infection that occurs in neonates as a result of organisms passing through the placenta from the woman to the fetus; includes toxoplasmosis, other agents, rubella, cytomegalovirus, and herpes simplex.	**N.** Uterine inversion

Multiple Choice

Read each item carefully, and then select the best response.

_____ 1. An abortion that occurs naturally and affects 10% to 25% of all pregnancies is called a(n):

A. spontaneous abortion.
B. septic abortion.
C. threatened abortion.
D. incomplete abortion.

_____ 2. What is the condition in which the placenta is implanted low in the uterus and, as it grows, it partially obscures the cervical canal?

A. Abruptio placenta
B. Molar pregnancy
C. Pseudocyesis
D. Placenta previa

_____ 3. Which of the following terms describes a woman who has had two or more pregnancies, irrespective of the outcome?

A. Multigravida
B. Primipara
C. Multipara
D. Parity

_____ 4. When the baby's head enters the birth canal, the __________ stage of labor begins.

A. fourth
B. third
C. second
D. first

_____ 5. The Apgar scoring system is an evaluation tool for the newborn's vital functions and is recommended to be taken at which intervals after birth?

A. 2 minutes and 10 minutes
B. 1 minute and 5 minutes
C. 5 minutes and 10 minutes
D. 1 minute and 2 minutes

_____ 6. __________ of blood loss, or more, after delivery is considered postpartum hemorrhage.

A. 1,000 mL
B. 150 mL
C. 750 mL
D. 500 mL

_____ 7. Which of the following medications can be used to control postpartum hemorrhage in the prehospital setting?

A. Oxytocin
B. Terbutaline
C. Magnesium sulfate
D. Diphenhydramine

_____ 8. An infection that occurs in neonates as a result of organisms passing through the placenta from woman to fetus is referred to as:

A. RSV.
B. toxoplasmosis.
C. hemolytic disease.
D. Down syndrome.

_____ **9.** The normal gestational period for an infant to develop in the uterus is how many weeks?

A. 30

B. 32

C. 38

D. 42

_____ **10.** A pregnant woman's heart rate gradually increases during pregnancy by an average of how many beats/min by term?

A. 15 to 20 beats/min

B. 5 to 10 beats/min

C. 20 to 25 beats/min

D. 15 to 30 beats/min

Labeling

Label the following diagram with the correct terms.

1. Structures of the pregnant uterus

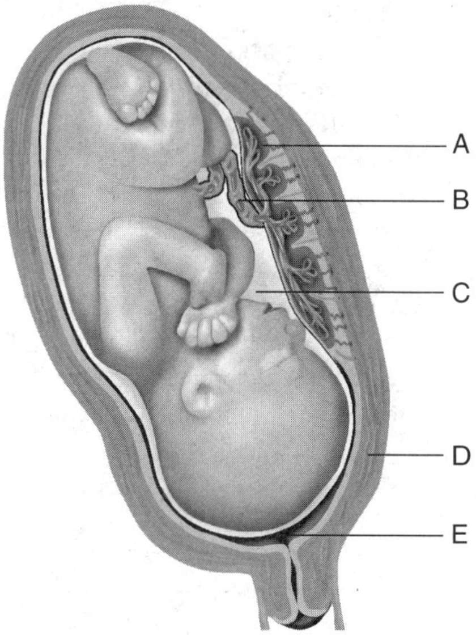

A. ______________________________

B. ______________________________

C. ______________________________

D. ______________________________

E. ______________________________

Fill in the Blank

Read each item carefully, and then complete the statement by filling in the missing word(s).

1. The __________ is a membranous bag that encloses the fetus in watery fluid.

2. The workload of the heart __________ significantly during both gestation and labor.

3. As maternal oxygen demand __________, the respiratory physiology changes.

4. __________ is the most serious of the hypertension disorders that occur during pregnancy.

5. __________ __________ develops after the 20th week of pregnancy in women with a normal blood pressure.

6. Some women experience recurrent miscarriages or _________ _________.

7. __________ __________ refers to a premature partial or incomplete separation of a normally implanted placenta from the uterus.

8. The __________ __________ of labor begins with the onset of labor.

9. In a(n) __________ presentation, the fetus lies crosswise in the uterus and may wave at the paramedic with one hand protruding from the vagina.

10. __________ __________ is a drug used in pregnancy as the principal management for eclampsia.

Identify

After reading the following case study, list the chief complaint, vital signs, and pertinent findings.

You are called to a private residence for a report of a pregnant patient who has vaginal bleeding. The patient is lying in bed. When you ask what is wrong, she tells you, "I am bleeding from my vagina." You see blood on the sheets. You and your partner start a primary survey. You then take the vital signs, and your partner obtains a SAMPLE history. The patient is 35 years old and states that she started to bleed about half an hour ago. Upon questioning, she tells you there is no pain, the blood was bright red, this is her third pregnancy, and she is in her eighth month. Both the previous pregnancies were full term and delivered by cesarean section. She states that she had strong contractions, but they have decreased. She feels weak and asks if she can have a drink of water. She has no allergies, is taking vitamin supplements per doctor's orders, has no significant past medical history, and had a light breakfast of toast and juice about 2 hours ago. Your partner reports the pulse to be 110 beats/min and thready, respirations are 24 breaths/min, blood pressure (BP) is 100/70 mm Hg, Spo_2 is 94%, and the patient is pale and diaphoretic. The patient tells you that the BP reading you just measured is lower than the pressure the doctor measured last week at her checkup appointment. You put the patient on 100% supplemental oxygen using a nonrebreathing mask, place a loose trauma pad over the vagina, prepare for immediate transport, start a large-bore IV line in the ambulance, contact medical control to discuss the use of magnesium sulfate (some emergency medical services [EMS] systems may use this medication in this kind of case), and notify the hospital so that personnel there can be properly prepared upon your arrival. You arrive at the receiving facility in 15 minutes and are told to go immediately to the delivery room. Later that evening while delivering another patient to the same hospital, you are informed that the mother delivered, and although the baby's birth weight is low, both the mother and the baby are expected to be fine.

1. Chief complaint:

____

____

2. Vital signs:

____

____

3. Pertinent findings:

____

____

Complete the Patient Care Report (PCR)

Reread the incident scenario in the preceding Identify exercise and then complete the following PCR for the patient.

EMS Patient Care Report (PCR)					
Date:	Incident No.:	Nature of Call:		Location:	
Dispatched:	En Route:	At Scene:	Transport:	At Hospital:	In Service:

Patient Information	
Age: Sex: Weight (in kg [lb]):	Allergies: Medications: Past Medical History: Chief Complaint:

Vital Signs				
Time:	BP:	Pulse:	Respirations:	SpO_2:
Time:	BP:	Pulse:	Respirations:	SpO_2:
Time:	BP:	Pulse:	Respirations:	SpO_2:

EMS Treatment (circle all that apply)				
Oxygen @ _____ L/min via (circle one): NC NRM Bag-mask device	Assisted Ventilation	Airway Adjunct	CPR	
Defibrillation	Bleeding Control	Bandaging	Splinting	Other:

Narrative

Ambulance Calls

The following case scenarios provide an opportunity to explore the concerns associated with patient management and paramedic care. Read each scenario, and then answer each question.

1. A 22-year-old woman calls for an ambulance because of vaginal bleeding. She states that she is "about 3 months pregnant" and that the bleeding started yesterday, when she thinks she passed some tissue. She has used about 10 sanitary napkins since then. On examination, her skin feels cool and wet. Her pulse is 120 beats/min and weak, and her BP is 90/60 mm Hg.

a. This woman is likely experiencing a(n) _____________ abortion.

A. threatened
B. imminent
C. incomplete
D. missed
E. septic

b. List the steps in the prehospital management of this patient.

(1)______________________________

(2)______________________________

(3)______________________________

(4)______________________________

(5)______________________________

(6)______________________________

(7)______________________________

2. A 32-year-old woman calls for an ambulance because she is "feeling poorly." She states that she is "about 6 months along" in a pregnancy. She has not had any prenatal care. She had some vaginal bleeding "early on," but it lasted only a few days and then stopped. Now, for several days, the patient has felt vaguely unwell. She has had a brownish vaginal discharge that smells rank, and "things are very quiet in there." On physical examination, the patient does not appear to be in any distress. Her pulse is 74 beats/min and regular, respirations are 18 breaths/min and unlabored, and BP is 120/80 mm Hg. On abdominal examination, you can feel the uterine fundus just above the pelvic brim; it feels quite hard. You are not able to hear fetal heart tones, but the room is noisy, so you are not sure what to make of that finding.

a. This woman is likely experiencing a(n) _____________ abortion.

A. threatened
B. imminent
C. incomplete
D. missed
E. septic

b. Describe the prehospital management required for this patient.

____

____

3. A 20-year-old primigravida calls for an ambulance because of vaginal bleeding. She states that she is in her fourth month of pregnancy and has been fine up to now, but this morning she noticed some bleeding. She denies abdominal pain or cramping. On physical examination, there are no abnormal findings.

a. This woman is likely experiencing a(n) _____________ abortion.

A. threatened
B. imminent
C. incomplete
D. missed
E. septic

b. Describe the prehospital management required for this patient.

____

____

4. You are called to a suburban home for a "sick girl." The patient is a 16-year-old girl with a high fever. She insists on giving you her history privately, without her parents in the room. After her parents exit, the girl tells you that she had gone that morning to "some hole in the wall" to have an abortion. A few hours after she got home, she started to feel sick, and she has been having a bad-smelling, bloody vaginal discharge ever since. On examination, she looks very ill. Her pulse is 120 beats/min and weak, respirations are 28 breaths/min and shallow, BP is 80/60 mm Hg, and oral temperature is 40°C (104°F).

a. This patient is likely experiencing a(n) ____________ abortion.

A. threatened
B. imminent
C. incomplete
D. missed
E. septic

b. List the steps in the prehospital management of this patient.

(1)____

(2)____

(3)____

(4)____

(5)____

(6)____

5. You are called to the home of a weeping 26-year-old woman in the 15th week of pregnancy. "It's happening again," she sobs, "I just know it's happening again." She tells you that she has had three miscarriages in the past and that this morning she started having severe abdominal cramps and bleeding, "just like all the other times." She has used six sanitary napkins since the bleeding started about 3 hours ago. On physical examination, she is very distraught. Her pulse is 110 beats/min and regular, respirations are 24 breaths/min and unlabored, BP is 110/70 mm Hg, and she is febrile. On palpating the abdomen, you can feel the uterine contractions.

a. This woman is likely experiencing a(n) ____________ abortion.

A. threatened
B. imminent
C. incomplete
D. missed
E. septic

b. List the steps in the prehospital management of this patient.

(1)____

(2)____

(3)____

(4)____

(5)____

6. You are called to the home of a 36-year-old grand multipara whose chief complaint is bleeding. She is in her 11th pregnancy and "due any day now." She states that the bleeding, a bright red blood, started a few hours ago without any warning. She has not had any cramps or other symptoms, and "the baby is still kicking like a soccer player." On physical examination, the woman looks a little pale and apprehensive. Her pulse is 124 beats/min and regular, respirations are 28 breaths/min and unlabored, and BP is 100/68 mm Hg; she is afebrile. On gentle palpation, you find the abdomen soft. The fundus is at the level of the xiphoid, and fetal heart tones are audible. The fetal heart rate is 140 beats/min.

a. List three possible causes of this woman's bleeding.

(1)____

(2)____

(3)____

b. Of those three causes, which do you think is the most likely cause in her case?

____

c. Which signs led you to this diagnosis?

(1)____

(2)____

(3)____

(4)____

d. List the steps you will take in managing this patient.

(1)____

(2)____

(3)____

(4)____

(5)____

(6)____

7. You are called to see a 28-year-old woman in her 35th week of pregnancy after she had a "fainting spell." The patient's husband greets you at the door and tells you, "We were just sitting there talking—Agnes was lying in bed, and I was sitting in the chair—and suddenly I look over, and I see that she's out cold. Not sleeping, just out." The patient has meanwhile regained consciousness. She says she feels rather dizzy and has a slight headache but otherwise feels well. She denies vaginal bleeding. On physical examination, her pulse is 104 beats/min and regular, her respirations are 24 breaths/min and unlabored, and her BP is 90/60 mm Hg. You have her roll onto her side and recheck her vital signs a few minutes later; her pulse is now 88 beats/min and her BP is 120/72 mm Hg. Her fundus is nearly at the level of the xiphoid, and fetal heart tones are present at a rate of 160 beats/min.

a. This woman is likely experiencing

A. an inevitable abortion.
B. preeclampsia.
C. eclampsia.
D. abruptio placenta.
E. supine hypotensive syndrome.

b. List the steps in the prehospital care of this patient.

(1)__________

(2)__________

(3)__________

(4)__________

(5)__________

8. You are called to a downtown department store, where an obviously pregnant woman has fallen and twisted her ankle. You find her surrounded by a knot of agitated people, none of them more agitated than the store manager. As you are checking the woman's pedal pulses, you notice that both ankles are swollen—not just the one she injured. You decide you had better get a set of vital signs because you vaguely remember learning that vital signs should be measured in every patient, especially every pregnant patient. In this woman, you find the pulse is 110 beats/min and regular, respirations are 20 breaths/min and unlabored, and BP is 150/90 mm Hg. As you are taking the radial pulse, you notice that the patient's hands seem puffy. It is too noisy in the store to even bother trying to listen for fetal heart tones, but the woman tells you that the baby is "kicking away."

a. This woman is likely experiencing:

A. an inevitable abortion.
B. preeclampsia.
C. eclampsia.
D. abruptio placenta.
E. supine hypotensive syndrome.

b. List the steps in the prehospital care of this patient.

(1)__________

(2)__________

(3)__________

c. En route to the hospital, you find yourself locked in a traffic jam on the freeway. Meanwhile, your patient starts complaining of cramping abdominal pains. "I've never had a baby before," she says, "but I think these are labor pains." While you look helplessly at the line of cars stretching endlessly in front of and behind the ambulance, the woman's eyes suddenly roll back, and she has a grand mal seizure. Which steps will you take now?

(1)__________

(2)__________

(3)__________

(4)__________

(5)__________

9. A 26-year-old woman in her 30th week of pregnancy was the driver of a car that skidded off the road and plowed head-on into a tree. The woman was wearing a shoulder/lap seat belt. Sitting in the passenger seat of the same car was a woman in her 28th week of pregnancy (they were returning together from a natural childbirth class), also wearing a seat belt. En route to the call, you try to review in your mind the injuries you will need to look for in particular because you remember that pregnancy makes a woman more vulnerable to trauma.

a. List five anatomic or physiologic changes of pregnancy that affect a woman's susceptibility or response to trauma.

(1)____

(2)____

(3)____

(4)____

(5)____

b. On reaching the scene of the accident, you find the driver of the car conscious, still sitting behind the wheel of the car. She complains of thirst. On physical examination, her skin is cool and moist. Her pulse is 120 beats/min and regular, respirations are 24 breaths/min and shallow, and BP is 110/68 mm Hg. There is a steering wheel bruise on the upper abdomen. The abdomen is not particularly tender, and it is not rigid. The conditions are too noisy to try to hear fetal heart tones. List the steps in managing this patient.

(1)____

(2)____

(3)____

(4)____

(5)____

(6)____

(7)____

c. The front-seat passenger is also fully conscious. She complains of "whiplash" but otherwise feels well. "At least the baby's okay," she says. "I can feel him moving around." On physical examination, her skin is warm and moist. Her pulse is 100 beats/min and regular, respirations are 20 breaths/min and unlabored, and her BP is 124/70 mm Hg. You do not find any evidence of injury. Can you conclude that there has been no injury to the fetus? Explain the reason for your answer.

____

____

____

____

10. For each of the following cases, indicate one of the following:
T There is time to transport the woman to the hospital for delivery.
D You will have to assist in emergency delivery in the field.
For each case that you decide requires prehospital delivery, indicate which, if any, complications you must anticipate.

________ **a.** A 20-year-old nullipara (gravida 1, para 0) in her first pregnancy. She says her water broke about 6 hours ago. Now her contractions are about 2 minutes apart, and she feels a need to move her bowels. You are 20 minutes from the hospital. Which, if any, complications may occur?

____

____

_______ **b.** A 32-year-old multipara (gravida 10, para 8) who has been in labor about 5 hours. Her contractions are 3 minutes apart. She says she thinks the baby's coming. You are 10 minutes from the hospital. What, if any, complications may occur?

____

____

_______ **c.** A 25-year-old nullipara (gravida 1, para 0) who has been in labor for 9 hours. Her contractions are 4 to 5 minutes apart. You are 20 minutes from the hospital. Which, if any, complications may occur?

____

____

_______ **d.** A 30-year-old multipara (gravida 4, para 3) who has been in labor for 6 hours. She had two of her three children by cesarean section. Her contractions are 2 minutes apart, and she is crowning. You are 5 minutes from the hospital. Which, if any, complications may occur?

____

____

_______ **e.** A 28-year-old nullipara (gravida 1, para 0) whose contractions started 24 hours ago. They do not come at regular intervals, and they have not gotten much more intense since they started. You are 25 minutes from the hospital. Which, if any, complications may occur?

____

____

_______ **f.** A 24-year-old multipara (gravida 3, para 2) who announces, as you enter her apartment, "Hurry, the twins are coming any minute!" She says she has been in labor "quite a while," and you time her contractions as coming less than 2 minutes apart. You are 20 minutes from the hospital. Which, if any, complications may occur?

____

____

11. You are assisting in the delivery of a baby in the lingerie section of a downtown department store.

a. The baby's head delivers spontaneously, and you notice that it is covered with a membrane. What should you do?

____

____

b. You deal with that problem successfully. The next thing you notice is that the umbilical cord is wound tightly around the baby's neck. What should you do about that?

____

____

c. List the steps in carrying out the remainder of the delivery (second and third stages).

(1)____

(2)____

(3)_____

(4)_____

(5)_____

(6)_____

(7)_____

(8)_____

(9)_____

12. During another one of your weekends off at the ski lodge, when you are cheerfully snowed in, one of the other guests arrives in the lounge and asks, "Does anyone here know anything about delivering a baby? My wife seems to be in labor." You shrivel up into a corner of your chair, hoping someone else will come forward, but there do not seem to be any obstetricians among the skiers. So, with a sigh, you stand up and follow the distraught husband to his room. There you find a woman in active labor, already crowning. Inspecting the presenting part, you note that it looks awfully smooth, and it has a sort of crack running down the middle.

a. What are you dealing with?

_____

_____

b. Describe how you will manage this case.

(1)_____

(2)_____

(3)_____

(4)_____

(5)_____

(6)_____

(7)_____

13. The day after you get back to work, your very first call is another "possible OB." The patient is a 24-year-old woman in her first pregnancy whose labor started about 10 hours earlier. "This wasn't supposed to happen for another month and a half," she tells you. The contractions are now about 2 minutes apart. When you inspect her to see whether she is crowning, you see a short length of umbilical cord protruding from her vagina. Describe how you will manage this case.

a. ______________________________

b. ______________________________

c. ______________________________

d. ______________________________

e. ______________________________

f. ______________________________

14. You are called to the home of a 30-year-old gravida 6, para 5, who has gone into labor. "It's twins," she announces as soon as you come in the door. "I'm carrying twins, and they're coming at any moment. I can feel it." And indeed, when you examine the woman, you find that she is crowning.

a. Describe the special measures necessary in this case.

(1)______________________________

(2)______________________________

b. After delivery of the placenta, the mother continues bleeding quite briskly from her vagina. Did this woman have any risk factors for postpartum hemorrhage? If so, what were they?

____

____

c. List three other risk factors for postpartum hemorrhage.

(1)______________________________

(2)______________________________

(3)______________________________

d. Describe how you will manage this situation.

(1)______________________________

(2)______________________________

(3)______________________________

(4)______________________________

(5)______________________________

(6)______________________________

True/False

If you believe the statement to be more true than false, write the letter "T" in the space provided. If you believe the statement to be more false than true, write the letter "F."

_______ **1.** If you are transporting a woman in labor, and she begins crowning when you are only a minute or two from the hospital, you should instruct her to cross her legs until you reach the emergency department (ED).

_______ **2.** If the fetal heart rate is less than 120 beats/min, the fetus is in danger.

_______ **3.** A woman should be discouraged from sitting up or squatting for delivery of her baby because those positions are counter to natural physiology and increase the demand on the mother's energy.

_______ **4.** If the baby is coming fast, it is more important to control the delivery than it is to drape the mother with sterile towels.

_______ **5.** If the cut ends of the umbilical cord are oozing blood, you should unclamp them and reapply the clamps more tightly.

_______ **6.** If the placenta has not delivered within 20 minutes of the baby's delivery, you should exert gentle traction on the umbilical cord while you vigorously massage the uterus.

_______ **7.** With the exception of buttocks breech, all other abnormal presentations must be delivered in the hospital.

Short Answer

Complete this section with short written answers using the space provided.

1. List the three abnormalities typically found in a child born with fetal alcohol syndrome.

a. ____

b. ____

c. ____

Fill in the Table

Fill in the missing parts of the following tables.

1. Fill in the amount of time needed for the three stages of labor for a nullipara and for a multipara.

The Stages of Labor: Nullipara Versus Multipara		
Stages of Labor	**Nullipara**	**Multipara**
First stage		
Second stage		
Third stage		

2. Fill in the missing information in distinguishing false labor from true labor.

False Labor Versus True Labor		
Parameter	**True Labor**	**False Labor**
Contractions		Irregularly spaced
Interval between contractions	Gradually shortens	
Intensity of contractions		Stays the same
Effects of analgesics	Do not abolish the pain	
Cervical changes		No changes

CHAPTER

42

Neonatal Care

© Jones & Bartlett Learning.

Don't milk the umbilical cord.

Matching

Part I

Match each of the definitions in the left column to the appropriate term in the right column.

______	1. A fissure or hole in the palate (roof of the mouth) that forms a communicating pathway between the mouth and nasal cavities.	A. Acrocyanosis
______	2. An abnormal defect or fissure in the upper lip that failed to close during development; often associated with cleft palate.	B. Apgar score
______	3. A narrowing or blockage of the nasal airway by membranous or bony tissue; a congenital condition, meaning it is present at birth.	C. Asphyxia
______	4. Blue discoloration of the skin due to the presence of deoxygenated hemoglobin in blood vessels near the skin surface.	D. Atrial septal defect
______	5. An injury of childbirth affecting the spinal nerves C8 to T1 of the brachial plexus.	E. Central cyanosis
______	6. An event where one part of the intestine folds into another part of the intestines, leading to a blockage.	F. Choanal atresia
______	7. A congenital condition in which part of the bowel is narrow.	G. Cleft lip
______	8. A congenital condition in which part of the bowel does not develop.	H. Cleft palate
______	9. Marked hypertrophy and hyperplasia of the two (circular and longitudinal) muscular layers of the pylorus.	I. Coarctation of the aorta
______	10. A hole in the atrial septal wall that allows oxygenated and deoxygenated blood to mix; patients with this hole have a higher incidence of stroke.	J. Congenital heart disease (CHC)
______	11. Condition of severely deficient supply of oxygen to the body, leading to end-organ damage.	K. Diaphragmatic hernia
______	12. Scale used to assess the status of a newborn 1 and 5 minutes after birth (range 0 to 10).	L. Erb palsy
______	13. Oxygen administered via oxygen tube and a cupped hand on the patient's face.	M. Fetal transition
______	14. A decrease in the amount of oxygen delivered to the extremities; the hands and feet turn blue because of narrowing of small arterioles toward the end of the arms and legs.	N. Foramen ovale
______	15. Pinching or narrowing of the aorta that obstructs blood flow from the heart to the systemic circulation.	O. Free-flow oxygen
______	16. An opening in the septum of the heart that closes after birth.	P. Gestation

______	**17.** The process through which the fluid in the fetal lungs is replaced with air, the ductus arteriosus constricts, and the newborn begins adequate oxygenation of its own blood.	**Q.**	Hypoplastic left heart syndrome
______	**18.** Lack of movement at the shoulder due to nerve injury resulting from the stretching of the cervical nerve roots during delivery of the newborn's head during birth; usually transient, but can be permanent.	**R.**	Hypotonia
______	**19.** Passage of loops of bowel with or without other abdominal organs, through a developmental defect in the diaphragm muscle; occurs as the bowel from the abdomen "herniates" upward through the diaphragm into the chest (thoracic) cavity.	**S.**	Hypoxic-ischemic encephalopathy
______	**20.** The most common birth defect; associated with hypoxia in the newborn period requiring intervention during the first months of life.	**T.**	Infantile hypertrophic pyloric stenosis (IHPS)
______	**21.** Damage to cells in the central nervous system (the brain and spinal cord) from inadequate oxygen.	**U.**	Intestinal atresia
______	**22.** Low or poor muscle tone (floppiness).	**V.**	Intestinal stenosis
______	**23.** Underdevelopment of the aorta, aortic valve, left ventricle, and mitral valve; this defect involves the entire left side of the heart.	**W.**	Intussusception
______	**24.** Period of time from conception to birth. For humans, the full period is normally 9 months (or 40 weeks).	**X.**	Klumpke paralysis

Part II

Match each of the definitions in the left column to the appropriate term in the right column.

______	**1.** A situation in which the ductus arteriosus does not transition after birth to become the ligamentum arteriosum; the connection between the pulmonary artery and the aorta remains, allowing some oxygenated blood to move back into the heart rather than all of it moving out of the aorta and into the systemic circulation.	**A.**	Malrotation
______	**2.** Decreased volume of amniotic fluid during a pregnancy; a risk factor associated with abnormalities of the urinary tract, postmaturity, and intrauterine growth retardation.	**B.**	Meconium
______	**3.** An infant within the first few hours after birth.	**C.**	Multifocal seizure
______	**4.** A congenital anomaly of rotation of the midgut, in which the small bowel is found predominantly on the right side of the abdomen; results in increased incidence of intestinal volvulus.	**D.**	Neonate
______	**5.** The pulse oximetry value obtained during neonatal resuscitation, which evaluates the oxygenation status of blood from the brachiocephalic artery, prior to the ductus arteriosus.	**E.**	Newborn
______	**6.** Any pregnancy that lasts more than 42 weeks.	**F.**	Oligohydramnios
______	**7.** An excessive amount of amniotic fluid; may cause preterm labor.	**G.**	Patent ductus arteriosus
______	**8.** Abnormally high red blood cell count.	**H.**	Persistent pulmonary hypertension
______	**9.** Abnormal location of the placenta in the lower part of the uterus, near or over the cervix.	**I.**	Pierre Robin sequence
______	**10.** Seizure activity that involves more than one site, is asynchronous, and is usually migratory.	**J.**	Placenta previa
______	**11.** An infant during the first month after birth.	**K.**	Polycythemia
______	**12.** A cardiac anomaly that consists of four defects: a ventricular septal defect, pulmonary stenosis, right ventricular hypertrophy, and an overriding aorta.	**L.**	Polyhydramnios
______	**13.** Describes a newborn delivered at 38 to 42 weeks' gestation.	**M.**	Postterm

______	**14.** An infant whose size and weight are considerably less than the average for infants of the same age.	**N.** Preductal oxygen saturation
______	**15.** A condition in which asphyxia continues after primary apnea, and the infant responds with a period of gasping respirations, falling pulse rate, and falling blood pressure.	**O.** Premature
______	**16.** A disease of the eye that affects premature infants, thought to be caused by disorganized growth of retinal detachment; can lead to blindness in serious cases.	**P.** Preterm
______	**17.** Describes an infant delivered at less than 37 completed weeks' gestation.	**Q.** Primary apnea
______	**18.** Underdeveloped; the condition of an infant born too soon; refers to infants delivered before 37 weeks from the first day of the last menstrual period.	**R.** Primigravida
______	**19.** Delayed transition from fetal to neonatal circulation.	**S.** Prolapsed cord
______	**20.** A condition present at birth marked by a small lower jaw; the tongue tends to fall back and downward, and there is a cleft soft palate.	**T.** Pulmonary hypertension
______	**21.** A dark green fecal material that accumulates in the fetal intestines and is discharged around the time of birth.	**U.** Pulmonary stenosis
______	**22.** Narrowing of the pulmonary valve.	**V.** Retinopathy of prematurity
______	**23.** Elevated blood pressure in the pulmonary arteries from constriction; causes problems with the blood flow in the lungs, and makes the heart work harder.	**W.** Secondary apnea
______	**24.** The condition in which the umbilical cord presents itself outside of the uterus while the fetus is still inside; an obstetric emergency during pregnancy or labor that acutely endangers the life of the fetus.	**X.** Small for gestational age
______	**25.** First pregnancy.	**Y.** Term
______	**26.** Apnea caused by oxygen deprivation; usually corrected with stimulation, such as drying or slapping the newborn's feet.	**Z.** Tetralogy of Fallot

Multiple Choice

Read each item carefully, and then select the best response.

______ **1.** As the baby is delivered, a rapid series of events must occur to enable the baby to breathe; this process is called fetal:

- **A.** transportation.
- **B.** transposition.
- **C.** transmission.
- **D.** transition.

______ **2.** A newborn delivered at less than 37 completed weeks of gestation is considered:

- **A.** preterm.
- **B.** term.
- **C.** postterm.
- **D.** None of the above

______ **3.** The Apgar score—named after Dr. Virginia Apgar, who developed this measure in 1953—helps record the condition of the newborn based on five signs. The Apgar score is typically recorded at __________ minutes after birth.

- **A.** 2 and 10
- **B.** 5 and 10
- **C.** 1 and 5
- **D.** 1 and 3

_____ **4.** Fewer than 1% of deliveries involve bradycardia that requires treatment with chest compressions or emergency medications. The most common etiology for bradycardia in a newborn is:
- **A.** fetal alcohol syndrome.
- **B.** maternal drug abuse.
- **C.** hypoxia.
- **D.** prolapsed cord.

_____ **5.** Infants do not normally pass stool before birth, but if they do and then inhale the meconium-stained amniotic fluid either in utero or at delivery, their airways may become plugged, and hypoxia may ensue. This, in turn, can lead to:
- **A.** atelectasis.
- **B.** pneumonitis.
- **C.** pneumothorax.
- **D.** All of the above

_____ **6.** Tetralogy of Fallot is a combination of four heart defects. These infants are born with each of the following, EXCEPT:
- **A.** hypoplastic left heart.
- **B.** ventricular septal defect.
- **C.** overriding aorta.
- **D.** pulmonary stenosis.

_____ **7.** Shock, hypoperfusion, sepsis, and cold stress may be indicators of which factor for hypoglycemia in a newborn?
- **A.** Prematurity
- **B.** Severe anemia
- **C.** Genetic disorders
- **D.** Disturbed oxidative metabolism

_____ **8.** A diagnosis of diaphragmatic hernia is suspected clinically in a newborn with:
- **A.** apnea.
- **B.** heart sounds shifted to the left.
- **C.** scaphoid abdomen.
- **D.** All of the above

_____ **9.** Primary apnea is often characterized by a short period of hypoxia and:
- **A.** rapid breathing, followed by apnea, and bradycardia.
- **B.** slow breathing, followed by apnea, and bradycardia.
- **C.** a lengthy period of apnea.
- **D.** a lengthy period of bradycardia.

_____ **10.** The lungs of a premature infant are weak, so the paramedic should use:
- **A.** the maximum allowable ventilatory pressure to expand lung tissue.
- **B.** mechanical devices to administer positive-pressure ventilation (PPV).
- **C.** small puffs from the paramedic's cheek with a pocket mask to ventilate.
- **D.** sufficient pressure to result in visible but not excessive chest rise.

Fill in the Blank

Read each item carefully, and then complete the statement by filling in the missing word(s).

1. Fetal circulation has three major blood flow deviations from that of an adult. These ________ occur at the ductus venosus, ______ ______, and ductus arteriosus.

2. Many newborns become centrally pink but have blue hands and feet. This is called ________.

3. Room air is preferred when resuscitating ________ infants, and the addition of supplemental oxygen may not be necessary.

4. The ________ ________ sequence is a series of developmental anomalies including a small chin and posteriorly positioned tongue.

5. In a newborn, it is important to provide the correct timing for ventilation at a rate of _____ to _______ breaths/min because breaths delivered at a higher rate can lead to __________, air trapping, or ___________.

6. Oral airways are rarely used for neonates, but they can be lifesaving if airway __________ leads to respiratory failure. Bilateral __________ __________ can be rapidly fatal but usually responds to placement of an oral airway.

7. Gastric __________ using a(n) __________ tube is indicated for prolonged bag-mask ventilation, if abdominal distention is impeding ventilation, or in the presence of a(n) __________ hernia.

8. Jitteriness is often confused with a(n) __________. Jitteriness is characteristically a disorder of the __________ and is rarely seen at a later age.

9. __________ is a congenital anomaly of rotation of the midgut.

10. Antiemetics should not be administered in the field. The infant may be dehydrated, however, and may need fluid __________. Dry mucous membranes, tachycardia, or a sunken __________ are clues that the patient needs hydration.

11. The _________ is the most frequently fractured bone in the newborn during even normal childbirth.

12. The most common cause of acute diarrhea in children is __________ __________.

Identify

In the following case studies, identify the appropriate resuscitation steps.

1. You are dispatched to the scene of a call for an infant with a seizure. The mother states that her baby daughter was "jerking her left arm and kicking her right leg for about a minute." At this point, the child is resting, and you note no irregularities during your primary survey.
   a. List five types of seizures that occur in infants.

      (1)____

      (2)____

      (3)____

      (4)____

      (5)____

   b. Based on the mother's description, which type of seizure did her child most likely have?

      ____

2. After assisting in the delivery of a full-term newborn boy, you bulb suction the infant's mouth and nose and dry and stimulate the baby.

a. After 30 seconds, the baby is centrally cyanotic of the trunk and mucous membranes. Which treatment would you now initiate?

(1)____________________

(2)____________________

b. After 30 seconds of adequate ventilation by PPV with 100% supplemental oxygen via a bag-mask device, the infant's pulse rate is less than 60 beats/min. Which treatment would you now initiate?

(1)____________________

(2)____________________

(3)____________________

Ambulance Calls

The following case scenarios provide an opportunity to explore the concerns associated with patient management and paramedic care. Read each scenario, and then answer each question.

1. You are called to attend a 38-year-old woman who is in active labor at home. She has not had any prenatal care. She tells you that "this baby is a month late according to my calendar and is sure a long time in coming." Her contractions started about 10 hours ago and are now 2 minutes apart. Her "bag of waters" broke 10 minutes before your arrival, and you notice greenish stains on the bedclothes. The woman says she feels as if she has to move her bowels.

a. Because birth is imminent, your partner sets up for delivery while you prepare for newborn resuscitation. List the categories of equipment that may be needed:

(1)____________________

(2)____________________

(3)____________________

(4)____________________

(5)____________________

(6)____________________

b. You immediately set up for delivery—and none too soon! You scarcely have your gloves on before the baby is crowning, and a moment later, the head is delivered. It is covered with a thick, greenish substance. List the steps you would take at this point.

(1)____________________

(2)____________________

c. The delivery went quickly. The infant is centrally blue and pale, has a pulse rate of 80, gives no response to flicking the bottom of the feet, and is limp, with slow and irregular respirations. Based on the information in the Apgar scoring table in your textbook, what is the Apgar score at this point, and how did you arrive at the score?

A ____________________

P ____________________

G ____________________

A ____________________

R ____________________

Total score at 1 minute = ____________________

d. What are the steps in the neonatal resuscitation pyramid that you will need to quickly follow with this newborn?

(1)______

(2)______

(3)______

(4)______

(5)______

2. You are called to a movie theater where a 23-year-old woman who is gravida 4, para 3, went into active labor while watching *Return of the Spider Monster.* You find the patient in a cold, drafty ladies' room, sitting on the floor, panting. "I'm only in my seventh month," she says. "This can't be happening." As she makes that statement, the baby's head delivers spontaneously. You scramble to the floor to control the rest of the delivery. Within seconds, you find yourself holding a very red, wrinkled little baby.

a. List in sequence the steps you would take at this point.

(1)______

(2)______

(3)______

(4)______

b. At which point would you clamp and cut the baby's umbilical cord? (Explain the reasoning behind your answer.)

______

______

______

c. Which steps can you take to prevent the baby from becoming hypothermic?

(1)______

(2)______

(3)______

(4)______

(5)______

3. You are called to a downtown apartment for a "sick woman." You arrive to find a teenage girl sitting on the toilet, having given birth only seconds before. The placenta has not yet delivered. You quickly remove the newborn from the toilet.

a. List the steps you would take at this point.

(1)______

(2)______

(3)______

(4)______

(5)______

b. What would be the indications for starting artificial ventilation on this baby?

(1)____________________

(2)____________________

(3)____________________

c. As it turns out, the baby has one of those indications, so you start artificial ventilation with a bag-mask device and 100% supplemental oxygen. After a minute, you reassess the baby and find that its heart rate is 84 beats/min. What should you do now?

____

____

____

d. After another minute or so, you reassess again. The baby's heart rate is now 56 beats/min. What should you do now?

____

____

____

____

e. Under which circumstance should you administer IV epinephrine to this baby?

____

True/False

If you believe the statement to be more true than false, write the letter "T" in the space provided. If you believe the statement to be more false than true, write the letter "F."

______ **1.** Jaundice that persists in a newborn beyond 2 to 3 weeks may indicate liver disease.

______ **2.** Even slight meconium staining of the amniotic fluid indicates a need to intubate the newborn immediately after delivery.

______ **3.** Administration of naloxone (Narcan) to a newborn who was just born of an addicted mother is routine clinical practice.

______ **4.** The typical umbilical cord has two arteries and one vein.

______ **5.** Infants may die of cold exposure at temperatures adults find comfortable.

______ **6.** Most newborns who require resuscitation will need cardiopulmonary resuscitation (CPR).

______ **7.** The umbilical vein is a large, thin-walled vessel usually found at the 4 o'clock position, as compared to the two thick-walled umbilical arteries usually found at 12 and 8 o'clock.

______ **8.** Newborns weighing less than 5.5 pounds (2,500 g) are considered low birth weight.

______ **9.** A normal number of stools per day for an infant is five to six, especially if the infant is breastfeeding, when infants often produce stool after every feeding.

______ **10.** Meconium-stained amniotic fluid, which is present in 10% to 15% of deliveries, carries a high risk of morbidity.

Short Answer

Complete this section with short written answers using the space provided.

1. Neonatal IV access under the best circumstances can be difficult and stressful. An important alternative is catheterization of the umbilical vein. Detail the steps necessary to perform this task.

   a. ______________________________

   b. ______________________________

   c. ______________________________

   d. ______________________________

   e. ______________________________

2. One of the most important skills that a paramedic must acquire and maintain is the ability to intubate neonates. Describe the steps necessary to properly intubate a neonate.

   a. ______________________________

   b. ______________________________

   c. ______________________________

   d. ______________________________

   e. ______________________________

Fill in the Table

1. Complete the following table by filling in the causes of neonatal seizures.

Causes of Neonatal Seizures
• Hypoxic-ischemic encephalopathy • ______________________________ • ______________________________ • ______________________________ • ______________________________ • ______________________________ • Development defects • Hypocalcemia • ______________________________ • ______________________________ • ______________________________

Problem Solving

Practice your calculation skills by solving the following math problems using the Apgar score. The Apgar scoring table is provided in your textbook.

You have just assisted in the delivery of a full-term newborn.

1. At 1 minute, the baby is centrally blue and pale, and the pulse rate is 100 beats/min; the baby grimaces, has some extremity flexion, and has a slow and irregular respiratory effort. The Apgar score is ______________.

2. At 5 minutes, the baby is pink with blue extremities, has a pulse rate of 120 beats/min, is actively crying with a strong effort, and has active motion. The Apgar score is ______________.

CHAPTER 43

Pediatric Emergencies

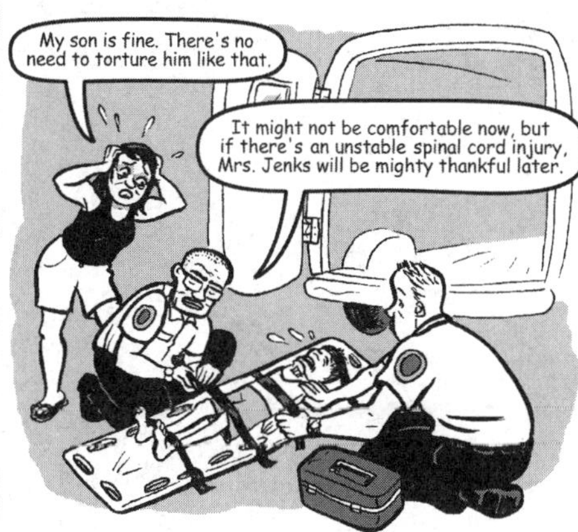

Matching

Part I

Match the following statements with the age group(s) most applicable to each. The statements may apply to more than one age group.

_____ **1.** Don't let your guard down regarding scene safety.

_____ **2.** They can be distracted by jangling keys and cooing noises.

_____ **3.** Give them appropriate choices and control whenever possible, and provide ongoing reassurance and encouragement.

_____ **4.** Assessment begins with observation of their interactions with the caregiver, vocalizations, and mobility, measured through the Pediatric Assessment Triangle.

_____ **5.** They should be examined on the parent's lap if stable.

_____ **6.** They can provide at least some of the history.

_____ **7.** They do not do very much other than eat, sleep, and cry.

_____ **8.** Tailor the physical exam to their age and developmental stage.

_____ **9.** Friends are key support figures, and this is a time of experimentation and risk-taking behaviors.

_____ **10.** Child abuse or maltreatment comes in many forms: physical abuse, sexual abuse, emotional abuse, and child neglect.

_____ **11.** They become much more analytic and capable of abstract thought. At this age, they can understand cause and effect.

_____ **12.** Use play and distraction techniques whenever possible.

_____ **13.** Make sure your hands and stethoscope are warm.

_____ **14.** Once secondary sexual characteristics have developed, they should be treated as an adult.

_____ **15.** They will be able to tell you what hurts and may have a story to share about the illness or injury.

A. Neonates and infants
B. Toddlers
C. Preschoolers
D. School-age children
E. Adolescents

Part II

Match the definitions in the left column with the most appropriate term in the right column.

_____ **1.** A condition seen in children younger than 2 years, characterized by dyspnea and wheezing.

_____ **2.** An unexpected sudden episode of color change, tone change, or apnea that requires mouth-to-mouth resuscitation or vigorous stimulation; formerly known as apparent life-threatening event (ALTE).

_____ **3.** A method of delivering oxygen by holding a face mask or similar device near an infant's or a child's face; used when a nonrebreathing mask is not tolerated.

_____ **4.** A group of congenital conditions that cause either accumulation of toxins or disorders of energy metabolism in the neonate; characterized by an infant's failure to thrive and by vague signs such as poor feeding.

_____ **5.** A condition in which the pituitary gland does not produce normal amounts of some or all of its hormones. It can be congenital; occur secondary to tumors, infection, or stroke; or develop after trauma or radiation therapy.

_____ **6.** A condition in which the heart muscle is unusually thick, forcing the heart to pump harder to get blood to leave.

_____ **7.** A short, low-pitched sound at the end of exhalation, present in children with moderate to severe hypoxia. It reflects poor gas exchange because of fluid in the lower airways and air sacs.

_____ **8.** A type of seizure characterized by manifestations that indicate involvement of both cerebral hemispheres.

_____ **9.** A tube that is surgically placed directly into the patient's stomach through the skin to provide nutrition or medications.

_____ **10.** An acute bacterial infection of the subglottic area of the upper airway that is complicated by copious thick, pus-filled secretions.

_____ **11.** Cyanosis of the extremities.

_____ **12.** A type of seizure characterized by a brief lapse of attention during which the patient may stare and not respond; formerly known as a petit mal seizure.

_____ **13.** The increased accumulation of cerebrospinal fluid within the ventricles of the brain.

_____ **14.** A bleeding disorder that is primarily hereditary, in which clotting does not occur or occurs insufficiently.

_____ **15.** Inflammation of the epiglottis.

_____ **16.** A condition in which the heart becomes weakened and enlarged, making it less efficient and causing a negative impact to the pulmonary, hepatic, and other systems.

_____ **17.** A genetic disease that primarily affects the respiratory and digestive systems.

_____ **18.** A type of child maltreatment in which a parent or guardian physically leaves a child, without regard for the child's health, safety, or welfare.

_____ **19.** Any improper or excessive action that injures or otherwise harms a child or infant.

_____ **20.** The community-based legal organization responsible for protection, rehabilitation, and prevention of child maltreatment and neglect; it has the legal authority to temporarily remove children from homes if there is reason to believe they are at risk for injury or neglect and to secure foster placement.

A. Abandonment

B. Absence seizures

C. Acrocyanosis

D. Bacterial tracheitis

E. Blow-by technique

F. Brief resolved unexplained event (BRUE)

G. Bronchiolitis

H. Bronchopulmonary dysplasia

I. Central venous catheter

J. Child abuse

K. Child protective services (CPS)

L. Complex febrile seizures

M. Complex partial seizures

N. Congenital adrenal hyperplasia (CAH)

O. Croup

P. Cystic fibrosis (CF)

Q. Dilated cardiomyopathy

R. Epiglottitis

S. Gastrostomy tube (G-tube)

T. Generalized seizures

_____	**21.** An unusual form of seizure that occurs in association with a rapid increase in body temperature.	**U.** Grunting
_____	**22.** A spectrum of lung conditions found in premature neonates who require long periods of high-concentration oxygen and ventilator support, ranging from mild reactive airway to debilitating chronic lung disease.	**V.** Hemophilia
_____	**23.** A catheter inserted into the vena cava to permit intermittent or continuous monitoring of central venous pressure and to facilitate obtaining blood samples for chemical analysis.	**W.** Hydrocephalus
_____	**24.** A common disease of childhood due to upper airway obstruction and characterized by stridor, hoarseness, and a barking cough.	**X.** Hypertrophic cardiomyopathy
_____	**25.** Inadequate production of cortisol and aldosterone by the adrenal gland.	**Y.** Hypopituitarism
_____	**26.** A type of seizure characterized by alteration of consciousness with or without complex focal motor activity.	**Z.** Inborn errors of metabolism (IEMs)

Part III

Match the definitions in the left column with the most appropriate term in the right column.

_____	**1.** The inadequate production or absence of the pituitary hormones, including adrenocorticotropic hormone, cortisol, thyroxine, luteinizing hormone, follicle-stimulating hormone, estrogen, testosterone, growth hormone, and antidiuretic hormone.	**A.** Intussusception
_____	**2.** An area where cartilage is transformed through calcification into a new area of bone.	**B.** Malrotation with volvulus
_____	**3.** A stiff or painful neck; commonly associated with meningitis.	**C.** Meckel diverticulum
_____	**4.** Refusal or failure on the part of the caregiver to provide life necessities to a child.	**D.** Meningitis
_____	**5.** A type of seizure that involves focal motor jerking or sensory abnormality in a patient who remains conscious.	**E.** Mottling
_____	**6.** A brief, self-limited, generalized seizure in a previously healthy child between ages 6 months and 6 years that is associated with the onset of or sudden increase in fever.	**F.** Myocarditis
_____	**7.** A disease that causes red blood cells to be misshapen, resulting in a poor oxygen-carrying capability and potentially resulting in lodging of the red blood cells in blood vessels or the spleen.	**G.** Neglect
_____	**8.** A pathologic state, usually in a febrile patient, resulting from the presence of invading microorganisms or their poisonous products in the bloodstream.	**H.** Nuchal rigidity
_____	**9.** A tube that is surgically placed directly into the patient's stomach through the skin to provide nutrition or medications.	**I.** Ossification center
_____	**10.** Hypertrophy (enlargement) of the pyloric sphincter of the stomach; ultimately leads to intestinal obstruction, often in infants.	**J.** Panhypopituitarism
_____	**11.** Pertaining to bruising of the skin.	**K.** Partial seizures
_____	**12.** An inflammation of the lungs caused by bacterial, viral, or fungal infections or infections with other microorganisms.	**L.** Pediatric Assessment Triangle (PAT)
_____	**13.** Inflammation of the myocardium.	**M.** Pertussis
_____	**14.** A condition of abnormal skin circulation, caused by vasoconstriction or inadequate perfusion.	**N.** Petechial
_____	**15.** Inflammation of the meningeal coverings of the brain and spinal cord; usually caused by a virus or bacterium. The viral type is less severe than the bacterial type; the bacterial type can result in brain damage, hearing loss, learning disability, or death.	**O.** Pneumonia

______	**16.** One of the most common congenital malformations of the small intestines, which presents with painless rectal bleeding.	**P.** Purpuric
______	**17.** A sign of respiratory distress characterized by skin pulling inward between and around the ribs and clavicles during inhalation.	**Q.** Pyloric stenosis
______	**18.** A virus that affects the upper and lower respiratory tracts. Disease (ie, pneumonia and bronchiolitis) is more prevalent in the lower respiratory tract.	**R.** Respiratory arrest
______	**19.** A clinical state of inadequate oxygenation, ventilation, or both.	**S.** Respiratory distress
______	**20.** A clinical state characterized by increased respiratory rate, effort, and work of breathing.	**T.** Respiratory failure
______	**21.** A condition that occurs when there is a twisting of the bowel around its mesenteric attachment to the abdominal wall.	**U.** Respiratory syncytial virus (RSV)
______	**22.** Telescoping of the intestines into themselves.	**V.** Retractions
______	**23.** Characterized by small purple, nonblanching spots on the skin.	**W.** Sepsis
______	**24.** An acute infectious disease characterized by a catarrhal stage, followed by a paroxysmal cough that ends in a whooping inspiration; also called whooping cough.	**X.** Sickle cell disease
______	**25.** An assessment tool that allows rapid formation of a general impression of the type and level of illness or injury in an infant or child without touching him or her; consists of assessing appearance, work of breathing, and circulation to the skin.	**Y.** Simple febrile seizures
______	**26.** A type of seizure that involves only one part of the brain.	**Z.** Simple partial seizures

Multiple Choice

Read each item carefully, and then select the best response.

______ **1.** Although child abuse can generate a big emotional response from the emergency medical services (EMS) crew, your primary focus as a paramedic should be:

- **A.** documenting the suspected abuse for further prosecution.
- **B.** separating the patient from the suspected abuser.
- **C.** the trauma assessment, management, and ensuring the safety of the child.
- **D.** properly securing the crime scene for investigators.

______ **2.** A child's developmental stage affects his or her response to injury. As a result:

- **A.** being strapped to a backboard may be considered fun.
- **B.** a paramedic could turn an activity as serious as immobilizing a child's spine on a backboard into a "game."
- **C.** being immobilized on a backboard may be terrifying and anxiety provoking.
- **D.** children should never be strapped or immobilized on a backboard.

______ **3.** All of the following injury patterns may be more common in pediatric patients, EXCEPT:

- **A.** blunt force trauma.
- **B.** falls.
- **C.** skull fractures.
- **D.** joint dislocations.

______ **4.** PAT is an acronym developed:

- **A.** from a popular children's book to help soothe a sick or injured child.
- **B.** to remember the proper methods of conducting a hands-on assessment of a child.
- **C.** to stand for the technique of palpating a tender abdomen.
- **D.** to stand for the Pediatric Assessment Triangle.

_____ **5.** One of the best ways to assess a pediatric patient's oxygenation status is to:
A. evaluate the child's respiratory rate.
B. evaluate the work of breathing.
C. auscultate the lung.
D. obtain the pulse.

_____ **6.** Abnormal positioning and retractions are physical signs of increased work of breathing that can easily be assessed without touching the patient. All of the following are signs of increased work of breathing, EXCEPT:
A. the sniffing position.
B. tripoding.
C. retractions.
D. All of the above are signs of increased work of breathing.

_____ **7.** Which of the following is a child with a serious mechanism of injury, who may need immediate transport to the emergency department (ED)?
A. A child with an unstable or compromised airway from a motor vehicle crash
B. A child with an isolated extremity fracture from a fall
C. A conscious, alert child who crashed his or her bicycle while wearing a helmet that cracked
D. A skateboarder with an obviously fractured wrist

_____ **8.** Paramedics may encounter children with special health care needs. These special needs may include:
A. physical, developmental, and learning disabilities.
B. tracheostomy tubes and artificial ventilators.
C. gastrostomy tubes (G-tubes).
D. All of the above

_____ **9.** The federally funded program that was created more than 25 years ago in an effort to reduce child disability and death caused by severe illness and injury is known as:
A. the DOT curriculum.
B. NHYSA.
C. EMSC.
D. TSA.

_____ **10.** Inserting an oral airway in a child is similar to inserting an airway in an adult, EXCEPT:
A. you use a different method for determining the proper size.
B. an oral airway should not be used in the presence of ingested caustics.
C. an oral airway is inserted in a child in an inverted manner, then flipped over into the correct position.
D. you must take care to avoid injuring the hard palate.

_____ **11.** When a parent or guardian physically leaves a child, without regard for the child's health or safety, this condition is referred to as:
A. physical abuse.
B. sexual abuse.
C. abandonment.
D. neglect.

_____ **12.** Which of the following is NOT a risk factor for child abuse?
A. Child with disability
B. Disorganized family structure
C. Parent was abused
D. Financial stability

_____ **13.** You are called to the scene of a 4-year-old child injured inside a residence. You enter the house and find the child and a parent. You assess the child and become suspicious about the injury. Your partner interviews the parent. Which of the following is a red flag for child abuse by a caregiver?

A. The caregiver overreacts to the child's condition.
B. The caregiver seems forthcoming about what happened.
C. The caregiver is enraged about care being provided by EMS.
D. The caregiver seems concerned.

_____ **14.** You have completed a call where there is a high suspicion of child abuse. When you write the patient care report, which type of information is helpful to include for child protective services when those personnel review the report?

A. Subjective analysis of the situation
B. Speculative view on what might be going on
C. Conjecture and results of your investigation
D. Verbatim comments in quotes

_____ **15.** You have been called to a residence where there is a 5-year-old boy who reportedly fell while running and hit his forehead. He has a bruise and an abrasion. While you do an assessment to determine if there are any additional injuries, you notice the boy has numerous bruises of different colors. Which location of bruises on the child would make you MOST suspicious of child abuse?

A. Knees
B. Arms
C. Lower legs
D. Back

Labeling

On the following diagram, indicate the technique for measuring the distance to insert a nasogastric (NG) or an orogastric (OG) tube.

A. ____________________

B. ____________________

C. ____________________

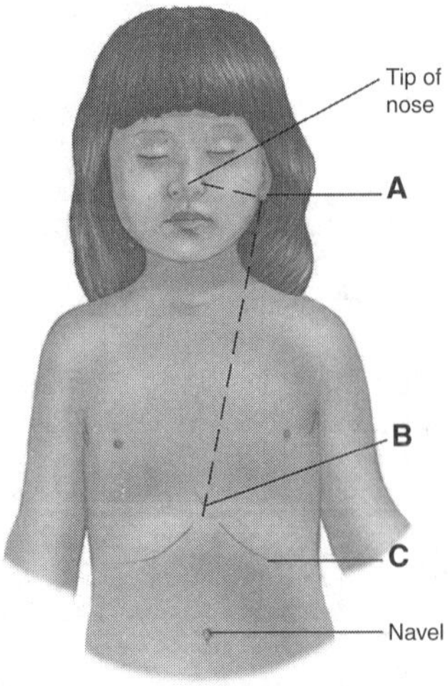

Fill in the Blank

Read each item carefully, and then complete the statement by filling in the missing word(s).

1. A nasopharyngeal airway is usually well __________ and is not as likely as the __________ airway to cause vomiting.

2. The __________ - __________ __________ can be used for a child with mild respiratory distress who will not tolerate a facial mask.

3. Bag-mask ventilation is always the first step in assisted __________, and it represents definitive __________ __________ for many patients.

4. Potential complications of pediatric intubation include damage to __________ and oral structures, __________ of gastric contents, and incorrect placement.

5. Because __________ can occur during intubation, the paramedic should apply a cardiac monitor and a(n) __________ __________.

6. The types of shock you may encounter are the same in adults and children: __________, __________, and __________.

7. A pediatric patient with __________ shock will often appear listless or lethargic and may have compensatory __________. The child may appear pale, __________, or cyanotic.

8. Further assessment of a pediatric patient in shock may identify signs of dehydration such as sunken eyes, dry __________ __________, poor skin __________, or __________ capillary refill, with cool extremities.

9. Complications associated with IO infusion may include __________ __________, growth plate injury, and bone inflammation caused by __________.

10. Cardiogenic shock is uncommon in the pediatric population but may be present in children with underlying __________ heart disease or __________ disturbances.

11. When you are confronted with a pediatric patient in __________ arrest, the most important consideration is to provide high-quality cardiopulmonary resuscitation (CPR). Attach a(n) ________ or defibrillator to determine the underlying cardiac rhythm.

12. Approximately 1,600 infants died of _______ in 2015. This condition is the leading cause of death among infants 1 to 12 months old.

Identify

After reading the following case studies, list the chief complaint, vital signs, and pertinent negatives.

1. It's about 0330 hours, and you are dispatched on a Priority 1 call for a 2-year-old child with difficulty breathing. As you approach the residence, you notice a family member frantically trying to wave you down. You think to yourself that this doesn't look good. You grab your pediatric gear and electrocardiogram (ECG) monitor and quickly enter the house. Once inside, you are told that the girl woke the whole household with a terrible barky cough. This child is now sitting on her mother's lap. The mother states that the child has been irritable for several days with symptoms consistent with an upper respiratory infection: coughing, runny nose, and sneezing. The child has audible stridor and a "seal-like" barking cough; she is conscious and alert. She has an oxygen saturation of 95% on ambient room air. She also has a normal capillary refill. When you attempt to take her blood pressure (BP), she begins to get agitated and clings to her mother.
   a. Chief complaint:

____

____

b. Vital signs:

____

____

c. Pertinent negatives:

____

____

2. Today is your shift on medivac duty. You are dispatched to intercept a ground ambulance about 25 minutes to the west. As you lift off, you discover that the patient is only 1 week old and was the survivor of a motor vehicle crash involving a fatality. You and your crew arrive on the scene several minutes before the ambulance arrives. The state police are on scene securing the landing zone. They advise you that the patient's mother was holding the baby; both were unrestrained in the vehicle and were ejected on impact. The mother suffered fatal injuries. You are thinking the worst and begin to set up your pediatric resuscitation equipment. When the ambulance arrives, you are quickly handed the neonatal trauma patient. The baby has oxygen in place, appears to be wrapped well, and is thoroughly secured with a vacuum splint conforming to his tiny body. The baby appears to be sleeping peacefully and has only a small forehead abrasion. You begin the primary survey during your flight to the trauma center. The assessment indicates an infant with no visible distress. The baby has an intact airway and is breathing at 30 breaths/min, he has an apical pulse rate at 150 beats/min, his skin color appears normal, and the skin is warm and dry. Lung sounds are clear and equal. Oxygen saturation is 96%. Remarkably, he does not appear to have any noticeable external bleeding. In fact, the assessment is totally unremarkable. After a "not so routine" mechanism of injury, the infant is safely delivered to the regional trauma center.

a. Chief complaint:

____

____

b. Vital signs:

____

____

c. Pertinent negatives:

____

____

3. While working in the advanced life support (ALS) "fly car," you are dispatched on a Priority 1 call for a mutual assist with a local basic life support (BLS) ambulance. The BLS team requests that you meet them while they begin the response to the local pediatric ED. They are treating a 2½-year-old girl in "status." You arrange a safe place to meet the ambulance and secure your vehicle. As you await the BLS crew's arrival, you prepare your pediatric ALS equipment and begin reviewing protocols. Once on the ambulance, you notice the small patient secured to the cot. The mother is in the front passenger's seat. The child has recently been sick with an upper respiratory infection and low-grade fever. The child suddenly appeared to go into convulsions after being given oral pediatric acetaminophen for an elevation in her fever. The BLS crew states that the patient was actively seizing on their arrival. They initiated high-flow supplemental oxygen with a pediatric nonrebreathing face mask, requested ALS assistance, and initiated transport. When you first encounter the child, she is postictal, with the following vital signs: ashen skin that is warm and dry and a rectal temperature of 100.3°F. The patient responds to pain. Her oxygen saturation is 98%. Pupils are sluggish but equal. The patient has equal bilateral breath sounds. The remainder of the exam is unremarkable. The patient's mother denies any other medications, history, or allergies to medications. She further denies any recent injury or trauma to the child.

a. Chief complaint:

____

____

b. Vital signs:

____

____

c. Pertinent negatives:

____

____

Complete the Patient Care Report (PCR)

Reread the first incident scenario in the preceding "Identify" exercises, and then complete the following PCR for the patient.

<table>
<tr><th colspan="6">EMS Patient Care Report (PCR)</th></tr>
<tr><td>Date:</td><td>Incident No.:</td><td colspan="2">Nature of Call:</td><td colspan="2">Location:</td></tr>
<tr><td>Dispatched:</td><td>En Route:</td><td>At Scene:</td><td>Transport:</td><td>At Hospital:</td><td>In Service:</td></tr>
<tr><th colspan="6">Patient Information</th></tr>
<tr><td colspan="3">Age:
Sex:
Weight (in kg [lb]):</td><td colspan="3">Allergies:
Medications:
Past Medical History:
Chief Complaint:</td></tr>
</table>

<table>
<tr><th colspan="5">Vital Signs</th></tr>
<tr><td>Time:</td><td>BP:</td><td>Pulse:</td><td>Respirations:</td><td>SpO_2:</td></tr>
<tr><td>Time:</td><td>BP:</td><td>Pulse:</td><td>Respirations:</td><td>SpO_2:</td></tr>
<tr><td>Time:</td><td>BP:</td><td>Pulse:</td><td>Respirations:</td><td>SpO_2:</td></tr>
<tr><th colspan="5">EMS Treatment
(circle all that apply)</th></tr>
<tr><td colspan="2">Oxygen @ ______ L/min via (circle one):
NC NRM Bag-mask device</td><td>Assisted Ventilation</td><td>Airway Adjunct</td><td>CPR</td></tr>
<tr><td>Defibrillation</td><td>Bleeding Control</td><td>Bandaging</td><td>Splinting</td><td>Other:</td></tr>
<tr><th colspan="5">Narrative</th></tr>
<tr><td colspan="5"></td></tr>
</table>

Ambulance Calls

The following case scenarios provide an opportunity to explore the concerns associated with patient management and paramedic care. Read each scenario, and then answer each question.

1. You are called to the scene of a collision in which a 6-year-old child was struck by a car as he darted into the street in front of his home. The child is lying in the street surrounded by a small group of people, including his very distraught parents.

a. Given the mechanism of injury (MOI), list at least three injuries you must look for in particular in this child.

(1)____

(2)____

(3)____

b. As you are kneeling beside the injured child, carefully going through the steps of the primary survey, the child's father (who looks like a pro wrestler) charges over and starts shouting at you: "What the h— do you think you're doing with my kid? Stop messing around and take him to a *hospital*. Can't you see he's hurt bad? He's going to die here while you dingbats muck about." [The father's actual comments are less polite but are not quoted verbatim in this workbook.]

(1) What are your feelings at this moment?

____

____

(2) How will you deal with this situation?

(a) ______________________________

(b) ______________________________

(c) ______________________________

(d) ______________________________

c. On checking the child's vital signs, you find the following: pulse is 120 beats/min and regular; respirations are 24 breaths/min and unlabored; BP is 90/60 mm Hg. Which of the following conclusions can be drawn from those vital signs?

(1) The child is going into shock.

(2) The child has increasing intracranial pressure.

(3) The vital signs are normal for a child of that age.

(4) There is probably significant intrathoracic injury.

(5) There is probably significant intra-abdominal bleeding.

2. You are called around 0100 hours for a child who "can't breathe." A haggard father greets you at the door and tells you that his 2-year-old Tammy has had "a little cold" for a couple of days but otherwise seemed fine. ("It didn't slow her down a bit.") Tonight, however, she began coughing, and the cough kept getting worse. Indeed, even as you are walking toward the child's room, you can hear a loud barking noise. On reaching Tammy's room, you see a very agitated 2-year-old struggling in her mother's lap. Her nostrils are flaring with each inhalation, and there are retractions of her neck muscles. Her lips are bluish. She flails and has a fit of dry coughing as you start to come near. Eventually, you manage to measure a pulse of 160 beats/min and a respiratory rate of 52 breaths/min. When you try to auscultate the child's chest, however, she grabs your stethoscope and yanks it out of your ears.

a. The vital signs are __________ (normal or abnormal?) for a child of this age.

b. The most likely diagnosis is ____________________.

c. Which steps will you take in managing this child?

(1)____

(2)____

(3)____

(4)____

(5)____

3. You are called for a 4-month-old infant in respiratory distress. His mother says that he has been "off his feed" for a couple of days and has been sneezing a lot. On examination, you notice that the baby seems to be breathing like a rabbit. The pulse is 180 beats/min, respirations are 60 breaths/min, and BP is 90/60 mm Hg. There is diffuse wheezing throughout the chest.

a. The vital signs are __________ (normal or abnormal?) for a child of this age.

b. The most likely diagnosis is ______________________________.

c. Which steps will you take in managing this child?

(1)____

(2)____

(3)____

(4)____

(5)____

(6)____

4. You are called for a 2½-year-old child having difficulty breathing. The mother says that she left little Bobby playing quietly in his room, and when she returned half an hour later, she found him in severe respiratory distress. She thinks he has had a slight respiratory infection, nothing serious: "You know, it's just one runny nose after another all winter with them. Each one gives it to the others, and I've got five little ones—so I can't always keep track of who has a runny nose."

You find Bobby in severe respiratory distress. He makes high-pitched squeaks when he tries to inhale, and his eyes look like they are popping out of his head. His lips are blue. You place the back of your hand on his forehead and note that the skin does not feel abnormally warm.

a. The most likely diagnosis is ______________________________.

b. Which steps will you take in managing this child?

(1)____

____

(2)____

____

(3)____

____

(4)____

____

(5)____

____

(6)____

____

(7)____

____

5. You are called to see a 4-year-old child who is "very sick." His mother says that he was fine until a few hours ago, when he began complaining of a sore throat. Since then, he would not eat or drink anything, and he is very feverish. You find the child sitting very still, bolt upright in bed, with his chin thrust forward. He does not reply to your questions but only nods or shakes his head slightly. Saliva is dribbling out of the corners of his mouth. His skin feels very hot. His pulse is 140 beats/min, respirations are 40 breaths/min and quiet, and BP is 90/60 mm Hg. The chest is clear.

a. The vital signs are __________ (normal or abnormal?) for a child of this age.

b. The most likely diagnosis is ______________________________.

c. Which steps will you take in managing this child?

(1)____

(2)____

(3)____

(4)____

(5)____

d. What is the special danger threatening this child?

____

____

6. You are called to a field about 6 miles outside of town where a 6-year-old child in the first-grade nature study class is having difficulty breathing. The teacher says that she noticed him lagging behind the others several times during the morning, and finally she found him sitting by himself under a tree, struggling to breathe. You find the child still sitting under the tree, but apparently dozing. It is difficult to wake him, and when he does open his eyes, he just stares at you blankly. When you ask him whether he has taken any medicine today, he just shakes his head and seems to doze again.

On examination, the child's pulse is 160 beats/min and somewhat weak, respirations are 52 breaths/min and shallow, and BP is 90/60 mm Hg on exhalation and 50 mm Hg systolic during inhalation. The lips look bluish. There is retraction of the neck muscles. The chest does not seem to move with respiration, and it sounds like an empty barrel when you tap on it. You can hardly hear any breath sounds at all. On the child's wrist is a medical identification bracelet inscribed "asthmatic."

a. List five signs that suggest this child is having a very serious asthmatic attack.

(1)____

(2)____

(3)____

(4)____

(5)____

b. List the steps you would take in managing this case.

(1)____

(2)____

(3)____

(4)____

(5)____

(6)____

7. The very same evening, you are called to see a child who is "short of breath." The child has been diagnosed with asthma in the past.

a. List five questions you would ask the child and his parents in taking the history.

(1)____

(2)____

(3)____

(4)____

(5)____

b. Your protocol calls for administering albuterol for an acute asthmatic attack.

(1) What are the relevant *contraindications* to albuterol?

____

____

(2) What are the possible adverse *side effects* of albuterol?

____

____

(3) What is the correct *dosage*, and how is the drug administered?

____

____

8. You are called to a downtown apartment for a "very sick baby." A frightened-looking young mother greets you at the door and hurries you into the bedroom, where a baby is lying very still in its crib. You observe at once that the baby's color is grayish and that it is not breathing. When you touch the baby to open the airway, you can feel that the skin is cold. Describe what you will do from this point on.

____

____

____

____

9. You are called for a 2-year-old child who is "having a fit." En route to the call, you review in your mind the possible causes of seizures in children.

a. List five causes of seizures in children.

(1)__________

(2)__________

(3)__________

(4)__________

(5)__________

b. List five questions you should ask in taking the child's history.

(1)__________

(2)__________

(3)__________

(4)__________

(5)__________

c. List five things you would look for in particular in examining the child.

(1)__________

(2)__________

(3)__________

(4)__________

(5)__________

d. You learn that the child has never experienced a seizure before. On examining him, you find that he is no longer seizing but is still somewhat drowsy. His skin is very hot, so you take an axillary temperature and get a reading of 39°C (102.2°F). The pupils are equal and reactive, the neck is supple, and the chest is clear. Describe how you would manage this case.

(1)__________

(2)__________

10. You are summoned to a local high school where a 14-year-old girl is having a seizure. The school nurse tells you that the child has never experienced a seizure in school before. This seizure came on while the girl was in the auditorium watching a movie. The seizure lasted about 5 minutes. One of the teachers then carried the girl to the nurse's office. The nurse was in the middle of trying to contact the girl's mother when the child had another grand mal seizure. Now, as you are speaking with the nurse, you witness a third grand mal seizure that lasts about 6 minutes.

a. List the steps in treating this patient.

(1)__________

(2)__________

(3)__________

(4)__________

(5)__________

(6)__________

(7)__________

b. Which drug is used in the emergency treatment of repeated seizures, and what are its contraindications?

____

____

11. You are called to attend to a 10-month-old baby who sustained burns to the foot when he "stepped on a cigarette." Something about the story sounds "fishy" to you, and you find yourself on the alert for evidence that the child has been abused.

a. What's "fishy" about the story?

____

____

b. List 10 possible clues that might substantiate your suspicion that a child has been abused.

(1)__________

(2)__________

(3)__________

(4)__________

(5)__________

(6)__________

(7)__________

(8)__________

(9)__________

(10)__________

c. By the time you finish examining the child, you are privately convinced that the baby was deliberately burned and that, furthermore, he has been burned and beaten in the past. How should you manage this case?

(1)__________

(2)__________

(3)__________

(4)__________

(5)__________

d. Suppose the child's parent refuses to allow the child to be transported to the hospital? What should you do then?

(1)__________

(2)__________

(3)__________

12. You are called to treat an 18-month-old baby who fell off a second-floor balcony to the ground 5 meters (about 15 feet) below. On examination, you find the baby conscious but drowsy. Vital signs are a pulse of 80 beats/min and regular, respirations are 16 breaths/min, and BP is 100/70 mm Hg. There is a bruise on the left forehead. The pupils are equal and reactive to light. The point of maximal impulse (PMI) is in the midclavicular line. Breath sounds are equal bilaterally. The abdomen does not appear distended. The baby is moving all extremities. List the steps in the prehospital management of this case.

a. ____

b. ____

c. ____

d. ____

e. ____

f. ____

13. You are called to the scene of a smoky house fire just as one of the firefighters is emerging from the building carrying a baby. "He was in the thick of it," the firefighter tells you. "Out cold when I found him." The baby still seems very drowsy.

a. Should this infant be intubated? Why or why not?

____

____

b. List five indications for the immediate intubation of an infant or small child who has been in a fire.

(1)____

(2)____

(3)____

(4)____

(5)____

14. You are all settled in to watch a football game on your day off when a neighbor comes running in, carrying her lethargic 2-year-old child. "Johnny's choking on peanuts!" she wails. "Did what?" you ask, not really wanting to know the answer.

"He's choking. Help, do something, he's turning blue!"

a. What is the recommended method to relieve a severe airway obstruction in a conscious child?

____

____

b. List the steps you would take to relieve the child's airway obstruction.

(1)____

____

(2)____

____

(3)____

(4)____

(5)____

(6)____

True/False

If you believe the statement to be more true than false, write the letter "T" in the space provided. If you believe the statement to be more false than true, write the letter "F."

______ **1.** A child who is seriously ill or injured will always be agitated and showing clear signs of distress.

______ **2.** A sunken anterior fontanel in an infant suggests meningitis or a head injury.

______ **3.** Neonates and infants can easily communicate their needs when they are in pain.

______ **4.** Grunting is a sign of respiratory distress in small children.

______ **5.** An infant falling from a height is most likely to sustain injury to the head.

______ **6.** RSV may be transmitted by direct contact with large droplets or indirect contact with contaminated hands.

______ **7.** To insert an oropharyngeal airway (OPA) in a small child, introduce the airway tip-upward, and then rotate it 180° and slide it into place.

______ **8.** Hypotension is an early response to blood loss in infants and small children.

______ **9.** The first step in assembling the equipment for pediatric intubation is to check the cuff on the endotracheal (ET) tube you have selected.

______ **10.** A straight blade is preferred for pediatric intubation.

______ **11.** Adrenal insufficiency can lead to distributive shock.

______ **12.** The narrowest point in an infant's airway is the opening between the vocal cords.

______ **13.** Initial burn management begins with removal of burning clothing and support of the ABCs.

______ **14.** Pediatric trauma victims must have a rigid cervical collar in place prior to transport.

______ **15.** Sinus tachycardia, referring to a pulse rate higher than normal for age, is common in children.

Short Answer

Complete this section with short written answers using the space provided.

1. List six signs suggestive of hypovolemic shock in infants and small children.

a. ____

b. ____

c. ____

d. ____

e. ______

f. ______

2. Upon completing the primary survey of any seriously injured person, of any age, the paramedic must make a decision whether to transport at once or to proceed to the secondary assessment. List five indications for immediate transport ("load-and-go") of injured infants and children.

a. ______

b. ______

c. ______

d. ______

e. ______

Fill in the Table

Fill in the missing parts of the following tables.

1. In examining an injured infant or child, you must know exactly what you are looking for so that each second spent on the physical examination is well invested. In the following table, indicate what, in particular, you would be looking for as you examine each part of the body areas mentioned.

Pediatric Physical Examination	
Body Area	**What I Am Looking for in Particular**
Head	• ______ • ______ • ______
Neck	• ______ • ______
Chest	• ______ • ______ • ______
Abdomen	• ______ • ______
Extremities	• ______ • ______ • ______

2. In the following table, provide the normal respiratory rate for each pediatric age group.

Pediatric Respiratory Rates	
Age	**Respiratory Rate (breaths/min)**
Infant	
Toddler	
Preschool-age child	
School-age child	
Adolescent	

Data from: American Heart Association (AHA). Vital signs in children. In: AHA. *Pediatric Advanced Life Support*. Dallas, TX: AHA; 2015.

3. In the following table, provide the normal pulse rate for each pediatric age group.

Pediatric Pulse Rates	
Age	**Pulse Rate (beats/min) [Awake]**
Infant	
Toddler	
Preschool-age child	
School-age child	
Adolescent	

Data from: American Heart Association (AHA). Vital signs in children. In: AHA. *Pediatric Advanced Life Support.* Dallas, TX: AHA; 2015.

4. In the following table, provide the normal blood pressure for each pediatric age group.

Normal Blood Pressure for Age	
Age	**Minimal Systolic Blood Pressure (mm Hg)**
Infant	
Toddler	
Preschool-age child	
School-age child	
Adolescent	

Data from: American Heart Association (AHA). Vital signs in children. In: AHA. *Pediatric Advanced Life Support.* Dallas, TX: AHA; 2015.

5. In the following table, describe what the letters in the CHILD ABUSE mnemonic represent.

CHILD ABUSE Mnemonic	
Mnemonic	**What the Letter Represents**
C	
H	History consistent with injuries
I	
L	Lack of supervision
D	
A	Affect
B	
U	Unusual injury patterns
S	
E	Environmental clues

Problem Solving

Practice your calculation skills by solving the following math problems.

1. For children 1 to 10 years old, you would calculate the lower limit of acceptable blood pressure for age using the following formula:

$$\text{Minimal systolic blood pressure} = 70 + (2 \times \text{age in years})$$

a. You are evaluating a pediatric trauma patient. His age is 6 years. What would you estimate a normal systolic BP to be?

b. This patient is a 10-year-old asthmatic. What would you estimate a normal systolic BP to be?

c. On arrival, you have an unconscious pediatric patient. You estimate his age to be 5 or 6 years. What would normal BP be for a patient this age?

2. You would calculate the ET tube size for a child older than 2 years as follows:

$$4 + (\text{Age in years} \div 4) = \text{Uncuffed tube size (in mm)}$$

a. Calculate the appropriate ET tube size for a 6-year-old child.

b. Calculate the appropriate ET tube size for a 9-year-old child.

3. You have been called to the scene for a 4-year-old child who is unconscious and unresponsive after being shocked by sticking his finger into an electrical outlet. He is also pulseless and apneic.

a. The child weighs 40 pounds. Appropriate two-person BLS is in progress on your arrival. You attach the patient to your defibrillator/monitor and notice ventricular fibrillation (VF). Which energy setting would you use to administer defibrillations?

b. How much energy should be used on subsequent defibrillations?

4. You have been called to the scene for a 6-year-old girl who has severe anaphylaxis after ingesting peanuts at a ball game. The child is anxious, and she has an increased work of breathing and poor circulation. She weighs 60 pounds.

a. As the paramedic in charge, you decide that among all your other treatment priorities, this patient requires epinephrine. How will you administer this drug and at which dose?

b. This patient further requires the administration of diphenhydramine (Benadryl). How will you administer this drug and at which dose?

c. Fortunately, your patient is beginning to improve, but she is still wheezing. Which drug would you consider and at which dose?

CHAPTER

Geriatric Emergencies

44

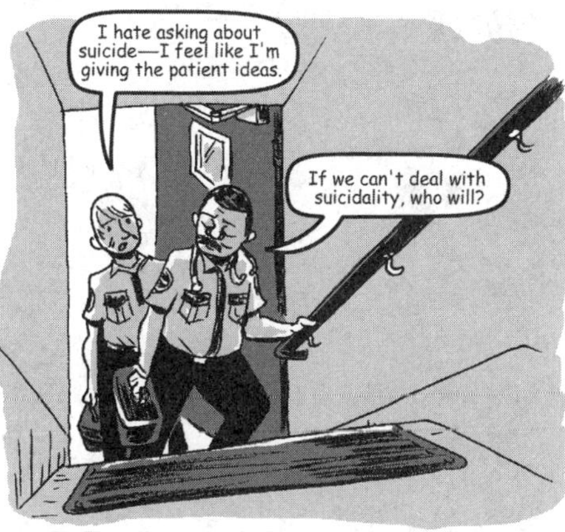

Matching

Match each of definitions in the left column to the appropriate term in the right column.

	Definition	Term
______	**1.** Inflammation of the joints.	**A.** Adult protective services (APS)
______	**2.** The assessment and treatment of disease in someone 65 years or older.	**B.** Alzheimer disease
______	**3.** A chronic deterioration of mental functions.	**C.** Arthritis
______	**4.** A progressive organic condition in which neurons die, causing dementia.	**D.** Bereavement
______	**5.** An ulcer that occurs when pressure is applied to the body tissue, resulting in a lack or perfusion and ultimately necrosis.	**E.** Cellulitis
______	**6.** An inflammatory disorder that affects the entire body and leads to degeneration and deformation of joints.	**F.** Delirium
______	**7.** A degenerative condition resulting in decreased mobility of vertebral joints and compression of neural elements.	**G.** Dementia
______	**8.** Swelling that presents around the sacral region of the spinal column.	**H.** Geriatrics
______	**9.** A disease state that results from the presence of microorganisms or their toxic products in the bloodstream.	**I.** Herpes zoster
______	**10.** An acute confusional state characterized by global impairment of thinking, perception, judgment, and memory.	**J.** Homeostasis
______	**11.** Sadness from loss; grieving.	**K.** Hospice
______	**12.** A disease in bone mass and density.	**L.** Old-age dependency ratio
______	**13.** An acute inflammation in the skin caused by a bacterial infection.	**M.** Osteoarthritis
______	**14.** An organization that investigates cases involving abuse and neglect and provides case management services in some cases.	**N.** Osteoporosis
______	**15.** Shingles; a contagious condition caused by the reactivation of the varicella virus or nerve roots.	**O.** Parkinson disease
______	**16.** A tendency toward constancy or stability in the body's internal milieu.	**P.** Polypharmacy
______	**17.** An organization that provides end-of-life care to patients with terminal illnesses and their families.	**Q.** Presbycusis
______	**18.** The ability to perceive the position and movement of one's body or limbs.	**R.** Pressure ulcer
______	**19.** A formula used to determine the number of older people in a society as compared with the number of potential workers who are theoretically capable of providing resources to sustain the whole population. It is the number of older people (65 years and older) for every 100 adults (potential caregivers) between the ages of 18 and 64 years.	**S.** Proprioception
______	**20.** The degeneration of a joint surface caused by wear and tear that leads to pain and stiffness.	**T.** Rheumatoid arthritis (RA)

______	**21.** A neurologic condition in which the portion of the brain responsible for production of dopamine has been damaged or overused, resulting in tremors.	**U.** Sacral edema
______	**22.** The use of multiple medications.	**V.** Sepsis
______	**23.** Progressive hearing loss, particularly in the high frequencies, along with lessened ability to discriminate between a particular sound and background noise.	**W.** Spondylosis

Multiple Choice

Read each item carefully, and then select the best response.

______ **1.** Geriatrics is the assessment and treatment of disease in someone __________ years or older.

- **A.** 55
- **B.** 65
- **C.** 75
- **D.** None of the above

______ **2.** A 35-year-old is aging just as fast as an 85-year-old, but the older person exhibits the cumulative results of a __________ process.

- **A.** longer
- **B.** shorter
- **C.** degenerative
- **D.** cumulative

______ **3.** In older adults, cardiac output during exercise may ________ by as much as 30% to 40%.

- **A.** increase
- **B.** strengthen
- **C.** decline
- **D.** weaken

______ **4.** Musculoskeletal changes, such as __________, may also affect pulmonary function by limiting lung volume and maximal inspiratory pressure.

- **A.** kyphosis
- **B.** osteoporosis
- **C.** decreased bone mass
- **D.** arthritis

______ **5.** Incontinence is not a normal part of aging and can lead to:

- **A.** skin irritation.
- **B.** skin breakdown.
- **C.** urinary tract infections.
- **D.** All of the above

______ **6.** __________ enables us to maintain postural stability by using a variety of receptors in the joints and information provided by the eyes. As these mechanisms fail with age, people become less steady on their feet, and the tendency to fall increases markedly.

- **A.** Balance
- **B.** Posture
- **C.** Proprioception
- **D.** Homeostasis

______ **7.** Older adults are much more vulnerable to the following temperature stresses, EXCEPT:

- **A.** heat exhaustion.
- **B.** hypothermia.
- **C.** the absence of a febrile response to illness.
- **D.** hormonal temperature effects.

______ **8.** Chronic obstructive pulmonary disease (COPD) includes all of the following, EXCEPT:
A. chronic asthma.
B. chronic bronchitis.
C. emphysema.
D. diuretic intolerant edema.

______ **9.** The extent of bone loss that a person undergoes is influenced by numerous factors, including:
A. genetics, smoking, and level of activity.
B. age, sex, and genetics.
C. age, skin condition, and diet.
D. smoking, age, and skin condition.

______ **10.** Some patients fear that mentioning a symptom will lead to a diagnosis or treatment that will jeopardize their independence. "If I mention those pains in my stomach," the older person may reason:
A. "They'll put me in that nursing home to die."
B. "My kids will think I'm going to die, and they'll start fighting over the money."
C. "They'll put me in the hospital, and I can't afford another hospitalization and more prescriptions."
D. "They'll put me in the hospital, and I may never come out of that place again."

Labeling

Label the components of the gastrointestinal (GI) system, and place an asterisk (*) next to the primary location(s) for GI bleeding.

1. Upper GI system

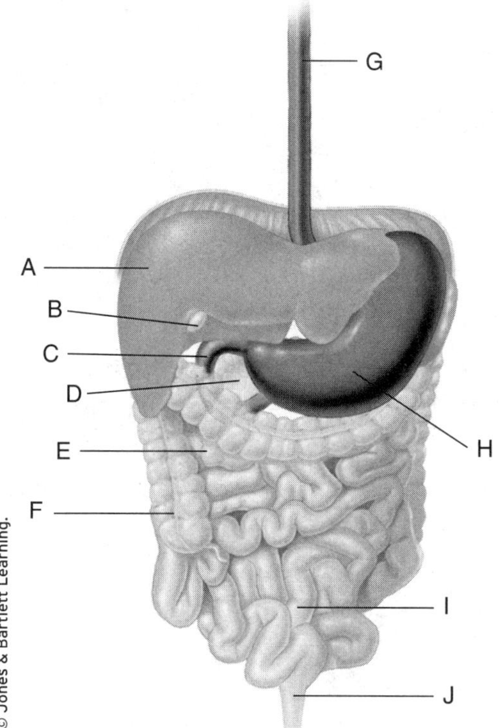

A. ______________________

B. ______________________

C. ______________________

D. ______________________

E. ______________________

F. ______________________

G. ______________________

H. ______________________

I. ______________________

J. ______________________

2. Lower GI system

A. ______________________________

B. ______________________________

C. ______________________________

D. ______________________________

E. ______________________________

F. ______________________________

G. ______________________________

H. ______________________________

I. ______________________________

J. ______________________________

Fill in the Blank

Read each item carefully, and then complete the statement by filling in the missing word(s).

1. __________ adults constitute an ever-increasing proportion of patients in the health care system, particularly the __________ care sector.
2. There is a widespread tendency to attribute genuine disease symptoms to "__________ __________ __________" and fail to provide proper treatment.
3. Some changes in __________ performance are probably not a direct consequence of ________, but rather reflect the ________ effect of sedentary lifestyle.
4. A person's __________ capacity also undergoes significant __________ with age, largely due to decreases in the elasticity of the lungs and in the size and strength of the respiratory muscles.
5. As a person ages, the kidneys shrink in size. This decline in weight results from a loss of functioning __________ __________, which translates into a smaller effective __________ surface.
6. The decrease in __________ may lead to malnutrition. Other changes in the mouth include a reduction in the volume of __________, with a resulting __________ of the mouth.
7. Narrowing of the __________ disks and __________ ____________of the vertebrae contribute to a decrease in __________ as a person ages, along with changes in posture.

8. A hearing-related impairment noted in the older adult population is __________ __________. Onset of symptoms usually occurs in early middle age, with symptoms presenting in __________ that last several __________ at a time.

9. __________ and loss of __________ of the skin are the most visible signs of aging. Wrinkling occurs because the skin becomes thinner, __________, less elastic, and more __________.

10. Heart attack or myocardial infarction is the major cause of __________ and __________ in people older than 65 years, and its potential for mortality increases significantly after a person reaches __________ years.

Identify

In the following case studies, list the chief complaint, vital signs, and pertinent negatives.

1. On arrival to the Adult Day Care Center, you discover an 84-year-old woman who has "fallen." She normally walks with the assistance of a cane or walker. She is lying on a deeply carpeted floor and is conscious, alert, and complaining of right-sided midthigh pain. The fall was reportedly not witnessed. Her aide was assisting another client when the fall occurred. Your patient does not have a good recollection of what happened. She denies chest pain, shortness of breath, dizziness, nausea, or vomiting. She also denies tripping and falling. The area appears clear of obstacles, rugs, or other obvious trip hazards. Your physical exam is as previously indicated. You notice some inward rotation and shortening of the extremity. Her pulse is 84 beats/min and very irregular. Her oxygen saturation is 88% on room air. Her blood pressure (BP) is 106/86 mm Hg. The patient's skin turgor is poor. Pupils are equal, round, regular in size, and reactive to light and accommodation (PERRLA). An electrocardiogram (ECG) shows a sinus rhythm with frequent premature ventricular contractions (PVCs) and short runs of ventricular tachycardia (VT) (with a pulse).
   a. Chief complaint:

   ____

   ____

   b. Vital signs:

   ____

   ____

   c. Pertinent negatives:

   ____

   ____

2. It's early afternoon on a clear and warm spring day. You are dispatched to the parking lot of a local supermarket for a reported motor vehicle crash. On arrival, you discover an elderly man who is 92 years old. He is the driver of a vehicle that struck several parked cars. Bystanders state that the patient appears to be either sleeping or unconscious. You find the patient to be conscious but not alert to person, place, time, or purpose. The police identify his home phone number and call it. A pleasant-sounding elderly woman answers and states that her husband left home over an hour ago to pick up some groceries. She states that he has a problem with "sugar" and wonders if he has his hearing aids in place. As you begin examining the patient and taking his history, it becomes obvious that he is not wearing hearing aids. There is minimally detectable damage to the vehicle as well as the vehicles that were struck. The patient was found not to be wearing his seat belt. He does have a medical identification bracelet on, and it indicates extensive cardiac and diabetic history. Vital signs indicate a blood glucose level of 66 mg/dL. His pulse rate is 92 beats/min and regular, and BP is 160/72 mm Hg. His skin is warm and moist, his capillary refill is normal, and he has an oxygen saturation of 96% on room air. The patient is able to maintain his own airway and gag reflex. He was initially assisted

with oral glucose by the emergency medical responders (EMRs) at the scene. He is becoming increasingly alert and oriented and denies any injury.

a. Chief complaint:

____

____

b. Vital signs:

____

____

c. Pertinent negatives:

____

____

Complete the Patient Care Report (PCR)

Read the first incident scenario in the preceding Identify exercises and then complete the following PCR for the patient.

EMS Patient Care Report (PCR)					
Date:	Incident No.:	Nature of Call:		Location:	
Dispatched:	En Route:	At Scene:	Transport:	At Hospital:	In Service:
Patient Information					
Age: Sex: Weight (in kg [lb]):			Allergies: Medications: Past Medical History: Chief Complaint:		
Vital Signs					
Time:	BP:	Pulse:	Respirations:	SpO_2:	
Time:	BP:	Pulse:	Respirations:	SpO_2:	
Time:	BP:	Pulse:	Respirations:	SpO_2:	
EMS Treatment (circle all that apply)					
Oxygen @ ______ L/min via (circle one): NC NRM Bag-mask device		Assisted Ventilation	Airway Adjunct	CPR	
Defibrillation	Bleeding Control	Bandaging	Splinting	Other:	
Narrative					

Ambulance Calls

The following case scenarios provide an opportunity to explore the concerns associated with patient management and paramedic care. Read each scenario, and then answer each question.

1. One way to try to ensure that you don't miss anything important in the patient's history is to ask some general screening questions, irrespective of the patient's chief complaint. Suppose an 80-year-old woman has called for an ambulance because she feels "tired and weak." List 10 general screening questions you would ask to assess the status of her major organ systems.

a. ____________________

b. ____________________

c. ____________________

d. ____________________

e. ____________________

f. ____________________

g. ____________________

h. ____________________

i. ____________________

j. ____________________

2. You are called to the apartment of a 78-year-old woman who fell down.

a. List six questions you would ask in taking the history of the present illness for an older patient who sustained trauma.

(1)____________________

(2)____________________

(3)____________________

(4)____________________

(5)____________________

(6)____________________

b. List the information you should obtain about the patient's past (other) medical history.

(1)____________________

(2)____________________

(3)____________________

(4)____________________

c. List six things that your environmental assessment should include:

(1)____________________

(2)____________________

(3)____________________

(4)________________________________

(5)________________________________

(6)________________________________

d. While conducting the physical examination, you will of course be alert for signs or symptoms of those injuries to which older people are particularly vulnerable. List three injuries to which older adult patients are more susceptible.

(1)________________________________

(2)________________________________

(3)________________________________

3. You are called to a shopping center where an older adult man tripped on a potted plant and fell, sustaining a minor laceration to his arm. As you are applying a dressing to the laceration, you notice that he seems very listless and depressed. List six factors of a "social assessment" you should consider.

a. ________________________________

b. ________________________________

c. ________________________________

d. ________________________________

e. ________________________________

f. ________________________________

True/False

The public (and also, regrettably, health care professionals) holds many widespread misconceptions about older adults and the process of aging that result in inaccurate stereotypes of older adults. If you believe the statement to be more true than false, write the letter "T" in the space provided. If you believe the statement to be more false than true, write the letter "F."

______ **1.** The rate of aging is the same in a 35-year-old as it is in an 85-year-old.

______ **2.** As the brain gets smaller and lighter, it loses its reserve capacity to store information.

______ **3.** Older adults are more likely than younger individuals to seek emergency care for minor, nonserious complaints.

______ **4.** The pain mechanism is often slowed among the older adults, causing burn injuries.

______ **5.** The possibility of hearing loss increases with age.

______ **6.** Sweat gland activity increases, hindering the ability to sweat and to regulate heat.

______ **7.** Tachypnea can be a sensitive indicator of acute illness in older people.

______ **8.** The older adult is at a higher risk of developing peripheral vascular disease.

______ **9.** The earliest stage of Alzheimer disease involves forgetting components of one's life history and difficulty writing letters.

______ **10.** One clue to elder abuse is unexplained injuries that do not fit the stated cause.

Short Answer

Complete this section with short written answers using the space provided.

1. Patients older than 65 years account for one-third of all ambulance calls today. As the population continues to age, that percentage can be expected to increase. It is therefore important for paramedics to understand the special problems and challenges posed by caring for the elderly. List five characteristics of the older adults that make it particularly challenging to diagnose their problems correctly and provide them with appropriate care.

   a. ______________________________

   b. ______________________________

   c. ______________________________

   d. ______________________________

   e. ______________________________

2. The process of aging in our society is nearly always accompanied by social and psychological stresses that may have an enormous impact on health. List two potentially stressful changes that tend to occur in a person's life as he or she approaches the "golden age."

   a. ______________________________

   b. ______________________________

3. The normal aging process produces changes in nearly every organ system of the body. It is important to know what constitutes a *normal* age-related change so that such a change will not be mistaken for a sign of disease (and, conversely, so that signs of disease will not be disregarded as "just part of getting old"). For each of the following organ systems, list two changes in structure or function that occur as a normal consequence of aging.

   a. Cardiovascular

   (1) ______________________________

   (2) ______________________________

   b. Respiratory

   (1) ______________________________

   (2) ______________________________

   c. Renal

   (1) ______________________________

   (2) ______________________________

   d. Digestive

   (1) ______________________________

   (2) ______________________________

   e. Musculoskeletal

   (1) ______________________________

   (2) ______________________________

f. Nervous

(1) ______________________________

(2) ______________________________

g. Homeostatic

(1) ______________________________

(2) ______________________________

4. In younger patients, the chief complaint often has considerable value in localizing the patient's underlying problem. A middle-aged man suffering an acute coronary syndrome, for example, will usually complain of pain or discomfort in his chest, whereas a young person with pneumonia usually will have a cough and a fever. Among the elderly, on the other hand, the response to serious illness tends to be less specific. List four responses to illness common among seriously ill elderly patients.

a. ______________________________

b. ______________________________

c. ______________________________

d. ______________________________

5. Obtaining an accurate history from an elderly patient requires considerable skill because there are a number of obstacles to history taking among older adults that do not exist when you talk with younger patients. List four obstacles to obtaining a medical history from an elderly person, and indicate what steps you can take to overcome each of them.

a. Obstacle:

____

____

What I can do to try to overcome the obstacle:

____

____

b. Obstacle:

____

____

What I can do to try to overcome the obstacle:

____

____

c. Obstacle:

____

____

What I can do to try to overcome the obstacle:

______

______

d. Obstacle:

______

______

What I can do to try to overcome the obstacle:

______

______

6. In a middle-aged patient, the clinical presentation of such conditions as acute myocardial infarction (AMI) or heart failure is usually straightforward. In an elderly person with the same problem, the clinical presentation may be much less clear-cut. List at least two signs or symptoms that are commonly part of the clinical presentation of AMI and of heart failure in the elderly.

Condition	Possible Signs and Symptoms in the Elderly
Acute myocardial infarction	
Heart failure	

7. One of the most common presenting symptoms among the elderly is an acute confusional state (delirium). Complete the list of conditions likely to present as delirium in the elderly, which are represented by the letters in the acronym DELIRIUMS that follows:

D: ______

E: ______

L: ______

I: ______

R: ______

I: ______

U: ______

M: ______

S: ______

Fill in the Table

Fill in the missing parts of the following tables.

1.

Causes of Falls in Older Adults	
Cause	Clues to Suggest This Cause
	Obvious environmental hazard at the scene, such as poor lighting, scatter rugs, uneven sidewalk, or ice or other slippery surface
	Sudden fall; patient found on the ground somewhat confused, often temporarily paralyzed and unable to get up; no premonitory symptoms
	Fall when getting up from a recumbent or sitting position (Check medications the patient is taking, and ask about occult blood loss, such as presence of black stools. Measure blood pressure in recumbent and sitting positions.)
	Marked bradycardia or tachydysrhythmias
	Other characteristic signs of stroke, such as hemiparesis, hemiplegia, or aphasia
	Patient felt something snap before falling

2.

Signs of Dehydration in Older Adults
Dry tongue
Dry mucous membranes
Confusion
Sunken eyes

CHAPTER

45

Patients With Special Challenges

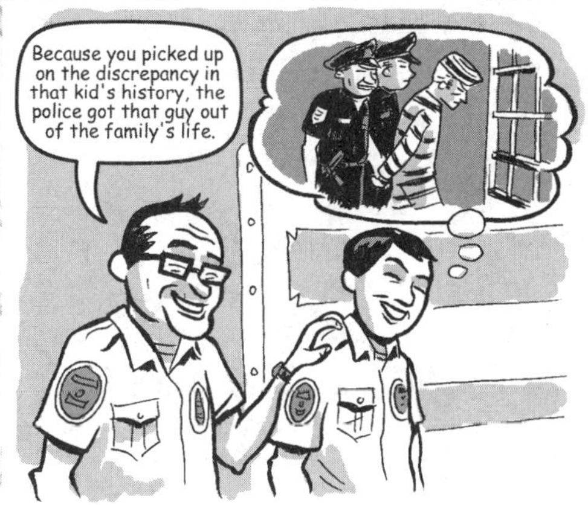

Matching

Part I

Match each of the terms in the right column to the appropriate definition in the left column.

_____	**1.** A type of hearing impairment due to problems with the middle ear bones' ability to conduct sounds from the outer ear to the inner ear.	**A.** Acute angle-closure glaucoma (AACG)
_____	**2.** Medical treatment aimed at symptom relief and providing comfort for the patient.	**B.** Apraxia
_____	**3.** A plastic pouch or bag attached over a colostomy to collect stool.	**C.** Auditory neuropathy
_____	**4.** The surgical establishment of an opening between the colon and the surface of the body for the purpose of providing drainage of the bowel.	**D.** Autism
_____	**5.** A tube placed in the body to relieve pressure by drawing excess cerebrospinal fluid from the brain or spinal cord.	**E.** Autism spectrum disorder
_____	**6.** The part of a tracheostomy tube that is used to stabilize the tube to the patient's neck.	**F.** Bariatrics
_____	**7.** A surgically created connection between an artery and a vein, usually in the arm, for dialysis access.	**G.** Cancer
_____	**8.** Having perforations, holes, or openings.	**H.** Central auditory processing disorder (CAPD)
_____	**9.** An area that a device was not intended to be inserted into—for example, a tracheostomy tube inserted into an area other than the trachea.	**I.** Cerebral palsy (CP)
_____	**10.** A form of abuse that may be verbal (such as ridicule, threats, blaming, or humiliation) or nonverbal (such as caregiver ignoring the victim or isolating the victim from others). The abuse causes a substantial change in the victim's behavior, emotional response, or cognitive function or may manifest as a variety of mental illnesses.	**J.** Cerebrospinal fluid shunt (CSF shunt)
_____	**11.** A developmental condition in which damage is done to the brain. It presents during infancy as a delay in walking or crawling and can take on a spastic form in which muscles are in a nearly constant state of contraction.	**K.** Colostomy
_____	**12.** A disorder in which patients have difficulty interpreting speech and differentiating it from other sounds that are present.	**L.** Colostomy bag
_____	**13.** Excessive growth and division of abnormal cells within the body that can occur in many body systems, tissues, and organs and that can progress rapidly and cause death in a relatively short period.	**M.** Comfort care

_____ **14.** The medical specialty dedicated to prevention and treatment of obesity.

_____ **15.** A group of complex disorders of brain development, characterized by difficulties in social interaction, repetitive behaviors, and verbal and nonverbal communication.

_____ **16.** A speech disorder caused by neuromuscular disturbance that causes speech to become slow and slurred.

_____ **17.** A genetic chromosomal defect that can occur during fetal development and that results in intellectual disability and certain physical characteristics, such as a round head with a flat occiput and slanted, wide-set eyes.

_____ **18.** Insufficient development of a portion of the brain, resulting in some level of dysfunction or impairment.

_____ **19.** A broad term that describes an infant or child's failure to reach a particular developmental milestone by the expected time.

_____ **20.** A genetic disorder of the endocrine system that makes it difficult for chloride to move through cells; primarily targets that respiratory and digestive systems.

_____ **21.** A developmental disorder characterized by impairments of social interaction; may include severe behavioral problems, repetitive motor activities, and impairments in verbal and nonverbal skills.

_____ **22.** A condition characterized by normal function of the structures of the ear without a corresponding stimulation of auditory centers of the brain; also called dyssynchrony.

_____ **23.** A neurologic impairment in which the brain is intermittently unable to carry out the command for speech or other tasks.

_____ **24.** Increased intraocular pressure that leads to ocular pain and decreased visual acuity. Sudden onset is a medical emergency.

_____ **25.** Medical treatment aimed at curing an illness.

_____ **26.** A psychological conditional in which stress or mental conflict is converted into physical complaints.

N. Conductive hearing loss
O. Conversion disorder
P. Curative care
Q. Cystic fibrosis (CF)
R. Developmental delay
S. Developmental disability
T. Down syndrome
U. Dysarthria
V. Emotional abuse
W. False lumen
X. Fenestrated
Y. Fistula
Z. Flange

Part II

Match each of the terms in the right column to the appropriate definition in the left column.

_____ **1.** A congenital condition characterized by failure of the optic nerve to completely develop, possibly resulting in optic nerve atrophy over time.

_____ **2.** An autoimmune disorder in which the extraocular muscles become weakened and are fatigued.

_____ **3.** A solid plug at the end of a tracheostomy.

_____ **4.** A condition in which a person's body mass index is greater than 30 kg/m^2.

_____ **5.** A developmental anomaly in which a portion of the spinal cord or meninges protrudes outside the spinal column or even outside the body, usually in the area of the lumbar spine; also called a spina bifida.

_____ **6.** A category of professional required by some states to report suspicions of child maltreatment. Prehospital professionals may be included.

_____ **7.** A type of disability in which difficulties with reading, spelling, or writing cause a person to fall behind expectations for a given age.

_____ **8.** A balloon that is inserted into the aorta and connected to a pump via a catheter. This therapy helps to increase the blood flow to the coronary arteries during diastole (inflation) and decrease afterload of blood from the left ventricle (deflation).

A. Hemodynamic monitoring
B. Heparinized solution
C. Hospice
D. Hydrocephalus
E. Ileus
F. Inner cannula
G. Intellectual disability
H. Intra-aortic balloon pump

______ **9.** A medical condition in which there is an abnormal buildup of cerebrospinal fluid in the skull; this can be acquired (occurring after birth) or congenital (developing before birth). — **I.** Language-based learning disability

______ **10.** An organization that provides end-of-life care to patients with terminal illnesses and their families. — **J.** Mandatory reporter

______ **11.** A saline solution mixed with heparin, an anticoagulant used to prevent blood clots from forming. — **K.** Muscular dystrophy

______ **12.** Monitoring and measurement of blood movement, volume, and pressure. — **L.** Myasthenia gravis

______ **13.** Paralysis of the upper and lower extremities. — **M.** Myasthenic crisis

______ **14.** The death of nerve fibers as a late consequence of polio. The syndrome is characterized by swallowing difficulties, weakness, fatigue, and breathing problems. — **N.** Myelomeningocele

______ **15.** A viral infection that attacks and destroys motor axons. The disease can cause weakness, paralysis, and respiratory arrest. Because an effective vaccine has been developed, the incidence of the disease is now rare. — **O.** Obesity

______ **16.** A form of abuse that involves an intentional act, such as throwing, striking, hitting, kicking, burning, or biting a vulnerable person. — **P.** Obturator

______ **17.** A category of disorders that impact a person's ability to produce sounds that combine into spoken words. — **Q.** Ocular myasthenia gravis

______ **18.** A complication of myasthenia gravis in which weakened respiratory muscles lead to respiratory failure. — **R.** Optic nerve hypoplasia

______ **19.** A condition in which the body generates antibodies against its own acetylcholine receptors, causing muscle weakness, often in the face. — **S.** Outer cannula

______ **20.** A broad term that describes a category of incurable genetic diseases that cause a slow, progressive degeneration of the muscle fibers. — **T.** Palliative care

______ **21.** A primarily cognitive disorder that appears during childhood and is accompanied by lack of adaptive behaviors, such as the ability to live and function independently or interact successfully with others; generally defined as an intelligence quotient below 70; formerly called mental retardation. — **U.** Paraplegia

______ **22.** The inner tube that is inserted into the outer cannula of a tracheostomy tube. — **V.** Phonologic process disorders

______ **23.** Disruption or loss of normal gastrointestinal motility. — **W.** Physical abuse

______ **24.** Paralysis of the lower extremities. — **X.** Poliomyelitis

______ **25.** Medical care aimed at relief of pain and suffering in terminally ill patients. — **Y.** Postpolio syndrome

______ **26.** The larger (outer) tube of a tracheostomy tube. — **Z.** Quadriplegia

Part III

Match each of the terms in the right column to the appropriate definition in the left column.

______ **1.** A person legally authorized to make health care decisions on behalf of a patient who is incapable of making or communicating the decision on his or her own. — **A.** Retinopathy

______ **2.** A developmental anomaly in which a portion of the spinal cord or meninges protrudes outside the spinal column or even outside the body, usually in the area of the lumbar spine (the lower third of the spine); also called myelomeningocele. — **B.** Semantic-pragmatic disorder

______ **3.** A form of cerebral palsy in which all four limbs are affected. — **C.** Sensorineural hearing loss

______ **4.** A chronic form of paralysis in which the affected muscles experience continued spasm. — **D.** Sexual abuse

_____	**5.** A surgically constructed opening for the urinary system.	**E.** Sexual exploitation
_____	**6.** A device that converts energy or pressure into electrical signals.	**F.** Spastic paralysis
_____	**7.** A plastic tube placed within the tracheostomy site (stoma).	**G.** Spastic tetraplegia
_____	**8.** A sickness that a patient cannot be cured of. Death is imminent.	**H.** Spina bifida
_____	**9.** A form of abuse that involves forcing a vulnerable person to perform or be involved in sexual acts, or to be involved in sexual activities, such as pornography, in return for something they need or want, such as money, food, or shelter.	**I.** Surrogate decision maker
_____	**10.** A form of abuse that involves a vulnerable person being forced into unwanted sexual acts, or into involvement in sexual activities such as pornography.	**J.** Terminal illness
_____	**11.** A permanent lack of hearing caused by a lesion or damage of the inner ear.	**K.** Tracheostomy tube
_____	**12.** A condition characterized by delayed language developmental milestones, resulting in the person repeatedly using irrelevant phrases out of context, confusing word pairs, and having trouble following conversations.	**L.** Transducer
_____	**13.** Any eye disorder in which the retina becomes diseased, leading to partial or total vision loss.	**M.** Urostomy

Multiple Choice

Read each item carefully, and then select the best response.

_____ **1.** Which of the following would be considered speech impairments?

A. Articulation disorders
B. Language disorders
C. Fluency disorders
D. All of the above

_____ **2.** Congenital causes of visual impairment would include each of the following, EXCEPT:

A. fetal exposure to cytomegalovirus.
B. cerebrovascular accident.
C. retinopathy of prematurity.
D. hydrocephalus.

_____ **3.** Bruises on the torso, ___________, and buttocks are suggestive of abuse.

A. ears
B. proximal arms
C. abdomen
D. All of the above

_____ **4.** The different types of paralysis include all of the following, EXCEPT:

A. spastic paralysis.
B. quadriplegia.
C. myasthenia gravis.
D. paraplegia.

_____ **5.** Which of the following is NOT typically tunneled under the skin and into the vena cava?

A. Hickman
B. Port-a-Cath
C. Vas-Cath/Permcath
D. Broviac

_____ **6.** Patients with a terminal illness who receive continued medical care, hoping for a statistically improbable recovery, are receiving:

A. comfort care.
B. acute care.
C. curative care.
D. palliative care.

_____ **7.** Chemotherapy medications are notorious for causing:

A. nausea and vomiting.
B. loss of appetite.
C. immune system compromise.
D. All of the above

_____ **8.** A potentially devastating, nonprogressive neurologic disorder resulting from brain tissue injury during brain development is a condition called:

A. epilepsy.
B. cerebral palsy.
C. cystic fibrosis.
D. multiple sclerosis.

_____ **9.** Which of the following devices serves as a long-term replacement for an endotracheal (ET) tube in a patient who has a chronic condition?

A. A ventricular assist device
B. A tracheostomy tube
C. An obturator
D. A stoma

_____ **10.** You are treating a 62-year-old man who is complaining of chest pain for the past 35 minutes. You have decided to administer aspirin, nitroglycerin, and oxygen and to start an IV. The patient has been receiving treatments through a long-term vascular access device in his chest. If there are still distal IV sites available, why should the paramedic *avoid* using the long-term device in the patient's chest?

A. The device may be inserted directly into the vena cava.
B. It may require a special needle to access the port.
C. The device may be maintained with a high dose of heparin.
D. All of the above

Labeling

Label the following diagrams with the correct terms.

1. American Sign Language (ASL) signs for common terms related to illness or injury

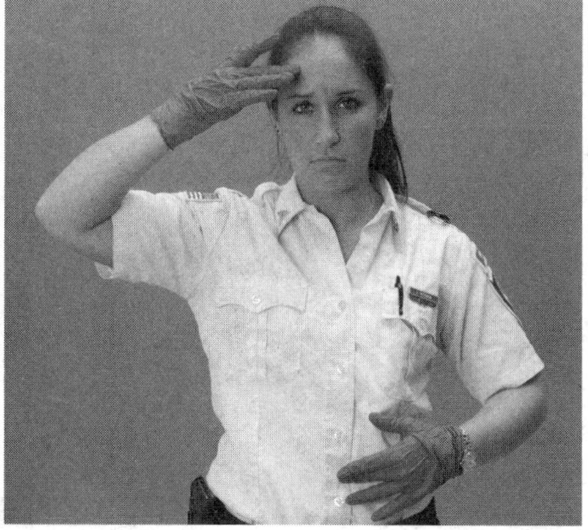

A. ______________________________

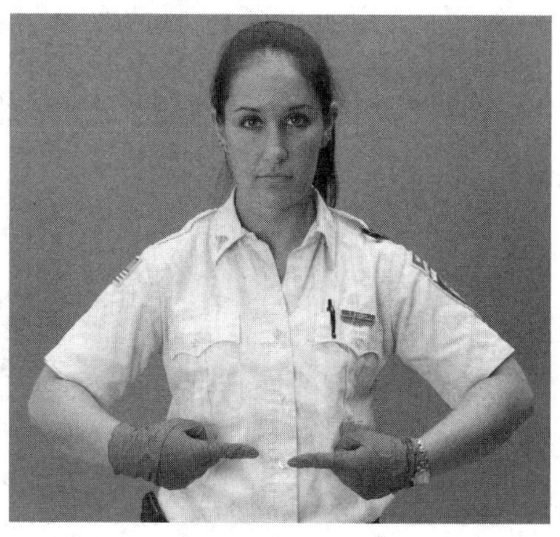

B. ______________________________

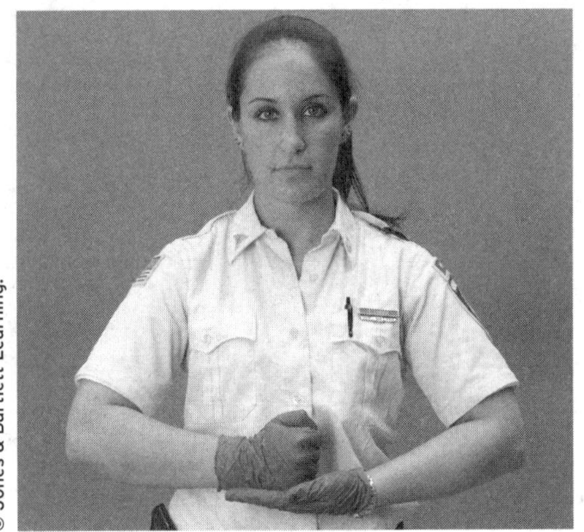

C. ____________________

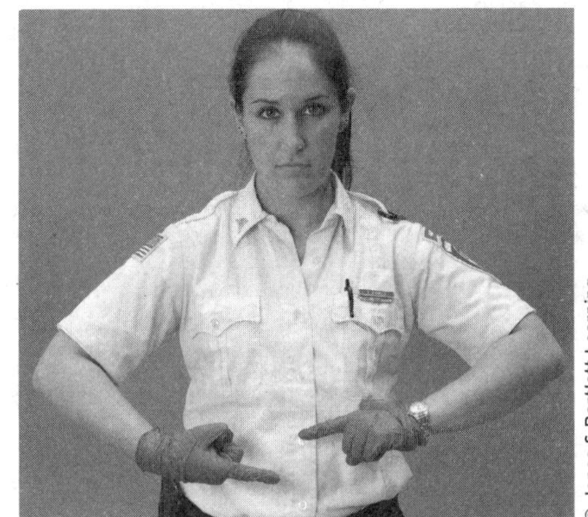

D. ____________________

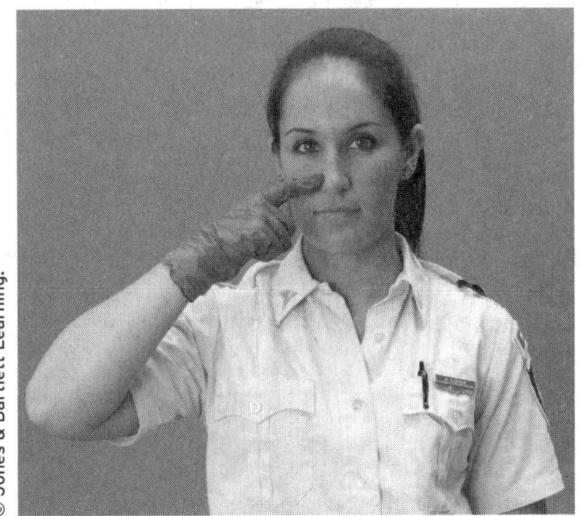

E1. ____________________

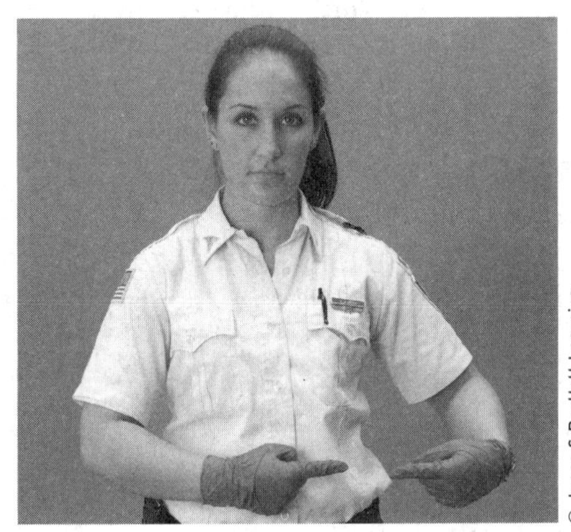

E2. ____________________

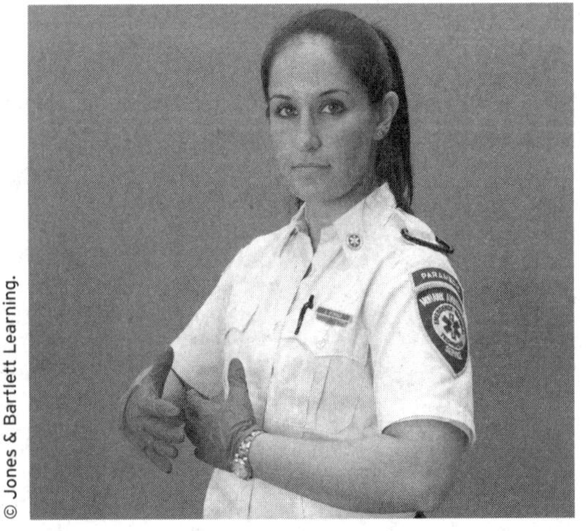

F. ____________________

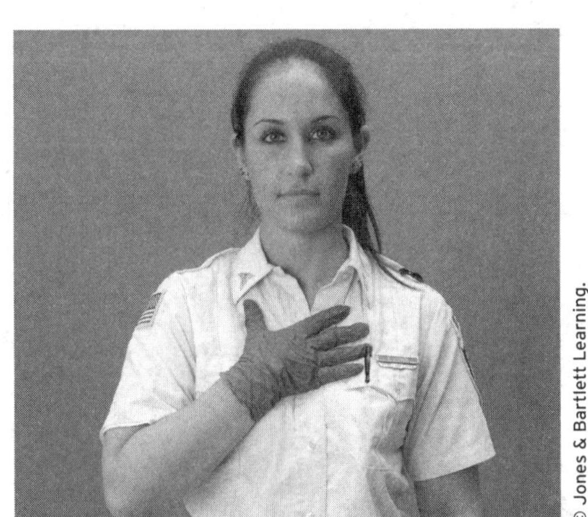

G. ____________________

H. 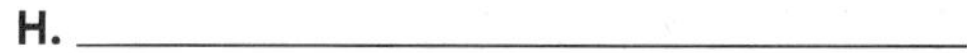

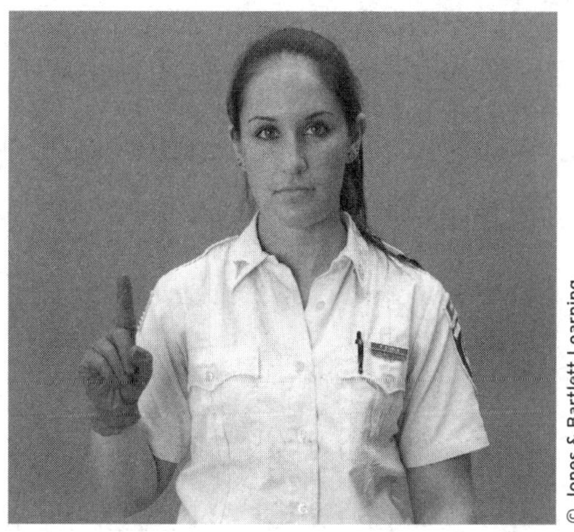

I. ______________________________

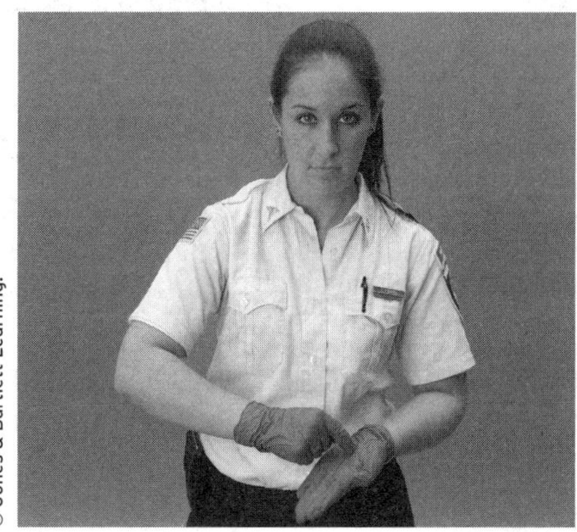

J. ______________________________

2. Parts of the tracheostomy tube

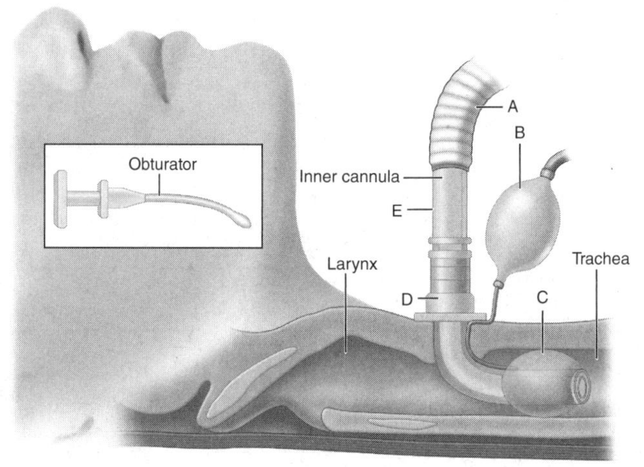

A. ______________________________

B. ______________________________

C. ______________________________

D. ______________________________

E. ______________________________

Fill in the Blank

Read each item carefully, and then complete the statement by filling in the missing word(s).

1. Hearing challenges are generally classified into two types: __________ and __________ deafness.
2. Hearing __________ may be __________ or acquired.
3. Speech impairment may be divided into disorders impacting __________, voice __________, fluency, and __________.
4. Autistic patients may present with a(n) __________-__________ disorder of speech.
5. Patients may receive a(n) __________ following __________ trauma or surgery.
6. The medical specialty of __________ has emerged in response to the widespread and profound incidence of adult and childhood __________.
7. Myelomeningocele, also known as __________ __________, is a birth defect caused by improper development of the __________ __________ tube consisting of the brain and spinal cord.
8. Infants and young children may be diagnosed with __________ __________ (__________), a genetic disorder that is characterized by increased production of mucus in the lungs and digestive tract. This disorder is caused by a(n) __________ __________ gene, inherited from each parent.
9. Cerebral palsy generally produces __________ __________ muscle function or __________.
10. Spina bifida, also known as ______________, is a birth defect caused by improper ______________ of the fetal neural tube consisting of the brain and ________ cord.

Identify

Read the following case studies, and then list the chief complaint, the history of the present illness, and other medical history.

1. You have been called to the scene by distraught family members. The patient is becoming increasingly disoriented and appears unresponsive. The patient is exhibiting an irregular breathing pattern with periods of apnea. His blood pressure (BP) is about 70/palp, and his pulse is very fast and erratic. Some family members have what appears to be a valid prehospital do not resuscitate (DNR) order.
   a. Chief complaint:

   ____

   ____

   b. History of the present illness:

   ____

   ____

   c. Other medical history:

   ____

   ____

2. You are responding to a call to an adult group home for adults with disabilities. The nature of the call is for a patient with seizures. On arrival, you are met by staff members who have the patient's complete chart. The patient has a history of Down syndrome and a seizure disorder. The patient is on multiple medications and has been given rectal diazepam (Diastat).

   a. Chief complaint:

   ____

   ____

   b. History of the present illness:

   ____

   ____

   c. Other medical history:

   ____

   ____

3. Your patient has a chief complaint of fever. The patient's home health aide states that the patient's urine has been cloudy and that he's suddenly developed a fever of 101.3°F. He is conscious and alert, and his vitals are a BP of 110/70 mm Hg and a heart rate of 108 beats/min. He is always confined to a wheelchair. He communicates with a writing board. He is a quadriplegic and has a Foley catheter, tracheotomy, colostomy, and feeding tube. He is taking an antibiotic and a steroid medicine.

   a. Chief complaint:

   ____

   ____

   b. History of the present illness:

   ____

   ____

   c. Other medical history:

   ____

   ____

Complete the Patient Care Report (PCR)

Read incident scenario 3 in the preceding Identify exercises, and then complete the following PCR for the patient.

<table>
<tr><th colspan="6">EMS Patient Care Report (PCR)</th></tr>
<tr><td>Date:</td><td>Incident No.:</td><td colspan="2">Nature of Call:</td><td colspan="2">Location:</td></tr>
<tr><td>Dispatched:</td><td>En Route:</td><td>At Scene:</td><td>Transport:</td><td>At Hospital:</td><td>In Service:</td></tr>
<tr><th colspan="6">Patient Information</th></tr>
<tr><td colspan="3">Age:
Sex:
Weight (in kg [lb]):</td><td colspan="3">Allergies:
Medications:
Past Medical History:
Chief Complaint:</td></tr>
<tr><th colspan="6">Vital Signs</th></tr>
<tr><td>Time:</td><td>BP:</td><td>Pulse:</td><td>Respirations:</td><td colspan="2">SpO_2:</td></tr>
<tr><td>Time:</td><td>BP:</td><td>Pulse:</td><td>Respirations:</td><td colspan="2">SpO_2:</td></tr>
<tr><td>Time:</td><td>BP:</td><td>Pulse:</td><td>Respirations:</td><td colspan="2">SpO_2:</td></tr>
<tr><th colspan="6">EMS Treatment
(circle all that apply)</th></tr>
<tr><td colspan="2">Oxygen @ ______ L/min via (circle one):
NC NRM Bag-mask device</td><td>Assisted Ventilation</td><td>Airway Adjunct</td><td colspan="2">CPR</td></tr>
<tr><td>Defibrillation</td><td>Bleeding Control</td><td>Bandaging</td><td>Splinting</td><td colspan="2">Other:</td></tr>
<tr><th colspan="6">Narrative</th></tr>
<tr><td colspan="6"></td></tr>
</table>

Ambulance Calls

The following case scenarios provide an opportunity to explore the concerns associated with patient management and paramedic care. Read each scenario, and then answer each question.

1. You receive an "alpha" response for a patient with chronic pain. On arrival, you note the wheelchair ramp in front of the apartment. Once inside, you recognize your patient. You have provided care for her in the past. She is 36 years old and is complaining of severe lower back pain and requesting transportation to the medical center. She is somewhat difficult to interact with and is not very polite. Despite that, you continue to be professional and initiate care. She has a history of spina bifida and is seated in her motorized wheelchair. She is covered in a blanket.
   a. What can you do to help alleviate her discomfort during transfer from her wheelchair to the cot?

   ____

   ____

   b. Based on your knowledge of spina bifida, what other medical issues may be present?

   ____

   ____

2. Tonight you are working a special event at the civic center. It's the concert of a popular country singer. The place is packed. Other than a couple of requests for ice packs and ear plugs, the event has been uneventful. Suddenly, security requests emergency medical services (EMS) to section 103 for a person having a seizure. Your patient is a 12-year-old girl with her mom. The patient has Down syndrome and a seizure disorder. The seizure is over by the time you arrive, but the patient appears postictal and has a large amount of saliva and snoring-type respirations.
   a. How would you go about treating the patient?

   ____

   ____

   b. What are the characteristic physical features of someone with Down syndrome?

   ____

   ____

True/False

If you believe the statement to be more true than false, write the letter "T" in the space provided. If you believe the statement to be more false than true, write the letter "F."

______ 1. Whatever the source of the challenge, patients with special needs will require you to adapt your assessment and management to accommodate their needs.

______ 2. A method of instilling a special solution through a catheter into the renal patient's abdomen is referred to as hemodialysis.

______ 3. A phonologic process disorder impacts a person's ability to produce sounds that combine into spoken words.

______ 4. Patients with nearsightedness have an impairment known as myopia.

______ 5. It is not necessary to modify patient assessment techniques for the patient with a cognitive impairment.

______ 6. Patients with mental impairments view all strangers, especially paramedics in uniform, in a friendly and calm manner.

______ 7. Cystic fibrosis is a chronic dysfunction of the endocrine system that targets multiple body systems but primarily the respiratory and digestive systems.

______ 8. Muscular dystrophy is an acquired muscular disease that causes degeneration of the muscle fibers. In many cases, the destroyed fibers are replaced by fat or connective tissue.

_____ **9.** Patients with myasthenia gravis have facial and throat muscles that could become so weak that the patient suffers an acute onset of respiratory failure.

_____ **10.** Patients with obesity may have a diminished respiratory reserve, causing hypoxia quickly.

_____ **11.** Speech is not possible unless expired air is allowed to pass around a tracheostomy tube and through the larynx.

Short Answer

Complete this section with short written answers using the space provided.

1. Many of the patients a paramedic encounters have hearing impairments. Sometimes this impairment is readily noticeable.

a. What clues would indicate to you that your patient has a hearing impairment?

(1) _____

(2) _____

(3) _____

b. List five ways you can go about communicating with someone with a hearing impairment.

(1) _____

(2) _____

(3) _____

(4) _____

(5) _____

2. Transporting obese patients can be particularly challenging for paramedic crews. List five strategies that would be helpful to the patient and the EMS providers.

a. _____

b. _____

c. _____

d. _____

e. _____

3. You respond to a car crash. On arrival, you discover a frightened but apparently uninjured rear-seat passenger. Everyone else appears to be out of the car and walking around. You discover that the passenger has a visual impairment.

a. What are some of the causes of visual impairments?

(1) _____

(2) _____

(3) _____

b. What can paramedics do to alleviate some of the fears felt by patients with visual impairments?

(1) ______________________________

(2) ______________________________

(3) ______________________________

(4) ______________________________

Fill in the Table

Fill in the missing parts of the tables.

1. A list of the known causes of developmental disabilities is found in the following table. Fill in the missing parts of the table.

Known Causes of Development Disabilities
Genetic abnormality
Maternal trauma, hemorrhage, or infection during fetal development
Malnutrition
Neurologic insult, injury, or infection
Toxic exposure
Near drowning
Trauma or hypoxia during delivery

Data from: Facts about developmental disabilities. Centers for Disease Control and Prevention website. https://www.cdc.gov/ncbddd/developmentaldisabilities/facts.html. Updated July 9, 2015. Accessed May 4, 2017; Pivalizza P, Lalani SR. Intellectual disability in children: evaluation for a cause. UpToDate website. http://www.uptodate.com/contents/intellectual-disability-in-children-evaluation-for-a-cause. Updated May 26, 2016. Accessed May 4, 2017; and Pivalizza P, Lalani SR. Intellectual disability in children: definition, diagnosis, and assessment of needs. UpToDate website. http://www.uptodate.com/contents/intellectual-disability-in-children-definition-diagnosis-and-assessment-of-needs?source=see_link. Updated August 15, 2016. Accessed May 4, 2017.

2. Complete the list of causes of obesity.

Causes of and Contributing Factors to Obesity
Poor dietary choices
Hormonal changes
Low basal metabolic rate
Cessation/reduction of cigarette smoking

Data from: Dare S, Mackay DF, Pell JP. Relationship between smoking and obesity: a cross-sectional study of 499,504 middle-aged adults in the UK general population. *PLoS One.* 2015;10(4):e0123579. https://www.ncbi.nlm.nih.gov/pmc/articles/PMC4401671/. Accessed May 4, 2017.

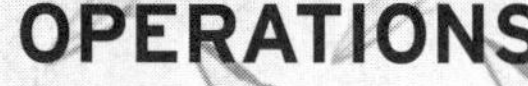

SECTION 10

OPERATIONS

CHAPTER 46 Transport Operations

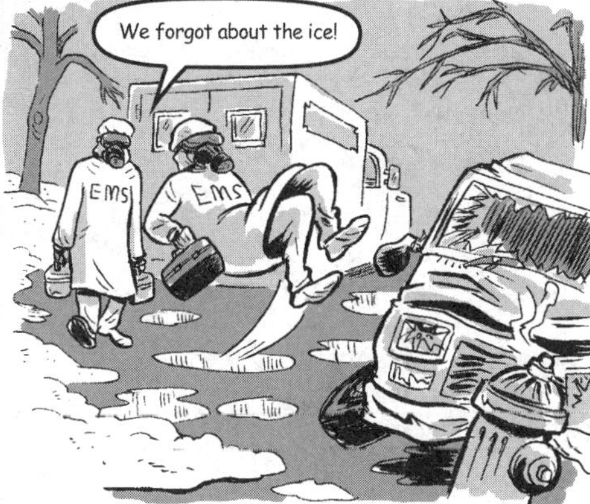

The size-up of the emergency scene is a critical process. . .

Matching

Part I

Match each of the numbered items to the appropriate type of ambulance transport.

Your air ambulance transports to a regional trauma center. Your ground ambulance transports to a community hospital. Choose the correct transportation for your patient.

A. Air ambulance

G. Ground ambulance

_____ **1.** 50-year-old in cardiac arrest

_____ **2.** 8-year-old having an asthma attack

_____ **3.** 22-year-old thrown from a rollover crash

_____ **4.** 44-year-old with amputation of the left hand

_____ **5.** 26-year-old mountain climber who fell approximately 50 feet

_____ **6.** 24-year-old with a breech presentation delivery

_____ **7.** 56-year-old with an active upper gastrointestinal bleed

_____ **8.** 18-year-old with a broken femur from an all-terrain vehicle crash

_____ **9.** 2-year-old submersion victim who fell through ice at the local pond

_____ **10.** 34-year-old with a broken ankle from a football game

Part II

Match each of the definitions in the left column to the appropriate term in the right column.

_____ **1.** A sensation that when an operator depresses the brake pedal, the steering wheel is being pulled to the left or the right.

_____ **2.** A person who assists a driver in backing up an emergency vehicle to compensate for blind spots at the back of the vehicle.

_____ **3.** A sensation of looseness or sloppiness in a vehicle's steering.

_____ **4.** A safe distance maintained between your vehicle and other vehicles on any side of you.

_____ **5.** Federal standards that regulate the design and manufacturing guidelines of emergency medical vehicles.

_____ **6.** A finding that when the operator lets go of the steering wheel, a vehicle consistently wanders to the left or right.

_____ **7.** The process of removing dirt, dust, blood, or other visible contaminants from a surface.

_____ **8.** Driving with awareness and responsibility for other drivers on the roadways when you are operating an emergency vehicle in the emergency mode, and making sure that other drivers are aware of your approach.

A. Aircraft transport

B. Belt noise

C. Blind spot

D. Brake fade

E. Brake pull

F. Cleaning

G. Cushion of safety

H. Decontaminate

______ 9. An extra-heavy-duty transport vehicle.
______ 10. Standard van, forward-control integral cab-body.
______ 11. Specialty van, forward-control integral cab-body.
______ 12. The killing of pathogenic agents by using potent means of disinfection.
______ 13. Medical or trauma evacuation of a patient by helicopter.
______ 14. Fixed-wing aircraft and helicopters that have been modified for medical care; used to evacuate and transport patients with life-threatening injuries to treatment facilities.
______ 15. A chirping or squealing sound, synchronous with engine speed.
______ 16. To remove or neutralize radiation, chemical, or other hazardous material from clothing, equipment, vehicles, and personnel.
______ 17. The killing of pathogenic agents by direct application of chemicals.
______ 18. An area of the road that is blocked from your sight by your own vehicle or mirrors.
______ 19. A sensation that an emergency vehicle has lost its power brakes.
______ 20. A time of day or day or week in which the call volume is at its highest.
______ 21. The placement of an emergency vehicle at a specific geographic location to cover larger areas of territory and reduce response times.
______ 22. A drift that is persistent enough that an operator can feel a tug on the steering wheel.
______ 23. A process, such as heating, that removes microbial contamination.
______ 24. The staging of emergency vehicles to strategic locations within a service area to allow for coverage of emergency calls.
______ 25. Conventional, truck-cab chassis with a modular body that can be transferred to a new chassis as needed.
______ 26. A vibration, synchronous with road speed, that can be felt in the steering wheel.
______ 27. A condition in which the tires of a vehicle may be lifted off the road surface as water "piles up" under them, making the vehicle feel as though it is floating.
______ 28. A designated location for the landing of aircraft.
______ 29. A common finding at low speeds when a vehicle has a bent wheel.

I. Disinfection
J. DOT KKK 1822
K. Drift
L. Due regard
M. Heavy-duty emergency vehicle
N. High-level disinfection
O. Hydroplaning
P. Landing zone
Q. Medevac
R. Peak load
S. Posting
T. Spotter
U. Steering play
V. Steering pull
W. Sterilization
X. Strategic deployment
Y. Type I emergency medical vehicle
Z. Type II emergency medical vehicle
AA. Type III emergency medical vehicle
BB. Wheel bounce
CC. Wheel wobble

Multiple Choice

Read each item carefully, and then select the best response.

______ 1. The design and manufacturing specifications outlined in KKK 1822 federal guidelines are developed by the:
- A. American Heart Association.
- B. General Services Administration.
- C. Bureau of Transport.
- D. National Fire Protection Association.

______ 2. Which of the following should be done at the beginning of each shift?
- A. Change the oil in the ambulance.
- B. Complete an ambulance equipment/supply checklist.
- C. Wash the ambulance.
- D. Repair the equipment tagged as faulty.

______ 3. When leaving the scene, what should you tell family members who are following you to the hospital?
- A. Drive as fast as you can with your flashers on.
- B. Follow the ambulance with your flashers on.
- C. Drive normally, and do not follow the ambulance.
- D. Don't come until the doctor has called you.

______ **4.** What can happen to the grass on the side of the road if you park the ambulance on it?

- **A.** Nothing.
- **B.** It can catch fire.
- **C.** It can die from the fumes of the ambulance.
- **D.** It can clog up the underside of the ambulance and cause the ambulance to stop running.

______ **5.** What should you use when backing up an ambulance?

- **A.** The mirrors
- **B.** The guidance system that beeps when you are about to run into something
- **C.** The mirrors and a spotter
- **D.** Never back up an ambulance; always park so that you can leave without backing up.

______ **6.** All of the following are considered advantages of using an air ambulance, EXCEPT:

- **A.** they can provide access to remote areas.
- **B.** they are used when rapid transport is needed.
- **C.** they can carry many caregivers.
- **D.** specialized equipment or skills are needed.

______ **7.** What size should the standard landing zone be for a typical helicopter?

- **A.** 50 × 50 feet
- **B.** 75 × 75 feet
- **C.** 100 × 100 feet
- **D.** 100 × 100 yards

______ **8.** What type of light should you use to mark a landing zone?

- **A.** A headlight facing downward, in each corner of the zone
- **B.** A strobe light in the center of the zone
- **C.** A spotlight shining straight up in the center of the zone
- **D.** Blue flares in the center of the zone

______ **9.** When should you approach the helicopter after it has landed?

- **A.** Only after the blades have come to a complete stop
- **B.** As soon as it touches down
- **C.** When the pilot or crew on the helicopter signal for you to approach
- **D.** Never approach; let the crew come to you.

______ **10.** Which of the following is NOT a key factor in staffing your ambulances?

- **A.** Unit cost of each run
- **B.** Taxpayer subsidies
- **C.** Response times
- **D.** The types of calls you will respond to

______ **11.** You had a very busy overtime shift and have not gotten any rest in the last 24 hours. You are feeling exhausted and still have 6 more hours to go. What should you do?

- **A.** Admit to yourself and your partner you are fatigued.
- **B.** Do not drive the ambulance.
- **C.** Ask your supervisor to place your unit out of service for a while.
- **D.** All of the above are appropriate.

______ **12.** If you are driving the ambulance to the hospital and notice that you are being tailgated very closely by another vehicle, what should you do?

- **A.** Get out and confront the driver.
- **B.** Notify your dispatcher to alert the police.
- **C.** Speed up to attempt to lose the tailgater.
- **D.** Slam on your brakes to try to scare the other driver.

Labeling

Label the following diagrams with the correct terms.

1. Locations of the landing zone
   - A. Where to post guard
   - B. Pilot's blind area
   - C. Pilot's area of vision

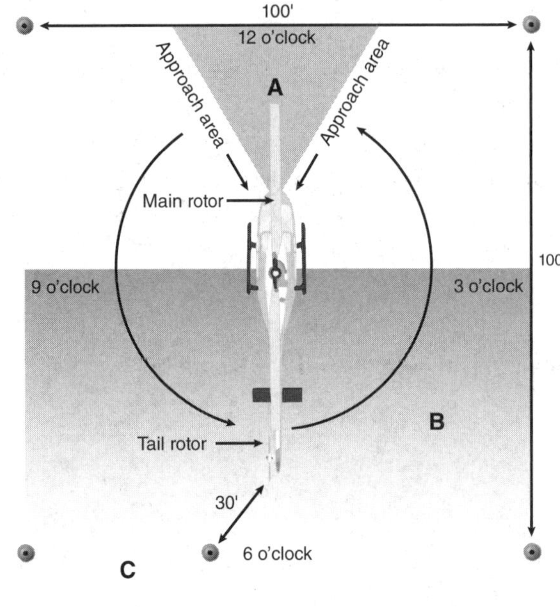

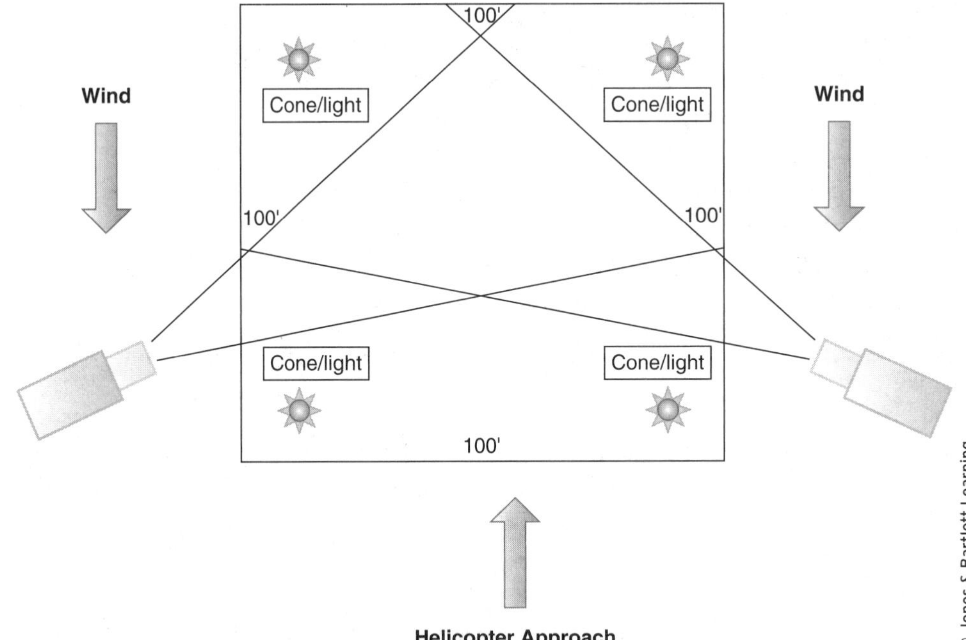

A. ______________________________

B. ______________________________

C. ______________________________

2. Helicopter hand signals

A B C

D E F

A. ______________________

B. ______________________

C. ______________________

D. ______________________

E. ______________________

F. ______________________

Fill in the Blank

Assume you have been called to the scene of a road crash. Among the equipment listed here, mark an X beside that which you would grab to take along on your first dash from the ambulance to the patient. If any equipment you need has been left off the list, add it at the end, and explain why you need it.

One sure way to *waste* time at the scene of a collision (or at any call) is to make a dozen trips back and forth to the ambulance to fetch equipment and supplies that you left behind. Well-organized paramedics take with them everything needed for the primary survey and first stages of management.

______ Long-leg air splint
______ Drug box
______ Portable suction unit
______ Oxygen cylinder
______ OB kit
______ Pocket mask
______ Oropharyngeal airways
______ Intravenous fluid bags
______ Dressing materials
______ Large-bore IV cannulas
______ Head immobilizer
______ Self-adhering roller bandage
______ Selection of board splints
______ Wheeled cot stretcher
______ ECG monitor
______ Contact lens remover
______ Stethoscope
______ Flashlight
______ Triangular bandages
______ Chemical cold packs
______ Cervical collar
______ Traction splint
______ Nonrebreathing mask
______ Long backboard/straps
______ Oral thermometer
______ Fire extinguisher
______ Bed pan
______ Heavy-duty scissors
______ Emesis basin
______ Handheld radio
______ Adhesive bandages

Other equipment that might be needed:

____

____

Identify

Read the following case study, and then list the chief complaint, vital signs, and pertinent negatives.

Walt and Dave respond to a two-vehicle crash. Their patient is a 41-year-old woman who tried to avoid a car that crossed the centerline on the highway. The sports utility vehicle (SUV) she was driving rolled twice and landed on its wheels. The back portion was struck by the oncoming car. Walt is able to gain access through a back door and performs manual stabilization. Dave begins an assessment on the patient. She is conscious and alert and remembers the entire collision. She is complaining of pain in her left shoulder area. The trauma assessment shows a deformity of the left collarbone and bruising beginning around the seat belt marks. Because of the collarbone, a cervical collar won't fit, and so Dave and Walt immobilize the woman on a backboard, pad the neck and head with towels, and then tape them down. Walt first applies supplemental oxygen because the Spo_2 is 94%, then begins baseline vital signs on the woman. He finds that her breathing is 22 breaths/min and shallow with decreased lung sounds on the left. Her pulse is 114 beats/min, and blood pressure (BP) is 132/84 mm Hg. The heart monitor shows sinus tachycardia with a few premature ventricular contractions (PVCs) every few minutes. The patient can feel her arms and legs and is rating her pain in the shoulder at a 9/10. Her pupils are equal, round, and reactive to light and accommodation (PERRLA). Skin is warm, but to help with shock, Dave turns the heat on in the unit and places a blanket over her. Walt starts an IV line, and they monitor her heart and breathing on the way to the trauma center. Walt does a secondary assessment and a physical exam that turns up a few small scrapes and bruises to her legs. He gets a SAMPLE history just as they pull into the regional trauma center.

a. Chief complaint:

____

____

b. Vital signs:

____

____

c. Pertinent negatives:

____

____

Complete the Patient Care Report (PCR)

Reread the case study in the preceding Identify exercise, and then complete the following PCR for the patient.

EMS Patient Care Report (PCR)

Date:	Incident No.:	Nature of Call:	Location:

Dispatched:	En Route:	At Scene:	Transport:	At Hospital:	In Service:

Patient Information

Age: Sex: Weight (in kg [lb]):	Allergies: Medications: Past Medical History: Chief Complaint:

Vital Signs

Time:	BP:	Pulse:	Respirations:	SpO_2:
Time:	BP:	Pulse:	Respirations:	SpO_2:
Time:	BP:	Pulse:	Respirations:	SpO_2:

EMS Treatment
(circle all that apply)

Oxygen @ ______ L/min via (circle one): NC NRM Bag-mask device		Assisted Ventilation	Airway Adjunct	CPR
Defibrillation	Bleeding Control	Bandaging	Splinting	Other:

Narrative

Ambulance Calls

The following case scenarios provide an opportunity to explore the concerns associated with patient management and paramedic care. Read each scenario, and then answer each question.

1. Unit 2 has been dispatched to a new subdivision for a man who fell off a second-story roof. When Cory and Bill arrive, they find a 22-year-old man unconscious and lying on a large pile of dirt. Cory and Bill don't really like each other much, and neither one is willing to concede to the other. They both sprint to the patient to try to be the "lead" medic on the scene. Neither one of them has bothered to take any equipment. The patient is lying on his back. Cory finally performs C-spine stabilization while Bill starts a secondary assessment, including a trauma assessment, but that is kind of hard because he has no equipment. Bill sends a worker from the scene to get his orange airway bag out of the squad. After the airway bag arrives, oxygen is applied, and Bill does his assessment. The patient doesn't seem to have any broken bones, but he is still out cold. One of the workers is trying to tell Cory what happened, but Cory won't listen. He lets the worker know that they are "here" now, and they will handle any medical problems. After about 15 minutes of being on scene, Bill finally has to go get a rigid cervical collar, scoop stretcher, and cot because the construction workers can't seem to find them even with Bill yelling at them. After they get the patient in the unit, they take vital signs, and they both try to grab the airway bag so that they can intubate. After a few seconds of arguing, they decide to do rock, paper, scissors to pick who gets to intubate. Cory wins and succeeds in intubating, and Bill decides to start a couple of IV lines. Bill gives Cory a high five after he sticks a 14-gauge in the left AC. After they get ready to roll, there is a discussion and another rock, paper, scissors contest to decide who is going to drive. Thirty-four minutes after reaching the scene, they are on the road to the closest hospital. Because their patient is starting to posture, they decide to turn around and head for the trauma center, another 15 minutes away.

a. What should Cory and Bill have done *prior* to arriving on the scene?

____

____

b. List six moves Cory and Bill made that were unprofessional while on the scene.

(1)____

(2)____

(3)____

(4)____

(5)____

(6)____

c. Discuss Cory and Bill's transport decision and what you would have done differently.

____

____

____

____

2. Jeff and Larry both show up just a few minutes late for their shift. Both of them were up late the night before watching the Monday night football game on TV. They both agree that because they are late and because they each have headaches, they will skip the morning check of the squad and go straight for the coffee and aspirin. Right away, they get a call for a woman who has fallen in front of the local grocery store. As they climb into the unit and take off, Jeff can hardly keep the squad on the road. It is doing a shimmy and shake down the road. When they arrive at the grocery store, the patient seems to be okay and doesn't want to go anywhere but home. She denies any pain and is alert. She states she just stepped off of the curb wrong and lost her balance. The store manager is the one who insisted on calling for an ambulance. Jeff turns off the squad when they decide this is a no-transport and grabs the paperwork for the patient to sign off on. After getting that all cleared up, they jump back into the squad to leave, but it won't start. They miss two calls while waiting for a tow truck. After they get the squad back to the service station, they are really embarrassed to find they were out of gas, and the shimmy they felt earlier was because of low pressure in a back tire. They finally make it back to the station around noon and are greeted by a very angry supervisor and a stressed-out crew number 2 who had to cover calls for Jeff and Larry.

a. Why should you check your emergency vehicle at the beginning of every shift?

____

____

b. What visual factors would you check before jumping in and running a call?

____

____

True/False

If you believe the statement to be more true than false, write the letter "T" in the space provided. If you believe the statement to be more false than true, write the letter "F."

_____ **1.** The standards for ambulances are determined by the Food and Drug Administration (FDA).

_____ **2.** Original guidelines called for ambulances to be painted orange and white.

_____ **3.** The DOT KKK 1822 standards developed the three main types of ambulances.

_____ **4.** The defibrillator and pulse oximeter do not need to be tested.

_____ **5.** Brake fade is tested before driving the ambulance.

_____ **6.** The Commission on Accreditation of Ambulance Services (CAAS) recommends that urban response time should be less than 8 minutes.

_____ **7.** One of the system status management (SSM) goals is to have a paramedic in every unit.

_____ **8.** It is the responsibility of every EMS agency to ensure that personnel are given emergency vehicle operation courses after they are hired.

_____ **9.** Due regard states that if you have your lights and sirens on, you have the right of way and can break the traffic laws.

_____ **10.** Patient cost is a disadvantage of using an air ambulance.

Short Answer

Complete this section with short written answers using the space provided.

When you are dispatched to an emergency, you must decide which route will be used to arrive at the scene safely. There are a number of ways to accomplish this. List three:

1. ______________________________

2. ______________________________

3. ______________________________

Fill in the Table

Fill in the missing parts of the table.

Advantages and Disadvantages of Using Helicopter Transport	
Advantages	**Disadvantages**
• Reduced transport time	• ____________
• ____________	• Altitude limitations
• ____________	• ____________
	• Aircraft cabin size limitations
	• Terrain that poses landing challenges
	• ____________
	• Patient condition that is not suited to helicopter transport
	• Restrictions on the number of responders
	• ____________

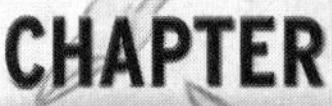

47

Incident Management and Mass-Casualty Incidents

Matching

Part I

Match each of the terms in the right column to the appropriate description in the left column.

_____ **1.** A Department of Homeland Security system designed to enable federal, state, and local governments and private-sector and nongovernmental organizations to effectively and efficiently prepare for, prevent, respond to, and recover from domestic incidents, regardless of cause, size, or complexity, including acts of catastrophic terrorism.

_____ **2.** An agreement between neighboring emergency medical services (EMS) systems to respond to mass-casualty incidents or disasters in each other's region when local resources are insufficient to handle the response.

_____ **3.** Any situation with more than one patient but that will not overwhelm available resources.

_____ **4.** In incident command, the person who works with area medical examiners, coroners, and law enforcement agencies to coordinate the disposition of dead victims.

_____ **5.** A group of operations in a unified command system, whose three designated sector positions are triage, treatment, and transport.

_____ **6.** A type of patient sorting used to rapidly categorize patients; the focus is on speed in locating all patients and determining an initial priority as their condition warrants.

_____ **7.** In incident command, the component that ultimately produces a plan to resolve any incident.

_____ **8.** In incident command, the section that is responsible for managing the tactical operations, including standard triage, treatment, and transport of patients.

_____ **9.** An ongoing or uncontained incident in which rescuers will have to search for patients and then triage or treat them. The situation may produce more patients. Examples include school shootings, tornadoes, a hazardous materials release, and rising floodwaters.

_____ **10.** A contained incident in which patients are found in one focal location, and the situation is not expected to produce more patients than are initially present.

_____ **11.** In incident command, the position that oversees the incident, establishes the objectives and priorities, and from there develops a response plan.

_____ **12.** A process that confronts responses to critical incidents and defuses them.

A. Closed incident

B. Command

C. Critical incident stress management (CISM)

D. Demobilization

E. Disaster

F. Extrication task force leader

G. Finance section chief

H. Freelancing

I. Hospital surge capacity

J. Incident action plan (IAP)

K. Incident commander (IC)

L. Incident command system (ICS)

______	**13.** The process of directing responders to return to their facilities when work at a disaster of mass-casualty incident has finished, at least for the particular responders.	**M.** Joint information center (JIC)
______	**14.** A situation declared by a locale, county, state, or the federal government for the purposes of providing additional resources and funds to those in need.	**N.** JumpSTART triage
______	**15.** In incident command, the person appointed to determine the type of equipment and resources needed for a situation involving extrication or special rescue; also called the rescue task force leader.	**O.** Liaison officer (LNO)
______	**16.** An emergency situation that can place a great demand on the equipment or personnel of the EMS system or has the potential to overwhelm available resources.	**P.** Logistics section
______	**17.** In incident command, the section that helps procure and stockpile equipment and supplies during an incident.	**Q.** Mass-casualty incident (MCI)
______	**18.** In incident command, the person who relays information, concerns, and requests among responding agencies.	**R.** Medical incident command
______	**19.** There is a minor adaptation for infants and children (including those with special needs) who cannot ambulate on their own.	**S.** Morgue unit leader
______	**20.** An area designated by the incident commander, or a designee, in which public information officers from multiple agencies disseminate information about the incident.	**T.** Multiple-casualty incident
______	**21.** In incident command, the position in an incident responsible for accounting of all expenditures.	**U.** Mutual aid response
______	**22.** When individual units or different organizations make independent and often inefficient decisions about the next appropriate action.	**V.** National Incident Management System (NIMS)
______	**23.** The capabilities of a receiving hospital to handle a large number of unexpected emergency patients, such as those seen in a mass-casualty incident.	**W.** Open incident
______	**24.** A system implemented to manage disasters and mass-casualty incidents in which section chiefs, including operations, finance, logistics, and planning, report to the incident commander.	**X.** Operations section
______	**25.** The overall leader of the incident command system to whom commanders or leaders of the incident command system divisions report.	**Y.** Planning section
______	**26.** An oral or written plan stating general objectives reflecting the overall strategy for managing an incident.	**Z.** Primary triage

Part II

Match each of the terms in the right column to the appropriate description in the left column.

______	**1.** Simple Triage And Rapid Treatment; a patient-sorting process that uses a limited assessment of the patient's ability to walk, respiratory status, hemodynamic status, and neurologic status.	**A.** Public information officer (PIO)
______	**2.** In incident command, the person who locates an area to stage equipment and personnel and tracks unit arrival and deployment from the staging area.	**B.** Rehabilitation group leader
______	**3.** In incident command, the subordinate positions under the commander's direction to which the workload is distributed; the supervisor-to-worker ratio.	**C.** Rescue task force leader
______	**4.** A command system in which one person is in charge, generally used with small incidents that involve only one responding agency or one jurisdiction.	**D.** Safety officer
______	**5.** In incident command, the person who keeps the public informed and relates any information to the press.	**E.** Secondary triage
______	**6.** In incident command, the person who establishes an area that provides protection for responders from the elements and the situation.	**F.** Single command system

______	**7.** A command system used in larger incidents in which there is a multiagency or multijurisdictional response to coordinate decision making and cooperation among the agencies.	**G.** Span of control
______	**8.** The person in charge of prioritizing patients, whose primary duty is to ensure that every patient receives initial triage.	**H.** Staging area manager
______	**9.** To sort patients based on the severity of their conditions and prioritize them for care accordingly.	**I.** START triage
______	**10.** In incident command, the person responsible for locating, setting up, and supervising the treatment area.	**J.** Termination of command
______	**11.** In incident command, the person who coordinates transportation and distribution of patients to appropriate receiving hospitals.	**K.** Transfer of command
______	**12.** A type of patient sorting used in the treatment sector that involves retriage of patients.	**L.** Transportation unit leader
______	**13.** In incident command, the person who gives the "go ahead" to plan or who may stop an operation when rescuer safety is an issue.	**M.** Treatment unit leader
______	**14.** In incident command, the person appointed to determine the type of equipment and resources needed for a situation involving extrication or special rescue; also called the extrication task force leader.	**N.** Triage
______	**15.** In incident command, when an incident commander turns over command to someone with more experience in a critical area.	**O.** Triage unit leader
______	**16.** The end of the incident command structure when an incident draws to a close.	**P.** Unified command system

Multiple Choice

Read each item carefully, and then select the best response.

______ **1.** The incident command system (ICS) is designed to control duplication of effort and:

- **A.** triaging.
- **B.** application of triage tags.
- **C.** freelancing.
- **D.** communication coding.

______ **2.** A large hazardous materials incident would require what kind of command system?

- **A.** Single command system
- **B.** Unified command system
- **C.** Rescue command system
- **D.** Medical command system

______ **3.** When sizing up the scene of a multiple-casualty incident (MCI), in addition to asking yourself "What do I have?" what other question is a part of the scene size-up?

- **A.** Why were we dispatched?
- **B.** What is the best response route?
- **C.** What resources do I need?
- **D.** How many police are responding?

______ **4.** What is the triage unit leader ultimately responsible for?

- **A.** Triage of every patient
- **B.** Movement of patients to a treatment sector
- **C.** Counting and prioritizing all patients
- **D.** Transportation to the hospitals

______ **5.** Where should the rehabilitation area be located?

- **A.** As close as possible to the treatment area
- **B.** Next to the media area
- **C.** Outside
- **D.** Away from the scene and the media

_____ **6.** What does the *D* stand for in the IDME mnemonic that applies to triage?
A. Delayed
B. Dead
C. Don't move
D. Decompensated shock

_____ **7.** Which of the following is NOT a special consideration during triage?
A. A hysterical and disruptive patient
B. An injured rescue worker
C. Death of a friend
D. Hazardous material exposure

_____ **8.** What color triage tag would you give a patient at an MCI who is breathing 4 breaths/min after you have opened the person's airway?
A. Green
B. Yellow
C. Red
D. Black

_____ **9.** When arriving on a scene to begin triage, what is a good thing to yell to the patients?
A. If you can walk, move across the street to the oak tree.
B. Stay where you are, and we will move all of you.
C. Everyone just lie still, and raise your hand if you think you are okay.
D. Run for your lives! Clear the area as fast as you can.

_____ **10.** What is your number-one priority at the scene of an MCI?
A. Triage of patients
B. Scene safety
C. Treatment of patients
D. Setting up the proper sectors

Labeling

Label the following diagrams with the correct terms.

1. Diagram of an MCI
Label the following areas:
A. Incident area
B. Extrication area
C. Triage area
D. Treatment area

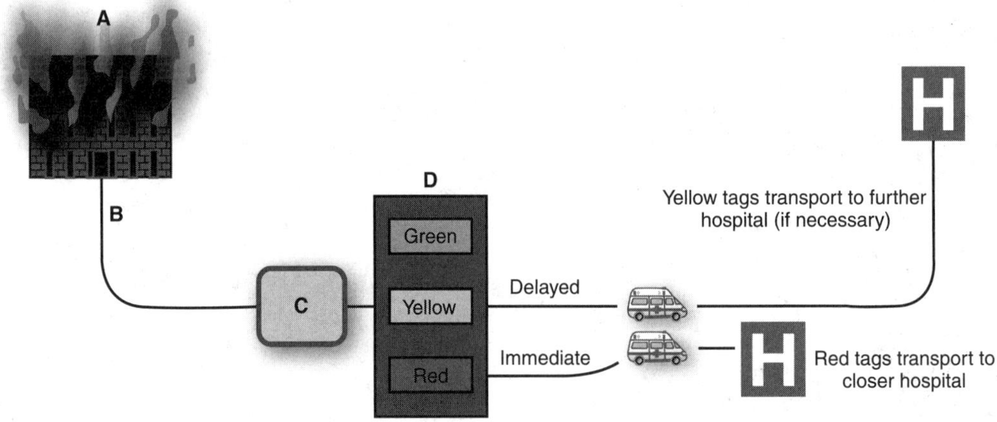

2. The JumpSTART pediatric MCI triage algorithm
Indicate if the following are deceased (black), immediate (red), or delayed (yellow).

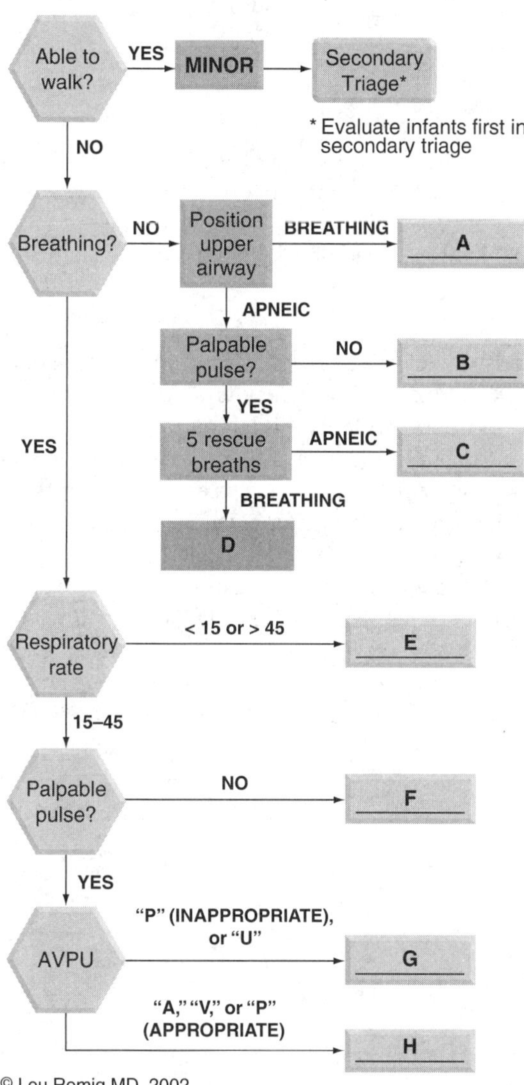

Fill in the Blank

Read each item carefully, and then complete the statement by filling in the missing word(s).

1. A(n) __________-__________ __________ refers to any situation with more than one patient but that will not overwhelm available resources.

2. One of the organizing principles of the ________ is limiting the ______ __ ______, the number expressed as a ratio of supervisors to responders.

3. The __________ section chief is responsible for documenting all expenditures at the incident that will need to be reimbursed.

4. The three officers that will help incident command (IC) the most are the __________, __________, and __________ officers.

5. __________ involves the decisions made and basic __________ done before an incident occurs.

6. The __________ unit leader coordinates and distributes patients to the appropriate hospitals.

7. Initial triage done in the field is known as __________, and then the __________ triage is done as the patients are brought to the treatment sector.

8. The *R* in the START triage system stands for __________.

9. __________START was developed for pediatric patients involved in an MCI.

10. The __________ area manager is in charge of parking vehicles and collecting supplies to be used at the scene.

Identify

Read the following case study, and then list the chief complaint, vital signs, and pertinent negatives.

You have responded to a blast at a local fertilizer plant. Your patient is a 32-year-old man who is found outside the blast area. He is lying on his side because he has a piece of wood impaled in his left buttock. He is conscious and alert. The wood is sticking out about 6 inches, and there is not much blood. He is unable to move because of the wood. Your partner starts the primary survey and secondary assessment as you apply oxygen. The trauma assessment shows small nicks and cuts on the man's back and legs, but they are all secondary injuries that are not life threatening. He says he was knocked to the ground when the explosion occurred. You are taking no chances and place him in a rigid cervical collar even though you won't be able to lay him flat. He is breathing 20 breaths/min, with an oxygen saturation of 97% and clear lung sounds. Pulse is 98 beats/min and regular, and blood pressure (BP) is 136/88 mm Hg. The patient rates his pain at a 7/10. His skin is warm and dry. You stabilize the wood in place and place the patient on a backboard and then use pillows to help stabilize him from rolling off his right side. You get him in the unit, place him on the electrocardiogram (ECG) monitor (which shows normal sinus rhythm), and then start an IV line on him. You give him 5 mg of morphine for the pain because it is really starting to hurt since you moved him. You opt for the regional trauma center even though it is 7 minutes farther away than the community hospital.

1. Chief complaint:

____

____

2. Vital signs:

____

____

3. Pertinent negatives:

____

____

Ambulance Calls

The following case scenarios provide an opportunity to explore the concerns associated with patient management and paramedic care. Read each scenario, and then answer each question.

1. It is a hot, stuffy day in June in your community of 1,600 people. You are on a volunteer rescue squad in your home community and work for a critical care ground transport company in the city 25 miles away. It is your day off, and you are enjoying the weather, but there have been tornado watches issued for your area. Later in the afternoon, the weather begins to get a little more serious, and you switch on your radio to get the latest updates. At 1630, the sirens indicating a tornado in the area go off, so you head down to the basement with your kids and the dog. Your wife is at work at the local nursing home. Before you know it, it sounds as if a freight train has hit your home. After everything is quiet, you fight your way out of the basement only to see total devastation of what used to be your community. You check with

your neighbors to see if they are okay and decide to leave your kids with them. Because your truck is nowhere to be found, you grab a bike lying in the street and head down to the fire department.

Okay, take a little break here to answer a few questions. Consider working in teams and comparing notes after you have answered your questions.

a. List 10 things you would like to have in your emergency kit to take with you.

(1)____

(2)____

(3)____

(4)____

(5)____

(6)____

(7)____

(8)____

(9)____

(10)_______________________________________

b. There is a lot of damage in the area, and people are gathering in the streets. What are you going to tell them to do as you ride by on your bicycle?

____

____

c. What type of hazards can you expect during the 2-mile ride to the fire station?

____

____

2. You finally arrive at the fire department as the rest of your crew gathers; there are 24 emergency responders present. It has been estimated that at least 100 homes were destroyed plus the nursing home, which houses 75 patients. This really worries you because you know your wife was there when the storm hit. The firehouse and the high school two blocks away have not been touched by the twister. You have three ambulances and six fire trucks. Emergency management has two pickups, and the sheriff's office has three cars available. Word has gone out to the surrounding communities, asking for all the help you can get.

a. Who should take command of this situation, and where should you set up the command post?

____

____

b. What type of buildings can be used for an emergency center for the walking wounded and displaced victims of the storm?

____

____

3. This is going to be a long night. Power is out all over town. You quickly begin to break into teams to begin searching for patients. There are many injuries at the nursing home as a result of the large number of people who were unable to get underground. You are sent there to work in the treatment center, and you see around 60 people with injuries over the next 6 hours. Your wife has made it through okay with only minor cuts. She is classified as walking wounded and actually pitches in to help with the patients who are worse. It takes 24 hours for all the homes to be searched, and your town suffers three deaths caused by this tornado. Three days later, most of the power has been restored to the houses that are still standing, and things start to calm down around town. There will be cleanup going on for the next few months, and it will take a couple of years to put everything back together. You are thankful that all the agencies in your town, even though they are small, work well together and have prepared for this type of emergency.
   a. List some outside agencies in your area that will be able to help you in the first 3 hours of this disaster.

   ____

   ____

True/False

If you believe the statement to be more true than false, write the letter "T" in the space provided. If you believe the statement to be more false than true, write the letter "F."

_______ 1. There will never be physicians on the scene of an MCI.

_______ 2. The planning section solves problems as they arise at an MCI.

_______ 3. Critical incident stress management should be available to responders, but its benefits are not evidence based.

_______ 4. An open incident is contained, with patients found in one focal point.

_______ 5. Command functions include triage and treatment functions.

_______ 6. The safety officer has the power to stop all rescue functions.

_______ 7. One function of the planning section is the development of an incident action plan.

_______ 8. Face-to-face communications are the best because of infrastructure problems at the scene of an MCI.

_______ 9. Yellow-tag patients are deemed immediate-priority patients because they have the best chance of survival.

_______ 10. The second step in the START process is triage of the nonwalking patients.

Short Answer

Complete this section with short written answers using the space provided.

1. Discuss the first step of the START triage system.

____

____

2. Discuss the second step of the START triage system.

____

____

3. Why is the JumpSTART triage system needed for a pediatric patient?

____

____

4. Why should you participate in the critical incident stress management in the rehabilitation sector?

____

____

Fill in the Table

Fill in the missing parts of the table.

MCI Equipment and Supplies	
Airway control	PPE (gloves, face shield, HEPA or N95 mask) ________________________ ________________________ Rigid-tip Yankauer and flexible suction catheters Laryngeal mask airway, i-gel or King LT airway, ET tubes[a] ________________________ Commercial tube holder, tape, syringes, stylet[a] $ETCO_2$ device
Breathing	________________________ Bag-mask device (adult and child), spare masks Oxygen delivery devices (nonrebreathing mask, cannula, extension tubing) ________________________ ________________________ Large-bore IV catheter for thoracic decompression[a]
Circulation	________________________ Sphygmomanometer, stethoscope Burn dressings, burn sheets, sterile water for irrigation ________________________ Hemolytic dressings 1,000-mL bags of normal saline, IV start kits, catheters[a]
Disability	________________________ Head beds, wide tape, backboard straps ________________________
Exposure	Space blanket to cover patients Scissors
Logistic/Command	Sector vests (triage, treatment, transport, staging, command, rescue) Pads of paper, pencils, pens, markers ________________________ Assessment cards Tarps: red, yellow, green, black

[a]These items could be packaged in an advanced life support (ALS) kit.

CHAPTER

48

Vehicle Extrication and Special Rescue

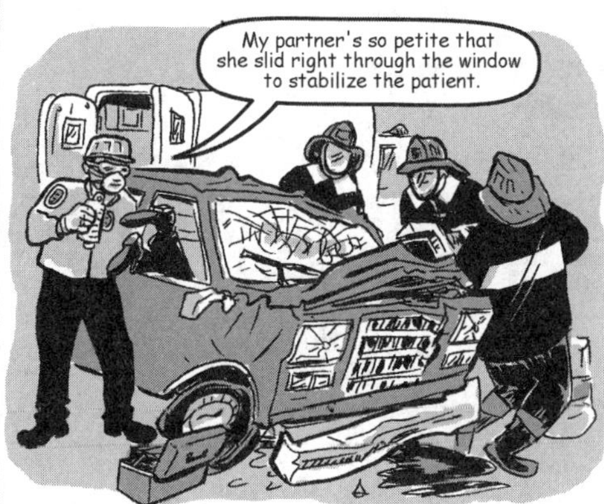

Matching

Part I

Match each of the definitions in the left column to the appropriate term in the right column.

	Definition	Term
_____	**1.** A rope rescue operation carried out on a mildly sloping surface (less than 45°) or on level ground. The ground is the rescuer's primary means of support, and the rope system is the secondary means of support.	**A.** Accountability system
_____	**2.** A type of window glazing that incorporates a sheeting material to keep the glass from breaking into shards. This kind of glass, often used for windshields, resists even deliberate breakage.	**B.** Alternative power vehicle
_____	**3.** An atmospheric concentration of any toxic, corrosive, or asphyxiant substance that poses an immediate threat to life or could cause irreversible or delayed adverse health effects. There are three general IDLH atmospheres: toxic, flammable, and oxygen deficient.	**C.** Awareness
_____	**4.** The area that directly surrounds an incident site and is considered immediately dangerous to life and health. All personnel working in the hot zone must wear all appropriate protective clothing and equipment. Entry requires approval by the incident commander (IC) or a designated sector officer. Complete backup, rescue, and decontamination teams must be in place at the perimeter before operations begin.	**D.** Belay
_____	**5.** A rope rescue operation in which the angle of the slope is greater than 45°. Rescuers depend on life safety rope rather than working from a fixed support surface, such as the ground.	**E.** Box crib
_____	**6.** A position used by a swift-water rescuer to avoid objects below the surface; the rescuer rolls into a faceup arched position, with the lower back higher than the feet (which are held together and face in the direction of travel—that is, feet first) and the arms at the sides.	**F.** Cold-protective response
_____	**7.** A collapse that occurs after the primary trench, excavation, or structural collapse.	**G.** Cold zone
_____	**8.** The process of locating a lost or overdue person and removing him or her from a hostile environment.	**H.** Complex access
_____	**9.** A cross between hill climbing and rock climbing used to ascend rocky surfaces and ridges.	**I.** Confined space
_____	**10.** The act of descending from a height on a fixed rope.	**J.** Cribbing

	Definition	Term
_____	**11.** A technique used to control a rope as it is fed out to climbers.	**K.** Disentanglement
_____	**12.** The first level of rescue training provided to all responders; emphasizes recognizing hazards, securing the scene, and calling for appropriate assistance. There is no use of actual rescue skills.	**L.** Entrapment
_____	**13.** A vehicle powered by energy other than petroleum-based fuel, or a vehicle that relies on a combination of petroleum and another fuel or energy source for power.	**M.** Hand tool
_____	**14.** A method of accounting for all personnel at an emergency incident and ensuring only those with specific assignments are permitted to work within the various zones.	**N.** High-angle operation
_____	**15.** Also known as a life vest, a water rescue device that allows the body to float.	**O.** Hot zone
_____	**16.** The act of preparing a patient for movement as a unit by means of a backboard or similar stabilization device.	**P.** Immediately dangerous to life and health (IDLH)
_____	**17.** The technical rescue training level geared toward working in the warm zone of an incident. Training at this level allows responders to directly assist those conducting the rescue operation and to use certain rescue skills and procedures.	**Q.** Laminated glass
_____	**18.** Any tool or piece of equipment operated by human power.	**R.** Low-angle operation
_____	**19.** A circumstance in which a patient is unable to extricate himself or herself from an impediment, such as debris or soil.	**S.** Operations
_____	**20.** Use of specialized tools and advanced techniques to free a patient from the area or object in which he or she is trapped.	**T.** Packaging
_____	**21.** A pallet-like framework used to shore up a heavy load.	**U.** Personal flotation device (PFD)
_____	**22.** A phenomenon associated with cold-water immersion in which the body reflexively lowers its metabolic rate in an effort to preserve basic bodily functions.	**V.** Rappelling
_____	**23.** A safe area for agencies involved in a rescue operation; the incident commander, command post, EMS providers, and other necessary support functions should be located in the cold zone.	**W.** Scrambling
_____	**24.** Complicated entry requiring special tools, advanced training, and the use of force, such as breaking windows.	**X.** Search and rescue (SAR)
_____	**25.** A space that is not meant for continuous occupancy and to which access is limited or restricted, such as a manhole, well, or tank.	**Y.** Secondary collapse
_____	**26.** A type of basic physical support, such as blocks or short lengths of wood, used to stabilize a vehicle during a rescue operation.	**Z.** Self-rescue position

Part II

Match each of the definitions in the left column to the appropriate term in the right column.

	Definition	Term
_____	**1.** A type of glass that is heat-treated so that it breaks into small, relatively dull pieces.	**A.** Shim
_____	**2.** The level of training necessary for a rescuer directly involved in a rescue operation; indicates a high level of competency in technical or hazardous materials rescue.	**B.** Shoring
_____	**3.** A group of rescuers expertly trained in the various disciplines of technical rescue.	**C.** Simple access
_____	**4.** A tapered shaft of wood or other material used to snug loose cribbing.	**D.** Special weapons and tactics (SWAT) team
_____	**5.** The area located between the hot and cold zones at an incident. Decontamination stations are located in the warm zone.	**E.** Spoil pile

______	**6.** A vehicle design with no formal frame structure. The body and frame are one piece, which is considered to be the structural integrity of the vehicle.	**F.** Step chock
______	**7.** The process of coordinating different partner agencies to detect, respond to, and clear traffic incidents as quickly as possible to reduce the impacts of incidents on safety and congestion, while protecting the safety of on-scene responders and the traveling public.	**G.** Supplemental restraint system
______	**8.** A complex rescue requiring specially trained personnel and sophisticated equipment and involving vehicle extrication; rescue from water, ice, or confined spaces; rescue following trench, structural, or other collapse; high-angle rescue; response to hazardous materials incidents; or wilderness search and rescue.	**H.** Tactical situation
______	**9.** A high-risk situation involving the potential for physical violence or armed combat typically involving law enforcement teams interacting with potentially dangerous criminal suspects.	**I.** Technical rescue incident (TRI)
______	**10.** A system of specialized devices, such as airbags and seat belt pre-tensioners, used to restrain a driver or passenger in the protected passenger compartment of a motor vehicle during a crash.	**J.** Technical rescue team
______	**11.** A slim, low-profile, wedgelike object used to snug loose cribbing under a load or to fill a void.	**K.** Technician
______	**12.** A hydraulic, pneumatic, or wood system to support a trench wall or reinforce building components such as walls, floors, or ceilings to prevent collapse.	**L.** Tempered glass
______	**13.** Access easily achieved with the use of simple hand tools or application of force.	**M.** Traffic incident management (TIM)
______	**14.** A specialized law enforcement tactical unit.	**N.** Unibody construction
______	**15.** A specialized cribbing assembly of wood or plastic blocks arranged in a step configuration.	**O.** Warm zone
______	**16.** The pile of dirt unearthed from an excavation. The pile may be unstable and prone to collapse.	**P.** Wedge

Multiple Choice

Read each item carefully, and then select the best response.

______ **1.** Which of the following is NOT considered a technical rescue incident?

- **A.** Trench collapse
- **B.** A fender-bender collision
- **C.** Water rescue
- **D.** Wilderness search and rescue

______ **2.** What is the first priority in a rescue situation?

- **A.** Mobilizing the correct teams
- **B.** Following the golden rule of public service
- **C.** Protecting the patient during the rescue
- **D.** Ensuring rescuer safety

______ **3.** Which of the following is NOT considered a step in a special rescue?

- **A.** Critique
- **B.** Access
- **C.** Disentanglement
- **D.** Removal

_____ **4.** You find the entry and rescue teams in the __________ zone(s).
A. cold
B. warm
C. hot
D. warm and hot

_____ **5.** Which of the following is NOT necessary to know when gathering information about a scene before you arrive?
A. The road conditions en route to the incident
B. The nature of the incident
C. The location of the incident
D. Hazards at the scene

_____ **6.** Who is in charge of having all of the utilities shut down at a scene?
A. Dispatcher
B. Incident command
C. Police chief
D. Fire chief

_____ **7.** Of the following means of powering a vehicle, which is NOT considered an alternative power source?
A. LPG
B. Diesel fuel
C. Ethanol and flex
D. Electric or hybrid

_____ **8.** On a vehicle, the "A" post is the post:
A. between the front seat and back seat.
B. between the middle seat and back seat.
C. that holds in the windshield.
D. that holds in the back window.

_____ **9.** When you need to stabilize a vehicle, you usually use the most basic physical support for vehicle stabilization, which is called:
A. a step block.
B. wedging.
C. a "C block."
D. cribbing.

_____ **10.** If you are unable to gain easy access by opening a door to the wrecked vehicle, what is the next best procedure?
A. Break the windshield
B. Displace the door
C. Peel back the roof
D. Break a side window

Labeling

Label the following diagrams with the correct terms.

1. Label the A, B, and C posts on the vehicle.

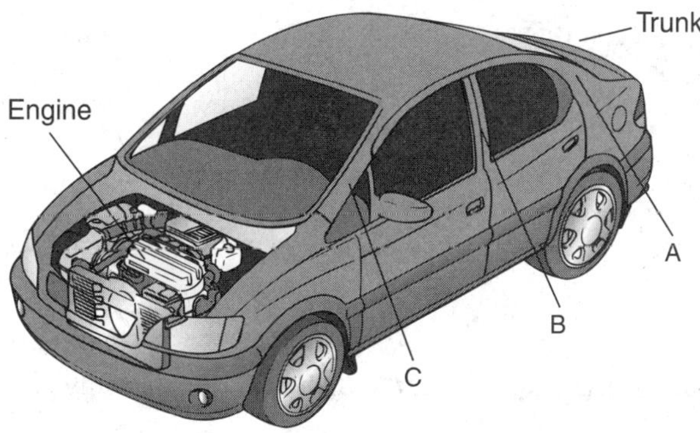

2. Label the following photos with the appropriate type of wood cribbing design.

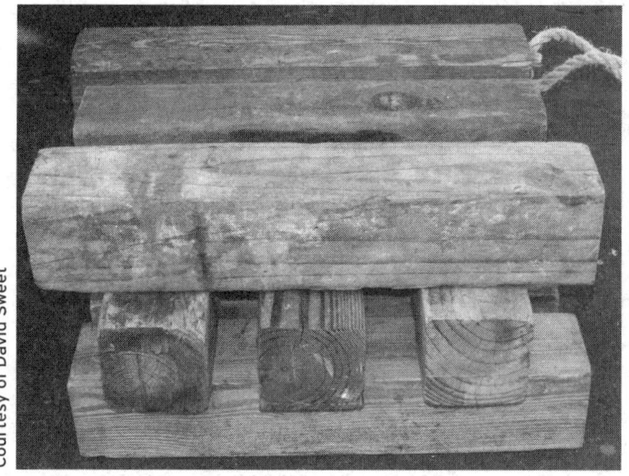

A. ______________________

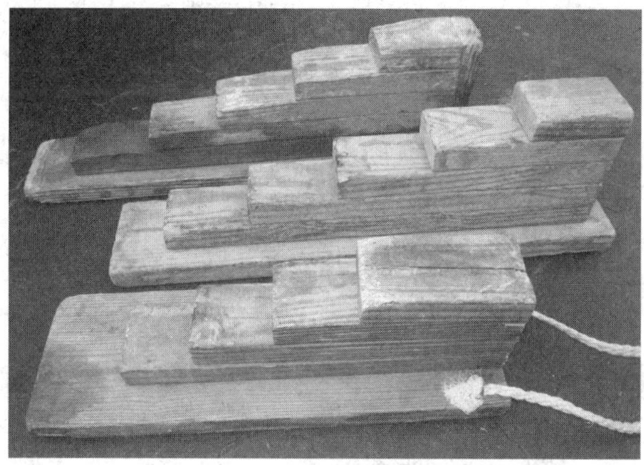

B. ______________________

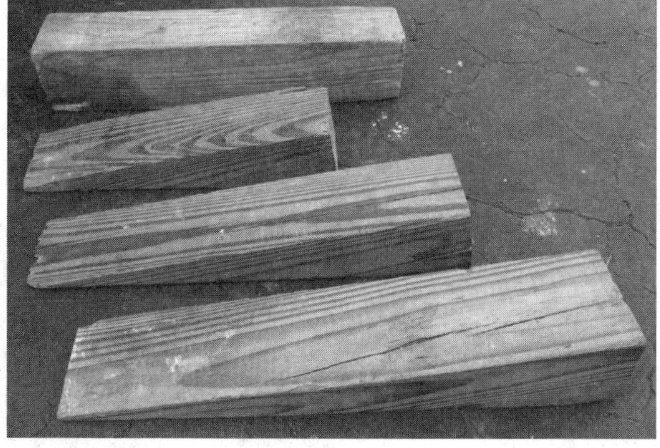

C. ______________________

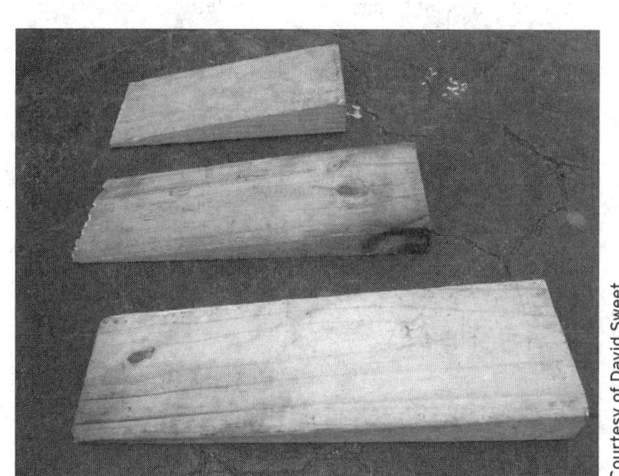

D. ______________________

Fill in the Blank

Read each item carefully, and then complete the statement by filling in the missing word(s).

1. A(n) ___________ that has deployed during a crash presents no safety ________ for the rescuer.
2. Do not attempt to cut a steering wheel if the _______ _______ contains an undeployed airbag.
3. During a(n) __________ collision, the vehicle's ________ may be pushed down or backward.
4. A(n) __________ __________ is a structure that is not designed for continuous occupancy.
5. __________ __________ is a gas that is released when bacteria break down organic material without oxygen. It is flammable, toxic, and colorless.
6. When dealing with an entrapment or trench collapse, the patient is dug out only after __________ has been put in place.
7. If you find yourself being swept away in fast water during a rescue, you should position yourself in the __________-__________ __________.
8. The first thing to do when attempting to help a person during a water rescue is to __________ __________ to the person.
9. In North America, the most common ________ water rescue scenario involves people who have attempted to __________ through floodwaters.
10. You respond to a rescue situation where the patient is down a slope that is less than 45°. This is known as a(n) __________-__________ operation.

Identify

Read the following case study, and then list the chief complaint, vital signs, and pertinent negatives.

You are called to a vehicle that has rolled down a 75-foot embankment. The rappelling team responded and has secured your patient on a backboard and then placed him in a Stokes basket. They pull the basket up the embankment for you to start working on the patient. He was wearing his seat belt when he lost control of the car and rolled. The patient, Jim, is conscious but unable to answer any questions except for providing his first name. Your partner applies high-flow supplemental oxygen, and you begin a trauma assessment while your partner takes the baseline vitals. Jim has multiple cuts on his face and head, with some blood coming from his left ear. You find instability in the pelvic region and a deformed left arm and collarbone. Jim's blood pressure (BP) is 102/68 mm Hg, and pulse is thready in the wrist at a rate of 116 beats/min. His oxygen saturation is 96%, and his breathing is shallow at 24 breaths/min. Lung sounds are slightly diminished on the left side. Jim is cool to the touch and appears very pale. His pupils are equal, round, and regular in size, but they do not react very quickly to light. You know that Jim needs to be at a regional trauma center, and you call for air medical transport. After hooking up the heart monitor, you find that Jim is in sinus tachycardia. Your partner does a halo test on the blood coming from his ear, and it is negative. Jim begins to come around a little more but doesn't remember any of the crash. Your partner starts two large-bore IV lines with normal saline while you do a secondary assessment. You find some rigidity in the lower abdomen. After you give a quick report to the helicopter personnel, Jim is flown to the closest regional trauma center.

1. Chief complaint:

____

____

2. Vital signs:

____

____

3. Pertinent negatives:

____

____

Complete the Patient Care Report (PCR)

Read the case study in the preceding Identify exercise, and then complete the following PCR for the patient.

<table>
<tr><th colspan="6">EMS Patient Care Report (PCR)</th></tr>
<tr><td>Date:</td><td>Incident No.:</td><td colspan="2">Nature of Call:</td><td colspan="2">Location:</td></tr>
<tr><td>Dispatched:</td><td>En Route:</td><td>At Scene:</td><td>Transport:</td><td>At Hospital:</td><td>In Service:</td></tr>
<tr><th colspan="6">Patient Information</th></tr>
<tr><td colspan="3">Age:
Sex:
Weight (in kg [lb]):</td><td colspan="3">Allergies:
Medications:
Past Medical History:
Chief Complaint:</td></tr>
<tr><th colspan="6">Vital Signs</th></tr>
<tr><td>Time:</td><td>BP:</td><td>Pulse:</td><td>Respirations:</td><td colspan="2">SpO_2:</td></tr>
<tr><td>Time:</td><td>BP:</td><td>Pulse:</td><td>Respirations:</td><td colspan="2">SpO_2:</td></tr>
<tr><td>Time:</td><td>BP:</td><td>Pulse:</td><td>Respirations:</td><td colspan="2">SpO_2:</td></tr>
<tr><th colspan="6">EMS Treatment
(circle all that apply)</th></tr>
<tr><td colspan="2">Oxygen @ ______ L/min via (circle one):
NC NRM Bag-mask device</td><td>Assisted Ventilation</td><td>Airway Adjunct</td><td colspan="2">CPR</td></tr>
<tr><td>Defibrillation</td><td>Bleeding Control</td><td>Bandaging</td><td>Splinting</td><td colspan="2">Other:</td></tr>
<tr><th colspan="6">Narrative</th></tr>
<tr><td colspan="6"></td></tr>
</table>

Ambulance Calls

The following case scenario provides an opportunity to explore the concerns associated with patient management and paramedic care. Read the scenario, and then answer each question.

1. You and your crew (two other paramedics) are called to the scene of a highway crash just outside of town. Arriving at the scene, you see a late-model sedan "accordioned" against a utility pole. The windshield is shattered. The driver is unconscious, bleeding, and tightly pinned between the steering wheel and the seat. There are no passengers.

a. List in order the steps you would take. Include details of how you would reach the patient.

(1)______________________________

____

(2)______________________________

____

(3)______________________________

____

(4)______________________________

____

(5)______________________________

____

(6)______________________________

____

(7)______________________________

____

(8)______________________________

____

b. List the actions you would take after the patient has been transferred to the care of emergency department (ED) personnel.

(1)______________________________

(2)______________________________

True/False

If you believe the statement to be more true than false, write the letter "T" in the space provided. If you believe the statement to be more false than true, write the letter "F."

______ **1.** In an extrication, the primary function of a paramedic is to direct the disentanglement of the patient from the wreckage.

______ **2.** Initial access to the patient may be limited because of safety hazards or physical restrictions.

______ **3.** Care of the car crash victim should start even before the patient is removed from the vehicle.

______ **4.** The paramedic should treat all downed wires as if they are charged until the power company turns them off.

______ **5.** To protect the scene and the rescuers, place a large emergency vehicle at an angle to provide a barrier against oncoming traffic.

______ **6.** A disabled vehicle that is upright on four wheels still needs to be stabilized before anyone enters it to reach the injured inside.

______ **7.** The windshield is another easy way to gain access.

______ **8.** The most common tool used to remove tempered glass is a flat-head axe.

______ **9.** Removal of the patient is referred to as disentanglement.

______ **10.** The side and rear windows are typically made of safety glass.

Short Answer

Complete this section with short written answers using the space provided.

1. Discuss the three phases of training that you might receive in technical rescue.

a. Awareness:

____

____

b. Operations:

____

____

c. Technician:

____

____

2. Discuss the four guidelines that are useful when working with a rescue team.

a. ______________________________

____

____

b. ______________________________

____

____

c. ______________________________

____

____

d. ______________________________

____

____

3. What gear is considered minimal for a water rescuer?

____

____

4. When breaking glass in an automobile, discuss the differences of the glass in the windows versus the windshield.

____

____

Fill in the Table

Fill in the missing parts of the table.

1. Write in the correct statement for the letters for the mnemonic "THREAT."

The Hartford Consensus: THREAT	
T	
H	
R	
E	
A	
T	

CHAPTER 49

Hazardous Materials

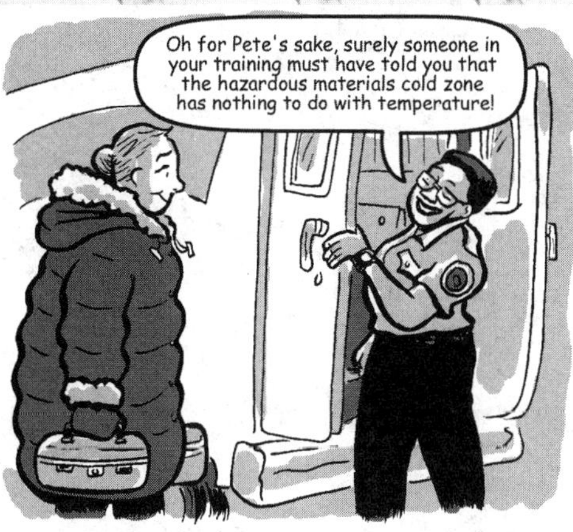

Matching

Part I

Match each of the items in the right column to the appropriate definition in the left column.

______	**1.** A glass, plastic, or steel nonbulk storage container, ranging in volume from 5 to 15 gallons (19 to 600 L).	**A.**	Absorption
______	**2.** A chemical asphyxiant that results in cellular respiratory failure; this gas ties up hemoglobin to the extent that oxygen in the blood becomes inaccessible to the cells.	**B.**	Asphyxiant
______	**3.** Computer-Aided Management of Emergency Operations; a tool to help predict downwind concentrations of hazardous materials based on the input of environmental factors into a computer model.	**C.**	Authority having jurisdiction (AHJ)
______	**4.** A chemical asphyxiant used in many industrial processes; exposure can occur from by-products of combustion at structure fires.	**D.**	Bill of lading
______	**5.** A class of chemicals with either high or low pH levels. Exposure can cause severe soft-tissue damage.	**E.**	CAMEO
______	**6.** Any vessel or receptacle that holds material, including storage vessels, pipelines, and packaging.	**F.**	Carbon monoxide
______	**7.** A document carried by drivers of commercial vehicles that should provide specific information about what is carried on the vehicle.	**G.**	Carboy
______	**8.** An organization, office, or person responsible for enforcing the requirements of a code or standard, or for approving equipment, materials, an installation, or a procedure.	**H.**	Cargo tank
______	**9.** Any gas that displaces oxygen from the atmosphere; can be deadly if exposure occurs in a confined space.	**I.**	Chemical asphyxiant
______	**10.** A type of decontamination that is done with large pads that the hazardous materials team uses to soak up liquid and remove it from the patient.	**J.**	CHEMTREC (Chemical Transportation Emergency Center)
______	**11.** Bulk packaging that is permanently attached to or forms a part of a motor vehicle or is not permanently attached to any motor vehicle, and that, because of its size, construction, or attachment to a motor vehicle, is loaded or unloaded without being removed from the motor vehicle.	**K.**	Container
______	**12.** A substance that interferes with the use of oxygen at the cellular level.	**L.**	Corrosives
______	**13.** A resource available to emergency responders via telephone on a 24-hour basis.	**M.**	Cyanide

_____ **14.** A portable, nonbulk, compressed gas container used to hold liquids and gases. Uninsulated compressed gas cylinders are used to store substances such as nitrogen, argon, helium, and oxygen. They have a range of sizes and internal pressures. — **N.** Cylinder

_____ **15.** Any substance that is toxic, poisonous, radioactive, flammable, or explosive and causes injury or death with exposure. — **O.** Decontamination corridor

_____ **16.** The minimum temperature at which a liquid or a solid releases sufficient vapor to form an ignitable mixture with air. — **P.** Dilution

_____ **17.** An expression of a fuel-air mixture, defined by upper and lower limits, that reflects an amount of flammable vapor mixed with a given volume of air. — **Q.** Disposal

_____ **18.** The removal or relocation of people who may be affected by an approaching release of a hazardous material. — **R.** Dose effect

_____ **19.** The process of removing the bulk of contaminants from a person without regard for containment. It is used in potentially life-threatening situations, without the formal establishment of a decontamination corridor. — **S.** Drum

_____ **20.** A mnemonic that stands for diarrhea, urination, miosis/muscle weakness, bradycardia/bronchospasm/bronchorrhea, emesis, lacrimation, seizures/ salivation/ sweating, which are the signs and symptoms that can be produced by exposure to organophosphate and carbamate pesticides or other nerve-stimulating agents. — **T.** Dry bulk cargo tank

_____ **21.** A controlled area within the warm zone where decontamination takes place. — **U.** DUMBELS

_____ **22.** A type of decontamination method that uses copious amounts of water to flush the contaminant from the skin or eyes. — **V.** Emergency decontamination

_____ **23.** A type of decontamination in which as much clothing and equipment as possible is disposed of to reduce the magnitude of the problem. — **W.** Evacuation

_____ **24.** The principle that the longer a hazardous material is in contact with the body or the greater the concentration, the greater the effect will most likely be. — **X.** Flammable range

_____ **25.** A barrel-like nonbulk storage vessel used to store a wide variety of substances, including food-grade materials, corrosives, flammable liquids, and grease. Drums may be constructed of low-carbon steel, polyethylene, cardboard, stainless steel, nickel, or other materials. — **Y.** Flash point

_____ **26.** A tank designed to carry dry bulk goods such as powders, pellets, fertilizers, or grain. Such tanks are generally V-shaped with rounded sides that funnel toward the bottom. — **Z.** Hazardous material

Part II

Match each of the items in the right column to the appropriate definition in the left column.

_____ **1.** The concentration of a material in air that, on the basis of laboratory tests (inhalation route) is expected to kill a specified number of the group of test animals when administered over a specified period. — **A.** HAZWOPER

_____ **2.** A dose that would be lethal to 50% of the test population. — **B.** Ignition temperature

_____ **3.** A type of signage at least 3.9 inches (9.9 cm) on each side that is often required on all four sides of individual packages and boxes that are being transported. — **C.** Immediately dangerous to life and health (IDLH)

_____ **4.** A bulk container that serves as both a shipping and a storage vessel. Such tanks hold between 5,000 and 6,000 gallons (18,900 to 22,700 L) of product and can be pressurized or nonpressurized. Intermodal tanks may be shipped by all modes of transportation. — **D.** Intermodal tank

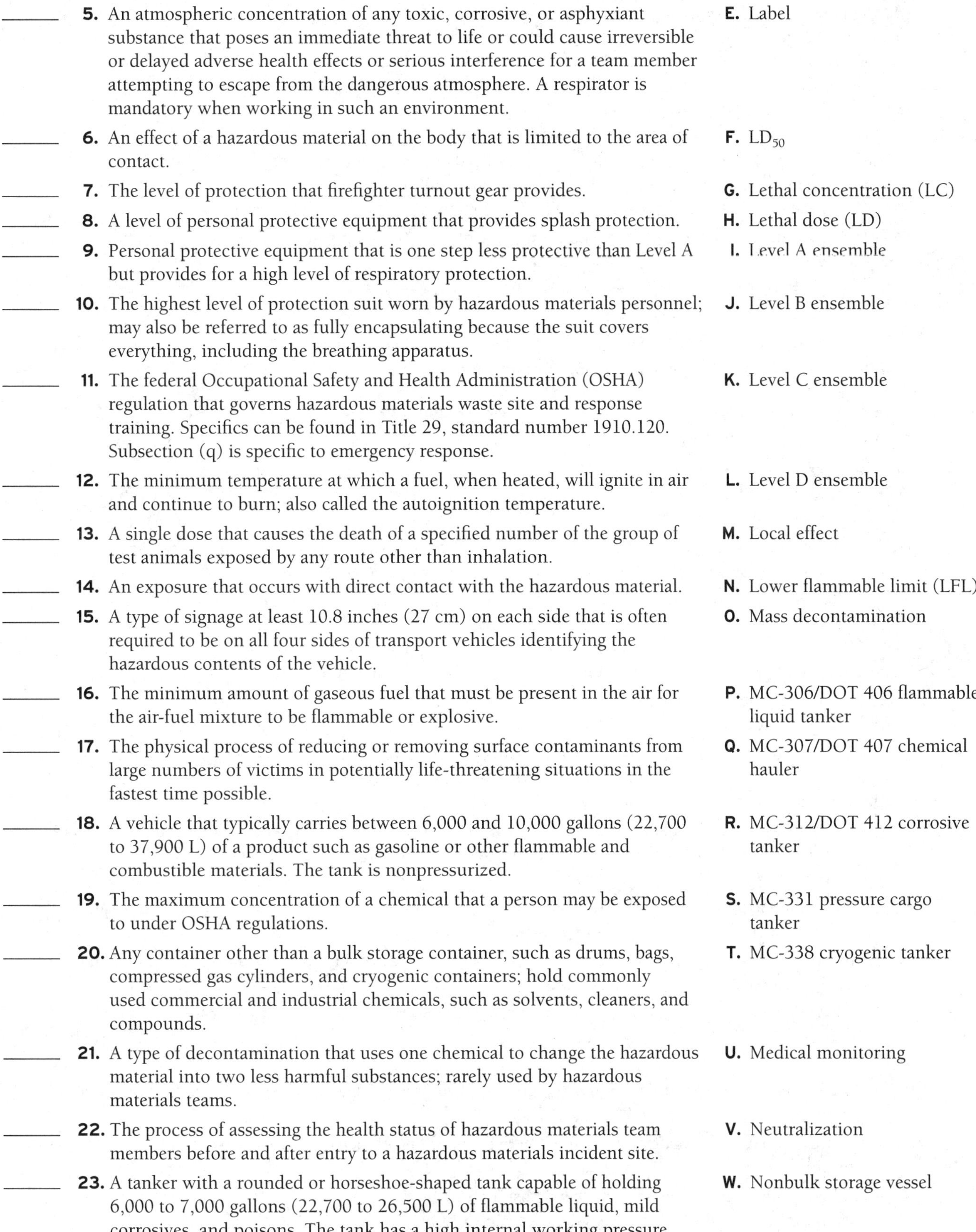

	Definition	Term
______	**5.** An atmospheric concentration of any toxic, corrosive, or asphyxiant substance that poses an immediate threat to life or could cause irreversible or delayed adverse health effects or serious interference for a team member attempting to escape from the dangerous atmosphere. A respirator is mandatory when working in such an environment.	**E.** Label
______	**6.** An effect of a hazardous material on the body that is limited to the area of contact.	**F.** LD_{50}
______	**7.** The level of protection that firefighter turnout gear provides.	**G.** Lethal concentration (LC)
______	**8.** A level of personal protective equipment that provides splash protection.	**H.** Lethal dose (LD)
______	**9.** Personal protective equipment that is one step less protective than Level A but provides for a high level of respiratory protection.	**I.** Level A ensemble
______	**10.** The highest level of protection suit worn by hazardous materials personnel; may also be referred to as fully encapsulating because the suit covers everything, including the breathing apparatus.	**J.** Level B ensemble
______	**11.** The federal Occupational Safety and Health Administration (OSHA) regulation that governs hazardous materials waste site and response training. Specifics can be found in Title 29, standard number 1910.120. Subsection (q) is specific to emergency response.	**K.** Level C ensemble
______	**12.** The minimum temperature at which a fuel, when heated, will ignite in air and continue to burn; also called the autoignition temperature.	**L.** Level D ensemble
______	**13.** A single dose that causes the death of a specified number of the group of test animals exposed by any route other than inhalation.	**M.** Local effect
______	**14.** An exposure that occurs with direct contact with the hazardous material.	**N.** Lower flammable limit (LFL)
______	**15.** A type of signage at least 10.8 inches (27 cm) on each side that is often required to be on all four sides of transport vehicles identifying the hazardous contents of the vehicle.	**O.** Mass decontamination
______	**16.** The minimum amount of gaseous fuel that must be present in the air for the air-fuel mixture to be flammable or explosive.	**P.** MC-306/DOT 406 flammable liquid tanker
______	**17.** The physical process of reducing or removing surface contaminants from large numbers of victims in potentially life-threatening situations in the fastest time possible.	**Q.** MC-307/DOT 407 chemical hauler
______	**18.** A vehicle that typically carries between 6,000 and 10,000 gallons (22,700 to 37,900 L) of a product such as gasoline or other flammable and combustible materials. The tank is nonpressurized.	**R.** MC-312/DOT 412 corrosive tanker
______	**19.** The maximum concentration of a chemical that a person may be exposed to under OSHA regulations.	**S.** MC-331 pressure cargo tanker
______	**20.** Any container other than a bulk storage container, such as drums, bags, compressed gas cylinders, and cryogenic containers; hold commonly used commercial and industrial chemicals, such as solvents, cleaners, and compounds.	**T.** MC-338 cryogenic tanker
______	**21.** A type of decontamination that uses one chemical to change the hazardous material into two less harmful substances; rarely used by hazardous materials teams.	**U.** Medical monitoring
______	**22.** The process of assessing the health status of hazardous materials team members before and after entry to a hazardous materials incident site.	**V.** Neutralization
______	**23.** A tanker with a rounded or horseshoe-shaped tank capable of holding 6,000 to 7,000 gallons (22,700 to 26,500 L) of flammable liquid, mild corrosives, and poisons. The tank has a high internal working pressure.	**W.** Nonbulk storage vessel

_____ **24.** A tanker that often carries aggressive (highly reactive) acids such as concentrated sulfuric and nitric acid. It is characterized by several heavy-duty reinforcing rings around the tank and holds approximately 6,000 gallons (22,700 L) of product.

_____ **25.** A tanker that carries materials such as ammonia, propane, Freon, and butane. This type of tank is commonly constructed of steel and has rounded ends and a single open compartment inside. The liquid volume inside the tank varies, ranging from the 1,000-gallon (3,800-L) delivery truck to the full-size 11,000-gallon (41,600-L) cargo tank.

_____ **26.** A low-pressure tanker designed to maintain the low temperature required by the cryogens it carries. A boxlike structure containing the tank control valves is typically attached to the rear of the tanker.

X. Permissible exposure limit (PEL)

Y. Placard

Z. Primary contamination

Part III

Match each of the items in the right column to the appropriate definition in the left column.

_____ **1.** A property that indicates that a material can be dissolved in water.

_____ **2.** A property that indicates that a material will undergo a chemical reaction (eg, explosion) when mixed with water.

_____ **3.** For the purpose of this chapter, the pressure associated with liquids held inside any type of closed container.

_____ **4.** The weight of an airborne concentration (vapor or gas) as compared with an equal volume of dry air.

_____ **5.** A high-volume transportation device made up of several individual compressed gas cylinders banded together and affixed to a trailer. Tube trailers carry compressed gases, such as hydrogen, oxygen, helium, and methane. One trailer may carry several different gases in individual tubes.

_____ **6.** Hazardous chemical compounds that are released when a material decomposes under heat.

_____ **7.** The concentration at which direct or airborne contact with a material could result in possible and significant exposure from absorption through the skin, mucous membranes, and eyes.

_____ **8.** The concentration of a substance that a worker can be exposed to for up to 15 minutes by no more than four times per day with at least 1 hour between each exposure.

_____ **9.** The maximum amount of gaseous fuel that can be present in the air if the air-fuel mixture is to be flammable or explosive.

_____ **10.** The maximum concentration of hazardous material to which a worker should not be exposed, even for an instant.

_____ **11.** A cargo document kept by the conductor of a train, also referred to as a consist.

_____ **12.** An engineered method to control spilled or released product if the main containment vessel fails.

_____ **13.** Exposure to a hazardous material by contact with a contaminated person or object.

_____ **14.** A method of safeguarding oneself or others' position during an emergency or event; in the context of a hazardous material, for example, by remaining in a safe atmosphere, usually inside structures.

_____ **15.** A substance that is capable of dissolving other substances.

_____ **16.** The concentration of a substance that is supposed to be safe for exposure of no more than 8 hours per day and 40 hours per week.

A. Safety data sheet (SDS)

B. Secondary containment

C. Secondary contamination

D. Shelter-in-place

E. Solvent

F. Specific gravity

G. Systemic effect

H. Technical decontamination

I. Threshold limit value (TLV)

J. Threshold limit value/ceiling (TLV/C)

K. Threshold limit value/short-term exposure limit (TLV-STEL)

L. Threshold limit value/skin

M. Toxic products of combustion

N. Tube trailer

O. Upper flammable limit (UFL)

P. Vapor density

______	**17.** A multistep process of carefully scrubbing and washing contaminants from a person or object, collecting runoff water, and collecting and properly handling all items.	**Q.** Vapor pressure
______	**18.** A physiologic effect on the entire body or one of the body's systems.	**R.** Water reactive
______	**19.** The measure that indicates whether a hazardous material will sink or float in water.	**S.** Water soluble
______	**20.** A document that provides a detailed product description and that is kept on site at workplaces for every potentially hazardous chemical at the workplace.	**T.** Waybill

Multiple Choice

Read each item carefully, and then select the best response.

______ **1.** You can learn a great deal from a pesticide label. Of the following, which would NOT be found on a label?

- **A.** The EPA registration number
- **B.** The UN Classification number
- **C.** The active ingredients
- **D.** The total amount of product in the container

______ **2.** A hazardous liquid, such as propane, is transported in which type of truck?

- **A.** The MC-331 pressure cargo tanker
- **B.** The MC-338 cryogenic tanker
- **C.** The MC-307/DOT 407 chemical hauler
- **D.** The MC-306/DOT 406 flammable liquid tanker

______ **3.** The threshold limit value (TLV) is the maximum concentration of a toxin that someone can be exposed to in ______________ over a typical 30-year career.

- **A.** 1 hour
- **B.** 24 hours
- **C.** 1 year
- **D.** a 40-hour work week

______ **4.** Emergency decontamination should be performed:

- **A.** at each and every hazardous materials incident.
- **B.** only if a qualified decontamination team is responding.
- **C.** only after appropriate personal protective equipment (PPE) has been donned.
- **D.** after a series of containment pools have been set up.

______ **5.** To prepare an ambulance for the transportation of contaminated patients, paramedics should do all of the following, EXCEPT:

- **A.** remove all unnecessary equipment, including the stretcher mattress.
- **B.** use as much disposable equipment as necessary.
- **C.** wrap the patient in a plastic barrier.
- **D.** line the interior of the ambulance with plastic sheets.

______ **6.** A paramedic should have a working knowledge of hazardous materials spills and properly providing care for injured patients. This knowledge should include training to which of the following levels?

- **A.** Technician
- **B.** Awareness
- **C.** Operations
- **D.** EMS operations

______ **7.** The safety data sheet (SDS) for a product provides a considerable amount of useful information to emergency responders. Of the following, which is NOT provided on the SDS?

- **A.** The product identifier
- **B.** The hazard identification
- **C.** The cost of the product
- **D.** The emergency telephone number

_____ **8.** Hazardous materials teams have many high-tech tools at their disposal. These tools include all of the following, EXCEPT:

A. Computer-Aided Management of Emergency Operations (CAMEO).
B. air-monitoring equipment.
C. colorimetric devices.
D. self-contained breathing apparatus (SCBA).

_____ **9.** Which of the following steps must be performed by paramedics who discover that a routine-sounding call is a hazardous materials incident?

A. Isolate the incident as much as possible using the guidelines in the *Emergency Response Guidebook* (ERG).
B. Remain in the hot zone to evacuate injured patients.
C. Approach and position your unit downwind from the incident.
D. Don Level A protection, and begin setting up the decontamination corridor.

_____ **10.** Paramedics need to balance the risk/benefit of invasive procedures for hazardous materials patients because:

A. IV lines may help contamination pass the skin barrier.
B. splints would become contaminated and have to be incinerated.
C. endotracheal (ET) tubes may cause upper airway obstruction as the plastic vaporizes.
D. There is no known risk; paramedics need to perform patient care as normal.

Fill in the Blank

Read each item carefully, and then complete the statement by filling in the missing word(s).

1. With __________ __________, you will not use rescue skills.

2. When you first arrive at a call and recognize a hazardous materials incident, your most important job will be to __________ __________ __________.

3. All emergency medical services (EMS) personnel should receive appropriate hazardous materials response training, based on the needs and requirements of the __________ __________ __________ and the local EMS agency.

4. Responding paramedics must gather as much __________ as possible when calling for the hazardous materials team.

5. If you are responding to an incident that involves a(n) __________ setting in which __________ may be in use or accidentally released, you should have a high index of suspicion of hazardous materials.

6. Other good sources of information for identifying hazardous materials include the __________ __________ __________, which should be carried by the truck driver in the cab, and the __________ or "consist" that is carried by the conductor of a train.

7. There are two basic types of contamination: __________ and __________.

8. __________ __________ is the direct exposure of a patient to a hazardous material.

9. __________ __________ takes place when a hazardous material is transferred to a person from another person or from contaminated objects.

10. A(n) __________ __________ may be described as a reddening of the skin or formation of blisters. Some chemicals may have a(n) __________ effect on your patient.

Identify

1. Respond to the following questions by basing your answers on the following *Emergency Response Guidebook* (ERG) information.

GUIDE 123 GASES - TOXIC AND/OR CORROSIVE ERG2004

POTENTIAL HAZARDS

HEALTH

- **TOXIC; may be fatal if inhaled or absorbed through skin.**
- Vapors may be irritating.
- Contact with gas or liquefied gas may cause burns, severe injury and/or frostbite.
- Fire will produce irritating, corrosive and/or toxic gases.
- Runoff from fire control may cause pollution.

FIRE OR EXPLOSION

- Some may burn, but none ignite readily.
- Vapors from liquefied gas are initially heavier than air and spread along ground.
- Cylinders exposed to fire may vent and release toxic and/or corrosive gas through pressure relief devices.
- Containers may explode when heated.
- Ruptured cylinders may rocket.

PUBLIC SAFETY

- **CALL Emergency Response Telephone Number on Shipping Paper first. If Shipping Paper not available or no answer, refer to appropriate telephone number listed on the inside back cover.**
- As an immediate precautionary measure, isolate spill or leak area for at least 100 meters (330 feet) in all directions.
- Keep unauthorized personnel away.
- Stay upwind.
- Many gases are heavier than air and will spread along ground and collect in low or confined areas (sewers, basements, tanks).
- Keep out of low areas.
- Ventilate closed spaces before entering.

PROTECTIVE CLOTHING

- Wear positive pressure self-contained breathing apparatus (SCBA).
- Wear chemical protective clothing that is specifically recommended by the manufacturer. It may provide little or no thermal protection.
- Structural firefighters' protective clothing provides limited protection in fire situations ONLY; it is not effective in spill situations where direct contact with the substance is possible.

EVACUATION

Spill

- See the Table of Initial Isolation and Protective Action Distances for highlighted substances. For non-highlighted substances, increase, in the downwind direction, as necessary, the isolation distance shown under "PUBLIC SAFETY".

Fire

- If tank, rail car or tank truck is involved in a fire, ISOLATE for 800 meters (1/2 mile) in all directions; also, consider initial evacuation for 800 meters (1/2 mile) in all directions.

Page 194

a. How dangerous of a substance is this?

____

____

b. What type of PPE should you be wearing if you are working in the "inner circle"?

____

____

c. Based on the preceding information, what should you do regarding your location and staging area?

____

____

2. Identify the four levels of PPE for hazardous materials scenes. Label each photo with the corresponding PPE level (A-D), then indicate their uses.

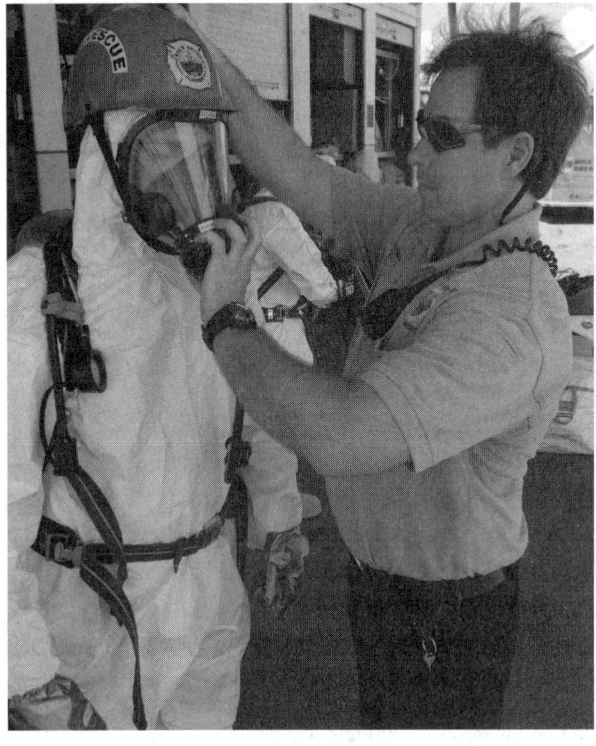

____

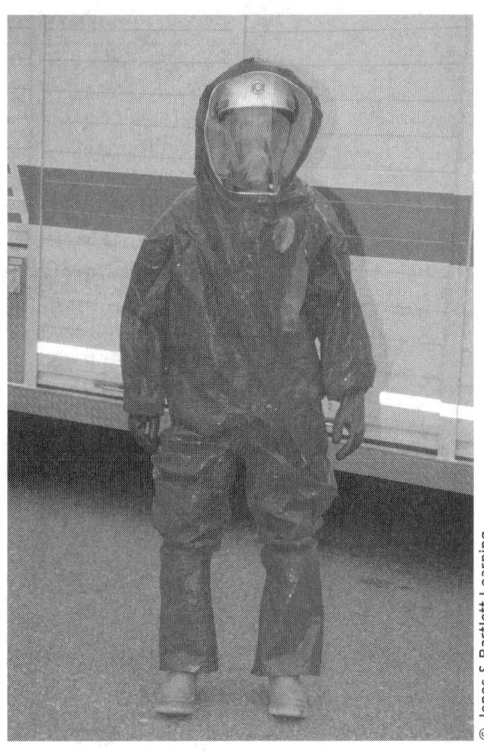

____

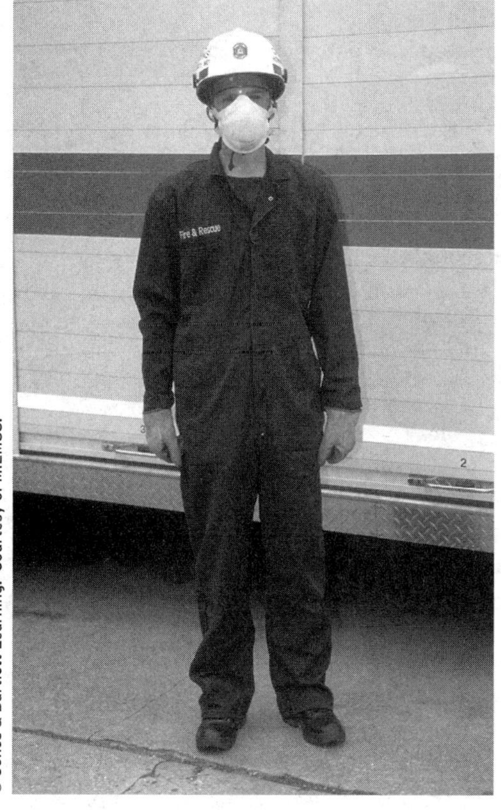

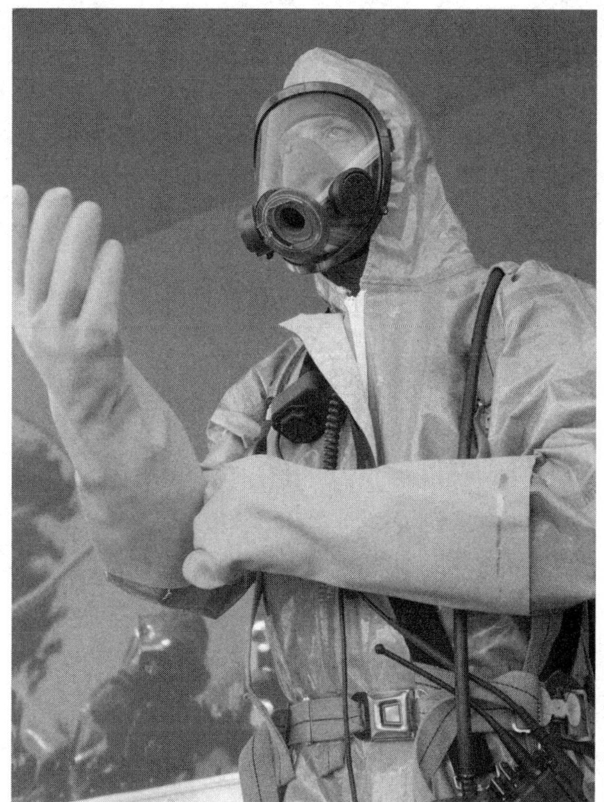

Level A:

Level B:

Level C:

Level D:

Ambulance Calls

The following case scenarios provide an opportunity to explore the concerns associated with patient management and paramedic care. Read each scenario, and then answer each question.

1. You are called to the infirmary of a local factory to see an employee who was injured in an unspecified "industrial accident." The plant manager who escorts you in explains, "There was a nasty accident. The valve on the tank of toluene wouldn't close. Jon was splashed in his face. I hope he's OK. He seems to have some trouble breathing. Our hazardous materials team had to go in and get him, and it took a few minutes for them to suit up and go in."

Before initiating patient contact, you take out your *ERG* and look up the chemical. The *ERG* lists guide number 130. You look up guide 130. Under Protective Clothing, it lists:

- Wear positive-pressure self-contained breathing apparatus (SCBA).
- Structural firefighters' protective clothing will provide only limited protection.

Under Health, it states:

- May cause toxic effects if inhaled or absorbed through skin.
- Inhalation or contact with material may irritate or burn skin and eyes.
- Fire will produce irritating, corrosive, and/or toxic gases.
- Vapors may cause dizziness or suffocation.
- Runoff from fire control or dilution water may cause pollution.

a. Is the scene safe? List considerations for your own immediate safety and patient decontamination.

(1)____

(2)____

(3)____

2. You are called to the scene of a railway incident in which the last 5 cars of a 12-car freight train derailed and toppled onto a highway below, crushing motor vehicles beneath them. Before approaching the derailed freight cars and the injured motorists underneath them, you want to make sure those train cars were not carrying a hazardous cargo.

a. List three potential sources of information regarding the nature of the train's cargo.

(1)____

(2)____

(3)____

b. You manage to determine that one of the derailed cars was carrying liquid chlorine, and as a matter of fact, you can already smell chlorine in the air. List the precautions you should be taking (assume that you are in the first public safety vehicle to reach the scene).

(1)____

(2)____

(3)____

(4)____

True/False

If you believe the statement to be more true than false, write the letter "T" in the space provided. If you believe the statement to be more false than true, write the letter "F."

1. You are called to the scene of a transportation crash in which a truck carrying radioactive waste (UN Class 7) overturned and caught fire. When you arrive, firefighters have just extinguished the fire, but there is still a lot of smoke. The driver of the truck is pinned inside the crushed cabin. Indicate which of the following statements about handling this call are true and which are false.

________ **a.** The ambulance should be parked upwind from the wrecked truck.

________ **b.** The ambulance does not need to be prepared in a special fashion before the driver transports to the hospital.

_______ **c.** The *ERG* should provide evacuation distances.
_______ **d.** The SDSs are helpful in managing hazardous materials.
_______ **e.** The bill of lading describes the contents carried within a vehicle.

2. Indicate which of the following statements regarding hazardous materials incidents are true and which are false.
_______ **a.** If there are no unusual odors at the scene of a transportation crash, it is safe to assume that hazardous materials are not involved.
_______ **b.** EMS personnel at a hazardous materials incident may become contaminated with toxic materials by touching a patient who is contaminated.
_______ **c.** In decontaminating a patient exposed to hazardous materials, one should use a brush to scrub the skin briskly with strong soap and lots of water.
_______ **d.** When decontamination is carried out at the scene, it is unnecessary to notify the receiving hospital that you are bringing in a hazardous materials case.
_______ **e.** It is preferable that an ambulance team that was not involved in treating and decontaminating the patient be summoned to transport the patient to the hospital.

Short Answer

Complete this section with short written answers using the space provided.

1. The *Emergency Response Guidebook* (*ERG*) can provide responders with the following information:

a. ______________________________

b. ______________________________

c. ______________________________

2. List other sources of information that may be useful to paramedics responding to a hazardous materials incident.

a. ______________________________

b. ______________________________

c. ______________________________

d. ______________________________

e. ______________________________

3. Although it's axiomatic in EMS that you never know what you may find at a call until you reach the scene, there are nonetheless certain types of calls that should start red lights flashing in the back of your brain: ALERT! Possible hazardous materials call! Listed here are some calls to 9-1-1 during a busy month. Determine whether each case is apt to involve hazardous materials, and if so, indicate what sort of hazardous materials might be involved.

a. Two-car collision downtown

____

b. Apartment-house fire

____

c. Three municipal workers collapsed in a sewer

____

d. Two police officers injured in a riot

____

e. Fire in a garden supply store warehouse

____

f. Semitrailer overturned on the interstate

____

g. Two "men down" on the maintenance staff of the municipal swimming pool

____

h. Freight train struck car on level crossing

____

i. Fire in a furniture factory

____

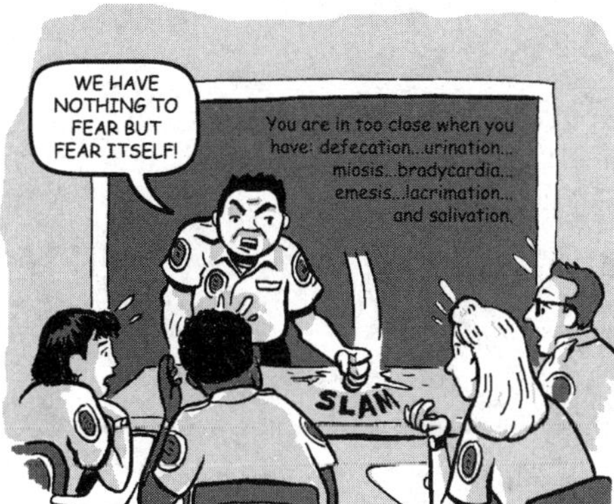

CHAPTER 50

Terrorism Response

Matching

Part I

Match each of the items in the right column to the appropriate definition in the left column.

______	**1.** Terrorism that is carried out by native citizens against their own country.	**A.** Alpha radiation
______	**2.** The means with which a terrorist will spread a disease—for example, by poisoning the water supply or aerosolizing the agent into the air or ventilation system of a building.	**B.** Ammonium nitrate
______	**3.** An infected animal that spreads a disease to another animal.	**C.** Anthrax
______	**4.** A bomb that is used as a radiologic dispersal device (RDD).	**D.** Apocalyptic violence
______	**5.** A natural process in which a material that is unstable attempts to stabilize itself by changing its structure.	**E.** Bacteria
______	**6.** A form of warfare in which a small group that is not part of the official military engages in combat that uses the element of surprise, such as raids and ambushes; sometimes used by terrorists to protect their training camps and bases of operation.	**F.** Beta radiation
______	**7.** A type of energy that is emitted from a strong radiologic source that is far faster and stronger than alpha and beta rays. These rays easily penetrate the human body and require several inches of either lead or concrete to prevent penetration; share key characteristics with x-rays.	**G.** Botulinum
______	**8.** Early nerve agents that were developed by German scientists in the period after World War I and into World War II. There are three such agents: sarin, soman, and tabun.	**H.** Buboes
______	**9.** A threat level in which a terrorist event is suspected, but there is no specific information about its timing or location.	**I.** Bubonic plague
______	**10.** A nerve agent antidote kit that contains a single injection of both atropine (2 mg) and 2-PAM chloride (pralidoxime chloride; 600 mg).	**J.** Chlorine
______	**11.** An agent that affects the body's ability to use oxygen. It is a colorless gas that has an odor similar to almonds. The effects begin on the cellular level and are very rapidly seen at the organ system level.	**K.** Communicability
______	**12.** Contamination of a person that results from coming into contact with another contaminated person, as opposed to coming into contact with the original source of contamination.	**L.** Contact hazard
______	**13.** An act in which the public safety community generally has no prior knowledge of the time, location, or nature of the attack.	**M.** Contagious
______	**14.** The characteristic of being communicable from one person to another person.	**N.** Covert

______	**15.** A hazardous agent that gives off little or no vapors and typically enters the body through the skin; also called a skin hazard.	**O.** Cross-contamination
______	**16.** A deadly bacterium (*Bacillus anthracis*) that lies dormant in a spore (protective shell); the germ is released from the spore when exposed to the optimal temperature and moisture. The route of entry is inhalational, cutaneous, or gastrointestinal (from consuming food that contains spores).	**P.** Cyanide
______	**17.** A commonly used industrial-grade fertilizer that is not in itself dangerous to handle or transport but forms an extremely explosive compound when mixed with fuel and other components.	**Q.** Decay
______	**18.** A type of energy that is emitted from a strong radiologic source. It is the least harmful penetrating type of radiation and cannot travel fast or through most objects.	**R.** Dirty bomb
______	**19.** A type of violence sought by some terrorists, such as violent religious groups and doomsday cults, in which they wish to bring about the end of the world.	**S.** Disease vector
______	**20.** Microorganisms that reproduce by binary fission. These single-cell creatures reproduce rapidly. Some can form spores (encysted variants) when environmental conditions are harsh.	**T.** Dissemination
______	**21.** The ease with which a disease spreads from one human to another human.	**U.** Domestic terrorism
______	**22.** The first chemical agent ever used in warfare. It has a distinct odor of bleach and creates a green haze when released as a gas. Initially, it produces upper airway irritation and a choking sensation.	**V.** DuoDote
______	**23.** An epidemic that spread throughout Europe in the Middle Ages, causing over 25 million deaths, also called the Black Death; transmitted by infected fleas and characterized by acute malaise, fever, and the formation of tender, enlarged, inflamed lymph nodes that appear as lesions, called buboes.	**W.** Elevated
______	**24.** Enlarged lymph nodes (up to the size of tennis balls) that are characteristic of people infected with the bubonic plague.	**X.** G agents
______	**25.** A very potent neurotoxin produced by bacteria; when introduced into the body, this neurotoxin affects the nervous system's ability to function and causes muscle paralysis.	**Y.** Gamma radiation
______	**26.** A type of energy that is emitted from a strong radiologic source. It is slightly more penetrating than alpha and requires a layer of clothing to stop it.	**Z.** Guerilla warfare

Part II

Match each of the items in the right column to the appropriate definition in the left column.

______	**1.** An area in the lymphatic system where infection-fighting cells are housed.	**A.** Imminent
______	**2.** A blistering agent that has a rapid onset of symptoms and produces immediate, intense pain and discomfort on contact. Its military abbreviation is L.	**B.** Improvised explosive device (IED)
______	**3.** The amount of an agent or substance that will kill 50% of people who are exposed to this level.	**C.** Incubation
______	**4.** Energy that is emitted in the form of rays or particles.	**D.** International terrorism
______	**5.** Terrorism that is carried out by those not of the host's country; also known as cross-border terrorism.	**E.** Ionizing radiation
______	**6.** Any container that is designed to disperse radioactive material.	**F.** LD_{50}
______	**7.** Any material that emits radiation.	**G.** Lewisite
______	**8.** A strategically placed facility that has been preestablished for the mass distribution of antibiotics, antidotes, and vaccinations, along with other medications and supplies.	**H.** Lymph node

______	**9.** A lung infection, also known as plague pneumonia, that is the result of inhalation of plague bacteria.	**I.** Lymphatic system
______	**10.** A blistering agent that has a rapid onset of symptoms and produces immediate, intense pain and discomfort on contact. Its military abbreviation is CX.	**J.** MARK 1
______	**11.** Biologic agents that are the most deadly substances known to humans. They include botulinum toxin and ricin.	**K.** Miosis
______	**12.** A class of chemicals called organophosphates that function by blocking an essential enzyme in the nervous system, which causes the body's organs to become overstimulated and burn out.	**L.** National Terrorism Advisory System (NTAS)
______	**13.** The US system for informing citizens of a potential terrorist threat; replaced the color-coded Homeland Security Advisory System.	**M.** Nerve agents
______	**14.** Bilateral pinpoint constricted pupils.	**N.** Neurotoxins
______	**15.** A nerve agent antidote kit containing two auto-injector medications, atropine, and 2-PAM chloride (pralidoxime chloride).	**O.** Neutron radiation
______	**16.** A passive circulatory system that transports a plasma-like liquid called lymph, a thin fluid that bathes the tissues of the body.	**P.** Off-gassing
______	**17.** A pulmonary agent that is a product of combustion, such as might be produced in a fire at a textile factory or house or at the site of metalwork or burning Freon; a very potent agent that has a delayed onset of symptoms, usually hours. Its military abbreviation is CG.	**Q.** Organophosphates
______	**18.** The length of time that a chemical agent will stay on a surface before it evaporates.	**R.** Patient collection point
______	**19.** The source that is causing people to become sick or injured.	**S.** Patient generator
______	**20.** The period between the person's exposure to the agent and the onset of symptoms.	**T.** Persistency
______	**21.** An explosive device built from unrestricted and often common equipment.	**U.** Phosgene
______	**22.** A threat level in which a terrorist event is known to be impending or will occur very soon.	**V.** Phosgene oxime
______	**23.** A location to which responders move patients to allow for safe assessment and treatment; also known as a casualty collection point.	**W.** Pneumonic plague
______	**24.** A class of chemical found in many insecticides used in agriculture and in the home. Nerve agents fall into this class of chemicals.	**X.** Point of distribution (POD)
______	**25.** The emitting of an agent after exposure, for example, from a person's clothes that have been exposed to the agent.	**Y.** Radioactive material
______	**26.** A type of energy that is emitted from a strong radiologic source. It is the fastest-moving and most powerful form of radiation. The particles easily penetrate lead and require several feet of concrete to stop them.	**Z.** Radiologic dispersal device (RDD)

Part III

Match each of the items in the right column to the appropriate definition in the left column.

______	**1.** A nerve agent that is one of the G agents; 36 times more persistent than sarin and approximately half as lethal. It has a fruity smell and is unique because the components used to manufacture the agent are easy to acquire, and the agent is easy to manufacture. Its military abbreviation is GA.	**A.** Ricin
______	**2.** The monitoring, usually by local or state health departments, of patients presenting to emergency departments and alternative care facilities and the recording of emergency medical services (EMS) call volume and the use of over-the-counter medications.	**B.** Route of exposure
______	**3.** A vesicant that is generally considered very persistent. It is a yellow-brown oily substance that has the distinct smell of garlic or mustard and, when released, is quickly absorbed into the skin and/or mucous membranes and begins an irreversible process of damaging the cells. Its military abbreviation is H.	**C.** Sarin

_____ **4.** A terrorist who wears or carries a weapon, such as an explosive, and triggers its detonation, killing himself or herself in the process.

_____ **5.** A small, suitcase-sized nuclear weapon that is designed to destroy individual targets, such as important buildings, bridges, tunnels, or large ships.

_____ **6.** Generally healthy people who seek medical treatment because they are concerned that they are exhibiting symptoms associated with a particular illness or incident they recently learned about.

_____ **7.** The creation of a weapon from a biologic agent generally found in nature and that causes disease. The agent is cultivated, synthesized, and/or mutated to maximize the target population's exposure to the germ.

_____ **8.** Any agent designed to bring about mass death, casualties, and/or massive damage to property and infrastructure (bridges, tunnels, airports, and seaports).

_____ **9.** The length of time that a chemical agent will stay on a surface before it evaporates.

_____ **10.** A germ that requires a living host to multiply and survive.

_____ **11.** A nerve agent that is one of the G agents; twice as persistent as sarin and five times as lethal. It has a fruity odor as a result of the type of alcohol used in the agent and is both a contact and an inhalation hazard that can enter the body through skin absorption and through the respiratory tract. Its military abbreviation is GD.

_____ **12.** A highly contagious disease that may be spread in an aerosolized form as an act of warfare or terrorism. It is most contagious when blisters begin to form.

_____ **13.** An additional explosive device used by terrorists that is set to explode after the initial bomb.

_____ **14.** A nerve agent that is one of the G agents; a highly volatile colorless and odorless liquid that turns from liquid to gas within seconds to minutes at room temperature. Its military abbreviation is GB.

_____ **15.** The manner by which a toxic substance enters the body.

_____ **16.** A group of diseases that includes the Ebola, Rift Valley, and yellow fever viruses, among others. This group of viruses causes the blood in the body to seep out from the tissues and blood vessels.

_____ **17.** A blister agent. The primary route of entry is through the skin.

_____ **18.** An agent that enters the body through the respiratory tract.

_____ **19.** A nerve agent that is one of the G agents; over 100 times more lethal than sarin and extremely persistent. It is a clear, oily agent that has no odor and looks like baby oil.

_____ **20.** A violent act dangerous to human life, in violation of the criminal laws of the United States, to intimidate or coerce a government, the civilian population, or any segment thereof, in furtherance of political or social objectives.

_____ **21.** A neurotoxin derived from mash that is left from pressing oil from a castor bean; causes pulmonary edema and respiratory and circulatory failure, leading to death.

D. Secondary device
E. Smallpox
F. Soman
G. Special atomic demolition munition (SADM)
H. Suicide bomber
I. Sulfur mustard
J. Syndromic surveillance
K. Tabun
L. Terrorism
M. VX nerve agent
N. Vapor hazard
O. Vesicant
P. Viral hemorrhagic fever (VHFs)
Q. Virus
R. Volatility
S. Weapon of mass destruction (WMD)
T. Weaponization
U. Worried well

Multiple Choice

Read each item carefully, and then select the best response.

_____ **1.** A virus that has been added to the water supply is called a(n) __________ weapon.

A. incendiary
B. chemical
C. biologic
D. explosive

______ **2.** The Department of Homeland Security rates the current terrorist threats using the National Terrorism Advisory System (NTAS). What does the term "imminent" mean in the NTAS system?

- **A.** There is a general risk of terrorist attack warning.
- **B.** There is currently no specific information about a terrorist attack.
- **C.** There is currently no risk of a terrorist attack.
- **D.** The threat is believed to be impending or expected soon.

______ **3.** A vesicant may produce all of the following, EXCEPT:

- **A.** seizures.
- **B.** large blisters.
- **C.** stridor.
- **D.** irritated eyes.

______ **4.** How long does it take for a patient to begin experiencing the signs and symptoms of sulfur mustard after being exposed?

- **A.** Minutes
- **B.** 2 to 4 hours
- **C.** 4 to 6 hours
- **D.** 6 to 8 hours

______ **5.** Which of the following agents causes chest tightness, severe cough, and shortness of breath?

- **A.** Vesicant agent
- **B.** Pulmonary agent
- **C.** Nerve agent
- **D.** All of the above

______ **6.** What does the "S" stand for in the medical mnemonic SLUDGEM?

- **A.** Salivation
- **B.** Signs and symptoms
- **C.** Stridor
- **D.** Seizures

______ **7.** Which of the following statements correctly distinguishes a smallpox rash from other types of rashes?

- **A.** The lesions will be in various stages of healing.
- **B.** The lesions will all be identical in their development.
- **C.** The lesions will start on the chest.
- **D.** The lesions will be different sizes and shapes.

______ **8.** Which of the following is NOT a route of exposure for the bubonic plague?

- **A.** Infected fleas
- **B.** Infected rodents
- **C.** Waste from infected rodents
- **D.** Infected birds

______ **9.** What is the most deadly substance known to humans?

- **A.** Anthrax
- **B.** Smallpox
- **C.** Neurotoxin
- **D.** Vesicant

______ **10.** What is the LEAST harmful form of radiation?

- **A.** Alpha
- **B.** Beta
- **C.** Gamma
- **D.** X-rays

Labeling

Label the three types of energy emitted from a strong radiologic source.

1. Alpha, beta, and gamma radiation

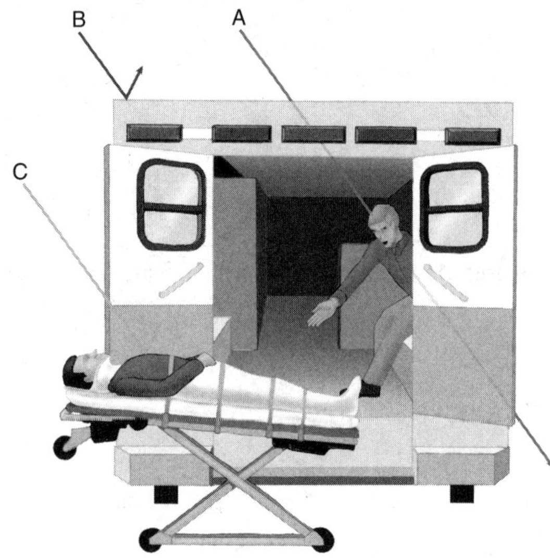

A. ______________________

B. ______________________

C. ______________________

Fill in the Blank

Read each item carefully, and then complete the statement by filling in the missing word(s).

1. __________ __________ __________ __________ is any agent designed to bring about mass death, casualties, and massive damage to property.
2. Most of the terrorist acts are __________, meaning the public has no previous knowledge of the attack.
3. Additional explosives set at a site that are intended to injure responders are known as __________ devices.
4. __________ __________ __________ is how an agent most effectively enters the body.
5. __________ __________ are the most deadly chemicals developed.
6. G agents were developed by __________ scientists in the early to mid-1900s.
7. Bubonic plague infects the __________ system.
8. __________ is a deadly bacterium that lies dormant in a spore.
9. Ricin is made from __________ __________.
10. __________ __________ __________ are strategically placed stockpiles of antibiotics, vaccinations, and other medications.

Identify

Read the following case study, and then list the chief complaint, vital signs, and pertinent negatives.

In your private vehicle, you respond to a vehicle crash about 2 miles from your home. Upon arriving at the scene, you see a truck that has rolled. The patient is outside of the truck, and bystanders are trying to help him. He is covered in white powder that has spilled from the truck. You walk up and take spinal precautions and start to assess the patient, knowing that your squad is about 3 minutes behind you. Jeff is 56 years old and is answering all your questions. You ask him what is in the truck because it is all over him, and now you have some on you also. He says it is some kind of chemical he was taking to a local plant. Jeff has some cuts on his arms. As your squad arrives, you yell at everyone to get back, and you call for the fire department. Unfortunately, you forgot the first rule of scene safety and didn't look around well enough before entering the scene. The chemical is raw organophosphate. You and Jeff get a wonderful water bath from the fire department before anyone can come and help you. Finally, you get Jeff in the squad and find that he is bradycardic with a heart rate of 50 beats/min, and his blood pressure (BP) is 98/66 mm Hg. He begins to lose consciousness, respirations are dropping quickly to 9 breaths/min, oxygen saturation is 88%, and he is drooling terribly. You realize that atropine is indicated in organophosphate poisoning. After starting an IV line, you give him 2 mg of atropine. You can give up to 5 mg, but you go with the lower dose because of his condition. You have your partner bagging him with 100% oxygen. After what seems like an eternity, he responds well with an increasing heart rate, BP, and respiratory rate. You run Priority 1 (Code 3) all the way to the hospital. You are also evaluated as soon as you get there to make sure you will be okay.

1. Chief complaint:

____

____

2. Vital signs:

____

____

3. Pertinent negatives:

____

____

Complete the Patient Care Report (PCR)

Reread the case study in the preceding Identify exercise, and then complete the following PCR for the patient.

<table>
<tr><th colspan="6">EMS Patient Care Report (PCR)</th></tr>
<tr><td>Date:</td><td>Incident No.:</td><td colspan="2">Nature of Call:</td><td colspan="2">Location:</td></tr>
<tr><td>Dispatched:</td><td>En Route:</td><td>At Scene:</td><td>Transport:</td><td>At Hospital:</td><td>In Service:</td></tr>
<tr><th colspan="6">Patient Information</th></tr>
<tr><td colspan="3">Age:
Sex:
Weight (in kg [lb]):</td><td colspan="3">Allergies:
Medications:
Past Medical History:
Chief Complaint:</td></tr>
<tr><th colspan="6">Vital Signs</th></tr>
<tr><td>Time:</td><td>BP:</td><td>Pulse:</td><td>Respirations:</td><td colspan="2">SpO_2:</td></tr>
<tr><td>Time:</td><td>BP:</td><td>Pulse:</td><td>Respirations:</td><td colspan="2">SpO_2:</td></tr>
<tr><td>Time:</td><td>BP:</td><td>Pulse:</td><td>Respirations:</td><td colspan="2">SpO_2:</td></tr>
<tr><th colspan="6">EMS Treatment
(circle all that apply)</th></tr>
<tr><td colspan="2">Oxygen @ ______ L/min via (circle one):
NC NRM Bag-mask device</td><td>Assisted Ventilation</td><td>Airway Adjunct</td><td colspan="2">CPR</td></tr>
<tr><td>Defibrillation</td><td>Bleeding Control</td><td>Bandaging</td><td>Splinting</td><td colspan="2">Other:</td></tr>
<tr><th colspan="6">Narrative</th></tr>
<tr><td colspan="6"></td></tr>
</table>

Ambulance Calls

The following case scenarios provide an opportunity to explore the concerns associated with patient management and paramedic care. Read each scenario, and then answer each question.

1. You are among the first ambulance personnel to reach the scene of a train derailment involving at least 60 casualties. Authorities on the scene think that this could be an act of terrorism.

a. As you recall, there are five categories of terrorist incidents. They are:

(1)____

(2)____

(3)____

(4)____

(5)____

b. You are directed to begin triage of the people trying to get clear of the wreckage. There seem to be a lot of people who are ambulatory, but you are located in a bean field with nothing around you to send the walking wounded toward. There is only one road close by, and it is jammed up with emergency vehicles. What can you do with the ambulatory people?

____

____

2. You respond to the local swimming pool right before it is scheduled to open. Dispatch says there are several kids coughing, and the lifeguards are having a hard time talking on the phone because of coughing spasms. As you arrive, you notice a green haze floating in the air around the pool house. There are about 50 kids standing around waiting for the pool to open.

a. What is the cause of this green haze?

____

____

b. Before you get out of the ambulance, what should you do?

____

____

c. You have a total of seven kids who are coughing hard, and you have two lifeguards who are really struggling to breathe. After help arrives, you begin treatment on one of the lifeguards. What type of problems should you expect?

____

____

True/False

If you believe the statement to be more true than false, write the letter "T" in the space provided. If you believe the statement to be more false than true, write the letter "F."

______ **1.** There are suits made for paramedics to shield them from radiation.

______ **2.** Radiologic material can be found at hospitals, power plants, and colleges.

______ **3.** Antibiotics will not help with bacteria.

______ **4.** A virus can live and thrive outside the host body.

______ **5.** The period of time between being exposed and showing signs and symptoms is known as the incubation period.

______ **6.** Ebola is a type of hemorrhagic fever.

______ **7.** Sarin is a vesicant.

______ **8.** In addition to men, women and children have also acted as suicide bombers.

______ **9.** The Oklahoma City Federal Building bombing was done by a domestic terrorist.

______ **10.** The greatest threats to a paramedic during an attack involving weapons of mass destruction (WMDs) are contamination and cross-contamination.

Short Answer

Complete this section with short written answers using the space provided.

1. List five examples of potential high-value targets for terrorists.

a. ______________________________

b. ______________________________

c. ______________________________

d. ______________________________

e. ______________________________

2. List four potential locations where sources of radiologic materials may be found.

a. ______________________________

b. ______________________________

c. ______________________________

d. ______________________________

Fill in the Table

Fill in the missing parts of the tables.

1. Nerve agents

Name	Code Name	Odor	Special Features	Onset of Symptoms	Volatility	Route of Exposure
________	________	Fruity	Easy to manufacture	Immediate	Low	Both contact and vapor hazard
________	________	None (if pure) or strong	Will off-gas while on victim's clothing	Immediate	High	Primarily respiratory vapor hazard; extremely lethal if skin contact is made
________	________	Fruity	Ages rapidly, making it difficult to treat	Immediate	Moderate	Contact with skin; minimal vapor hazard
________	________	None	Most lethal chemical agent; difficult to decontaminate	Immediate	Very low	Contact with skin; no vapor hazard (unless aerosolized)

2. Chemical agents

Class	Military Designation	Odor	Lethality	Onset of Symptoms	Volatility	Primary Route of Exposure
________	Mustard (H) Lewisite (L) Phosgene oxime (CX)	________ ________	Causes large blisters to form on victims; may severely damage upper airway if vapors are inhaled; severe, intense pain and gray skin discoloration (L, CX)	________ ________	Very low (H, L) Moderate (CX)	Primarily contact; with some vapor hazard
________	Chlorine (CL) Phosgene (CG)	________ ________	Causes irritation; choking (CL); severe pulmonary edema (CG)	________ ________	Very high	Vapor hazard
________	Tabun (GA) Sarin (GB) Soman (GD) VX agent (VX)	________	Most lethal chemical agents can kill within minutes; effects are reversible with antidotes	________	Moderate (GA, GD) Very high (GB) Low (VX)	Vapor hazard (GB) Both vapor and contact hazard (GA, GD) Contact hazard (VX)
________	Hydrogen cyanide (AC) Cyanogen chloride (CK)	________ ________	Highly lethal chemical gases; can kill within minutes; effects are reversible with antidotes	________	Very high	Vapor hazard

3. Symptoms of persons exposed to nerve agents

Mnemonic: SLUDGEM	
S	Salivation
L	________________
U	Urination
D	________________
G	Gastrointestinal (GI) distress
E	________________
M	Miosis
Mnemonic: Killer Bs	
B	Bradycardia
B	________________
B	Bronchospasm

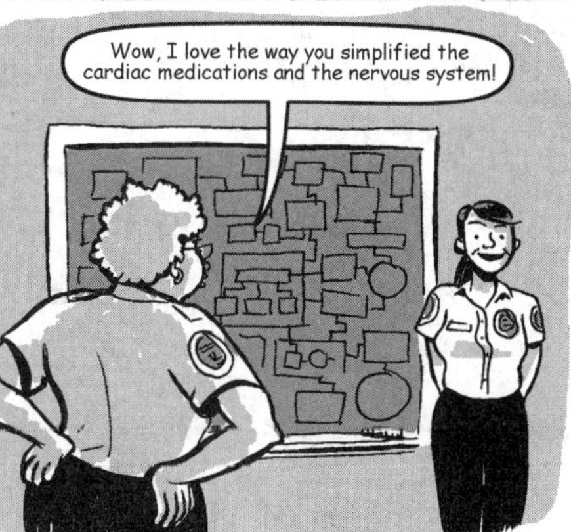

CHAPTER 51

Disaster Response

Matching

Match each of the terms in the right column to the appropriate description in the left column.

______	**1.** Blasts from flowing or standing lava that can have a wide dispersal circumference, spewing ash and magma.	**A.** 6-feet rule
______	**2.** A strategically placed facility that has been preestablished for the mass distribution of antibiotics, antidotes, and vaccinations, along with other medications and supplies.	**B.** After-action report (AAR)
______	**3.** An illness or disease that affects a high proportion of the population over a broad or potentially worldwide geographic area.	**C.** All-hazards approach
______	**4.** A situation in which a reservoir overflows its borders.	**D.** Ashfall
______	**5.** Documents that preplan how you will access help from other areas when needed.	**E.** Casualty collection points
______	**6.** A command system used in larger incidents in which there is a multiagency response or multijurisdictional response to coordinate decision making and cooperation among the agencies.	**F.** Cold stress
______	**7.** Debris from satellites and other man-made objects that reenter the earth's atmosphere.	**G.** Continuity of operations plan (COOP)
______	**8.** A method of safeguarding oneself or others' position during an emergency event or event involving a hazardous material; includes measures such as remaining in a safe atmosphere, usually inside structures, or other simple measures such as shutting the windows, going to the cellar, or turning off the heating and air-conditioning systems.	**H.** Critical infrastructure
______	**9.** Depression that can affect people in long periods of bad weather, usually winter.	**I.** Directed area
______	**10.** Heavy canvas bags that can be hung from trees containing water in amounts from 40 to 100 gallons (151 to 379 L).	**J.** Disaster
______	**11.** A guideline to follow regarding the distance to place between oneself and a person who sneezes or coughs, to avoid exposure to germs.	**K.** Disaster management
______	**12.** A system implemented to manage disasters and mass-casualty incidents in which section chiefs, including operations, finance, logistics, and planning, report to the incident commander.	**L.** Dust suffocation
______	**13.** A team, usually staffed with physicians, nurses, and emergency medical services (EMS) providers, that performs minor surgical procedures and debridements in the field, taking some of the load from the hospital facility.	**M.** Emergency operations center (EOC)

______	**14.** An illness or disease that affects or tends to affect a disproportionately large number of people within a specific population, community, or region at the same time.	**N.**	Epidemic
______	**15.** A central command and control facility, found at all government levels, responsible for strategic overview; tactical decisions are left to incident commanders.	**O.**	Forward surgical team
______	**16.** The external foundation in communities made up of structures and services critical in the day-to-day living activities of humans; energy sources, fuel, water, sewage removal, food, hospitals, and transportation systems.	**P.**	Incident command system (ICS)
______	**17.** The detailed plan describing the functioning of the agency in situations that disrupt normal operations.	**Q.**	Lister bags
______	**18.** A psychologic condition that can develop in people who are exposed to cold weather for long periods of time, even if sheltered.	**R.**	Mutual aid agreements
______	**19.** Areas where slightly injured or noninjured displaced people can be gathered together and transported by bus or truck for further treatment.	**S.**	Overtopping
______	**20.** The residue left behind from a volcanic eruption.	**T.**	Pandemic
______	**21.** A phenomenon that can occur during an earthquake, in which particles of dust and debris are loosened and released into the air, producing a toxic and hypoxic atmosphere.	**U.**	Point of distribution (POD)
______	**22.** A planned, coordinated response to a disaster that involves cooperation of multiple responders and agencies and enables effective triage and provision of care according to triage decisions.	**V.**	Pyroclastic explosions
______	**23.** A sudden, calamitous event, such as an accident or catastrophe, that causes great damage, loss, or destruction.	**W.**	Seasonal affective disorder (SAD)
______	**24.** An area away from the command post or emergency operations center, considered by engineering expertise to be a safe place to stage until directed otherwise.	**X.**	Shelter-in-place
______	**25.** The act of conducting comprehensive preplanning that will apply to any disaster.	**Y.**	Space junk
______	**26.** The official internal report of the entire event, such as a disaster, which should contain the facts of the incident reflected in a chronologic, accurate manner.	**Z.**	Unified command system

Multiple Choice

Read each item carefully, and then select the best response.

______ **1.** The critical infrastructure includes the food and hospitals as well as which of the following?

- **A.** Communications systems
- **B.** Electrical power grid
- **C.** Sewage removal
- **D.** All of the above

______ **2.** Disaster response preplanning includes assessing each of the following, EXCEPT:

- **A.** geography of response areas.
- **B.** number of paramedics on each ambulance.
- **C.** immunizations of personnel.
- **D.** training standards.

______ **3.** In planning for disasters, which nongovernmental organization should be included to assist with disaster relief?

- **A.** Homeland Security Agency
- **B.** The Red Cross
- **C.** Federal Emergency Management Agency (FEMA)
- **D.** National Highway and Traffic Safety Administration (NHTSA)

_____ **4.** When planning for sheltering, what will your plan need to consider?
A. Adult supervision for children
B. Access to automated teller machines (ATMs)
C. Facilities for mass decontamination
D. Housing for wild animals

_____ **5.** Which of the following is NOT considered a high priority for after a disaster event?
A. Physical examination of personnel
B. Stress reaction review
C. Mobilization of personnel
D. Finance and reimbursement

_____ **6.** Each of the following is considered a natural disaster, EXCEPT:
A. flooding.
B. a tanker crash.
C. a pandemic.
D. a landslide or avalanche.

_____ **7.** During an earthquake, the release of particles of debris into the air can cause:
A. dust suffocation.
B. a landslide.
C. flooding.
D. magma release.

_____ **8.** In which of the following incidents should you consider sheltering-in-place?
A. An earthquake nearby
B. A drought in the valley this season
C. A sandstorm or dust storm
D. Prolonged cold weather and power outages

_____ **9.** When people are exposed to cold weather for long periods of time, even though sheltered, they can develop a condition called:
A. trench foot.
B. frostbite.
C. walking pneumonia.
D. cold stress.

_____ **10.** Which of the following is NOT a man-made disaster?
A. A hazardous materials incident
B. A pandemic
C. A civil disturbance
D. An IT (cyber) disruption

Fill-in-the-Blank

Read each item carefully, and then complete the statement by filling in the missing word(s).

1. The act of conducting comprehensive __________ for all types of disasters is called a(n) __________-__________ approach.

2. EMS is normally accustomed to __________ __________ __________ that allow EMS agencies and fire departments in neighboring jurisdictions to cover emergency calls.

3. The __________ supervisor must maintain a(n) __________ of all patients and the hospitals to which they are transported.

4. You must keep the __________ updated on field conditions so that they can __________ their priorities, if necessary.

5. Consider a press __________ location and provide prompt __________ so that all the facts that you are allowed to release about the incident can be communicated through the __________.

6. The __________-__________ __________ is your official internal report of the entire event.

7. You may need to help set up field hospitals and first-aid stations at __________ __________ __________.

8. EMS may be represented in the __________ __________ __________ or in the unified command center.

9. During a heat wave, small, more frequent meals are better than large ones. Eat foods that are __________ in fluids, such as __________, fruits, and salads.

10. A(n) __________ is illness that affects a disproportionately large geographic area and number of people. A(n) __________ is an extensive one.

Identify

Read the following case study, and then list the chief complaint, vital signs, and pertinent negatives.

You have responded to a structure fire involving a strip mall with eight stores in a row. The suspected arsonist had a grudge against the owner of the Software Plus store and pried open the rear door and started a fire with gasoline. It was around midnight, and all the stores were closed, so aside from the potential danger to the firefighters, there were no victims in the buildings. While you are standing by in the rehab sector, you are notified that the police found the suspected arsonist hiding in a nearby alleyway. They bring him to your EMS unit because most of the front of his clothing has been burned, and he is disoriented and in a lot of pain. Your patient is a 22-year-old man who at first inspection has burns to his hands, arms, and the front of his chest, and his beard has been mostly burned off. Apparently, the fire got out of control before he was able to exit the building, and the gasoline had splashed the front of his clothing. He is conscious and alert, but you note that he has a raspy voice and is in extreme pain. (He reports a 20 on the 10 scale!) He did remember the grade-school lesson to "stop, drop, and roll," managing to put the fire on his clothing out by rolling around in a puddle in the alley.

Your partner starts the primary survey and secondary assessment as you apply oxygen with a nonrebreathing mask. The rapid trauma exam shows only partial-thickness burns on the hands and arms, but his chest is a full-thickness burn. You are most concerned with the potential for a respiratory burn and know this patient will end up in a burn bed this morning. As you remove his watch and rings and give them to the officer, your partner gets some vital signs. He is breathing 24 breaths/min and shallow, with an oxygen saturation of 96% and clear lung sounds. Pulse is 110 beats/min and regular, and blood pressure (BP) is 108/68 mm Hg. His pupils are equal, round, and reactive to light and accommodation (PERRLA) and fortunately were not burned. The patient rates his pain at a 10/10. His skin, in the noninjured areas, is pale, cool, and moist. You remove his remaining clothing and have him lie down on a burn sheet that was placed on your stretcher. The patient denies taking any medications and denies any allergies. He says he is normally as healthy as a horse. You get him in the unit, place him on the heart monitor (which shows sinus tachycardia with no ectopic beats), and then start a large-bore IV line in a vein in an area that was not burned. You decide to administer plenty of fluids for the burns and fentanyl for pain due to his dropping BP. After consultation with medical control, the decision is to transport him to the local high school soccer field, where a landing zone has been set up for the regional medevac helicopter crew to pick him up and transport him to the regional burn center.

1. Chief complaint:

____

____

2. Vital signs:

____

____

3. Pertinent negatives:

____

____

Ambulance Calls

The following case scenario provides an opportunity to explore the concerns associated with patient management, paramedic care, and preparation for major incidents in your community. Read the scenario, and then answer each question.

1. It is a hot, stuffy day with high humidity in July in your community. You are on the medic unit today and state to your partner, "This makes 10 straight days of 90-degree temps." You have been running calls all morning, mostly patients with respiratory complaints. At 1500 hours, you get a call for the Fairwood Nursing Home for an unresponsive patient. On arrival, you find a five-floor facility that normally houses 200 patients. It is extremely hot inside the lobby. As you are led to room 105 by a nursing aide, your partner notices that there are a number of patients in a community room who look unconscious on the couch with the TV blasting. The aide tells you that the air conditioner has been broken all week, and the place only has two aides for each floor and one nurse in the office. Some doctors stop by in the mornings, but they are not there today. As you walk into the patient's room, you note it is a semiprivate room, and both occupants are restrained in a seated position in chairs. That sure makes it difficult for them to keep drinking fluids when they can't even get up out of their chairs. Further, they are wearing flannel nightgowns! The aide, who has been very talkative, says he thinks there are a lot of patients getting sicker; he certainly is not feeling well. He also states that the windows have never been opened. There is a large fan in the hallway, basically blowing hot air around the hallways.

As your partner begins to assess the patient in room 105, you decide to pick up the phone and discuss this situation with your supervisor, who promptly alerts dispatch to assign a group of ambulances, the police, the fire department (for ventilation), and the Special Operations Unit.

This story is based on an actual incident that occurred in the heat wave of 1978 in Queens, New York. It could happen in your community, too, if you live in a warmer climate.

a. List four problems and potential solutions to issues that occur during a heat wave.

(1) ____

____

(2) ____

____

(3) ____

____

(4) ____

____

b. What are five examples of the illnesses that you may be treating in a nursing home during a heat emergency similar to the one described in the scenario?

(1)__________

(2)__________

(3)__________

(4)__________

(5)__________

True/False

If you believe the statement to be more true than false, write the letter "T" in the space provided. If you believe the statement to be more false than true, write the letter "F."

______ **1.** Woodland fires have a much higher death rate than structural fires.

______ **2.** The trend of increasing frequency and severity of extreme weather is expected to continue in the foreseeable future.

______ **3.** When it is very cold out, you should dress in loose clothing and multiple layers.

______ **4.** A hurricane can occur anywhere, but they tend to happen in the northern states and inland regions.

______ **5.** Tsunamis can come in a series.

______ **6.** The biggest immediate danger from an earthquake is structural collapse.

______ **7.** Cave-ins can release sewer and chemical gases.

______ **8.** The media should not be a concern during a disaster.

______ **9.** Your agency's designated infection control officer should be aware of each member's immunization status.

______ **10.** If a crew is sent to another area, it may need to be self-sustaining for 48 to 72 hours.

Short Answer

Complete this section with short written answers using the space provided.

1. List the three phases of any plan of response to a disaster.

a. __________

b. __________

c. __________

2. List the considerations during a disaster.

____

____

____

Fill-in-the-Table

Fill in the missing parts of the table.

1. Examples of natural and man-made disasters

Natural Disasters	Man-Made Disasters
Forest and brush fires	____________________
____________________	Construction failures and building collapse
Tornadoes	____________________
____________________	Riots, civil disturbances, and stampedes
Tsunamis	____________________
____________________	Sniper, shooter, and hostage situations
Landslides, avalanches, mudslides	____________________
____________________	Information technology (cyber) disruptions
Volcanic eruptions	____________________
____________________	Hazardous materials incidents
Sandstorms and dust storms	
____________________	
Drought	
____________________	
Meteors and space debris	
____________________	

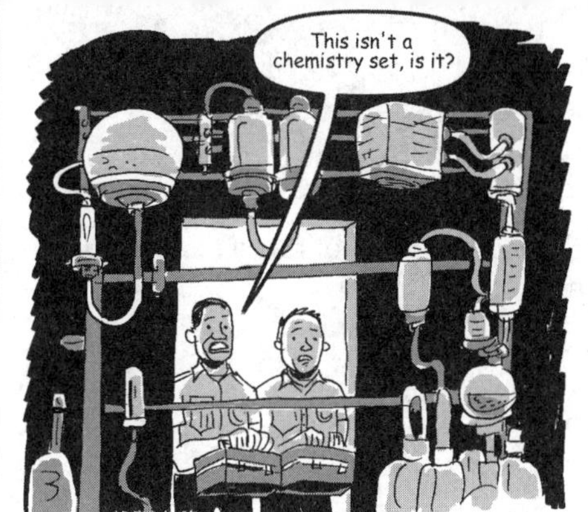

CHAPTER 52

Crime Scene Awareness

Matching

Match each of the items in the right column to the appropriate definition in the left column.

______	1. Any other means of egress, including windows and rear doors.	A.	Active shooter
______	2. The main means of escape should violence erupt. This is usually the door you used to enter the building.	B.	Clandestine drug laboratories
______	3. A gunman who has begun to fire on people and is still at large.	C.	Concealment
______	4. The evidence that ties a suspect or victim to a crime. It may include body materials, objects, and impressions.	D.	Contact and cover
______	5. Protection from being seen.	E.	Cover
______	6. Locations where illegal drugs, such as methamphetamine, lysergic acid diethylamide (LSD), ecstasy, and phencyclidine hydrochloride (PCP), are manufactured.	F.	Physical evidence
______	7. A situation in which a paramedic becomes so completely involved with patient care that he or she fails to see the possibility of physical harm to the patient or other care providers.	G.	Primary exit
______	8. The oral documentation by a witness of his or her perceived facts of a criminal act.	H.	Secondary exit
______	9. Knowing your surroundings, the people and groups in your environment, and the climate of violence or strife.	I.	Situational awareness
______	10. A technique that involves one paramedic making contact with the patient to provide care while the second paramedic obtains patient information, gauges the level of tension, and warns his or her partner at the first sign of trouble.	J.	Tactical paramedics
______	11. Obstacles that are difficult or impossible for bullets to penetrate.	K.	Testimonial evidence
______	12. Specially trained paramedics who provide medical care for special weapons and tactics (SWAT) team members conducting operations, barricaded patients, patients being held hostage, and other special operations.	L.	Tunnel vision

Multiple Choice

Read each item carefully, and then select the best response.

______ 1. For maximum safety when arriving at incidents with a single vehicle in which the potential danger is high, your vehicle should be positioned a minimum of how many feet behind the stopped vehicle?

- A. 50
- B. 15
- C. 21
- D. 10

_____ **2.** When approaching a passenger vehicle (sedan), you should stop at which column (post) of the vehicle to look in the rear and side windows?

A. A

B. B

C. C

D. D

_____ **3.** When announcing your arrival at the front door of a residence, where should you stand?

A. To the doorknob side of the door

B. To the hinged side of the door

C. In front of the door

D. Ten to 15 feet back from the door

_____ **4.** When you enter a structure, the door you use to enter the building is referred to as the _________ exit.

A. tertiary

B. secondary

C. primary

D. general

_____ **5.** Which of the following is considered concealment when you are confronted by violence?

A. Curb

B. Depression in the ground

C. Utility pole

D. Shrubbery

_____ **6.** You are dispatched to a residence for a possible sick person. En route to the call, the dispatcher informs you that the caller hung up before all the information could be collected. When you are suspicious that something is not right, prior to announcing your arrival at the door, you should do all the following, EXCEPT:

A. listen for loud noises.

B. look for neighbors to talk with.

C. glance through a window for signs of a struggle.

D. listen for threatening voices.

_____ **7.** You have entered a residence that you initially thought was safe, but once inside, you and your partner are suspicious that there might be trouble. You approach the patient to start the assessment, and your partner starts to look around to see if there is any immediate danger and gather information relevant to providing care. What is this technique called?

A. Assess and act

B. Contact and cover

C. Respond and react

D. Link and look

_____ **8.** In a hostage situation, you should assume all of the following, EXCEPT:

A. other hostages may look to you for guidance.

B. your captors could kill you at any moment.

C. your captors will be lenient on you because your uniform is an image of authority.

D. removing pieces of your uniform may make you less threatening to the captors.

_____ **9.** In all potentially violent situations, the paramedic's best (and often only) defense is:

A. a hidden weapon.

B. police backup.

C. the portable radio.

D. situational awareness.

______ **10.** You respond to a stabbing. While treating the patient and packaging for transport, you observe some footprints in the patient's blood, and you try to work quickly with minimal disruption to the evidence. The footprints are considered __________ evidence.

A. physical
B. testimonial
C. circumstantial
D. substantiated

Fill in the Blank

Read each item carefully, and then complete the statement by filling in the missing word(s).

1. Becoming completely involved with patient care and failing to see possible physical harm is called __________ __________.

2. For maximum safety when arriving at an incident with a single vehicle in which the potential for danger is high, position your vehicle at least __________ feet behind the stopped vehicle at a(n) __________-degree angle.

3. When there are two or more paramedics in the unit and you come to the scene of a motor vehicle crash, the person riding in the right front seat of the ambulance is the __________ __________.

4. When you approach a van in a situation where safety is a concern, move 10 to 15 feet away from the passenger side, and then belly-in and walk parallel until you are approximately 45° forward of the __________ post.

5. When you enter a structure, pick a(n) __________ exit and a(n) __________ exit to keep one means of escape accessible at all times.

6. To enter a scene where violence is suspected, one technique is for one paramedic to start providing patient care and the other to obtain information and warn the partner at the first sign of trouble. This technique is called __________ and __________.

Identify

Read the following case study, and then list the possible errors in handling scene safety, warning signs of danger, and potential evidence.

You are assigned to respond to a call for an injured person in a residence in a middle-class neighborhood. You are provided no additional information by the dispatcher because the caller hung up before more questions could be asked. You approach the house and hear a loud conversation inside, and without announcing yourself, you stand in front of the door and knock. You enter through the front door (primary exit), and without looking around, you ask what is happening. You find a woman on the couch, with bruising to the face, holding her right arm. She appears to be in considerable pain. Both you and your partner go to the patient and do not pay much attention to the person on the other side of the room, who is still arguing with the patient. You see a ceramic object in pieces on the floor and brush it out of the way with your foot as you approach the patient. You start to assess the patient, and your partner cuts and rips through the bloody shirt sleeve to examine the arm. You decide the person standing on the other side of the room is a potential threat and realize that he is between you and the front door. You notice there are a number of tables with drawers and a fire poker in a stand next to the fireplace. Just as you and your partner become anxious about the potential threats, two police officers come through the front door.

1. Errors in handling scene safety:

____

____

____

____

2. Warning signs of danger:

3. Potential evidence:

Ambulance Calls

The following case scenarios provide an opportunity to explore the concerns associated with patient management and paramedic care. Read each scenario, and then answer each question.

1. You respond to a residence that has previously had calls for domestic violence, but the dispatcher informs you that the information provided was for a medical problem including severe difficulty breathing, and no information indicated danger or that responders would be at risk. You are told the police will not arrive for another 5 minutes after you are on the scene. When you arrive at the residence, you are suspicious. What precautions might you take to help ensure that there is no immediate violence that would place you at risk?

2. You and your paramedic partner, who is driving the ambulance, are the first emergency personnel to arrive at the scene where a car ran off the road into a guardrail. When you arrive on the scene, you see no activity around the vehicle, and you see only one person in the driver's seat of the car. You are initially suspicious.
   a. How should you park and approach the scene?

   b. What precautions should you take to identify the car?

   c. Who should be the incident commander, and how should that person proceed?

3. You receive a call for a sick child. You arrive on the scene of the call, and someone is outside waiting for you. You are led into the house to find a wheezing pediatric patient who, you are told, is 7 years old. She is an asthmatic, and her family members report that they can't find her inhaler. You and your partner signal each other to use "contact and cover." You start to treat the patient, and your partner obtains information from the person who met the ambulance. Your partner's observations lead her to believe this residence is a clandestine drug laboratory.
   a. What does "contact and cover" mean?

   ____

   ____

   b. What actions should you and your partner take?

   ____

   ____

   c. What are your concerns?

   ____

   ____

4. Upon arrival at the scene of a shooting, you find a young patient shot in the leg and lying in a pool of blood. You and your partner do a rapid assessment and provide care quickly. The patient is prepared for transport, placed on the stretcher, and loaded into the ambulance. What are your primary concerns when trying to preserve evidence?

   ____

   ____

   ____

   ____

True/False

If you believe the statement to be more true than false, write the letter "T" in the space provided. If you believe the statement to be more false than true, write the letter "F."

_____ 1. Physical evidence is oral documentation by witnesses of facts.

_____ 2. The most popular substance manufactured in clandestine labs is methamphetamine.

_____ 3. The secondary exit is the door that you use to enter the building.

_____ 4. When standing at the door to a residence, you should stand on the hinged side of the door.

_____ 5. When there are two paramedics in an ambulance and you arrive on the scene where a vehicle needs to be checked out, the incident commander is the driver of the ambulance.

_____ 6. Some agencies have developed standard operating procedures that guide how to handle potentially violent situations.

_____ 7. When checking out a vehicle where the back seat is occupied, do not pass the C column/post until you are sure that it is safe to do so.

_____ 8. When you arrive at the scene of a single-vehicle crash with potential danger, the ambulance should be parked at least 10 feet behind the vehicle.

_____ 9. Many gangs use graffiti to mark off their territories.

_____ 10. Clandestine drug laboratories are not hazardous and present no danger to emergency medical services personnel.

Short Answer

Complete this section with short written answers using the space provided.

1. You are on the scene of a call that, because of unsafe circumstances, dictates your retreat to a safe area. After you have backed away from the danger zone and are in a safe area, you supply the dispatcher with your unit identifier, your location, and the location of the injured. What additional information would you want to provide to the dispatcher?

   a. ____________________

   b. ____________________

   c. ____________________

   d. ____________________

   e. ____________________

2. What three immediate hazards present dangers to emergency responders in regard to a clandestine drug laboratory?

   a. ____________________

   b. ____________________

   c. ____________________

3. When approaching a motor vehicle, a paramedic should always be attentive to impending danger. In which locations in a vehicle could a weapon be concealed?

   a. ____________________

   b. ____________________

   c. ____________________

   d. ____________________

   e. ____________________

   f. ____________________

   g. ____________________

4. When you enter a structure, the primary exit is usually the door you used to enter. What is a secondary exit, and why should it be identified?

   ____

   ____

5. What is the difference between *cover* and *concealment*?

   ____

   ____

6. Give three examples each of cover and concealment that you can use when there is danger from a shooter.

   a. Cover

      (1)____________________

      (2)____________________

      (3)____________________

   b. Concealment

      (1)____________________

      (2)____________________

      (3)____________________

7. If you are taken hostage by a subject with a gun, what should you assume during the capture stage?

   ____

   ____

8. There are two general classifications of evidence. Name and provide a brief description of each.

   a. ____________________

   b. ____________________

CAREER DEVELOPMENT

CHAPTER 53

Career Development

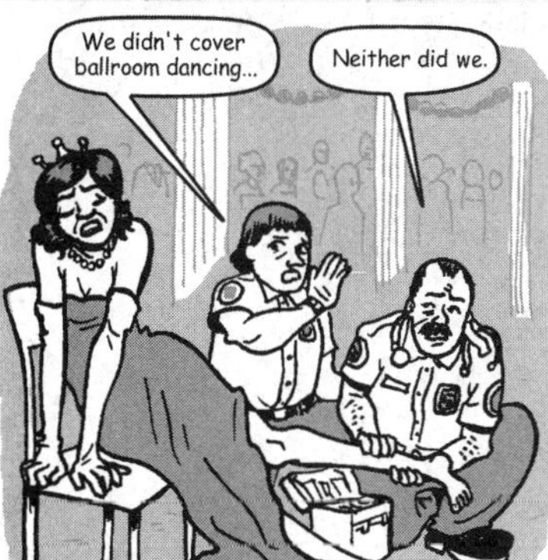

Each sport has common mechanisms of injury...

Matching

Match each of the items in the right column to the appropriate definition in the left column.

_____ 1. Paramedics who may work in military combat settings or civilian settings as part of special response teams such as special weapons and tactics (SWAT) teams.

_____ 2. Paramedics who provide trauma care and other emergency services in remote and frontier areas.

_____ 3. Paramedics who work as part of an air rescue team that provides either on-scene care in remote field settings or interfacility transports from one clinical setting to another.

_____ 4. Paramedics whose primary role is to assist patients, such as those who frequently use the emergency medical services (EMS) system for health care needs that can be managed outside the emergency department, in managing their health care needs more effectively.

_____ 5. A specialty role for paramedics, in which the paramedic is trained to provide advanced care and transport for critically injured or ill patients; also called a critical care transport professional (CCTP).

A. Critical care paramedic (CCP)

B. Flight paramedics

C. Mobile integrated health care providers/community paramedics (MIHPs/CPs)

D. Tactical paramedics

E. Wilderness paramedics

Multiple Choice

Read each item carefully, and then select the best response.

_____ 1. According to the US Bureau of Labor Statistics, which occupation will be the fastest growing in the next 10 years?
- **A.** Accountants
- **B.** Registered nurses
- **C.** Emergency medical technician (EMT) and paramedic
- **D.** Auto mechanics

_____ 2. Ultimately, the primary goal of an MIHP/CP is to get the right patient to the:
- **A.** right resource.
- **B.** right treatment.
- **C.** right tools.
- **D.** All of the above

_____ **3.** The training program for the MIHP/CP focuses primarily on pathophysiology, public health, prevention, and:
- **A.** transport ventilators.
- **B.** tactical weapons.
- **C.** social assessment needs.
- **D.** hemodynamic monitoring.

_____ **4.** The International Board of Specialty Certification or other local regulatory bodies often administer certification exams for:
- **A.** MIHP/CPs.
- **B.** CCTPs.
- **C.** tactical paramedics.
- **D.** bicycle response teams.

_____ **5.** A career as a flight paramedic may require any of the following skills, EXCEPT:
- **A.** trauma management.
- **B.** neurologic emergency management.
- **C.** cycling fundamentals for all terrains.
- **D.** advanced airway management.

_____ **6.** Paramedics who are specially trained to provide medical care within the "hot zone" are usually referred to as:
- **A.** bicycle emergency response.
- **B.** flight paramedics.
- **C.** critical care paramedics.
- **D.** tactical paramedics.

_____ **7.** Responsibilities of the wilderness paramedic may include any of the following, EXCEPT:
- **A.** general environmental medicine.
- **B.** providing wellness checks.
- **C.** improvised medicine.
- **D.** expedition medicine.

_____ **8.** An EMT or paramedic with experience in patient transportation and EMS care is an ideal candidate to serve as a(n):
- **A.** transportation coordinator.
- **B.** emergency management coordinator.
- **C.** hospital EMS coordinator.
- **D.** tactical paramedic.

_____ **9.** One of the best ways to maintain interest in your profession is to train and educate others to:
- **A.** be tactical paramedics in your community.
- **B.** provide the same level of care you provide.
- **C.** be EMS researchers in academic settings.
- **D.** be mobile integrated health care providers.

_____ **10.** If you were searching for an organization that can provide you with help in your interest in becoming a flight paramedic it would make sense to check the website:
- **A.** http://wms.org.
- **B.** nemsma.org.
- **C.** www.nasemso.org.
- **D.** www.iafccp.org.

Fill in the Blank

Read each item carefully, and then complete the statement by filling in the missing word(s).

1. Tactical paramedics may also serve as training instructors for the law enforcement agency in areas such as ____________ and __________.
2. The wilderness paramedic role may not only be ______ demanding due to extended length of time between injury and illness and _________ care, but could also be _______ demanding.
3. Emergency _________ ___________ assist hospitals with disaster planning, drills, and training on the concepts of a hospital __________ command system.
4. Visualize and _________ your career ________ in EMS.
5. When doing home visits the MIHP/CP may be trained to provide: ________ checks, obtain patient __________ inventory and determine _________ to recommended guidelines.
6. A _________ paramedic must be in _____ physical condition and able to ________ long-term fitness.

Ambulance Calls

The following case scenarios provide an opportunity to explore the concerns associated with patient management and paramedic care. Read each scenario, and then answer each question.

1. You respond to a shopping mall for a fight in which at least two individuals have been injured. On your arrival, there are shoppers who are running out the mall door stating, "Someone has a gun and is shooting people." What should you do right away, and which type of specialty training would have been helpful for you as a paramedic?

   ____

   ____

   ____

   ____

2. You and your paramedic partner just worked a 70-year-old male who was in cardiac arrest. The patient had return of spontaneous circulation (ROSC), and you transported him to a community hospital because he was not stable. The emergency department (ED) physician has decided it would be appropriate to transport the patient to the regional cardiac care center because he is a candidate for percutaneous coronary intervention (PCI).
   a. What type of specialty training would be helpful for the transport of this critical patient?

   ____

   ____

   b. The patient is on multiple IV drips to maintain his blood pressure (BP). What specific skills would be helpful for those paramedics doing this transport?

   ____

   ____

3. You receive a call for a diabetic patient who has an altered level of mental status. You have been to this location at least three times this week, and it seems the patient and family could use some help with monitoring the patient's diabetes.
   a. What type of specialty training could be helpful on calls like this as well as to prevent these calls from occurring in the first place?

   ____

   ____

   b. What specific responsibilities are included in this specialty training that would be helpful in this situation?

   ____

   ____

True/False

If you believe the statement to be more true than false, write the letter "T" in the space provided. If you believe the statement to be more false than true, write the letter "F."

_____ 1. The rise in violent crime is a reason for needing more EMS providers in the next decade.

_____ 2. Career development begins with your self-assessment.

_____ 3. The stabilization and evacuation of patients in hostile and austere environments are a key component of the MIHP/CP.

_____ 4. When the career options for paramedics increase, the opportunities for EMS educators will decrease.

_____ 5. There are roles for EMS providers in developing community programs to help prevent injury and illness.

_____ 6. The CCP is focused on functioning in nontraditional settings and providing nonemergency care with a preventive and long-term focus.

_____ 7. Learning how to use sonography and medical diagnostic tools may be a part of the training of a CCP.

_____ 8. Field sanitation, hygiene, and preventive medicine are often components of the training of the wilderness paramedic.

Short Answer

Complete this section with short written answers using the space provided.

1. List five examples of the factors influencing the need for paramedics in the next decade.

   a. ______________________________

   b. ______________________________

   c. ______________________________

   d. ______________________________

   e. ______________________________

2. List five examples of organizations for EMS providers for career development.

   a. ______________________________

   b. ______________________________

   c. ______________________________

   d. ______________________________

   e. ______________________________

3. When completing your training as a paramedic, it is advisable to have some short- and long-term career goals. Becoming a paramedic may be an achievement of one of your goals already! Take the time to think about and write down your short- and long-term goals. Next, discuss these goals with your instructor(s) and mentors, and obtain some advice on an action plan to help achieve your goals.

   a. Short-term goal: ______________________________

   b. Short-term goal: ______________________________

   c. Short-term goal: ______________________________

   d. Short-term goal: ______________________________

   e. Short-term goal: ______________________________

   f. Long-term goal: ______________________________

   g. Long-term goal: ______________________________

   h. Long-term goal: ______________________________

i. Long-term goal: ______________________________

____

____

j. Long-term goal: ______________________________

____

____

Instructor/Mentor Comments and Advice:

____

____

____

APPENDIX A

Case Studies and Answers

Case Studies

Case Study 1

It is 0900 hours, and you have been dispatched to a Priority 1 (Charlie response) call for a serious injury. As you arrive at 0908 hours, the police have just arrived and are calling you to come to the side of the house right away. The scene is safe, although there is a blood trail from a basement window to the spot where the patient is lying, holding his right leg and screaming out in pain. His airway is obviously open! You don appropriate personal protective equipment (PPE) and approach the patient to find a 20-year-old man who states he tried to kick open the basement window and managed to cut the back of his knee. He said it has continued to spurt bright red blood all over the place. Quickly, you open the trauma kit and apply direct pressure with gauze to the large laceration to the artery behind the right knee. Meanwhile, your partner determines that the patient, who is screaming that he is in a lot of pain (10/10), is alert and restless. The patient reports no other injuries. His vital signs are taken and are found to be as follows: respirations of 26 breaths/min, deep and full; pulse of 100 beats/min, thready and weak at the wrist. His blood oxygen saturation (Spo_2) is 94%. His skin is pale, cool, and clammy. The patient denies any other injuries and states he feels thirsty, weak, and dizzy at this point. You are busy trying to control the bleeding, following all the appropriate methods you learned in your paramedic training. Meanwhile, your partner applies a nonrebreathing mask with 100% oxygen to the patient as you prepare to load him on the stretcher. You both decide to do the secondary assessment en route to the hospital because the patient's condition is serious. As you load him into the ambulance, you note that the time is now 0916 hours.

1. What is the appropriate order of initial management of this patient?

____

____

____

____

____

____

2. How will you manage the continued bleeding from the patient's injury?

____

____

____

____

____

____

3. What is the appropriate intravenous (IV) fluid resuscitation regimen for this patient?

4. What is the difference between a crystalloid and a colloid solution?

5. What is the purpose of performing a secondary assessment?

6. Complete the PCR.

EMS Patient Care Report (PCR)					
Date:	Incident No.:	Nature of Call:		Location:	
Dispatched:	En Route:	At Scene:	Transport:	At Hospital:	In Service:

Patient Information	
Age: Sex: Weight (in kg [lb]):	Allergies: Medications: Past Medical History: Chief Complaint:

Vital Signs				
Time:	BP:	Pulse:	Respirations:	SpO_2:
Time:	BP:	Pulse:	Respirations:	SpO_2:
Time:	BP:	Pulse:	Respirations:	SpO_2:

EMS Treatment (circle all that apply)				
Oxygen @ ______ L/min via (circle one): NC NRM Bag-mask device		Assisted Ventilation	Airway Adjunct	CPR
Defibrillation	Bleeding Control	Bandaging	Splinting	Other:

Narrative

Case Study 2

It is 1700 hours, and you have been dispatched to a Priority 1 (Charlie response) call for an elderly woman with breathing difficulty. As you arrive, at 1707 hours, the fire department is just pulling up in front of the house. There is a family member, most likely the patient's daughter, who meets you at the front door of the residence. The scene is safe, and you have enough help. You don your PPE as you enter the bedroom in the rear of the second floor. The patient is sitting in bed, propped with about four pillows, and is in obvious respiratory distress. She is pale with blue lips, and her skin is warm and clammy to touch. She is confused but tries to talk to you in two-word sentences. Her level of consciousness (LOC), which is altered, is a V on the AVPU scale. Her daughter begins to fill you in as your partner determines that her airway is open and clear and tries to assess her respirations. The daughter states that her mother, Millie, is 72 years old and has a long history of smoking two packs a day until she was diagnosed with emphysema a few years ago. Now she only smokes one pack a day. She is on a long list of medications, which do not seem to be working today, and she has had a fever of 101.5°F all day. She called you because Millie's breathing has continued to get worse, and now she is acting very confused. The last time she was this bad, she spent 2 weeks in a critical care unit on a respirator. Your partner reports that Millie's respirations are 28 breaths/min, labored, and shallow; her pulse is about 120 beats/min and irregular; her blood pressure (BP) is 130/90 mmHg and her Spo_2 is 88%; and she does feel like she is burning up.

As you begin to set up for a nebulizer treatment, you ask the daughter whether Millie has any allergies. Your partner applies the electrodes for an electrocardiogram (ECG), which reveals an atrial rhythm that is irregularly irregular. Next, her breath sounds are found to be wheezes on expiration in all lung fields. She looks like she is tiring out, so you decide to assist her breathing and "bag in the treatment" with a bag-mask device as your partner starts an IV line. Once the IV line is in place and the first treatment is on board, the next decision will likely involve a nasal intubation, or better yet, perhaps continuous positive airway pressure (CPAP) and transportation. You both decide to do the rest of the secondary assessment en route to the hospital because the patient's condition is serious. The daughter hands you a long list of medications to take along to the hospital, which includes albuterol (Ventolin), digoxin (Lanoxin), methyldopa (Aldomet), and warfarin (Coumadin). As you load Millie into the ambulance, you note that the time is now 1720.

1. What initial management is indicated for this patient?

2. What is your interpretation of this cardiac rhythm?

3. What is your field impression of this patient?

4. Are the patient's vital signs and SAMPLE history consistent with your field impression?

5. What specific treatment is required for this patient's condition?

6. Is further treatment required for this patient?

7. Are there any special considerations for this patient?

8. Complete the PCR.

EMS Patient Care Report (PCR)					
Date:	Incident No.:	Nature of Call:		Location:	
Dispatched:	En Route:	At Scene:	Transport:	At Hospital:	In Service:
Patient Information					
Age: Sex: Weight (in kg [lb]):			Allergies: Medications: Past Medical History: Chief Complaint:		
Vital Signs					
Time:	BP:	Pulse:	Respirations:	SpO_2:	
Time:	BP:	Pulse:	Respirations:	SpO_2:	
Time:	BP:	Pulse:	Respirations:	SpO_2:	
EMS Treatment (circle all that apply)					
Oxygen @ ______ L/min via (circle one): NC NRM Bag-mask device	Assisted Ventilation	Airway Adjunct	CPR		
Defibrillation	Bleeding Control	Bandaging	Splinting	Other:	
Narrative					

Case Study 3

It is 1900 hours, and you have been dispatched to a Priority 1 (Charlie response) call for an elderly woman who fell in the hallway of the nursing home. As you arrive at 1908, an aide meets you to escort you to the location where the patient was found. Apparently, Mrs. Smith wandered out of her room and was found on the floor in the hallway near the dining room. A family member has been called and will be meeting you at the local hospital's emergency department (ED). The scene is safe, and you have enough help. You don your PPE as you approach the patient, who is lying on her back on the floor and looking very uncomfortable. The patient's right leg seems to be twisted laterally, which leads you to suspect she may have injured her hip when she fell. She is a bit confused but glad that help has arrived at her side. According to the aide, Mrs. Smith is 68 years old and has a history of diabetes and osteoarthritis. She takes medications for both conditions and has no known allergies. You ask her a few questions and determine that she is verbally responsive, and you note that she has an open airway and is breathing adequately. She is pale and clammy, and her radial pulse is fast and irregular. Your partner provides manual stabilization of the cervical spine as you do a quick head-to-toe exam on the patient. Moments later, your supervisor arrives on the scene and assists in placing the cervical collar and then securing the patient on the scoop stretcher.

Vital signs reveal the following: Respirations are 24 breaths/min and regular, her pulse is about 100 beats/min and irregular, BP is 110/70 mm Hg, and her Spo_2 is 98%. You decide to place a board between the legs to secure the possible fractured hip, then do a quick test of her blood glucose because the aide says she is usually alert and very talkative. Your partner places ECG electrodes and confirms sinus tachycardia with occasional premature ventricular contractions (PVCs) as well as a blood glucose of 70 mg/dL. You have decided that she should be moved to the stretcher and kept in a supine position, which has been a bit difficult due to the kyphosis of her spine, so giving sugar by mouth might be difficult. You therefore start an IV line and quickly administer 10% dextrose (D_{10}). Once you document another set of vital signs and note that her mental status is now alert, you decide that hypoglycemia was part of the cause of the fall. Now it is time to get rolling to the hospital because there is a potential for internal bleeding from the hip fracture, which you realize older patients do not compensate for very well. You will be reassessing the blood glucose, monitoring vital signs, listening to her lungs, carefully administering fluid, and acquiring a 12-lead ECG on the way to the hospital. As you load Mrs. Smith into the ambulance, you note that the time is now 1920.

1. What are common contributing factors to falls in the geriatric population?

___

___

___

___

___

___

2. What are some common causes of altered mental status in the geriatric population?

___

___

___

___

___

___

3. What is kyphosis? How will you immobilize this patient's spine and hip?

4. How does aging affect the body's ability to compensate for shock?

5. Complete the PCR.

EMS Patient Care Report (PCR)					
Date:	Incident No.:	Nature of Call:		Location:	
Dispatched:	En Route:	At Scene:	Transport:	At Hospital:	In Service:
Patient Information					
Age: Sex: Weight (in kg [lb]):			Allergies: Medications: Past Medical History: Chief Complaint:		
Vital Signs					
Time:	BP:	Pulse:	Respirations:	SpO_2:	
Time:	BP:	Pulse:	Respirations:	SpO_2:	
Time:	BP:	Pulse:	Respirations:	SpO_2:	
EMS Treatment (circle all that apply)					
Oxygen @ ______ L/min via (circle one): NC NRM Bag-mask device		Assisted Ventilation	Airway Adjunct	CPR	
Defibrillation	Bleeding Control	Bandaging	Splinting	Other:	
Narrative					

Case Study 4

It is 2200 hours, and you have been dispatched to a Priority 1 (Charlie response) call for a serious injury from a bar fight. The police are already on the scene, and they are looking for you to respond directly to the alleyway behind the tavern. As you arrive at 2206, the police are assisting a 23-year-old man to your ambulance. You barely open the doors to get your equipment out when the patient is already passing out on the ground just behind the ambulance. A firefighter begins to hold the head and neck while you note that the patient has a slash wound to his face and lots of blood on the front of his shirt. You note that the airway is patent, but he is having difficulty breathing. You assign a rescuer to control the bleeding to the face while you remove the patient's shirt and listen to his lungs. He has equal breath sounds, but you note a stab wound in the anterior chest on the left side, way too close to the heart. You seal the wound with an occlusive dressing and note that he has jugular venous distention (JVD). Your partner states that he has a barely palpable radial pulse, so the decision is to put him on a scoop stretcher, begin assisting his ventilations, and do the rest while en route to the trauma center.

Once in the ambulance, a full set of vital signs reveals the following: weak pulse of 108 beats/min, respirations of 26 breaths/min and shallow, BP of 90/60 mm Hg, and Spo_2 of 94%. You are assisting his ventilations with a bag-mask device and 100% oxygen while a large-bore IV line is inserted. A reassessment of vital signs shows a barely palpable radial pulse, and the BP is now 78/64 mm Hg. You make a quick call to the ED and tell them you suspect his heart was nicked by the knife because his pulse pressure is narrowing, his neck veins are distended, and the location of the wound is close to the heart. There is too much noise with the siren blaring to listen for muffled heart sounds. The ED appreciates the early warning so they can be prepared to crack his chest upon your arrival. As you pull up at the ED, you note that the time is now 2222.

1. What immediate care is required for this patient?

____

____

____

____

____

____

2. What does JVD in this patient suggest?

3. What additional signs may accompany JVD in a patient with penetrating chest trauma?

4. What specific treatment is required to treat this patient's condition?

5. Complete the PCR.

EMS Patient Care Report (PCR)			
Date:	Incident No.:	Nature of Call:	Location:

Dispatched:	En Route:	At Scene:	Transport:	At Hospital:	In Service:

Patient Information	
Age:	Allergies:
Sex:	Medications:
Weight (in kg [lb]):	Past Medical History:
	Chief Complaint:

Vital Signs				
Time:	BP:	Pulse:	Respirations:	SpO_2:
Time:	BP:	Pulse:	Respirations:	SpO_2:
Time:	BP:	Pulse:	Respirations:	SpO_2:

EMS Treatment (circle all that apply)			
Oxygen @ ______ L/min via (circle one): NC NRM Bag-mask device	Assisted Ventilation	Airway Adjunct	CPR

Defibrillation	Bleeding Control	Bandaging	Splinting	Other:

Narrative

Case Study 5

It is 0630 hours, and you have been dispatched to a Priority 2 (Bravo response) call for a sick child. As you arrive at 0640, the father is waiting at the front door of the residence. He leads you to the nursery where the 18-month-old daughter sleeps. She has not been sleeping all night, and the father states that her mom has been up with her because she was so irritable and crying. The scene is safe, and you decide to don PPE upon entering the room because the mother states her daughter is running a fever and has been vomiting. She believes she has a headache and a neck ache, and she has never seen her so irritable before. You decide that because there is no obvious immediate life threat, the child can stay in her mom's lap during your assessment.

The airway is open and clear. The breathing is slightly elevated, but skin color is good, and the tidal volume seems adequate. It is obvious that the child, whose name is Jessica, has a fever, and you decide that masks and eye shields are appropriate in addition to the gloves. As you examine the child, you see some petechiae on the extremities, but no purpura is present, and there is no obvious trauma. Jessica is alert according to the mom but still very irritable. You decide that oxygen would be helpful but do not want to get the child any more agitated than she is already, so you let Mom administer blow-by with a pediatric nonrebreathing mask. Your partner gets a full set of vital signs, and you compare them to the vital signs in the pocket guide in your pediatric kit. The pulse is fast, BP is slightly low, and respirations are on the high side of the normal range. After talking with the mother, you find this is a normally healthy child who has been sick for the last day and unable to keep any food down. The child takes no medications and has no allergies.

After consulting with your partner and the family, the plan is to wrap the child up so that she is warm and transport to the local pediatric ED. If the respirations become depressed, you will switch to bag-mask ventilations, and if the mental status changes or pulse further increases, you will consider venous access by IV or intraosseous (IO) line and then administer 20-mg/kg boluses to improve the perfusion. As you load Jessica into the ambulance, you note that the time is now 0650.

1. What is your initial treatment for this child?

____

____

____

____

____

____

2. What is your field impression of this child?

____

____

____

____

____

____

3. What are petechiae and purpura? What do they indicate?

4. What treatment will you provide to this child en route to the hospital?

5. Complete the PCR.

EMS Patient Care Report (PCR)					
Date:	Incident No.:	Nature of Call:		Location:	
Dispatched:	En Route:	At Scene:	Transport:	At Hospital:	In Service:
Patient Information					
Age: Sex: Weight (in kg [lb]):			Allergies: Medications: Past Medical History: Chief Complaint:		
Vital Signs					
Time:	BP:	Pulse:	Respirations:	SpO_2:	
Time:	BP:	Pulse:	Respirations:	SpO_2:	
Time:	BP:	Pulse:	Respirations:	SpO_2:	
EMS Treatment (circle all that apply)					
Oxygen @ ______ L/min via (circle one): NC NRM Bag-mask device		Assisted Ventilation	Airway Adjunct	CPR	
Defibrillation	Bleeding Control	Bandaging	Splinting	Other:	
Narrative					

Answers and Summary

Case Study 1

1. What is the appropriate order of initial management for this patient?

Management for the critically injured patient is based on what is going to kill the patient first. In most cases, airway management takes priority over all else; however, this is not always the case. The following represents the appropriate order of initial management for *this* patient:

- **Bleeding control**
  - The bright red blood spurting from the injury behind the patient's knee suggests a severed or partially severed popliteal artery. If not immediately controlled, severe arterial bleeding can result in death within a matter of minutes.
  - In the case of *this particular patient,* bleeding control takes priority over airway management. Because the patient is screaming in pain, he obviously has a patent airway.
- **100% supplemental oxygen**
  - The patient's respirations, although increased, are producing adequate tidal volume. Therefore, 100% oxygen via nonrebreathing mask is appropriate.
  - This patient is displaying signs of shock (ie, restlessness, tachycardia, diaphoresis). Therefore, 100% supplemental oxygen should be administered as soon as possible.
  - Monitor the patient for signs of inadequate breathing (eg, shallow depth, decreased mental status), and be prepared to provide ventilatory assistance.
- **Shock management**
  - Place the patient in the supine position (unless not in your local protocol).
  - The supine position will not only help control bleeding from the lower extremity wound but also will facilitate venous return to the right side of the heart (increased preload), increasing cardiac output and maintaining perfusion to the vital organs of the body.
- **Thermal management**
  - Place a blanket on the patient to help maintain body temperature. Patients in shock do not have the amount of oxygen needed to produce energy and maintain body temperature.
  - Hypothermia interferes with the body's clotting mechanisms and may worsen the patient's bleeding.

2. How will you manage the continued bleeding from the patient's injury?

Initial management of severe bleeding involves applying direct pressure to the wound. Direct pressure, in the majority of cases, adequately controls the bleeding. A pressure dressing should then be applied over the wound to maintain constant pressure. If bleeding continues, place additional dressings over the pressure dressing. The site should be closely monitored for signs of continued bleeding, as evidenced by blood soaking through the pressure dressing. The popliteal fossa is a difficult place to secure an adequate pressure dressing. Be prepared to proceed to the next step in bleeding control should direct pressure fail.

There are occasions when the wound continues to bleed despite the application of direct pressure. This is common when large arteries (eg, femoral, radial, popliteal) are damaged or in areas of the body where maintenance of adequate pressure is difficult (eg, popliteal fossa). If the wound continues to bleed despite initial bleeding-control measures, consider the use of a hemostatic dressing or an arterial tourniquet.

It should be noted that continuing to apply additional dressings to a severely bleeding wound will prove ineffective. Although the blood is contained within the additional dressings, the patient is still losing blood externally. If the wound continues to bleed uncontrollably, apply a tourniquet to the extremity proximal to the site of bleeding (high and tight). This may not be possible if the bleeding is coming from the proximal humerus or proximal thigh—two locations where the application of a tourniquet proximal will not be feasible because of the shoulder and hip, respectively. However, for bleeding at the level of the elbow or distal in the upper extremity or at the level of the knee and distal in the lower extremity (as in the current situation), correct tourniquet application is almost always an effective means of controlling bleeding.

Another method for controlling severe bleeding if initial methods fail is to remove all dressings, locate the site of the bleeding, and apply a hemostatic dressing directly to the site.

In the worst-case scenario, when all attempts to control bleeding fail, immediately transport the patient to the closest hospital while continuing bleeding-control efforts en route.

IV therapy would clearly be of no benefit to the patient with severe, uncontrolled bleeding. Remember to focus your efforts on treating what will kill the patient *first*.

3. What is the appropriate IV fluid resuscitation regimen for this patient?

The goal of IV therapy in the shock trauma patient is to maintain adequate perfusion, regardless of whether the patient is bleeding internally or externally. Optimally, lost blood should be replaced with blood. However, because blood must be refrigerated, typed, and cross-matched, and because it has a short shelf life, it is not practical for use in the prehospital setting.

Crystalloid solutions, such as normal saline or lactated Ringer, are more practical for use in the prehospital setting than blood. They are well-balanced solutions that closely resemble the electrolyte concentration of plasma. Additionally, they are less expensive and have a longer shelf life than blood.

As previously discussed in other case studies within this book, IV therapy for the patient with internal bleeding should be somewhat conservative, infusing just enough IV fluid to maintain adequate perfusion (eg, good mental status, systolic BP of 90 mm Hg). Because internal bleeding cannot be controlled in the prehospital setting, rapid IV fluid infusions may interfere with the body's hemostatic processes, thus resulting in increased internal hemorrhage and deterioration of the patient's condition.

External bleeding, however, can be controlled in the prehospital setting; therefore, IV fluid resuscitation in the hypotensive patient should be more aggressive. After you have controlled all external bleeding, and when you have no reason to suspect internal hemorrhage, infuse 1,000 mL of a crystalloid solution, and then reassess the patient. Continue to administer fluid boluses as needed until you have stabilized the patient's BP at 90 mm Hg and/or systemic perfusion has improved (eg, improved mental status, stronger peripheral pulses).

Because two-thirds of crystalloid solutions leave the intravascular space within 1 hour of administration, you must administer 3 mL of crystalloid solution for every 1 mL of estimated blood loss.

Crystalloid solutions improve tissue perfusion by increasing circulating volume and facilitating the transport of oxygen-carrying red blood cells that remain in the vascular space; however, they do not carry oxygen themselves. Additionally, because excessive crystalloid administration may result in hemodilution of the blood, administration of more than 2 L in the prehospital setting should be reserved for situations where perfusion cannot be maintained by any other means.

The paramedic should follow locally established protocols or contact medical control as needed regarding IV fluid resuscitation for the shock patient.

4. What is the difference between crystalloid and colloid solutions?

Crystalloid solutions, which are the primary solutions used for prehospital fluid resuscitation, contain electrolytes and water. However, because crystalloids lack proteins and larger molecules, their presence in the vascular space, once administered, is of relatively short duration. Furthermore, crystalloids, unlike whole blood, do not have the ability to carry oxygen.

The three main types of crystalloid solutions are classified by their tonicity (number of particles per unit volume) relative to that of blood plasma:

- **Isotonic crystalloids**
  - Tonicity is equal to that of blood plasma; therefore, in a normally hydrated patient, they will not cause a significant shift in fluids or electrolytes.
  - Examples of isotonic crystalloids include 0.9% sodium chloride (normal saline) and lactated Ringer.
- **Hypertonic crystalloids**
  - These have a higher solute concentration than that of the cells; therefore, when administered to a normally hydrated patient, they cause fluid to shift out of the intracellular space and into the extracellular space.
  - An example of a hypertonic crystalloid is 50% dextrose in water ($D_{50}W$).
- **Hypotonic crystalloids**
  - These have a lower solute concentration than that of the cells; therefore, when administered to a normally hydrated patient, they cause fluid to shift from the extracellular space and into the intracellular space.
  - Examples of hypotonic crystalloids include 0.45% sodium chloride (half normal saline) and 5% dextrose in water (D_5W).

As previously discussed, normal saline and lactated Ringer are the most commonly used IV crystalloids in the prehospital setting because of their ability to expand circulating volume immediately and rapidly.

Colloid solutions contain large proteins and molecules that cannot pass through the capillary membrane; therefore, relative to crystalloids, they remain in the vascular space for a longer period of time. Additionally, the osmotic properties of colloids attract water into the vascular space; therefore, a small amount of colloid can significantly increase intravascular volume. The following are examples of colloid solutions:

- **Plasmanate (plasma protein fraction).** The principal protein in Plasmanate is albumin, which is suspended in a saline solution.

- **Dextran.** Not a protein; however, it contains large sugar molecules with osmotic properties similar to those of albumin.
- **Hetastarch (Hespan).** Similar to dextran in that it contains large sugar molecules with osmotic properties similar to those of proteins.
- **Salt-poor albumin.** Contains only human albumin. Each gram of albumin administered causes retention of approximately 18 mL of water in the vascular space.

Although colloids maintain vascular volume better than crystalloids, their use in the prehospital setting is not practical. Colloids have a short shelf life, are costly, and have specific storage requirements—attributes that make them more suitable for the hospital setting. Like crystalloids, the colloids listed do not have the ability to carry oxygen.

5. What is the purpose of performing a secondary assessment?

The secondary assessment is a comprehensive head-to-toe examination that is performed on patients who are either critically injured or unresponsive. It encompasses all of the components of the primary survey; however, it is more in-depth and methodical, and it takes more time to perform.

The purpose of the secondary assessment is to detect injuries or conditions that were either not evident during earlier assessments or did not require immediate emergency care.

With critically ill or injured patients, you will seldom have time to perform this time-consuming examination on the scene because you will often be preoccupied with performing reassessments and rendering emergency treatment. If the patient's condition deteriorates while en route to the hospital, you should immediately repeat a primary survey and address any newly developed life-threatening conditions. Because this may occur several times throughout transport, you will likely not have time to perform a secondary assessment.

If, however, your transport time to the hospital is lengthy, and you have addressed all life-threatening injuries or conditions, a secondary assessment should be performed.

It is most appropriate to perform a secondary assessment of your patient in the back of the ambulance while en route to the hospital. Remaining at the scene to perform a thorough examination on a critically ill or injured patient would clearly delay definitive care and increase the possibility of a poor patient outcome.

Summary

During the primary survey of your patient, all airway, breathing, and circulation problems must be corrected immediately. Invasive procedures, such as IV therapy or intubation, are of no value to the patient if there is uncontrolled bleeding or a nonpatent airway.

The patient in this case study had an obviously patent airway; however, he had an uncontrolled arterial hemorrhage. Therefore, controlling the bleeding had priority over applying oxygen. If, however, sufficient help were available (eg, emergency medical responder [EMR], law enforcement), then bleeding control and oxygen therapy could have been accomplished simultaneously. Remember that the order in which you manage your patient's injuries or condition is based on what will be the ***most rapidly*** fatal. A severe, uncontrolled arterial hemorrhage will kill the patient before you can even prefill the reservoir of a nonrebreathing mask!

Once a patent airway has been established and all external bleeding has been controlled, the patient should be rapidly assessed for signs of shock. If signs of shock are present, immediately transport the patient, and perform all interventions, such as IV therapy and cardiac monitoring, en route to the hospital.

In addition to 100% oxygen and thermal management, shock caused by external blood loss should be treated with aggressive IV infusions of an isotonic crystalloid solution (eg, normal saline, lactated Ringer). The goal of IV therapy is to maintain adequate perfusion (eg, systolic blood pressure of 90 mm Hg, improved mental status). Because crystalloid solutions quickly leave the vascular space, you must infuse 3 mL for each 1 mL of estimated blood loss. Because excessive crystalloids may hemodilute the blood, more than 3 liters should not be administered in the prehospital setting unless absolutely necessary to maintain perfusion.

Continually monitor the patient en route to the hospital, and be prepared to infuse additional IV fluids for BP maintenance, assist ventilations for inadequate breathing, or perform CPR if the patient develops cardiac arrest.

Show the PCR to your instructor, and ask for some feedback!

Case Study 2

1. What initial management is indicated for this patient?

Positive-pressure ventilations (bag-mask device or pocket-mask device) are indicated. This patient has multiple signs of inadequate breathing, including confusion, rapid and labored respirations, inability to speak in full sentences, and perioral cyanosis.

Tidal volume is needed and can be provided only with the use of positive-pressure ventilatory support.

Consider placing a nasopharyngeal airway if the patient's LOC further decreases.

2. What is your interpretation of this cardiac rhythm?

The cardiac rhythm described is *atrial fibrillation*, which is characterized by an irregularly irregular rhythm and the absence of discernible P waves.

Atrial fibrillation is caused by multiple ectopic foci in the atria that discharge in a chaotic fashion. Many of the impulses are blocked at the AV junction, whereas others are allowed to pass through. This randomized impulse passage through the AV junction causes the ventricular rhythm in atrial fibrillation to be irregularly irregular.

Atrial fibrillation is often seen with conditions such as heart failure and chronic obstructive pulmonary disease (COPD; eg, emphysema) and is commonly caused by pulmonary hypertension with subsequent atrial dilation.

3. What is your field impression of this patient?

This patient is experiencing an *acute exacerbation of emphysema* and is quickly approaching complete respiratory failure. The following assessment findings support this field impression:

- History of emphysema, no doubt attributed to her history of cigarette smoking
- Recent flu-like symptoms, which indicate a possible respiratory tract infection, the most common precursor to acute exacerbation of COPD
- Temperature of 101.5°F, which confirms the presence of an infection
- Acute worsening of her shortness of breath, which is classic in COPD exacerbation following an acute respiratory tract infection

Emphysema falls within a myriad of conditions collectively called COPD. Other forms of COPD include chronic bronchitis and, to a lesser degree, asthma, which is more of an episodic disease than a chronic one.

Emphysema is a progressive, irreversible pulmonary disease that is most often attributed to a history of long-term cigarette smoking or repeated exposure to other toxic substances. The incidence of emphysema is much higher in men than in women.

Emphysema results in gradual destruction of the alveolar walls due to a loss of pulmonary surfactant, which decreases the surface area of the alveolar membrane and interferes with gas exchange in the lungs. Additionally, the number of pulmonary capillaries decreases, which increases the resistance to pulmonary blood flow. This process ultimately causes pulmonary hypertension, which may lead to right-sided heart failure (cor pulmonale). Because the right side of the heart must pump against a high-pressure gradient, atrial dilation may occur, thus resulting in atrial fibrillation.

Emphysema also weakens the walls of the small bronchioles, which, in combination with alveolar wall destruction, decreases the ability of the lungs to recoil effectively during exhalation. This causes air to become trapped in the lungs, giving the person's chest a characteristic barrel-shaped appearance. Frequent pulmonary infections further the degree of air trapping because of inflammation and mucus production within the bronchioles.

The destruction of lung tissue causes the alveoli to collapse (atelectasis). The patient attempts to compensate for this by breathing through pursed lips, thus creating an effect similar to that of positive end-expiratory pressure (PEEP).

As the degenerative process of emphysema continues, the partial pressure of oxygen in the arterial blood ($Pa{O_2}$) decreases and remains chronically low. This stimulates red blood cell production, perhaps even to excessive levels (polycythemia), which would explain why the patient's skin remains pink (pink puffer) despite inadequate pulmonary gas exchange. The presence of cyanosis, therefore, would indicate severe hypoxia in patients with emphysema, more so than if it were present in an otherwise healthy person.

Patients with COPD tend to retain carbon dioxide and, therefore, have a chronically elevated partial pressure of arterial carbon dioxide ($Pa{CO_2}$). Chemoreceptors that monitor the levels of oxygen in carbon dioxide in the body eventually become accustomed to this, and the respiratory center in the brain (medulla oblongata) stops using increased $Pa{CO_2}$ levels to regulate breathing, as it does in an otherwise healthy person. This activates a mechanism called the hypoxic drive, which increases breathing stimulation when $Pa{O_2}$ levels fall and inhibits breathing stimulation when $Pa{O_2}$ levels increase. In rare cases, the administration of high-concentration oxygen, which can quickly increase $Pa{O_2}$ levels, may cause the chemoreceptors to stop stimulating the respiratory centers, resulting in hypoventilation or even apnea. If this occurs, simply assist the patient's ventilations. **Never** withhold oxygen from a hypoxic patient, even in the face of this potential—although highly uncommon—threat.

Patients with emphysema are predisposed to lower respiratory tract infections such as pneumonia because of their diminished ability to expel secretions from the lungs effectively. In addition, hypoxia-related cardiac dysrhythmias may occur.

Patients with emphysema and COPD in general learn to live with their chronic illness on a daily basis and grow accustomed to the normal respiratory distress and physical limitations that accompany it. When they call emergency medical services (EMS), something has changed for the worse.

4. Are the patient's vital signs and SAMPLE history consistent with your field impression?

The patient's vital signs do not reinforce a field impression of COPD exacerbation as much as her medical history does. In particular, the recent flu-like symptoms that preceded an acute exacerbation of her respiratory distress make this a classic case.

Because this patient takes numerous medications, each of which is used to treat different conditions, it would be worthwhile to review each of them briefly.

- **Albuterol (Ventolin, Proventil).** A selective beta$_2$ agonist that dilates the bronchioles and is thus used to treat diseases associated with bronchiole constriction and/or inflammation, such as asthma, emphysema, and bronchitis
- **Digoxin (Lanoxin, digitalis).** A cardiac glycoside that is used for, among other conditions, ventricular rate control in patients with chronic atrial fibrillation
- **Warfarin (Coumadin).** An anticoagulant commonly prescribed as prophylactic therapy to patients with atrial fibrillation who are prone to developing microemboli (small clots) when blood stagnates in the poorly contracting atria
- **Methyldopa (Aldomet).** A centrally acting antiadrenergic used in the treatment of hypertension. Its active metabolite, alpha-methylnorepinephrine, lowers the blood pressure by stimulating central inhibitory alpha-adrenergic receptors and reducing plasma levels of renin. Renin is a proteolytic enzyme of the kidney that plays a major role in the release of angiotensin, a potent vasoconstrictor.

5. What specific treatment is required for this patient's condition?

- **Endotracheal intubation.** If the paramedic has difficulty providing effective ventilations utilizing basic means (bag-mask device, pocket-mask device), endotracheal (ET) intubation should be performed to facilitate administration of 100% oxygen directly into the patient's lungs and more definitively protect the patient's airway.

  As evidenced by the patient's falling oxygen saturation level and markedly diminished LOC, it is clear that bag-mask ventilation is not providing adequate oxygenation.

  Because of the patient's already diminished LOC, a hypnotic-sedative drug (Versed, etomidate) may be all that is required to facilitate intubation. If sedation alone is not effective, however, a neuromuscular blocker (paralytic) may be needed to perform rapid sequence intubation (RSI).

  When inducing paralysis with medications, succinylcholine (Anectine) is the preferred initial agent to use. Succinylcholine has a duration of action of only 3 to 5 minutes, which means that if intubation is unsuccessful, you will not have to ventilate the patient with a bag-mask device for a prolonged period of time. Succinylcholine does, however, depolarize potassium ions, which produces muscular fasciculations (generalized muscle twitching). Therefore, use of a nondepolarizing paralytic, such as vecuronium (Norcuron) in a premedication (priming) dose prior to inducing a full neuromuscular blockade with succinylcholine is advisable. Once intubation is *successfully performed and confirmed*, the neuromuscular blockade can be maintained with a longer-acting paralytic, especially if your transport time will be prolonged. Again, vecuronium, which has a 45-minute duration of action, would be an appropriate drug to use.

  Follow locally established protocols regarding the use and doses of neuromuscular blockers for RSI.
- **Pharmacologic interventions.**
  - *Aerosolized bronchodilators* can be administered endotracheally with a small-volume inline nebulizer. The following medications can be given alone or in combination:
    - Selective beta$_2$-adrenergic agonists, such as albuterol (Ventolin, Proventil), metaproterenol (Alupent), or isoetharine (Bronkosol)
    - Anticholinergic bronchodilators such as ipratropium (Atrovent)

  When used in combination with beta-agonists, the beta-agonist must be administered first, followed by a 5-minute interval prior to administering Atrovent.

  Aerosolized bronchodilators, because of their rapid onset of action (3 to 5 minutes), would be the preferred initial pharmacologic intervention because of the severity of the patient's condition. The significant bronchoconstriction, which is impairing effective positive-pressure ventilation in this patient, must be reversed as soon as possible. Follow locally established protocols regarding the dose of ET-administered bronchodilators.

- *IV glucosteroids*:
  - Methylprednisolone (Solu-Medrol): Reduces acute and chronic inflammation and potentiates the relaxation of bronchiole smooth muscle caused by beta-adrenergic agonists
  - Solu-Medrol has an onset of action of approximately 1 to 2 hours. The adult dose varies, usually ranging from 40 to 125 mg IV.

The goal in treating patients with acute COPD decompensation—or any lower airway disorder, for that matter—is to correct hypoxemia and relieve the bronchoconstriction that is causing the hypoxemia. These actions will prevent respiratory failure and subsequent cardiac arrest.

Administration of 100% supplemental oxygen is the first and most important intervention, given the Spo_2. Oxygen may be given with a nonrebreathing mask or via positive-pressure ventilatory support if the patient's respiratory effort is inadequate.

Medications, administered by aerosol or IV line or both, are needed to relax the smooth muscles of the lower airways, thus improving ventilation and facilitating oxygenation.

6. Is further treatment required for this patient?

By improving this patient's oxygenation status, her LOC may improve. The patient may fight the ET tube, making it safer to consider removal. Because of the potential for vomiting and aspiration following removal of the ET tube and the possibility that her condition could worsen, she should remain intubated. Extubation in the field (unless done by the patient) is not commonly performed. For patient comfort and to prevent field extubation by the patient, consider administering additional doses of a long-acting paralytic (eg, Norcuron) and/or keeping the patient sedated with the appropriate medications (Versed, Valium).

Although her oxygen saturation of 88% was low, it may not come up to 98% due to her chronic condition. An improvement from 88% to 92% might be as good as she gets in the field. Continue to monitor her ventilatory status, oxygen saturation, and ECG. She is still prone to cardiac dysrhythmias.

7. Are there any special considerations for this patient?

As previously mentioned, patients with COPD have chronically low Pao_2 levels and are stimulated to breathe based on these levels (hypoxic drive).

If high concentrations of oxygen are administered, the respiratory centers in the brain may be fooled into thinking that the patient is adequately oxygenated and will therefore send messages to the respiratory muscles to decrease the rate and strength of breathing. Oxygen-induced hypoventilation or apnea occurs in a very limited number of instances. Should this rare event occur, simply provide positive-pressure ventilatory support. Never withhold oxygen from a hypoxic patient!

Summary

When patients with chronic respiratory disease call EMS, a significant change has occurred in their condition. Otherwise, your assistance would not have been requested.

Due to the nature of their illness, patients with COPD typically have a baseline respiratory distress; however, they cannot live with *severe* hypoxia any better than a healthy person could.

An acute lower respiratory tract infection, such as pneumonia, in which the patient cannot effectively expel secretions from the lungs, is the most common precursor to exacerbation of COPD. The mucus production and bronchiole inflammation that accompany many respiratory infections only worsen the patient's hypoxia.

You must perform a careful, systematic assessment of the patient and provide the appropriate treatment in a timely manner. It is critical that you recognize the difference between an adequately and an inadequately breathing patient.

Prehospital care focuses on ensuring adequate oxygenation and ventilation and pharmacologically reversing bronchoconstriction. Definitive care includes treating the underlying cause of the exacerbation, which usually involves antibiotics to treat the underlying infection. If the patient begins to show signs of respiratory failure, such as a rapidly falling oxygen saturation level or decreasing LOC, use sedating agents and neuromuscular blocking medications to intubate the patient without delay.

Show the PCR to your instructor, and ask for some feedback!

Case Study 3

1. What are common contributing factors to falls in the geriatric population?

Falls are a common cause of injury in geriatric patients and can result in serious problems. Injuries from falls are the leading cause of accidental death in the elderly.[1] Additionally, falls are the most common cause of nonfatal trauma-related hospital admissions among older adults.[2] Such injuries can have a profound impact on the patient's quality of life. Children and young adults have a higher incidence of falls than geriatric people; however, unlike geriatric people, their injuries are not associated with a high mortality rate.

Falls in older people are caused by intrinsic (patient-related) factors, extrinsic (environmental) factors, or a combination of both (multifactorial). Extrinsic factors include torn or loose rugs, poor lighting, furniture obstructions, wet floors, and high steps on stairways.

Intrinsic factors may be age related or the result of an acute or prior medical condition. Age-related changes include impaired balance and coordination (gait impairment), decreased muscle and bone strength, impaired vision and depth perception, and decreased proprioception (perception of body position and movement).

Common acute medical conditions include acute myocardial infarction (AMI), stroke, hypoglycemia, and infection with associated dehydration. Prior medical illnesses—such as stroke, cataracts, and Parkinson disease—can impair the older patient's balance and coordination, leading to falls.

The use of certain medications can also predispose the older patient to falls. These medications include anxiolytics such as temazepam (Restoril) and diazepam (Valium), antidepressants such as amitriptyline (Elavil) and paroxetine (Paxil), and antihypertensives such as propranolol (Inderal) and metoprolol (Lopressor). Medication-related falls are often the result of nervous system impairment, drug-to-drug interaction, or inadvertent overdose. Many older patients take multiple medications (polypharmacy) for different medical conditions, and it is often impossible to determine how one drug will interact with another.

The cause of falls in older adults is often multifactorial. An overmedicated patient may trip on a loose rug or fall down steps, or the patient may experience a syncopal episode and strike his or her head on an end table while falling.

Through a careful and systematic assessment of the patient, the paramedic must attempt to determine the cause of the patient's fall. In many cases, a fall may be the only presenting sign of an acute illness. Unfortunately, the patient's fall may be the result of physical abuse, which should be suspected when the injury sustained does not coincide with the mechanism described.

2. What are some common causes of altered mental status in the geriatric population?

You should assume that any alteration in mental status is abnormal until proven otherwise, regardless of the patient's age. Advanced age does not automatically equate to an altered mental status. Older patients are frequently capable of highly creative and productive thought processes.

By the time a person reaches the age of 80 years, brain size has decreased by approximately 10%; however, this decrease in brain size does not affect the person's intelligence. The following slight changes, which are not present in all patients, are commonly associated with the aging process:

- Forgetfulness
- Psychomotor slowing
- Decreased reaction time
- Difficulty remembering recent events

When assessing an older patient with altered mental status, you must first determine the patient's baseline mental status. According to the aide, your patient is normally well oriented. This confirms the presence of a new onset of altered mentation.

Older patients are predisposed to several neurologic disorders that can produce alterations in mentation. It may not be possible to determine the exact cause in the prehospital setting, which is why these patients should be evaluated in the ED.

One in three Americans over the age of 65 years will develop dementia.[3] Dementia is defined as a progressive impairment of cognitive function. Alzheimer disease, a common cause of dementia, is a degenerative disease of the brain that results in impaired memory, thinking, and behavior. Approximately 5.5 million Americans were affected by Alzheimer disease in 2017.[4] Brain tumors, which typically grow slowly, are another possible cause of dementia.

In the prehospital setting, dementia is often difficult to differentiate from delirium, especially in the absence of a friend or family member who is familiar with the patient's normal mental state. Unlike dementia, delirium is characterized by an acute onset of cognitive impairment and is frequently caused by a life-threatening medical condition. Delirium can be reversed if the underlying cause is rapidly identified and promptly treated.

Once it has been established that the altered mental status is a new onset, the paramedic should carefully and systematically assess the patient in an attempt to identify and treat the underlying cause. Routine actions include evaluating for signs of trauma, obtaining a blood glucose reading, and considering the administration of naloxone (Narcan) if a drug overdose is suspected.

Again, do not become complacent and assume that an altered mental status in the geriatric patient is simply the result of advanced age.

3. What is kyphosis? How will you immobilize this patient's spine and hip?

Kyphosis is an exaggerated curvature (concave ventral) of the spine that results in a rounded or hunched back. Kyphosis can occur for many reasons and at any age; however, in older adults, it is most commonly caused by osteoporosis. As the bones of the spine weaken and thin, they begin to deteriorate and compress. This results in deformation of the spine, most commonly in the upper thoracic region.

Because of the age-related deterioration of bone structure (eg, osteoporosis), fractures of the spine can occur with even minor mechanisms of injury (MOIs). Therefore, spinal precautions are recommended for this patient (thus the scoop).

Immobilizing this patient's kyphotic spine will require modification of the spinal immobilization technique. Additionally, as evidenced by the lateral rotation and shortening of her left leg, you should suspect and treat this patient for a hip fracture.

When immobilizing the spine of kyphotic patients, several pillows or blankets may be required to provide support to the head and upper back. Padding of these areas is necessary to provide support because the kyphotic patient's back will not completely conform to the scoop stretcher.

Hip fractures are actually fractures of the proximal portion of the femur near or at the site of articulation with the acetabulum. Commonly, fractures of the proximal femur can occur between the femoral head and the trochanteric region (femoral neck fractures), between the greater and lesser trochanters (intertrochanteric), or below the lesser trochanter (subtrochanteric).

Hip fractures are commonly splinted by placing pillows or other padding under the injured extremity to support the fracture site in the deformed position. Splinting the extremity in the position in which it was found will minimize the risk of further injury as well as reduce the patient's pain.

An orthopedic (scoop) stretcher can be used to immobilize a fractured hip. These devices will allow the patient and the splinting material to be properly secured. Traction splints are not recommended for immobilizing hip fractures. Because it is not possible to determine the exact location of the fracture in the prehospital setting, it is not possible to assess the integrity of the pelvis accurately. If the fracture involves the pelvis, applying a traction splint could actually be detrimental and result in further displacement and potential injury. Furthermore, the risk of injury to the skin and other soft tissues with the application of traction splints in older people is potentially higher. Thus, the use of these devices in older hip fracture patients should be avoided unless alternatives are inadequate or otherwise inappropriate.

4. How does aging affect the body's ability to compensate for shock?

Even at rest, the aging body's physiologic functions are diminished. Therefore, the ability of the older person to compensate for a low cardiac output, hypoxia, and shock effectively is markedly diminished. The respiratory, nervous, and cardiovascular systems are the key body systems that compensate during shock; therefore, age-related changes that occur with each of these systems will be discussed.

The aging process adversely affects ventilatory function, thus impairing the older person's ability to compensate for hypoxia. The smooth muscles of the lower airway weaken with age. When increases in tidal volume are needed (eg, hypoxia, shock), the patient attempts to breathe deeply; however, the walls of the lower airway collapse. This reduces tidal volume.

Loss of respiratory muscle mass, increases in the stiffness of the thoracic cage, and a decreased surface area available for air exchange contribute to a decrease in vital capacity (volume of air exchanged after maximal inhalation and exhalation) of up to 50%. Decreased vital capacity causes an increase in residual volume, which is the amount of air remaining in the lungs following a maximal exhalation. This leaves more stagnant air in the alveoli, which impairs effective gas exchange.

With aging, the body's chemoreceptors become less sensitive. Chemoreceptors, which are located in the aortic arch, sense changes in arterial oxygen and carbon dioxide and send signals to the brainstem to regulate breathing accordingly. Additionally, nerve impulse transmission from the brainstem to the diaphragm and the nerves of the intercostal muscles is decreased. The net effect is a decreased ability to increase respirations quickly in response to conditions that cause hypoxia (ie, shock).

The cardiovascular system undergoes, to varying degrees, age-related deterioration that decreases its ability to compensate for shock. The vasculature loses its elasticity, which causes an increase in systolic blood pressure and afterload (the force against which the heart must pump). As a result, the wall of the left ventricle becomes enlarged (hypertrophy) and thickens. The myocardium also loses its ability to stretch effectively (Frank-Starling effect), thus decreasing ventricular filling and contractility. Hypertrophy of the mitral and tricuspid valves also occurs, which impedes blood flow into and out of the heart. These myocardial changes cause a natural decrease in stroke volume and cardiac output. Furthermore, the ability to increase cardiac output to meet the increased demands of the body is decreased.

Baroreceptors, which are located in the aortic arch and carotid sinus, become less sensitive to changes in blood volume with age. These receptors, which sense changes in arterial blood pressure, send messages to the adrenal glands, causing them to secrete the hormones epinephrine and norepinephrine, which causes increases in heart rate, myocardial contractility, and blood pressure. The heart's response to epinephrine and norepinephrine decreases with age; therefore, the older person is less able to compensate for blood loss and decreases in blood volume quickly and effectively.

Due to age-related decreases in elastin and collagen in the vascular walls, blood vessel elasticity can be reduced by as much as 70% in the older person. Therefore, compensation in shock is significantly reduced because the peripheral vasculature must be able to constrict and dilate accordingly to maintain blood pressure and adequate perfusion.

Summary

Falls are a leading cause of accidental death in patients over the age of 65 years.[1] Contributing factors to falls in older adults can be intrinsic (eg, age-related changes, acute or prior illness), extrinsic (eg, loose rugs, poor lighting), or a combination of both. When assessing the older patient who has fallen, the paramedic must attempt to determine the cause of the fall. Because of osteoporosis, spinal fractures can occur with even minor mechanisms of injury; therefore, the geriatric patient who has fallen should be immobilized, with modifications made as needed for the patient with a kyphotic spine.

Hip fractures account for 300,000 hospital admissions in people over the age of 65 in the United States each year.[5] Approximately 75% of hip fractures occur in women, and the likelihood of sustaining a hip fracture increases with age.[5] The elderly are prone to fractures because of osteoporosis, which makes the bones very fragile. Patient outcome is significantly worse in older patients with pelvic fractures than in younger patients.[6] In the acute setting, death following a hip fracture is usually caused by pneumonia, AMI, or pulmonary embolus. Long-term, common causes of death include pulmonary embolus and sepsis.

Mental status changes do not occur in all patients with age. Many older patients maintain effective cognitive processes. Any change in mentation must be assumed to be abnormal until proven otherwise. The paramedic should determine, by talking with friends or family members, whether the patient's mental status has changed and, if so, to what degree. Common causes of altered mental status in older adults include hypoglycemia, medication-related issues, and stroke. Any patient with an altered mental status should be given supplemental oxygen or assisted ventilations as needed.

Age-related changes reduce the older person's ability to compensate for hemodynamic compromise (eg, blood loss) quickly and effectively. The muscles of the respiratory system weaken, and the chemoreceptors become less sensitive to changes in oxygen and carbon dioxide levels in the blood. Due to hypertrophy and thickening of the ventricular myocardium, stroke volume decreases, resulting in a decreased cardiac output, both at rest and in times of increased demand. Blood vessel elasticity decreases, making the peripheral vasculature less able to constrict and dilate in response to the body's demands.

Show the PCR to your instructor, and ask for some feedback!

Case Study 4

1. What immediate care is required for this patient?

This patient has multiple significant MOIs. Each one must be addressed based on severity (ie, what will kill the patient first). Continue to have the firefighter maintain manual stabilization of the patient's head while you and your partner perform the following interventions:

- **Control of external hemorrhage**
  - All external bleeding must be stopped immediately. Your partner can accomplish this while you tend to the patient's airway.
  - The stab wound to the left anterior chest should be covered with an occlusive dressing. Any open wound to the chest could indicate underlying pulmonary injury and an open pneumothorax (sucking chest wound).
- **100% supplemental oxygen**
  - Although increased, this patient's respiratory effort is adequate (good tidal volume), and his SpO_2 is 94%; therefore, 100% supplemental oxygen via a nonrebreathing mask should be applied.
  - Monitor this patient's respiratory effort carefully, and be prepared to initiate positive-pressure ventilatory support if his breathing becomes inadequate (eg, reduced tidal volume, profoundly labored).

Teamwork between you and your partner is critical to providing effective patient care. Had the firefighters not been present to assist with spinal immobilization (meaning that your partner would have to), your first priority would have been to control the external bleeding. Only after the external bleeding is controlled would you apply oxygen. You must treat injuries in the order in which they would kill the patient. Severe external bleeding can cause death within a few seconds if not immediately controlled. Delaying oxygen therapy for the 1 or 2 minutes that it takes to control the severe bleeding will not kill the patient.

2. What does JVD in this patient suggest?

The stab wound to the left side of the chest and JVD should make you suspicious of a ***pericardial tamponade***. The presence of bilaterally equal breath sounds rules out a tension pneumothorax, another potential cause of JVD.

The heart is encased in a fibrous, inelastic membrane called the pericardium. The pericardial space, which is actually a potential space that normally contains 20 to 30 mL of lubricating fluid, exists between the pericardium and the heart. Blood can enter the pericardial space if small myocardial blood vessels (eg, coronary arteries) are torn or if direct penetration of the myocardium occurs. As a result, a condition called hemopericardium occurs. As more blood enters the pericardial space, a pericardial tamponade can develop.

Pericardial tamponade is most commonly associated with stab wounds to the chest. Larger penetrating injuries, such as gunshot wounds, often create a large enough hole in the pericardium for blood to exit the pericardial space and are typically associated with exsanguination into the thoracic cavity rather than pericardial tamponade.

Because the tough, fibrous pericardium does not stretch, accumulating blood puts pressure on the heart, affecting both the systolic and the diastolic phases of the cardiac cycle. Pressure on the heart impairs venous return to the heart (preload) and limits right ventricular filling. As venous pressure increases, the jugular veins become distended.

3. What additional signs may accompany JVD in a patient with penetrating chest trauma?

In the adult patient, the pericardial space can hold 200 to 300 mL of blood before signs of a pericardial tamponade become evident; however, smaller volumes of blood can still significantly reduce cardiac output. Progression of a pericardial tamponade depends on how fast blood is filling the pericardial space.

As previously discussed, pericardial tamponade causes an increase in venous pressure and JVD. In addition, right ventricular expansion (and filling) is impaired, which compromises output through the pulmonary arteries and subsequent venous return to the left side of the heart. This causes a *decreased cardiac output and systemic hypotension*. A *reflex tachycardia* attempts to (but cannot) compensate for the low cardiac output.

Because myocardial contractility is compromised, the patient's systolic blood pressure decreases. Additionally, decreased ability of the myocardium to relax fully causes an increase in the diastolic BP. These factors result in a *narrowed pulse pressure* (the difference between the systolic and diastolic BP).

Pulsus paradoxus, which is characterized by a drop in systolic BP of greater than 10 mm Hg during inspiration, may also occur and is caused when the expanding lungs literally stop the heart momentarily by putting additional pressure on the already compressed myocardium. Pulsus paradoxus can be determined clinically by noting a diminished or even disappearing radial pulse upon inspiration.

Increasing amounts of blood in the pericardium may also cause *muffled or distant heart sounds*; however, these are often difficult to hear, especially in a loud environment such as the back of a moving ambulance.

Beck triad, a classic finding in pericardial tamponade, is characterized by three clinical signs: (1) JVD, (2) muffled heart sounds, and (3) a narrowing pulse pressure. However, all three of these clinical signs may not be present, especially if the patient is hypovolemic from other injuries (eg, pelvic fracture).

4. What specific treatment is required to treat this patient's condition?

Patients with pericardial tamponade require rapid transport to a trauma center with continuous monitoring of airway, breathing, and circulation en route. As with any critical trauma patient, unnecessary delays must not occur in the field. Treatment for patients with pericardial tamponade includes removing blood from the pericardium by a procedure called *pericardiocentesis*. This procedure, however, is almost exclusively performed in the ED and is only a temporizing intervention until bleeding control and surgical repair of the injury can occur in the operating room. Refer to locally established protocols in regard to performing pericardiocentesis in the prehospital setting.

Ensure airway patency, and administer 100% supplemental oxygen. If the patient's respiratory effort is inadequate (eg, reduced tidal volume), assisted ventilations with 100% oxygen will be necessary.

Provide spinal immobilization if the MOI suggests spinal trauma, using the scoop stretcher and a cervical collar should work just fine.

Crystalloid IV fluids should be administered (en route to the ED) to increase venous return to the right atrium (preload). By increasing preload, the full and vigorously contracting atrium will force blood into the ventricles, thus stretching its walls. Stretching of the ventricular wall enhances contractility and the force with which it ejects blood out to the body. Increased cardiac contractility due to stretching of the myocardial wall is called the *Frank-Starling mechanism*; by administering IV fluids, the Frank-Starling mechanism will be enhanced and can maintain cardiac output until a pericardiocentesis can be performed.

Continuous cardiac monitoring is essential in the management of a patient with pericardial tamponade. Decreased cardiac output and hypoperfusion can result in life-threatening dysrhythmias. Pericardial tamponade is also associated with pulseless electrical activity (PEA), a condition in which a cardiac rhythm is present on the cardiac monitor but a palpable pulse is not present.

Summary

Pericardial tamponade is a condition in which blood accumulates in the pericardium and causes hemodynamic compromise. It is most often the result of penetrating trauma—specifically, stab wounds to the chest. A small tear in a myocardial blood vessel or direct penetrating trauma to the myocardium causes blood to seep into the myocardium, which puts pressure on the heart and impairs its performance. The progression of a pericardial tamponade depends on the rate at which blood is accumulating within the pericardium.

Patients with pericardial tamponade typically present with signs of shock (eg, tachycardia, hypotension, diaphoresis) as well as JVD, muffled heart sounds, and a narrowing pulse pressure (Beck triad). If the patient is severely hypovolemic from other injuries, however, JVD may not be present.

Complications associated with pericardial tamponade include cardiac dysrhythmias, such as ventricular fibrillation (VF) or pulseless ventricular tachycardia (VT), or cardiac arrest with PEA.

A rapid, systematic assessment of the patient is required to identify the signs of pericardial tamponade and to initiate the most appropriate treatment. Prehospital management consists of ensuring a patent airway, administering 100% oxygen (or ventilatory support if needed), immobilizing the spine if spinal trauma is suspected, infusing IV crystalloids to increase venous return, and rapidly transporting the patient to a trauma center. Cardiac monitoring en route is essential in being able to identify and treat life-threatening cardiac dysrhythmias.

A pericardiocentesis is required to remove blood from the pericardium, thus improving cardiac output. However, this is almost exclusively performed in the ED by a physician and is only a temporizing intervention until the injury can be repaired surgically.

Show the PCR to your instructor, and ask for some feedback!

Case Study 5

1. What is your initial treatment for this child?

- **Minimize the child's anxiety.** Although the child is clearly ill, your findings in the primary survey do not warrant immediate separation of her from her mother. If possible, continue your assessment of the child while her mother is holding her. This will minimize the child's anxiety and may facilitate a more accurate assessment.
- **Administer 100% supplemental oxygen.** As needed, use a pediatric nonrebreathing mask or the blow-by technique.

Although the child's respirations are increased, they are unlabored and are producing adequate tidal volume; therefore, ventilatory assistance is not indicated at this point. Administer passive oxygenation in a nonthreatening manner to avoid increasing the child's anxiety. If she becomes more irritable after applying a nonrebreathing mask, have the mother hold oxygen tubing near her nose and mouth.

Continue to monitor the child's respiratory effort, and closely observe for signs of inadequate ventilation, such as a shallow depth of breathing (reduced tidal volume) or a decreasing mental status. Be prepared to assist ventilations with a bag-mask device if signs of inadequate breathing are observed.

2. What is your field impression of this child?

This child's clinical presentation is highly suggestive of meningitis. The following signs, symptoms, and historic findings support this field impression:

- **Fever.**
- **Headache.** Young children will often grab the sides of the head or place their hands on the head when they are experiencing a headache. Older children are usually able to tell you that they have a headache.
- **Irritability.** Irritability is a very common sign of meningitis in smaller children. You should be especially suspicious if the child tends to become more irritable when she is picked up (paradoxical irritability); this indicates increased pain as traction is pulled on the inflamed meninges surrounding the spinal cord.
- **Apparent nuchal rigidity (neck stiffness).** The fact that the child will not move her head suggests that she is experiencing nuchal rigidity—a classic sign of meningitis. Nuchal rigidity may not be a reliable sign in children less than 18 to 24 months of age.

Meningitis, also referred to as spinal meningitis, is an inflammation of the meningeal layers that surround and protect the brain and spinal cord. The infection can be bacterial, viral, or even fungal in origin. In many cases, meningitis is preceded by upper respiratory infection symptoms. In the prehospital setting, it is not possible to determine the etiologic pathogen causing the disease (eg, bacterial, viral, fungal); therefore, you should assume the disease to be bacterial in origin (the most life threatening) until proven otherwise.

Approximately 10% to 15% of cases of meningococcal disease are fatal.[7] Approximately 11% to 19% of survivors have long-term disabilities.[7] Long-term disabilities include nervous system problems, brain damage, deafness, and loss of limb(s).[7]

Relative to viral (aseptic) meningitis, which typically does not pose the risk of permanent neurologic damage, bacterial meningitis is a potentially life-threatening infection. It is often associated with an altered mental status, seizures, and increased intracranial pressure (ICP). If left untreated, bacterial meningitis can result in severe sepsis, permanent neurologic damage, and even death.

Prior to 1990, *Haemophilus influenzae* type b (Hib) was the most common cause of bacterial meningitis; however, because a vaccine for Hib is now administered to children as part of their routine immunizations, the occurrence of *H. influenzae* has decreased. According to the Centers for Disease Control and Prevention (CDC), the incidence of Hib-related meningitis between 1980 and 1990 was approximately 40 to 50 per 100,000 children under 5 years of age.[8] Since vaccinations against Hib began, the incidence has decreased by more than 99%.[8] *Neisseria meningitidis* (also called meningococcal meningitis) and *Streptococcus pneumoniae* (also called pneumococcal meningitis) are usually the causes of bacterial meningitis in children greater than 1 month of age. In neonates (birth to 1 month of age), meningitis is usually caused by *Escherichia coli* (*E. coli*), group B streptococcus, or *Listeria monocytogenes*.

Classic signs and symptoms of bacterial meningitis include high fever, headache, and nuchal rigidity. In infants, the clinical presentation is commonly that of increased irritability, poor feeding, vomiting, a bulging fontanelle (sign of increased ICP), and inconsolability. Because infants and children less than 18 to 24 months of age often lack adequately developed neck musculature, nuchal rigidity may not manifest; therefore, it is an unreliable sign in this age group. Only in children older than 18 to 24 months are headache and nuchal rigidity reliable manifestations of meningitis.

The signs and symptoms of meningitis can develop over several hours or a few days and may vary depending on the child's age. For example, infants may present with increased irritability, poor feeding, and difficulty in being consoled; older children are often unable to maintain a comfortable position secondary to muscle stiffness.

In older children, the inability to extend the legs with the hips flexed (Kernig sign) and/or involuntary flexion of the hip, knee, or ankle when the neck is passively flexed (Brudzinski sign) are suggestive of meningeal irritation. However, the absence of these clinical findings does not rule out meningitis.

Bacterial meningitis is a contagious disease. The primary mode of transmission is via the airborne droplet route, such as the exchange of respiratory secretions (eg, coughing, sneezing, kissing). Unlike the common cold or flu, however, the bacteria are not spread via casual contact with an infected person. Nonetheless, the appropriate standard precautions—gloves and facial protection—must be strictly followed when caring for a patient with suspected meningitis.

3. What are petechiae and purpura? What do they indicate?

Petechiae are small (< 0.05 cm) circumscribed areas of superficial bleeding into the skin. Initially, they appear as red pinpoint-sized spots and then turn purple or dark blue. A petechial rash is not a disease itself but a manifestation of an underlying problem. The presence of petechiae indicates a low platelet count (thrombocytopenia) and is associated with a severe systemic infection (sepsis).

Some children with meningococcal meningitis develop an erythematous (red) maculopapular rash followed by petechiae or purpura, most commonly located on the extremities. Purpura, also a manifestation of thrombocytopenia, appears as purple circumscribed skin lesions greater than 0.5 cm in size.

Although petechiae and purpura are classically seen in children with meningococcal meningitis, they can also occur in conjunction with other infectious diseases, viral or bacterial.

4. What treatment will you provide to this child en route to the hospital?

Children with suspected meningitis must be closely monitored for the presence of increased ICP, seizures, and signs of septic shock. Because infants and small children have relatively immature immune systems, they are particularly vulnerable to sepsis.

If respiratory depression develops (suggestive of increased ICP), assist the child's ventilations with a bag-mask device and 100% oxygen. ET intubation may be necessary if you are unable to provide effective bag-mask ventilations or your transport time to the hospital will be lengthy.

Provided the child remains hemodynamically stable, allow him or her to remain with the caregiver. Continue oxygen therapy as tolerated, and promptly transport the child to the hospital. If signs and symptoms of septic shock are present, obtain IV or IO access and administer 20-mL/kg boluses of normal saline or lactated Ringer as needed to maintain adequate perfusion. If the child is hemodynamically stable, consider deferring IV therapy until the child is in the ED. Remember, you should avoid any unnecessary procedures; these will likely increase the child's anxiety and could cause acute deterioration of his or her clinical condition.

If the child experiences a seizure, administer a benzodiazepine drug such as diazepam (Valium) or midazolam (Versed). If IV or IO access is not available, diazepam can be given via the rectal route; midazolam can be given intramuscularly if needed. Follow locally established protocols or contact medical control as needed regarding the pediatric doses of these drugs.

If the child remains hypotensive despite two or three crystalloid fluid boluses, medical control may order an infusion of one of the following vasoactive drugs, both of which should be titrated as necessary to improve perfusion:

- Epinephrine: 0.1 to 1 mcg/kg per minute
- Dopamine: 5 to 20 mcg/kg per minute (usual starting dose is 5 to 10 mcg/kg/min.)

Definitive treatment for a child with meningitis and septic shock involves the administration of antibiotics—an intervention that cannot be provided in the prehospital setting. Therefore, rapid transport to an appropriate medical facility is essential.

Summary

Meningitis remains a significant cause of mortality and morbidity in children. *N. meningitidis* (also called meningococcal meningitis) and *S. pneumoniae* (also called pneumococcal meningitis) are the most common causes of bacterial meningitis in children older than 1 month of age. *H. influenzae* type b (Hib) has been virtually eradicated as a cause of bacterial meningitis in children due to Hib vaccinations that began in the late 1980s. If left untreated, bacterial meningitis may result in septic shock, permanent neurologic impairment, or death.

Meningitis should be suspected in any child who presents with fever, headache, and nuchal rigidity; however, headache and nuchal rigidity are most reliably assessed in children older than 18 to 24 months of age. Other signs and symptoms include nausea and vomiting, irritability, photophobia, signs of increased ICP, seizures, and a petechial or purpuric rash. In infants, common signs include paradoxical irritability, poor feeding, a bulging fontanelle, and inconsolability.

Prehospital care for a child with meningitis begins by taking the appropriate standard precautions, including gloves and facial protection; bacterial meningitis is a contagious disease that is spread by the airborne droplet route. Obtain and maintain the child's airway, and provide supplemental oxygen or assisted ventilation as needed. If signs of hypoperfusion are present, 20-mL/kg IV or IO crystalloid fluid boluses should be given. Vasopressor therapy (eg, epinephrine, dopamine) may be required for fluid-refractory hypoperfusion. If the child is hemodynamically stable, consider deferring IV therapy to avoid causing unnecessary anxiety. Promptly transport the child to an appropriate medical facility while closely monitoring his or her ABCs en route. Meningitis is diagnosed in the ED with a lumbar puncture (spinal tap) and is treated definitively with antibiotic therapy.

Show the PCR to your instructor, and ask for some feedback!

References

1. 10 leading causes of injury deaths by age group highlighting unintentional injury deaths, United States—2015. Centers for Disease Control and Prevention website. https://www.cdc.gov/injury/wisqars/LeadingCauses.html. Accessed September 27, 2017.
2. Falls prevention facts. National Council on Aging website. https://www.ncoa.org/news/resources-for-reporters/get-the-facts/falls-prevention-facts/. Accessed June 13, 2016.
3. 2017 Alzheimer's disease facts and figures. Alzheimer's Association website. http://www.alz.org/facts/. Accessed October 2, 2017.
4. Alzheimer's Association. 2017 Alzheimer's disease facts and figures. *Alzheimers Dement*. 2017;13:325-373.
5. Hip Fractures Among Older Adults. Centers for Disease Control and Prevention website. https://www.cdc.gov/homeandrecreationalsafety/falls/adulthipfx.html. Updated September 20, 2016. Accessed October 2, 2017.
6. Henry SM, Pollak AN, Jones AL, et al. Pelvic fracture in geriatric patients: a distinct clinical entity. *J Trauma*. 2002;53(1):15-20.
7. Meningococcal disease: technical and clinical information. Centers for Disease Control and Prevention website. https://www.cdc.gov/meningococcal/clinical-info.html. Updated July 6, 2017. Accessed October 2, 2017.
8. Centers for Disease Control and Prevention. *Epidemiology and prevention of vaccine-preventable diseases*. Hamborsky J, Kroger A, Wolfe S, eds. 13th ed. Washington, DC: Public Health Foundation; 2015:123.

APPENDIX B

Skill Review

Note: Not every chapter includes skills. Skills are listed in order of chapter sequence.

Chapter 11

Skill Drill 11-1 Performing a Rapid Full-Body Scan

Step 1 Inspect and palpate head for open/closed findings and crepitus.

Step 2 Inspect and palpate neck for open/closed findings, jugular venous distention (JVD), tracheal deviation, and crepitus. In trauma patients, consider applying a cervical spinal immobilization device. Assess neck *before* covering it with a cervical collar.

Step 3 Inspect and palpate chest for open/closed findings, paradoxical motion, and crepitus. Listen to breath sounds on both sides of chest.

Step 4 Inspect and palpate abdomen for open/closed findings, rigidity (firm or soft), and distention.

Step 5 Inspect and palpate pelvis for open/closed findings. If there is no pain, gently compress pelvis downward and inward to look for tenderness and instability.

Step 6 Inspect and palpate four extremities for open/closed findings. Assess bilaterally for distal pulses and motor and sensory functions.

Step 7 Inspect and palpate back and buttocks for open/closed findings. In all trauma patients, maintain in-line stabilization of spine while rolling patient on his or her uninjured side in one smooth motion. If you place patient on a backboard, check back before you finish log rolling patient onto board. If you use a scoop stretcher, you won't be able to inspect or palpate lower thoracic and lumbar spine.

Skill Drill 11-2 Performing Percussion

Step 1 Place your hand lightly against surface to be examined.

Step 2 Hyperextend your middle finger, and apply firm pressure to surface to be percussed.

Step 3 Directly strike middle phalanx of your middle finger with one or two fingertips of your other hand. Apply same force over each area of body to accurately compare sounds produced by percussion.

Skill Drill 11-3 Performing the Full-Body Exam

Step 1 Examine face for obvious lacerations, bruises, fluids, and deformities.

Step 2 Inspect area around eyes and eyelids.

Step 3 Examine eyes for redness and for contact lenses. Use a penlight to assess pupils.

Step 4 Look behind ears for bruising (Battle sign).

Step 5 Use penlight to look for drainage of spinal fluid or blood in ears.

Step 6 Examine head for bruising and lacerations. Palpate for tenderness, skull depressions, and deformities.

Step 7 Palpate zygomas for tenderness, symmetry, and instability.

Step 8 Palpate maxillae.

Step 9 Check nose for blood and drainage.

Step 10 Palpate mandible.

Step 11 Assess mouth and nose for cyanosis, foreign bodies (eg, loose or broken teeth or dentures), bleeding, lacerations, and deformities.

Step 12 Check for unusual odors on patient's breath.

Step 13 Inspect neck for obvious lacerations, bruises, and deformities. Observe for jugular venous distention and/or tracheal deviation.

Step 14 Palpate front and back of neck for tenderness and deformity.

Step 15 Inspect chest for obvious signs of injury before you begin palpation. Watch for movement of chest with respiration. Assess work of breathing.

Step 16 Gently palpate over ribs to assess structural integrity and elicit tenderness. Avoid pressing over obvious bruises and fractures.

Step 17 Listen for breath sounds over midaxillary and midclavicular lines—a minimum of four fields if you check anterior chest, six fields if you are assessing posterior chest.

Step 18 Assess lungs including bases and apexes of lungs. At this point, also assess back for tenderness and deformities, so you log roll patient only once. Remember, if you suspect a spinal cord injury, use spinal precautions as you log roll patient.

Step 19 Look for obvious lacerations, bruising, and deformity of abdomen and pelvis. Gently palpate abdomen for tenderness. Begin by palpating quadrant diagonal from where any pain is located. If patient indicates his or her pain is localized to one quadrant, palpate that area last. Contraction of abdominal muscles in response to palpation is seen with underlying conditions such as appendicitis and is described as "guarding." When contraction persists throughout abdominal musculature, abdomen is described as "rigid," a condition seen with severe abdominal inflammation such as peritonitis.

Step 20 Gently compress pelvis from sides to assess for tenderness.

Step 21 Gently press iliac crests to elicit instability, tenderness, and/or crepitus.

Step 22 Inspect all four extremities for any lacerations, bruises, swelling, deformities, or medical alert jewelry. Also, assess distal pulses and motor and sensory functions in all extremities. Compare right and left sides whenever possible.

Skill Drill 11-4 Using a Glucometer to Assess Blood Glucose Level

Step 1 Identify need to obtain a blood glucose level, normal parameters for blood glucose level, contraindications, and possible complications. Take standard precautions. Clearly explain procedure to patient. Select, check, and assemble equipment (glucometer, test strip, needle or spring-loaded puncture device, alcohol prep pads). Turn on glucometer and insert a test strip. Cleanse fingertip with an alcohol prep pad.

Step 2 Puncture prepped site with lancet needle or puncture device, drawing capillary blood.

Step 3 Dispose of lancet needle in a sharps container.

Step 4 Express a blood sample and transfer it to test strip. Insert test strip into glucometer and activate device per manufacturer's instructions.

Step 5 Dress fingertip wound with pressure and an alcohol prep pad, and place a bandage over puncture site. Record reading from glucometer and document appropriately.

Skill Drill 11-5 Assessing the Head

Step 1 Visually inspect and palpate head for open/closed findings and crepitus.

Step 2 Palpate top and back of head to locate any subtle abnormalities. Use a systematic approach, going from front to back, to ensure nothing is missed.

Step 3 Part hair in several places to examine condition of scalp. Identify any lesions beneath hair.

Step 4 Palpate structure of face, note any open/closed findings and crepitus. Pay attention to condition of skin, hair distribution, and shape of face.

Skill Drill 11-6 Examining the Eye

Step 1 Examine exterior portion of eye. Carefully inspect and palpate upper and lower orbits, starting at nose and working toward lateral edge. Look for any obvious trauma or deformity. Ask about general problems (eg, any pain or redness, altered vision, vision loss, diplopia, photophobia, blurring, discharge, sensitivity to light, and corrective lens use). Note periorbital ecchymosis (raccoon eyes).

Step 2 Measure visual acuity by having patient count number of fingers you are holding up at varying distances (usually 6 feet [2 m], 3 feet [1 m], and 1 foot [0.3 m] away from patient). Perform this exam on each eye independently. If corrective lenses are normally worn, check visual acuity with correction in place.

Step 3 Examine pupils for size (in millimeters), shape, and symmetry. They should be equal. Test pupils for reactivity to light in as dark an environment as possible. Both pupils should constrict when exposed to light, and they should be equal in response.

Step 4 Test for cranial nerve function by asking patient to follow your fingers in a "Z" or "H" pattern. Eyes should move smoothly and symmetrically, tracking your finger movement. Evaluate whether eyes move in sync (conjugate gaze) and whether they can track in all fields (up, down, left, right). Note any abnormal movement of eyes. A visual field exam assesses retina's ability to perceive light. This is done by checking patient's peripheral vision, examining each eye separately.

Step 5 Inspect eyelids, lashes, and tear ducts for evidence of trauma, or discharge. Turn up lids to look for foreign bodies, and inspect conjunctivae and sclera. Sclera ought to be white, not jaundiced or injected (red). Painless subconjunctival hemorrhage is a common but benign presentation. Conjunctivae should be pink—not cyanotic, pale, or overly reddened. Cornea and lens will be difficult to examine without additional assessment tools, although in a trauma situation, you should note whether globe is patent. Next, examine anterior chamber and iris for clarity, noting any cloudiness or bleeding.

Skill Drill 11-7 Examining the Neck

Step 1 If spinal trauma is suspected, take precautions to protect cervical spine in accordance with your protocol. Assess for usage of accessory muscles during respiration.

Step 2 Palpate neck to find any structural abnormalities or subcutaneous air and to ensure trachea is midline. Begin at suprasternal notch and work your way toward head. Be careful when applying pressure to area of carotid arteries because doing so may stimulate a vagal response.

Step 3 Assess lymph nodes and note any swelling, which may indicate infection.

Step 4 Assess jugular veins for distention, which may indicate a problem with venous return to heart.

Skill Drill 11-8 Examining the Chest

Step 1 Ensure patient's privacy as best you can. Assess chest, inspecting and palpating for open/closed findings, paradoxical motion, and crepitus. Observe chest wall for respiratory effort, and document respiratory rate, depth, and rhythm. If you find any open wounds, dress them appropriately.

Step 2 Compare two sides of chest for symmetry. Note shape of chest—it can give you clues to many underlying medical conditions, such as emphysema. Look for any surgical scars (eg, midline "zipper" scar, which may be result of pacemaker implantation or a previous cardiac surgery). Palpate chest to reveal any air under skin (as occurs in subcutaneous emphysema).

Step 3 Auscultate lung fields. Note any abnormal lung sounds. Auscultate for heart tones. Always auscultate directly to patient's skin, not through his or her clothing. Listening over fabric will result in breath sounds being muted by clothing. With each stethoscope placement, listen to at least one full inhalation and exhalation. If patient is able to cooperate, have him or her breathe through an open mouth to help emphasize lung sounds.

Step 4 Percuss chest to detect any abnormalities. Repeat appropriate portions of exam for posterior aspect of thorax.

Skill Drill 11-9 Examining the Abdomen

Step 1 Inspect and palpate abdomen for open/closed findings, rigidity (firmness), tenderness, distention, swelling, or bruising. Look at skin as well as contour and overall appearance of abdominal wall. Note any surgical scars because they may be clues to an underlying illness, previous trauma, or surgeries. Look for symmetry and distention. Look for a rash or other signs of an allergic reaction. Finally, note any wounds, striae, dilated veins, or generalized distention or localized masses.

Step 2 Auscultate abdomen for bowel sounds (if time and noise level permit). Note presence or absence of bowel sounds. Note frequency and character of any hyperactive sounds.

Step 3 Before palpating abdomen, ask patient to point to area of greatest discomfort. Avoid touching that area until last. Systematically palpate four quadrants of abdomen, beginning with quadrant farthest from patient's complaint. Work slowly, and avoid quick movements. Perform percussion as appropriate. Pay special attention to patient's expressions because they may yield valuable information.

Skill Drill 11-10 Examining the Musculoskeletal System

Step 1 Beginning with upper extremities, inspect skin overlying muscles, bones, and joints for soft-tissue damage. Note any deformities or abnormal structures.

Step 2 Inspect and palpate hands and wrists. Note any open/closed findings and crepitus.

Step 3 Inspect and palpate elbows. Ask patient to flex and extend elbow to establish range of motion. Note any abnormalities.

Step 4 Check for adequate distal pulse, motor function, and sensation in each extremity.

Step 5 Ask patient to flex and extend joints of fingers, hands, and wrist to establish range of motion. If patient experiences any discomfort, immediately stop that portion of exam.

Step 6 Ask patient to turn his or her hand from palm-down position to palm-up position and back again.

Step 7 Inspect and palpate shoulders. Ask patient to shrug shoulders and raise and extend both arms.

Step 8 Inspect and palpate bony structures to establish range of motion. Ask patient to point and bend his or her toes.

Step 9 Ask patient to rotate ankle to check for pain or restricted range of motion.

Step 10 Inspect and palpate knee joints and patella to establish range of motion. Ask patient to bend and straighten both knees.

Step 11 Check for structural integrity of pelvis by applying gentle pressure to iliac crests, pushing in and then down.

Step 12 Ask patient to lift both legs, bend at hip, and turn legs inward and outward. Note any abnormalities.

Skill Drill 11-11 Examining the Peripheral Vascular System

Step 1 As you examine upper extremities, note any abnormalities in radial pulse, skin color, temperature, or condition.

Step 2 If you note abnormalities in distal pulse, work your way proximally, check those pulse points, and note your findings.

Step 3 Palpate epitrochlear and brachial nodes of lymphatic system. Note any swelling or tenderness.

Step 4 Examine lower extremities, noting any abnormalities in size and symmetry of legs. Evaluate temperature of each leg relative to rest of body and to each other.

Step 5 Inspect skin color and condition, noting any abnormal venous patterns or enlargement.

Step 6 Check distal pulses, noting any abnormalities.

Step 7 Palpate inguinal nodes for swelling or tenderness.

Step 8 Evaluate for pitting edema in legs and feet.

Skill Drill 11-12 Examining the Spine

Step 1 Inspect cervical, thoracic, and lumbar curves for any abnormalities.

Step 2 Evaluate height of shoulders and iliac crests. Differences between one side and other may indicate abnormal spinal curvature.

Step 3 Palpate posterior portion of cervical spine, noting any point tenderness or structural abnormalities.

Step 4 In nontrauma patient, and in absence of reported pain, ask patient to move his or her head forward, backward, and from side to side.

Step 5 Palpate each vertebra with thumbs.

Step 6 In absence of pain or trauma, ask patient to bend at waist in each direction to establish range of motion.

Skill Drill 11-13 Examining the Nervous System

Step 1 Use AVPU scale to assess patient's mental status. Note patient's posture. Evaluate cranial nerve function.

Step 2 Evaluate patient's coordination by performing finger-to-nose test using alternating hands.

Step 3 If appropriate, test patient's gait and balance by having him or her walk heel-to-toe or take a heel-to-shin stance.

Step 4 Perform pronator drift test by asking patient to close his or her eyes and hold both arms out in front of body. There should not be a difference in movement on either side.

Step 5 Evaluate patient's sensory function by checking his or her responses to both gross and light touch. If appropriate, check for deep tendon reflexes.

Skill Drill 11-14 Evaluating Deep Tendon Reflexes

Step 1 Place patient in a sitting position.

Step 2 Flex patient's arm at elbow to a 45° angle. Locate biceps tendon in antecubital fossa. Place your thumb over tendon, with your fingers behind elbow. Strike your thumb with reflex hammer, note flexion of elbow.

Step 3 With patient's arm remaining at a 45° angle, rest patient's forearm on your arm, with hand slightly pronated. Strike patient's brachioradialis tendon proximal to wrist, note flexion of elbow.

Step 4 Flex patient's arm at elbow to a 90° angle, and rest his or her hand against body. Locate and strike triceps tendon, noting contraction of triceps or extension of elbow.

Step 5 Flex patient's knee to a 90° angle, allowing leg to dangle. Support upper leg with your hand, and strike patellar tendon just below patella. Note contraction of quadriceps and extension of lower leg.

Step 6 With patient's leg in same position, hold heel of patient's foot in your hand. Strike Achilles tendon, noting plantar flexion of foot.

Chapter 14

Skill Drill 14-1 Spiking the Bag

Step 1 Take standard precautions. Ensure you've chosen correct administration set (primary or piggyback), tubing is not tangled, and protective covers are in place. Ensure you have proper solution, that it is clear and has not expired, and that protective tail port covers are in place. Move roller clamp to off position.

Step 2 Remove protective covering found on end of IV bag. Bag is still sealed and will not leak until piercing spike punctures this port. Remove protective cover from piercing spike (remember, this spike is sterile and sharp!), and slide spike into IV bag port until it is seated against bag.

Step 3 Squeeze drip chamber to fill to line marking chamber, then run fluid into line to flush air out of tubing.

Step 4 Twist protective cover of opposite end of IV tubing to allow air to escape. Do not remove this cover yet because cover keeps tubing end sterile until it is needed. Let fluid flow until air bubbles are removed from line before turning roller clamp wheel to stop flow or setting drip rate per required dose.

Step 5 Next, go back and check drip chamber; it should be only half-filled. Fluid level must be visible to calculate drip rates. If fluid level is too low, then squeeze chamber until it fills; if chamber is too full, with roller clamp in off position, invert bag and chamber and squeeze chamber to empty fluid back into bag. Hang bag in an appropriate location with end of IV tubing easily accessible.

Skill Drill 14-2 Obtaining Vascular Access

Step 1 Choose appropriate fluid, and examine bag for clarity and expiration date. Ensure no particles are floating in fluid and that fluid is appropriate for patient's condition and not expired.
Choose appropriate drip set, and attach it to fluid. A macrodrip set (eg, 10 gtt/mL) should be used for a patient who needs volume replacement; a microdrip set (eg, 60 gtt/mL) should be used for a patient who needs a medication infusion. If an IV extension set is available, then attach it to end of tubing to assist hospital staff in manipulating IV tubing at hospital. Fill drip chamber by squeezing it.

Step 2 Flush or "bleed" tubing to remove any air bubbles by opening roller clamp. Ensure no errant bubbles are floating in tubing.

Step 3 Before venipuncture, tear tape needed to secure site and collect and open antiseptic swabs, gauze pads, and anything else needed for vascular access per local practice.

Step 4 Take standard precautions before making contact with patient. Palpate a suitable vein. Veins should be "springy" when palpated. Avoid areas that are hard when palpated.

Step 5 Apply constricting band above intended IV site. It should be placed approximately 4 to 8 inches (10 to 20 cm) above intended site.

Step 6 Clean area using aseptic technique. Use an alcohol pad to cleanse in a circular motion from inside out. Use a second alcohol pad to wipe straight down center.

Step 7 Choose appropriately sized catheter, and twist catheter to break seal. Do not advance catheter upward because this may cause needle to shear catheter. Examine catheter, and discard it if you discover any imperfections. Occasionally you will find "burrs" on edge of catheter. Loosen catheter hub.

Step 8 Advise patient to expect a needlestick. While applying distal traction at site with one hand, insert catheter at an angle of approximately 45° with bevel up.

Step 9 Feel for a "pop" as stylet enters vein and observe for "flashback" as blood enters catheter. Clear chamber at top of catheter should fill with blood when catheter enters vein. If you note only a drop or two, then you should gently advance catheter farther into vein, approximately ⅛ to ¼ inches (0.3 to 0.6 cm).
Apply pressure to site to occlude catheter and prevent blood from leaking while removing stylet. Hold hub while withdrawing needle so as not to pull catheter out of vein.

Step 10 Immediately dispose of all sharps in proper container.

Step 11 Attach prepared IV line. Hold hub of catheter while connecting IV line.

Step 12 Remove constricting band.

Step 13 Open IV line to ensure fluid is flowing and IV is patent. Observe for any swelling or infiltration around IV site. If fluid does not flow, then check whether constriction band has been released. If infiltration is noted, then immediately stop infusion and remove catheter while holding pressure over site with a piece of gauze to prevent bleeding.

Step 14 Secure catheter with tape or a commercial device.

Step 15 Secure IV tubing and adjust flow rate while monitoring patient.

Skill Drill 14-3 Gaining Intraosseous Access with an EZ-IO Device

Step 1 Check selected IV fluid for proper fluid, clarity, and expiration date. Look for discoloration and for particles floating in fluid. If particles are found in fluid, then discard bag and choose another bag of fluid.

Select appropriate equipment (ie, intraosseous [IO] needle, syringe, saline, extension set, antiseptic swabs, and gauze pads).

A three-way stopcock may also be used to facilitate easier fluid administration.

Select proper administration set. Connect administration set to bag. Prepare administration set. Fill drip chamber and flush tubing. Ensure all air bubbles are removed from tubing.

Prepare syringe and extension tubing. Ensure tubing is not tangled.

Cut or tear tape and prepare bulky dressings. This can be done at any time before IO puncture.

Step 2 Take standard precautions. This must be done before IO puncture.

Step 3 Identify proper anatomic site for IO puncture. Palpate landmarks and then prepare site.

- **Tibia placement.** This site is reserved for EZ-IO and BIG.
- **Humerus placement.** Humeral placement is typically reserved for adults when using EZ-IO or BIG.

Step 4 Cleanse site appropriately. Follow aseptic technique by cleansing in a circular manner from inside out.

Step 5 Attach needle to EZ-IO gun, and remove protective cover. Examine needle. If you find any imperfections, then discard needle and select another one.

Step 6 Perform IO puncture by first stabilizing tibia, then placing a folded towel under knee, and finally holding extremity in a manner to keep your fingers away from site of puncture. For humeral placement, continue to apply pressure on anterior and inferior aspects of humerus.

Insert needle at a 90° angle to insertion site. Advance needle with a twisting motion until a "pop" is felt. Unscrew cap, and remove stylet from needle.

Step 7 Remove stylet from catheter.

Step 8 Attach syringe and extension set to IO needle. Pull back on syringe to aspirate blood and particles of bone marrow to ensure proper placement. Absence of marrow does not mean access failed. Check site for other signs of extravasation.

Slowly inject saline to ensure proper placement of needle. Responsive patients should receive 1% lidocaine prior to infusion of fluids. Watch for extravasation, and stop infusion immediately if it is noted. It is possible to fracture bone during insertion of IO needle. If this happens, then remove IO needle and switch insertion site.

Connect administration set and adjust flow rate as appropriate. Fluid does not flow as rapidly through an IO catheter as through an IV line; crystalloid boluses should be given with a syringe in children and a pressure infuser device in adults.

Secure needle with tape, and support it with a bulky dressing. Stabilize in place in same manner that an impaled object is stabilized. Use bulky dressings around catheter, and tape securely in place. Be careful not to tape around entire circumference of leg because this could impair circulation and potentially result in compartment syndrome.

Dispose of needle in proper container.

Skill Drill 14-4 Administering Medication via a Nasogastric Tube

Step 1 Take standard precautions. Confirm proper gastric tube placement. Attach a 60-mL cone-tipped syringe to gastric tube, and slowly inject air as you or your partner auscultates over epigastrium. To further confirm proper placement, withdraw plunger of syringe, and observe for return of gastric contents in tube. Leave gastric tube open to air.

Step 2 Draw up 30 to 60 mL of normal saline into syringe, and irrigate gastric tube. If you meet resistance, ensure tube is not kinked.

Step 3 Draw up appropriate amount of medication, ensure it is correct medication and amount, and slowly inject medication into gastric tube.

Step 4 Inject 30 to 60 mL of normal saline into gastric tube following administration of medication. This will ensure tube is flushed and patient has received entire dose of medication.

Step 5 Clamp off proximal end of gastric tube. Do not attach gastric tube to suction because this will result in removal of medication from stomach. Monitor patient for adverse reactions. Document: medication given, route, dose, administration time, and patient condition and response. Repeat medication dose if indicated.

Skill Drill 14-5 Drawing Medication from an Ampule

Step 1 Check medication, ensuring expiration date has not passed and that it is correct drug and concentration.

Shake medication into base of ampule. If some of drug is stuck in neck, then gently thump or tap stem.

Step 2 Using a 4-inch × 4-inch (10-cm × 10-cm) gauze pad, an alcohol prep, or an ampule breaker, grip neck of ampule and snap it off where ampule is scored. If ampule is not scored and an attempt is made to break it, some sharp edges may be present. Drop stem in sharps container.

Step 3 Insert a filtered needle into ampule without touching outer sides of ampule. Draw solution into syringe, and dispose of ampule in sharps container.

Step 4 Hold syringe with needle pointing up, and gently tap barrel to loosen air trapped inside and cause it to rise.

Step 5 Press gently on plunger to dispel any air bubbles. Recap needle using one-handed method. Dispose of needle in sharps container, and attach a standard hypodermic needle to syringe if necessary to administer medication.

Skill Drill 14-6 Drawing Medication from a Vial

Step 1 Check medication, ensuring expiration date has not passed and that it is correct drug and concentration.

Remove sterile cover, or clean top with alcohol if vial was previously opened.

Step 2 Determine amount of medication that you will need, and draw that amount of air into syringe. Allow a little extra room to expel some air while removing air bubbles.

Step 3 Invert vial, clean rubber stopper with an alcohol prep, and insert needle through rubber stopper into medication. Expel air in syringe into vial, and then withdraw amount of medication needed.

Step 4 Once you have correct amount of medication in syringe, withdraw needle from vial, and expel any air in syringe.

Step 5 Recap needle using one-handed method. Label syringe if it is not immediately given to patient.

Skill Drill 14-7 Administering Medication via the Subcutaneous Route

Step 1 Take standard precautions. Determine need for medication based on patient presentation. Obtain a history, including any drug allergies and vital signs. Follow standing orders, or contact medical control for permission. Check medication to ensure that it is correct, that it is not cloudy or discolored, and that expiration date has not passed, and determine appropriate amount and concentration for correct dose.

Step 2 Advise patient of potential discomfort while explaining procedure.

Assemble and check equipment needed: alcohol preps and a 3-mL syringe with a 24- to 26-gauge needle. Draw up correct dose of medication and dispel air while maintaining sterility.

Step 3 Cleanse area for administration (usually upper arm or thigh) using aseptic technique.

Step 4 Pinch skin surrounding area, advise patient of a stick, and insert needle at a 45° angle. Inject medication and remove needle. Immediately dispose of needle and syringe in sharps container.

Step 5 To disperse medication through tissue, rub area in a circular motion with your gloved hand (unless contraindicated for medication). Properly store any unused medication. Monitor patient's condition, and document medication given, route, administration time, and patient response.

Skill Drill 14-8 Administering Medication via the Intramuscular Route

Step 1 Take standard precautions. Determine need for medication based on patient presentation. Obtain a history, including any drug allergies and vital signs. Follow standing orders, or contact medical control for permission.

Check medication to ensure that it is correct, that it is not cloudy or discolored, and that expiration date has not passed, and determine appropriate amount and concentration for correct dose.

Advise patient of potential discomfort while explaining procedure.

Assemble and check equipment needed (eg, alcohol preps and a 3- to 5-mL syringe with a 21-gauge, 1-inch or 2-inch [4-cm or 5-cm] needle). Draw up correct dose of medication, and dispel air while maintaining sterility.

Step 2 Cleanse area for administration (usually upper arm or hip) using aseptic technique.

Step 3 Stretch skin over cleansed area, advise patient of a stick, and insert needle at a 90° angle.

Pull back on plunger to aspirate for blood (presence of blood in syringe indicates you may have entered a blood vessel). In such a case, remove needle, and hold pressure over site. Discard syringe and needle in sharps container. Prepare a new syringe and needle, and select another site.

If there is no blood in syringe, then inject medication and remove needle.

Step 4 Immediately dispose of needle and syringe in sharps container. Store any unused medication properly. Monitor patient's condition, and document: medication given, route, administration time, and response of patient.

Skill Drill 14-9 Administering Medication via the Intravenous Bolus Route

Step 1 Take standard precautions. Determine need for medication based on patient presentation. Obtain a history, including any drug allergies and vital signs.

Follow standing orders, or contact medical control for permission.

Check medication to ensure that it is correct, that it is not cloudy or discolored, and that expiration date has not passed, and determine appropriate amount and concentration for correct dose.

Explain procedure to patient and need for medication. Assemble needed equipment, and draw up medication. Expel any air in syringe. Draw up 20 mL of normal saline to use as a flush for medication.

Cleanse injection port with alcohol, or remove protective cap if using needleless system.

Step 2 Insert needle into port, and pinch off IV tubing proximal to administration port. Failure to shut off line will result in medication taking pathway of least resistance and flowing into bag instead of into patient.

Administer correct dose of medication at appropriate rate. Some medications must be administered quickly, whereas others must be pushed slowly to prevent adverse effects.

Step 3 Place needle and syringe into sharps container.

Unclamp IV line to flush medication into vein. Allow it to run briefly wide open, or flush with a 20-mL bolus of normal saline.

Readjust IV flow rate to original setting.

Properly store and label any unused medication.

Monitor patient's condition, and document medication given, route, time of administration, and patient response.

Skill Drill 14-10 Administering a Medication via Intravenous Piggyback Infusion

Step 1 Take standard precautions. Ensure established IV line is patent.

Step 2 Determine need for medication based on patient presentation. Obtain a history, including any drug allergies and vital signs. Follow standing orders, or contact medical control for permission. Identify concentration, then determine appropriate dose and rate of infusion. Check medication to ensure that it is correct, that it is not cloudy or discolored, and that expiration date has not passed, and determine appropriate amount and concentration for correct dose. Explain procedure to patient and/or parent and need for medication.

Step 3 Assemble needed equipment. Check medication clarity and expiration date. Ensure you have proper IV solution and that it is clear, sterile, and not expired. Ensure you have correct administration set and correct drip rating. Check for tangling and that protective covers are on ends. Flow clamp should be closed.

Step 4 Cleanse injection port of secondary IV bag (into which medication will be infused) with alcohol. Inject medication into second IV bag, and then place syringe into sharps container. Gently swirl IV bag to mix injected medication into solution. Note: Drawing up medications may not be necessary if manufacturer attaches medication to second IV bag (IV antibiotics, some antidysrhythmics, etc).

Step 5 Remove protective cover on secondary IV bag. Insert tubing spike into second IV bag tail port. Turn bag with medication upright. Squeeze drip chamber until it is half full. Maintain sterility.

Step 6 Unclamp line from secondary IV bag to dispel air from it, or utilize infusion pump to accomplish this step. Maintain sterility. While removing air, try to minimize loss of fluid. Clamp line after all air bubbles have been removed.

Step 7 If applicable, program IV infusion pump with appropriate dose and rate. Place cartridge from secondary IV bag in pump.

Step 8 Cleanse a port on primary IV line. Attach distal end of secondary IV line to a port on primary IV line. Begin flow and ensure that rate is appropriate. Maintain sterility.

Step 9 Label secondary IV bag. Monitor patient's condition, and document: medication given, route, concentration, dose, date time, and your initials. Document patient's response to medication.

Skill Drill 14-11 Administering Medication via the Intraosseous Route

Step 1 Take standard precautions. Determine need for medication based on patient presentation. Obtain a history, including any drug allergies and vital signs. Follow standing orders, or contact medical control for permission. Check medication to ensure that it is correct, that it is not cloudy or discolored, and that expiration date has not passed, and determine appropriate amount and concentration for correct dose.

Explain procedure to patient and/or parent and need for medication.

Assemble needed equipment, and draw up medication. Also draw up 20 mL of normal saline for a flush.

Step 2 Cleanse injection port of extension tubing with alcohol, or remove protective cap if using needleless system.

Step 3 Insert needle into port, and clamp off IV tubing proximal to administration port. This is usually managed with a three-way stopcock. Failure to shut off line will result in medication taking pathway of least resistance and flowing into bag instead of into patient.

Administer correct dose of medication at proper push rate. Some medications must be administered quickly, whereas others must be pushed slowly to prevent adverse effects.

Step 4 Place needle and syringe into sharps container. Unclamp IV line to flush medication into site. Flush with at least a 20-mL bolus of normal saline. Readjust IV flow rate to original setting. Store any unused medication properly.

Monitor patient's condition, and document: medication given, route, time of administration, and response of patient.

Skill Drill 14-12 Administering Medication via the Sublingual Route

Step 1 Take standard precautions. Determine need for medication based on patient presentation. Obtain a history, including any drug allergies and vital signs. Follow standing orders, or contact medical control for permission. Check medication to ensure that it is correct and that its expiration date has not passed, and determine appropriate amount for correct dose.

Step 2 Ask patient to rinse his or her mouth with a little water if mucous membranes are dry. Explain procedure, and ask patient to lift his or her tongue.

Place tablet or spray dose under tongue, or ask patient to do so. Advise patient not to chew or swallow tablet but to let it dissolve slowly.

Monitor patient's condition, and document: medication given, route, administration time, and patient's response.

Skill Drill 14-13 Administering Medication via the Intranasal Route

Step 1 Take standard precautions. Determine need for medication based on patient presentation. Obtain a history, including any drug allergies and vital signs. Follow standing orders, or contact medical control for permission. Check medication to ensure it is correct and its expiration date has not passed, and determine appropriate amount for correct dose.

Step 2 Ask patient to rinse mouth with a little water if mucous membranes are dry. Explain procedure, and ask patient to lift his or her tongue.

Place tablet or spray dose under tongue, or ask patient to do so. Advise patient not to chew or swallow tablet but to let it dissolve slowly.

Monitor patient's condition, and document: medication given, route, administration time, and patient's response.

Step 3 Attach mucosal atomizer device to syringe, maintaining sterility.

Step 4 Explain procedure to patient (or to a relative if patient is unresponsive) and need for medication. Stop ventilation of patient if necessary; remove any mask. Insert mucosal atomizer device into larger and less deviated or less obstructed nostril.

Step 5 Quickly spray half of medication dose into a nostril.

Step 6 Dispose of atomizer device and syringe in appropriate container.

Step 7 Monitor patient's condition. Document medication given, route, time of administration, and patient response.

Skill Drill 14-14 Assisting a Patient With a Metered-Dose Inhaler

Step 1 Take standard precautions. Obtain an order from medical control, or follow local protocol. Assemble needed equipment.

Ensure you have right medication, right patient, right dose, right route, and that medication is not expired.

Ensure patient is alert enough to use inhaler. Check to see whether patient has already taken any doses. Obtain baseline breath sounds for comparison after a few minutes of inhaler use. Ensure inhaler is at room temperature or warmer.

Step 2 Shake inhaler vigorously several times. Stop administering supplemental oxygen, and remove any mask from patient's face. Ask patient to exhale deeply and, before inhaling, to put his or her lips around opening of inhaler.

Step 3 If patient has a spacer, then attach it to allow more effective use of medication.

Have patient depress handheld inhaler as he or she begins to inhale deeply.

Instruct patient to hold his or her breath for as long as he or she comfortably can to help lungs absorb medication.

Step 4 Continue administering supplemental oxygen.

Allow patient to breathe a few times, then give second dose per direction from medical control or according to local protocol. Monitor patient's condition, and document: medication given, route, administration time, and patient response.

Skill Drill 14-15 Administering a Medication via a Small-Volume Nebulizer

Step 1 Take standard precautions. Determine need for an inhaled bronchodilator based on patient presentation. Obtain a history, including any drug allergies and vital signs.

Follow standing orders, or contact medical control for permission. Check medication and its expiration date. Make sure that you have right medication and that it is not cloudy or discolored. Assemble and check needed equipment.

Step 2 If medication is in a premixed package, then add it to bowl of nebulizer. If it is not premixed, then add medication to bowl and mix with specified amount of normal saline, usually 2.5 to 3 mL.

Step 3 Connect "T" piece with mouthpiece to top of bowl, or mask to bowl, and connect it to oxygen tubing.

Set flowmeter at 6 L/min to produce a steady mist. Remove oxygen mask from patient if oxygen is being administered.

Step 4 With metered-dose inhaler (MDI) or handheld nebulizer in position, instruct patient on proper way to breathe. Have patient breathe as deeply as possible and hold his or her breath for 3 to 5 seconds before exhaling. Continue to coach patient as needed.

Monitor patient's condition, and document medication given, route, time of administration, and response of patient to medication.

Cardiac monitoring is essential when administering a beta agonist. If cardiac dysrhythmias are noted, then stop administering medication, manage in accordance with current resuscitation guidelines, and contact medical control.

Skill Drill 14-16 Accessing a Tunneling Device

Step 1 Use aseptic technique. Prepare all appropriate equipment: empty 10- to 20-mL syringe (nothing less than a 10-mL syringe should be used), 10-mL normal saline flush, sterile gloves, alcohol prep, 10-gtt administration set, 500 mL normal saline.

Ensure all lumens are clamped. Air embolism is a serious risk with these patients because many of these devices go directly into vena cava. That is why central lines must be clamped whenever they are not in use.

Use an alcohol prep to prepare lumen that will be used.

Step 2 Attach empty syringe, and withdraw a minimum of 10 mL of blood from lumen. Discard this immediately into sharps container. Do not withdraw too forcefully. If you meet some resistance, then gently flush and withdraw. Ask patient to turn his or her head in opposite direction of central line.

Step 3 After you have withdrawn 10 mL of blood, attach 10-mL syringe filled with normal saline and slowly administer it.

Step 4 Attach prepared IV drip set and set it up for at least 10 mL/h. Depending on size of catheter, you can infuse at a rate of 125 to 250 mL/h. The line must be running continuously because heparin is not available.

Administer IV medications through attached IV drip set.

Monitor patient's condition, and document: medication given, route, administration time, and patient response.

Chapter 15

Skill Drill 15-1 Removing an Upper Airway Obstruction With Magill Forceps

Step 1 With patient's head in sniffing position, open patient's mouth and insert laryngoscope blade.

Step 2 Visualize obstruction and retrieve object with Magill forceps.

Step 3 Remove object with Magill forceps.

Step 4 Attempt to ventilate patient.

Skill Drill 15-2 Using CPAP

Step 1 Take standard precautions. Assess patient for indications and contraindications of continuous positive airway pressure (CPAP). Confirm patient's BP, and explain procedure to him or her. Check your equipment, then connect circuit to CPAP device.

Step 2 Connect face mask to circuit tubing. After system is connected, look for an on/off button or switch. Some models have this feature. Confirm device is powered on and working before you apply CPAP to patient.

Step 3 Connect tubing to oxygen tank.

Step 4 Place mask over patient's mouth and nose, creating as much of an airtight seal as possible. Place patient in a high Fowler position to facilitate breathing, and coach him or her through initial application of mask. To reduce some of stress and anxiety associated with application of CPAP, it may be beneficial to initially allow patient to hold mask to his or her face. Allow patient to get used to mask.

Step 5 After mask is placed on face and patient adjusts to it, use strapping mechanism to secure it to patient's head. Ensure seal between mask and face remains intact. Consult manufacturer's guidelines for specific strapping instructions.

Step 6 Adjust positive end-expiratory pressure (PEEP) valve and FIO_2 level according to manufacturer's recommendations to maintain adequate oxygenation and ventilation. With CPAP in place, patient's oxygenation saturation level should improve, work of breathing should decrease, ease of speaking should increase, and breath sounds should improve. Constantly reassess patient for signs of clinical deterioration and/or complications (ie, pneumothorax).

Skill Drill 15-3 Inserting a Nasogastric Tube in a Responsive Patient

Step 1 Explain procedure to patient, and oxygenate him or her if necessary and possible. Ensure patient's head is in a neutral or slightly flexed position. Suppress gag reflex with a topical anesthetic spray.

Step 2 Constrict blood vessels in nares with a topical alpha-agonist, if available.

Step 3 Measure tube for correct depth of insertion (nose to ear to xiphoid process).

Step 4 Lubricate tube with a water-soluble gel.

Step 5 Advance tube gently along nasal floor.

Step 6 Encourage patient to swallow or drink to facilitate passage of tube into esophagus.

Step 7 Advance tube into stomach.

Step 8 Confirm proper placement: Auscultate over epigastrium while injecting 20 to 30 mL of air into tube, and/or observe for gastric contents in tube. There should be no reflux around tube.

Step 9 Apply suction to tube to aspirate stomach contents, and secure tube in place. Blue extension of gastric tube should remain open to air.

Skill Drill 15-4 Inserting an Orogastric Tube in an Unresponsive Patient

Step 1 Position patient's head in a neutral or slightly flexed position. Measure tube for correct depth of insertion (mouth to ear to xiphoid process).

Step 2 Lubricate tube with a water-soluble gel.

Step 3 Introduce tube at midline, and advance it gently into oropharynx. Advance tube into stomach.

Step 4 Confirm proper placement: Auscultate over epigastrium while injecting 20 to 30 mL of air and/or observe for gastric contents in tube. There should be no reflux around tube. Afterwards, auscultate over lung fields to confirm ET tube has not been dislodged.

Step 5 Apply suction to tube to aspirate stomach contents.

Step 6 Secure tube in place.

Skill Drill 15-5 Suctioning of a Stoma

Step 1 Take standard precautions.

Step 2 Inject 3 mL of sterile saline through stoma and into trachea.

Step 3 Instruct patient to exhale (if he or she is responsive), and insert catheter without providing suction until resistance is felt (no more than 12 cm).

Step 4 Suction while withdrawing catheter.

Skill Drill 15-6 Ventilating Through a Stoma Using a Resuscitation Mask

Step 1 Position patient's head in a neutral position with shoulders slightly elevated.

Step 2 Locate and expose stoma site.

Step 3 Place resuscitation mask over stoma, and ensure an adequate seal. For best results, use a pediatric mask.

Step 4 Maintain patient's neutral head position, and ventilate patient by exhaling directly into resuscitation mask. Assess patient for adequate ventilation by observing his or her chest rise and feeling for air leaks around mask.

Step 5 If air leakage is evident, then seal patient's mouth and nose and ventilate.

Skill Drill 15-7 Ventilating a Stoma With a Bag-Mask Device

Step 1 With patient's head in a neutral position, locate and expose stoma.

Step 2 Place bag-mask device (with a pediatric mask) over stoma, and ensure an adequate seal. Ventilate patient by squeezing bag-mask device, and assess for adequate ventilation by observing chest rise and feeling for air leaks when using a mask. Seal mouth and nose if an air leak is evident from upper airway.

Step 3 Auscultate over lungs to confirm adequate ventilation.

Skill Drill 15-8 Replacing a Dislodged Tracheostomy Tube With a Temporary Endotracheal Tube

Step 1 Take standard precautions. Assemble equipment.

Step 2 Lubricate same-sized tracheostomy tube or an ET tube (at least 5.0 mm) with a water-soluble gel.

Step 3 Instruct patient to exhale, and gently insert tube approximately 0.5 to 0.75 inches (1 to 2 cm) beyond balloon cuff.

Step 4 Inflate balloon cuff.

Step 5 Ensure patient is comfortable, and confirm patency and proper placement of tube by listening for air movement from tube and noting patient's clinical status. Ensure that a false lumen (placement of tube into soft tissue of neck, rather than in trachea) was not created.

Step 6 Auscultate lungs to confirm correct tube placement.

Skill Drill 15-9 Performing Orotracheal Intubation Using Direct Laryngoscopy

Step 1 Take standard precautions. If you suspect trauma, then maintain manual in-line stabilization of head.

Step 2 Measure for proper size, and insert an oropharyngeal airway (OPA).

Step 3 Ventilate patient with a bag-mask device at a rate of 10 to 12 breaths/min with sufficient volume to produce chest rise. Preoxygenate for 2 to 3 minutes with 100% oxygen.

Step 4 Check, prepare, and assemble your equipment.

Step 5 Place patient's head in sniffing position.

Step 6 Remove OPA, then insert blade into right side of patient's mouth, and displace tongue to left.

Step 7 Gently lift long axis of laryngoscope handle until you can visualize glottic opening and vocal cords.

Step 8 Insert ET tube through right corner of mouth.

Step 9 Visualize entry of ET tube between vocal cords.

Step 10 Remove laryngoscope from patient's mouth.

Step 11 Note depth of ET tube (in centimeters) at patient's teeth, and remove stylet from ET tube.

Step 12 Inflate distal cuff of ET tube with 5 to 10 mL of air, and immediately detach syringe from inflation port.

Step 13 Attach $ETCO_2$ detector (waveform capnography preferred) to ET tube.

Step 14 Attach $ETCO_2$ detector to cardiac monitor/defibrillator and observe for a capnographic waveform and numeric CO_2 reading.

Step 15 Attach ventilation device and ventilate. Listen over epigastrium and over both lungs.

Step 16 Secure ET tube with a commercial device or tape. Ventilate patient at proper rate while monitoring capnography and pulse oximetry.

Skill Drill 15-10 Performing Orotracheal Intubation Using Video Laryngoscopy

Step 1 Take standard precautions. If you suspect trauma, then maintain manual in-line stabilization of head.

Step 2 Measure for proper size, and insert an OPA.

Step 3 Ventilate patient with a bag-mask device at a rate of 10 to 12 breaths/min with sufficient volume to produce chest rise. Preoxygenate for 2 to 3 minutes with 100% oxygen.

Step 4 Check, prepare, and assemble your equipment. Turn on video laryngoscope, and ensure light and camera are functioning.

Step 5 Remove OPA and place patient's head in sniffing position.

Step 6 Insert video laryngoscope blade into right side of patient's mouth. Sweep tongue to left (displacing laryngoscope) or midline of mouth (nondisplacing laryngoscope). Visualize epiglottis, vocal cords, and arytenoid cartilage.

Step 7 Visualize entry of ET tube between vocal cords on video monitor.

Step 8 Remove laryngoscope from patient's mouth.

Step 9 Remove stylet from ET tube (if used).

Step 10 Inflate distal cuff of ET tube with 5 to 10 mL of air, and immediately detach syringe from inflation port.

Step 11 Attach $ETCO_2$ detector (waveform capnography preferred) to ET tube.

Step 12 Attach $ETCO_2$ detector to cardiac monitor/defibrillator and observe for a capnographic waveform and numeric CO_2 reading.

Step 13 Attach ventilation device and ventilate. Auscultate over epigastrium and over both lungs.

Step 14 Secure ET tube with a commercial device or tape.

Step 15 Ventilate patient at proper rate while monitoring capnography and pulse oximetry.

Skill Drill 15-11 Performing Nasotracheal Intubation

Step 1 Take standard precautions.

Step 2 Preoxygenate whenever possible with a bag-mask device and 100% oxygen. Auscultate patient's breath sounds to confirm adequate ventilation.

Step 3 Check, prepare, and assemble your equipment.

Step 4 Place patient's head in a neutral position.

Step 5 Preform nasotracheal tube by bending it in a circle.

Step 6 Administer nasal spray to cause vasoconstriction of nasal mucosa

Step 7 Lubricate tip of nasotracheal tube with a water-soluble gel.

Step 8 Gently insert nasotracheal tube into more compliant nostril, with bevel facing toward nasal septum, and advance tube along nasal floor. Pause to ensure that tip of tube is positioned just superior to vocal cords. Observe for condensation in tube, and note audible breath sounds from proximal end of tube.

Step 9 Advance nasotracheal tube through vocal cords as patient inhales. BAAM® device can be helpful in this step. Ensure that patient is aphonic (unable to speak).

Step 10 Inflate distal cuff with 5 to 10 mL of air, and immediately detach syringe.

Step 11 Attach $ETCO_2$ detector (waveform capnography preferred) to nasotracheal tube.

Step 12 Attach $ETCO_2$ detector to cardiac monitor/defibrillator.

Step 13 Attach bag-mask device, ventilate, and auscultate over epigastrium and over both lungs. Ensure proper tube placement with waveform capnography. Secure nasotracheal tube. Ventilate patient at appropriate rate while monitoring capnography and pulse oximetry.

Skill Drill 15-12 Performing Transillumination Intubation

Step 1 Take standard precautions.

Step 2 Preoxygenate for 2 to 3 minutes with a bag-mask device and 100% oxygen.

Step 3 Check, prepare, and assemble your equipment.

Step 4 Insert lighted stylet into ET tube.

Step 5 Bend ET tube by placing a slight curve at its distal end (like a hockey stick), and turn on lighted stylet.

Step 6 Lift patient's tongue and mandible anteriorly.

Step 7 Insert ET tube into midline of patient's mouth and slowly advance toward larynx, but stop before passing through vocal cords.

Step 8 Observe for a tightly circumscribed light at midline of neck, and advance ET tube approximately
1 to 1.5 inches (2 to 4 cm) farther.

Step 9 Remove stylet from ET tube.

Step 10 Inflate distal cuff of ET tube with 5 to 10 mL of air, and immediately detach syringe.

Step 11 Attach $ETCO_2$ detector (waveform capnography preferred) to ET tube.

Step 12 Attach ventilation device, ventilate, and auscultate over apices and bases of both lungs and over epigastrium. Ensure proper tube placement with waveform capnography.

Step 13 Secure ET tube, and recheck breath sounds.

Skill Drill 15-13 Performing Retrograde Intubation

Step 1 Take standard precautions. Place patient supine. Ventilate patient with 100% oxygen via appropriate device while preparing equipment and patient. Cleanse anterior part of neck from laryngeal prominence to just below cricoid ring, and position a fenestrated drape. A fenestrated drape is a sheet with a round or slit-like opening in center that is positioned over site where incision will be made.

Step 2 If patient is responsive, then consider numbing area over cricothyroid membrane using a local anesthetic.

Step 3 Puncture cricothyroid membrane using a large needle aligned with airway and pointed approximately 30° cephalad (toward head), perpendicular at level of cricothyroid membrane.

Step 4 Identify tracheal lumen by aspirating air into syringe attached to needle.

Step 5 Pass 28-inch (70-cm) guide wire through catheter until it appears in oropharynx.

Step 6 Grasp guide wire with a clamp/Magill forceps, and pull wire partially out of mouth, ensuring that distal end is still emerging from neck and wire is pulled taut.

Step 7 Insert guide wire, emerging from mouth, through lumen of ET tube.

Step 8 Advance ET tube into trachea.

Step 9 Verify tube placement by auscultating lungs bilaterally and over epigastrium. Attach an $ETCO_2$ detector (waveform capnography preferred) to ensure proper tube placement.

Step 10 After tube placement is confirmed, remove guide wire by pulling on distal end emerging from neck, then advance tube approximately 1 inch (2 to 3 cm) further.

Step 11 If tube placement is incorrect, then remove tube and attempt to ventilate. If ventilating adequately, then continue to ventilate with high-flow oxygen and reassess. Determine whether additional attempts at retrograde intubation are warranted or whether another means of securing airway is necessary (such as cricothyrotomy).

Step 12 Secure ET tube in place, and continue to ventilate.

Skill Drill 15-14 Performing Tracheobronchial Suctioning

Step 1 Check, prepare, and assemble your equipment.

Step 2 Lubricate suction catheter.

Step 3 Preoxygenate patient.

Step 4 Detach ventilation device and inject 3 to 5 mL of sterile water down ET tube.

Step 5 Gently insert catheter into ET tube until you feel resistance.

Step 6 Suction in a rotating motion while withdrawing catheter. Monitor cardiac rhythm and oxygen saturation level during procedure.

Step 7 Reattach ventilation device and resume ventilation and oxygenation.

Skill Drill 15-15 Inserting a King LT Airway

Step 1 Take standard precautions.

Step 2 Preoxygenate with a bag-mask device and 100% oxygen.

Step 3 Gather your equipment. Choose proper size of King LT airway for patient. Test cuffs for proper inflation. Ensure all air is removed from cuffs before insertion. Lubricate tip of device with a water-soluble gel for easy insertion and minimal airway damage.

Step 4 Place patient's head in a neutral position, unless contraindicated (use jaw-thrust maneuver if trauma suspected). In your dominant hand, hold King LT at connector. With your other hand, hold patient's mouth open while positioning head. Insert tip of King LT airway into midline of mouth.

Step 5 Advance tip beyond base of tongue. If you meet resistance, then rotate device slightly, change your angle, and advance it again. Continue to gently advance device until base of connector is aligned with patient's teeth or gums. Do not use excessive force. Inflate cuffs with recommended amount of air or just enough to seal device.

Step 6 Attach tube to ventilation device, and confirm tube placement by auscultating lungs and epigastrium and attaching waveform capnography. Add additional air to cuffs to maximize airway seal, if needed; however, avoid exceeding manufacturer's recommended maximum amount of air. After placement is confirmed, continue to ventilate patient.

Skill Drill 15-16 Inserting an LMA

Step 1 Take standard precautions. Check cuff of LMA by inflating it with 50% more air than is required for size of airway to be used.

Step 2 Deflate cuff completely so that no folds appear near tip. Deflation is best accomplished by pressing device, cuff facing down, on a flat surface to remove all wrinkles from cuff.

Step 3 Lubricate outer rim of device.

Step 4 Preoxygenate before insertion. Do not interrupt ventilation for more than 30 seconds to accomplish airway placement. Place patient in sniffing position.

Step 5 Proper insertion of LMA depends on holding device properly. Insert your finger between cuff and tube. Place index finger of your dominant hand in notch between tube and cuff. Open patient's mouth. Lift jaw with one hand, and begin to insert device with other hand.

Step 6 Insert LMA along roof of mouth. The key to proper insertion is to slide convex surface of airway along roof of mouth. Use your finger to push airway against hard palate. After it slides past tongue, LMA will move easily into position.

Step 7 Inflate cuff with amount of air indicated for airway being used. If LMA is properly positioned, then it will move out of airway slightly 0.5 to 0.75 inches (1 to 2 cm) as it moves into position (a good indication that LMA is in correct position).

Step 8 Begin to ventilate patient. Confirm chest rise and presence of breath sounds. Ensure proper tube placement with waveform capnography. Continuously and carefully monitor patient's condition.

Skill Drill 15-17 Inserting an i-gel Supraglottic Airway

Step 1 Take standard precautions.

Step 2 Lubricate back, sides, and front of cuff with a thin layer of water-soluble gel.

Step 3 Preoxygenate before insertion. Do not interrupt ventilation for more than 30 seconds to accomplish airway placement. Place patient in sniffing position.

Step 4 Open airway with tongue-jaw lift maneuver, and position i-gel so that cuff outlet is facing toward patient's chin.

Step 5 Introduce leading soft tip of i-gel into patient's mouth, directing it toward hard palate.

Step 6 Glide i-gel downward and backward along hard palate with a continuous but gentle push until a definitive resistance is felt.

Step 7 Begin to ventilate patient. Confirm chest rise and presence of breath sounds. Ensure proper tube placement with waveform capnography. Continuously and carefully monitor patient's condition.

Step 8 Secure i-gel in place with provided strap.

Skill Drill 15-18 Performing an Open Cricothyrotomy

Step 1 Take standard precautions.

Step 2 Check, assemble, and prepare equipment. Place a 90° bend in a 6.0-mm ET tube (with a stylet inserted), just proximal to cuff.

Step 3 With patient's head in a neutral position, palpate for and locate cricothyroid membrane.

Step 4 Cleanse area with an iodine-or chlorhexidine-containing solution.

Step 5 Stabilize larynx, and make a vertical incision (approximately 0.5 to 0.75 inch [1 to 2 cm]) over cricothyroid membrane.

Step 6 Puncture cricothyroid membrane.

Step 7 Make a horizontal incision (approximately 0.5 inch [1 cm]) in each direction from midline. Insert scalpel handle into opening and rotate it.

Step 8 Insert tube into trachea as you remove scalpel handle.

Step 9 Manually stabilize ET tube between your thumb and index finger, carefully remove stylet, and inflate distal cuff.

Step 10 Attach an $ETCO_2$ detector between tube and ventilation device.

Step 11 Ensure proper tube placement with waveform capnography. Attach $ETCO_2$ detector to monitor. Ventilate patient.

Step 12 Confirm correct tube placement by auscultating apices and bases of both lungs and over epigastrium.

Step 13 Secure tube with a commercial device or tape. Reconfirm correct tube placement, and resume ventilations at appropriate rate.

Skill Drill 15-19 Performing Needle Cricothyrotomy and Translaryngeal Catheter Ventilation

Step 1 Take standard precautions.

Step 2 Attach a 14- to 16-gauge IV catheter to a 10-mL syringe containing approximately 3 mL of sterile saline or water.

Step 3 With patient's head in a neutral position, palpate for and locate cricothyroid membrane.

Step 4 Cleanse area with an iodine-containing solution.

Step 5 Stabilize larynx, and insert needle into cricothyroid membrane at a 45° angle toward feet.

Step 6 Aspirate with syringe to determine correct catheter placement.

Step 7 Slide catheter off of needle until hub of catheter is flush with patient's skin.

Step 8 Place syringe and needle in a puncture-proof container.

Step 9 Connect one end of oxygen tubing to catheter and other end to jet ventilator. Maintain manual stabilization of catheter until it has been secured in place to avoid dislodgment with jet ventilation.

Step 10 Press or occlude ventilation valve on jet ventilator for 1 second while observing for chest rise. Release ventilation valve for 2 to 3 seconds to allow for exhalation.

Step 11 Auscultate apices and bases of both lungs and over epigastrium to confirm correct catheter placement.

Step 12 Secure catheter with a 4-inch × 4-inch (10-cm × 10-cm) gauze pad and tape. Continue ventilations while frequently reassessing for adequate ventilations and potential complications.

Chapter 17

Skill Drill 17-1 Performing Cardiac Monitoring

Step 1 Take standard precautions. Check your equipment. Ensure there are no loose pins in end of ECG cable and that cable/lead wires are intact. Ensure monitor has an adequate paper supply. Connect ECG cable to machine. Connect lead wires to ECG cable (if not already connected). Turn on power to monitor. Adjust screen contrast if necessary.

Step 2 Explain procedure to patient. To minimize distortion of ECG tracing, prepare skin for electrode placement by briskly rubbing it with a dry gauze pad to remove skin oils and improve impulse transmission. If you are applying electrodes to patient's chest, rather than to his or her limbs, then ensure good contact by shaving small amounts of chest hair if needed.

Step 3 Attach electrodes to lead wires before placing them on patient.

Step 4 One at a time, remove backing from each electrode and apply it to patient.

Step 5 If you plan to obtain a 12-lead tracing as well, then place limb leads. Limb-lead electrodes are usually placed on wrists and ankles but may be positioned anywhere on appropriate limb. To reduce muscle tension, ensure patient's limbs are resting on a supportive surface. Do not apply electrodes over bony areas, broken skin, joints, skin creases, scar tissue, or rashes.

Step 6 Turn on monitor and select desired lead, which is typically lead II. Adjust ECG size if necessary to ensure machine detects patient's QRS complexes. Feel patient's pulse, and compare it with heart rate indicator on monitor. If not already preset, then set heart rate alarms on monitor according to your agency's policy.

Step 7 Record tracings.

Step 8 Label each strip.

Skill Drill 17-2 Performing Transcutaneous Pacing

Step 1 Select, check, and assemble all necessary equipment, including a monitor/defibrillator with pacing capability, ECG electrodes, pacing pads, medication for pain or sedation (to be used if necessary), oxygen, and an appropriate oxygen administration device. Take standard precautions. Apply ECG electrodes, and assess patient's vital signs. Ensure patient is oxygenated adequately, and establish a patent IV line.

Step 2 Identify rhythm and confirm transcutaneous pacing (TCP) is warranted. Obtain a baseline rhythm strip.

Step 3 Ensure scene and environment are safe; evaluate risk of sparks, combustibles, oxygen-rich atmosphere. Explain need for procedure to patient and family. Apply pacing pads to patient according to manufacturer's recommendations. Sedation or analgesia may be needed to minimize discomfort associated with this procedure. Ask patient about any medication allergies before administering medications.

Step 4 Switch on power to pacer.

Step 5 Set pacing rate to desired number of paced pulses per minute (ppm). A rate between 60 and 80 beats/min is usually selected.

Step 6 Set current (milliamps) to be delivered to minimum setting. While watching monitor screen, slowly but steadily increase current until you achieve electrical capture (each pacer spike is followed by a wide QRS complex).

Step 7 Evaluate mechanical capture by assessing patient's pulse and BP. Reassess patient's mental status, Spo_2, color, and level of discomfort.

Step 8 Obtain rhythm strips for documentation, and continuously monitor patient's condition.

Skill Drill 17-3 Performing Synchronized Cardioversion

Step 1 Select, check, and assemble all necessary equipment, including a monitor/defibrillator with defibrillation pads, ECG electrodes, medication for pain or sedation (to be used if necessary), oxygen, and an appropriate oxygen administration device. Take standard precautions. Assess patient's vital signs. Ensure patient is oxygenated adequately, and establish a patent IV line.

Step 2 Place ECG electrodes in same position as you would when performing cardiac monitoring. Obtain a baseline rhythm strip. Identify rhythm and confirm that cardioversion is warranted. If patient is responsive, you should consider appropriate medication to sedate patient. Ask about medication allergies before administering sedation.

Step 3 Ensure environment is safe (evaluate risk of sparks, combustibles, oxygen-rich atmosphere). Explain need for procedure to patient and family. Apply defibrillation pads to patient according to manufacturer's recommendations. Turn on power to defibrillator.

Step 4 Connect pads to monitor.

Step 5 Select appropriate energy setting. Turn synchronize switch on machine to on position.

Step 6 Observe ECG rhythm. Confirm that a sense marker appears near middle of each QRS complex. If sense markers are not visible or appear in wrong location (eg, on T wave), adjust ECG size or select another lead until machine reads QRS complexes appropriately. Clear area by announcing, "All clear!"; ensure everyone is clear of patient.

Step 7 Depress *Shock* buttons. Keep them depressed until defibrillator discharges.

Step 8 Reassess ECG rhythm and patient (pulse and BP). If tachycardia persists, ensure machine is in sync mode before delivering another shock. If rhythm changes to ventricular fibrillation (VF), ensure patient has no pulse. If no pulse is present, ensure sync control is off, and proceed with defibrillation.

Skill Drill 17-4 Performing Manual Defibrillation

Step 1 Select, check, and assemble all necessary equipment, including a monitor/defibrillator with defibrillation pads, oxygen, and an appropriate oxygen administration device. Take standard precautions, and ensure scene and environment are safe (evaluate risk of sparks, combustibles, oxygen-rich atmosphere).

Step 2 If available (and possible without interrupting care), ask bystanders about events surrounding arrest. Check responsiveness. Request additional help, if needed.

Step 3 Assess patient for breathing while simultaneously checking for a carotid pulse.

Step 4 Begin chest compressions if patient is not breathing or is only gasping and has no pulse. Ensure an adequate depth and rate, use correct compression-to-ventilation ratio, allow chest to recoil completely, deliver an adequate volume for each breath, and keep interruption of chest compressions to 10 seconds or less throughout resuscitation effort.

Step 5 Turn on power to defibrillator. If EMS providers have been using machine in AED mode before your arrival, switch machine to manual mode.

Step 6 Remove clothing from patient's upper body. With gloves, remove any medication paste or patches from patient's chest, and wipe away any residue.

Step 7 If using standard paddles, place pre-gelled defibrillator pads on patient's chest (or apply defibrillator gel to electrode surface of paddles). If using adhesive electrodes, place one electrode just to right of sternum just below clavicle, and place other on left lower chest area with top of pad 2 to 3 inches below armpit (or position electrodes according to manufacturer's instructions). Do not place electrodes on top of breast tissue. If necessary, lift breast out of way and place electrode underneath.

Step 8 Stop CPR, identify rhythm, and confirm that defibrillation is warranted. After verifying that a shockable rhythm is present, set defibrillator to proper energy setting.

Step 9 Charge defibrillator.

Step 10 Clear area. Announce, "All clear!"; ensure no one is touching patient. Press *Shock* button on machine if using a hands-free system. If using paddles, depress *Shock* button on each paddle at same time, and hold until defibrillator discharges. Resume CPR immediately.

Skill Drill 17-5 Performing Defibrillation with an AED

Step 1 Select, check, and assemble all necessary equipment, including AED, AED pads, oxygen, and an appropriate oxygen administration device. Take standard precautions, and ensure scene and environment are safe (evaluate risk of sparks, combustibles, oxygen-rich atmosphere).

Step 2 If available (and possible without interrupting care), ask bystanders about events surrounding arrest. Check responsiveness. Request additional help, if needed.

Step 3 Assess patient for breathing while simultaneously checking for a carotid pulse.

Step 4 If CPR is already in progress, then assess effectiveness of chest compressions. If patient is not breathing or is only gasping and has no pulse, and CPR has not been started, then begin chest compressions and rescue breaths. Ensure an adequate depth and rate, use correct compression-to-ventilation ratio, allow chest to recoil completely, deliver an adequate volume for each breath, and keep interruption of chest compressions to 10 seconds or less throughout resuscitation effort. Continue until an AED arrives and is ready for use.

Step 5 Turn on AED. Remove clothing from patient's upper body. With gloves, remove medication paste or patches from patient's chest, if present, and wipe away any residue.

Step 6 Follow machine's prompts; apply AED pads to patient's bare chest according to manufacturer's recommendations. Attach pads to AED.

Step 7 Stop CPR and press *Analyze* button (some AEDs will begin analyzing patient's rhythm automatically). Ensure everyone is clear of patient. Wait for AED to analyze cardiac rhythm. If no shock is advised, then resume CPR, starting with chest compressions. Perform five cycles (about 2 minutes) of CPR, and then reanalyze cardiac rhythm. If a shock is advised, then recheck that all are clear, and press *Shock* button.

Step 8 After shock is delivered, immediately resume CPR, beginning with chest compressions. Do not interrupt chest compressions for more than 10 seconds. Do not turn off AED during CPR. Continue to follow AED prompts. To reduce likelihood of rescuer fatigue, rotate position of chest compressor and ventilator during AED's analysis phase.

Skill Drill 17-6 Acquiring a 12-lead ECG

Step 1 Take standard precautions. Check your equipment. Ensure end of ECG cable has no loose pins and that cable or lead wires are intact. Ensure monitor has an adequate paper supply. Connect ECG cable to machine. Connect lead wires to ECG cable (if not already connected).

Step 2 Explain procedure to patient. Prepare patient's skin for electrode placement; shave and cleanse patient's skin as needed before placing monitoring electrodes.

Step 3 Attach electrodes to leads before you place them on patient.

Step 4 Position electrodes on patient. Connect four limb electrodes. Place them on arms and legs. Do not place electrodes on trunk of body, as is sometimes done for ECG monitoring. Double-check to confirm correct electrode has been positioned on each limb (LA electrode on left arm, RA electrode on right arm, and so on). Once limb electrodes have been secured, connect and apply electrodes for precordial leads:

- V_1—Fourth intercostal space (ICS) to right of sternum
- V_2—Fourth ICS to left of sternum
- V_3—Directly between leads V_2 and V_4
- V_4—Fifth ICS at left midclavicular line
- V_5—At level of lead V_4 at left anterior axillary line
- V_6—At level of lead V_4 at left midaxillary line

Step 5 Connect cables to monitor. Ensure patient is sitting or lying still, extremities are not crossed, and he or she is breathing normally and is not talking. Turn on power to monitor, and adjust screen contrast if necessary. Ensure all electrodes and cables are still connected and that no error message is displayed.

Step 6 Press *12-Lead Analyze* button.

Step 7 Obtain 12-lead ECG recording.

Step 8 Examine tracing for acceptable quality. Interpret 12-lead ECG, label it, and determine whether additional views of right and posterior walls (15- or 18-lead tracings) are needed. Obtain a 12-lead ECG every 5 to 10 minutes in high-risk patients and post-treatment.

Chapter 19

Skill Drill 19-1 Examining the Eye with an Ophthalmoscope

Step 1 Darken environment as much as possible. Ask patient to look straight ahead and focus on a distant object.

Step 2 Set light on ophthalmoscope to a setting no brighter than necessary and lens to 0, unless another setting works better for your eyes. Use your right hand and eye to examine patient's right eye; use your left hand and eye to examine patient's left eye.

Step 3 Place scope to your eye, and look into patient's pupil from 10 to 20 inches (25 to 51 cm) away at a 45° angle to eye. You should see retina as a "red reflex" or a bright orange glow. Slowly move toward patient to appreciate structures of fundus. Adjust lens as needed to improve focus. Locate a blood vessel, and follow it back to disk. Use this blood vessel as a point of reference.

Step 4 Inspect for size, color, and clarity of disk. Note integrity of blood vessels and any lesions present on retina. Move nasally to observe macula. Repeat process with other eye.

Skill Drill 19-2 Examining the Ear with an Otoscope

Step 1 Select an appropriately sized speculum. Dim lights as much as possible. Ensure ear is free of foreign bodies. Place your hand firmly against patient's head, and gently grasp auricle. Move ear to best visualize canal, usually upward and backward in an adult patient.

Step 2 To avoid damaging ear, instruct patient not to move during exam. Turn on otoscope, and insert speculum into ear. Do not insert speculum deeply into canal.

Step 3 Inspect canal for any lesions or discharge. A small amount of cerumen (earwax) is normal. Visualize tympanic membrane (eardrum), and inspect it for integrity and color. It should be translucent or a pearly gray color. Note any signs of inflammation, including swelling or discoloration (a pink-tinged or red ear canal or tympanic membrane).

Chapter 28

Skill Drill 28-1 Restraining a Patient

Step 1 Law enforcement officers should bring down patient into prone position. Then, acting at same time, secure patient in supine or left lateral position with wrist and ankle restraints. Some services require use of backboard for restraint so that a patient who becomes unconscious or who vomits can be turned onto his or her side quickly to manage airway.

Step 2 Use stretcher straps or sheets to secure legs.

Step 3 Fasten remaining stretcher straps.

Step 4 Continue to verbally reassure and calm patient following chemical/physical restraint. Regularly check circulation to extremities.

Chapter 30

Skill Drill 30-1 Managing External Hemorrhage

Step 1 Take standard precautions. Maintain airway with cervical spine immobilization if mechanism of injury (MOI) suggests possibility of spinal injury. Apply direct, even pressure over wound with a dry, sterile dressing.

Step 2 If bleeding stops, apply a pressure dressing and/or splint. Hold pressure dressing in place using gauze.

Step 3 If direct pressure does not rapidly control bleeding on an extremity injury, apply a tourniquet above level of bleeding.

Step 4 Tighten tourniquet until bleeding stops. Position patient supine unless contraindicated. Apply oxygen as necessary. Keep patient warm, transport promptly, monitor serial vital signs, and watch diligently for developing shock.

Skill Drill 30-2 Applying a Commercial Tourniquet (Combat Application Tourniquet)

Step 1 Hold direct pressure over bleeding site, and place tourniquet proximal to injury, preferably at groin or axilla. Wrap band around limb, and fasten it to buckle.

Step 2 Pull band tightly, and secure band back on itself. Ensure that tips of three fingers cannot fit between band and limb.

Step 3 Tighten rod (windlass) until bleeding stops.

Step 4 Secure rod inside clip. Ensure bleeding is still controlled, and assess for a distal pulse.

Step 5 Wrap rest of band through clips. Secure rod with strap labeled *TIME:*, and document time.

Skill Drill 30-3 Managing Internal Hemorrhage

Step 1 Take standard precautions. Maintain airway with cervical spine immobilization if mechanism of injury (MOI) suggests possibility of spinal injury. Administer supplemental oxygen as needed, and assist ventilation if necessary.

Step 2 Control all obvious external bleeding, and treat suspected internal bleeding using a splint if possible. Apply a tourniquet for severe bleeding from an extremity that cannot be controlled with direct pressure.

Step 3 Depending on local protocols, if a pelvic fracture is suspected, use a pelvic binder or sheets to bind pelvic area.

Step 4 Monitor and record vital signs at least every 5 minutes.

Chapter 34

Skill Drill 34-1 Performing Spinal Immobilization of a Supine Adult Patient

Step 1 Take standard precautions, and then begin manual in-line stabilization from a kneeling position at patient's head. Hold head firmly with both hands. The provider at head directs all patient movement.

Support lower jaw with your index and middle fingers, and support head with your palms. If patient's head is not facing forward, gently move it until patient's eyes are looking straight ahead and head and torso are in alignment (neutral alignment). Never twist, flex, or extend head or neck excessively. Do not remove your hands from patient's head until patient is properly secured to a backboard and head is immobilized.

Evaluate patient's reliability in giving a history.

Step 2 Assess distal pulses and motor and sensory function in each extremity.

Step 3 Apply a well-fitting cervical collar as previously discussed.

Step 4 Other team members should position immobilization device (backboard) beside patient and place their hands on patient's far side to increase their leverage while kneeling. Instruct them to use their body weight, shoulders, and back muscles to ensure a smooth, coordinated pull. The pull should concentrate on heavier portions of body.

Step 5 On count/command from paramedic at patient's head, rescuers should roll patient toward themselves until patient is balanced on his or her side. This prevents patient from twisting as he or she is pulled down by gravity and up by provider. One rescuer should then quickly examine back while patient is rolled on side, and then slide backboard behind and under patient. The team should then roll patient back onto board, avoiding rotation of head, shoulders, and pelvis.

Step 6 Ensure patient is centered on board. Alternatively, patient may be moved onto board as follows: board is placed beside patient with foot end at level of patient's hips. The patient is log rolled, then patient is pulled onto board along axis of spine to a centered position. This alternative method results in only moving patient twice (one roll and one slide).

Step 7 Apply padding as necessary to fill voids between patient and device. When possible, prepare blanket rolls ahead of time, and have them ready to go. When you have blankets prepared, you need only seconds to place them. Use of blanket rolls has been shown to dramatically improve effectiveness of immobilization.

Step 8 Center patient on backboard.

Step 9 Secure upper torso to board after patient has been centered on backboard.

Step 10 Secure pelvis and upper legs, using padding as needed. For pelvis, use straps over iliac crests and/or groin loops (leg straps).

Step 11 Pad behind patient's head and neck as needed to maintain a neutral in-line position.

Step 12 Immobilize head to board with a commercial immobilization device per manufacturer's instructions. Secure head to board only after entire torso has been secured. If head is secured first and body shifts, spine may be compromised. Securing most of body weight first creates better protection.

Step 13 Secure patient's lower legs to board.

Step 14 Secure patient's arms with a single strap.

Step 15 Check and readjust straps as needed to ensure that entire body is snugly secured and will not slide during movement of board or during patient transport. Reassess distal pulse, motor function, and sensation (PMS) function in each extremity and repeat periodically.

Skill Drill 34-2 Using a Scoop Stretcher

Step 1 With scoop stretcher separated, measure length of scoop and adjust to proper length.

Step 2 Position stretcher, one side at a time. Lift patient's side slightly by pulling on far hip and upper arm while your partner slides stretcher into place.

Step 3 Lock stretcher ends together by engaging their locking mechanisms one at a time, and continue to lift patient slightly as needed to avoid pinching patient or your fingers.

Step 4 Apply and tighten straps to secure patient to scoop stretcher before transferring to stretcher.

Skill Drill 34-3 Performing Spinal Immobilization of a Seated Adult Patient

Step 1 Take standard precautions, and direct your assistant to place and maintain head in a neutral in-line position. Stabilize head and neck with manual in-line stabilization until patient is secured to long backboard. Evaluate patient's reliability as a historian. Assess distal pulse and motor and sensory function in each extremity.

Apply a well-fitting cervical collar. Because cervical collar does not completely stabilize cervical spine, continue manual stabilization of head and neck until patient is fully immobilized on a backboard.

Step 2 Insert immobilization device between patient's upper back and seat back.

Step 3 Open board's side flaps (if present), and position them around patient's torso, snug to armpits.

Step 4 When device is properly positioned, secure upper torso straps.

Step 5 Position and fasten both groin/leg straps. Pad groin as needed. Check all torso straps, and make sure they are secure. Make any necessary adjustments without excessively moving patient.

Step 6 Pad any space between patient's head and device. Secure forehead strap or tape head securely, and then fasten lower head strap around rigid cervical collar. Reevaluate patient to assure that he or she is adequately immobilized. Reassess distal pulses and motor and sensory function in each extremity.

Step 7 Place long backboard next to patient's buttocks, perpendicular to trunk.

Step 8 Turn patient parallel to long board, and slowly lower him or her onto it. Lift patient and vest-type board together as a unit (without rotating patient), and slip long backboard under patient and device. Slide patient onto backboard as a unit using any handles that may be built into device. Release leg straps and loosen chest strap to allow legs to straighten and give chest room to fully expand.

Step 9 Secure short board and long backboard together. Do not remove vest-type board from patient. Reassess distal pulse and motor and sensory function in all four extremities. Note your findings on PCR and prepare for transport.

Chapter 35

Skill Drill 35-1 Needle Decompression (Thoracentesis) of a Tension Pneumothorax

Step 1 Assess patient to ensure that presentation matches that of a tension pneumothorax. Look for difficult ventilation despite an open airway, jugular venous distention (JVD; may not be present with associated hemorrhage), absent or decreased breath sounds on affected side, hyperresonance to percussion on affected side, tracheal deviation away from affected side (late sign, not always present), pulsus paradoxus, and tachycardia.

Step 2 Prepare and assemble all necessary equipment, including a large-bore IV catheter, preferably 14- to 16-gauge and at least 3.25 inches (8 cm) long (this ensures ability of needle to reach intended depth to relieve pressure); alcohol or povidone iodine (Betadine) preps; a flutter valve (cut off one finger of a glove to use as a substitute if you do not have a commercial device available); and adhesive tape. A two-way or three-way stopcock can also be used to seal or relieve pressure should it begin to build within thoracic cavity. Obtain medical control if required by regional protocols.

Step 3 Locate appropriate site. Find second or third rib. Insert needle just above third rib into intercostal space at midclavicular line on affected side. If there is significant trauma to anterior portion of chest, or chest wall is too deep, use intercostal space between fourth and fifth ribs at midaxillary line on affected side.

Step 4 Cleanse appropriate area using aseptic technique.

Step 5 Make a one-way valve, or flutter valve, by inserting catheter through end of finger of a medical glove, cut off from glove. Alternatively, use a commercially prepared device.

Step 6 Insert needle at a 90° angle, and listen for release of air. Insert needle just superior to third rib, midclavicular line, or just above sixth rib, midaxillary line. (To avoid nerves, arteries, and veins, run along inferior borders of each rib.)

Step 7 Remove needle, and properly dispose of needle in sharps container.

Step 8 Secure catheter in place in same manner you would use to secure an impaled object. Monitor patient closely for recurrence of tension pneumothorax. This procedure may need to be repeated several times before arrival at ED.

Chapter 37

Skill Drill 37-1 Performing a Motor Function and Sensory Exam

Step 1 Have patient flex his or her arms at elbow to test musculocutaneous nerve motor function.

Step 2 Have patient extend arms at elbow to test radial nerve motor function.

Step 3 Have patient extend thumbs (thumbs up) to test radial nerve motor function.

Step 4 Have patient make an "okay" sign to test median nerve motor function.

Step 5 Have patient spread his or her fingers apart to test ulnar nerve motor function.

Step 6 Instruct patient to extend his or her legs at knee to test femoral nerve motor function.

Step 7 Have patient flex his or her feet and ankles downward (plantarflex) to test tibial nerve motor function.

Step 8 Instruct patient to flex feet and ankles upward (dorsiflex) to test deep peroneal nerve motor function.

Step 9 Lightly touch lateral surface of shoulder (over deltoid) to test axillary nerve sensory function using corner of a bandage or tissue to make contact with skin.

Step 10 Lightly touch anterolateral surface of forearm to test musculocutaneous nerve sensory function.

Step 11 Lightly touch dorsal surface of web space of thumb to test radial nerve sensory function.

Step 12 Lightly touch volar surface of distal thumb, index, and middle fingers to test median nerve sensory function.

Step 13 Lightly touch distal volar surface of small finger to test ulnar nerve sensory function.

Step 14 Lightly touch anteromedial surface of thigh to test femoral nerve sensory function.

Step 15 Lightly touch plantar surface of toes to test tibial nerve sensory function.

Step 16 Lightly touch web space between great toe and second toe to test peroneal nerve sensory function.

Chapter 39

Skill Drill 39-1 Performing Two-Rescuer Adult CPR

Step 1 Take standard precautions, and ensure scene safety. Move to patient's head and establish unresponsiveness while your partner moves to patient's side to be ready to deliver chest compressions.

Step 2 If patient is unresponsive, then simultaneously check for breathing and palpate for a carotid pulse; take no more than 10 seconds to do this. If patient has no pulse and is either not breathing or only gasping, then apply an AED if available.

Step 3 If an AED is unavailable, begin chest compressions at a ratio of 30:2. After an advanced airway is inserted, rescuers should switch from cycles of CPR to continuously delivered compressions at a rate of 100 to 120/min.

Step 4 If patient has a pulse, position patient to open airway according to your suspicion of spinal injury. If breathing is adequate, then place patient in recovery position, and monitor breathing and pulse.

Step 5 If patient has a pulse but is not breathing adequately, then deliver rescue breaths at a rate of 10 breaths/min (1 breath every 6 s).

Step 6 If CPR was started, then compressor and ventilator should switch positions after 2 min. Switch time should take no longer than 5 s. If a third rescuer is available, then position him or her at chest opposite compressor. If only two rescuers are available, then switch mid-cycle during compressions.

Step 7 Reassess patient every few minutes. Each assessment should last no more than 10 s. Depending on patient's condition, continue CPR, continue rescue breathing only, or place patient in recovery position, monitoring breathing and pulse.

Note: After an advanced airway has been inserted, compressions and ventilations are no longer performed in cycles. Instead, they are performed individually, are not timed, and do not require waiting for other rescuer to pause (asynchronous). Compressor provides between 100 and 120 compressions/min without pausing for breaths, and ventilator gives 10 breaths/min (1 breath every 6 s). Because compressor will inevitably get tired, switch compressors every 2 min, but minimize break in compression cycle to approximately 5 s.

Skill Drill 39-2 Performing CPR on a Child

Step 1 Take standard precautions, and ensure scene safety. Move to child's head and establish unresponsiveness while your partner moves to patient's side to be ready to deliver chest compressions. If patient is unresponsive, then simultaneously check for breathing and palpate for a pulse; take no more than 10 seconds to do this. If patient has no pulse and is either not breathing or only gasping, then apply an AED if available.

Step 2 Place child on a firm surface. Prepare to place heel of one or both hands in center of chest, in between nipples, avoiding xiphoid process.

Step 3 Compress chest one-third anterior-posterior diameter of chest (approximately 2 in. [5 cm] in most children) at a rate of 100 to 120/min. In between compressions, allow chest to fully recoil; do not lean on chest. Compression and relaxation time should be same duration. Use smooth movements. Hold your fingers off child's ribs, and keep heel of your hand(s) on sternum.

Step 4 Coordinate compressions and ventilations in a 30:2 ratio for one rescuer and 15:2 for two rescuers, making sure chest rises with each ventilation. At end of each cycle, pause for two ventilations.

Step 5 Continue cycles of compressions and ventilations until an AED becomes available or patient shows signs of spontaneous breathing. If child resumes effective breathing, then place him or her in a position that allows for frequent reassessment of airway and vital signs during transport.

Step 6 If child remains in cardiac arrest, continue CPR. Rotate compressors every 2 minutes of CPR.

Note: After an advanced airway has been inserted, compressions and ventilations are no longer performed in cycles. Instead, they are performed continuously at a rate of at least 100 breaths/min, without pauses for ventilation. Ventilations should be delivered at breath every 6 to 8 s (8 to 10 breaths/min). Because compressor will inevitably get tired, switch compressors every 2 min but limit break in compressions to approximately 5 s.

Skill Drill 39-3 Infant CPR

Step 1 Take standard precautions, and ensure scene safety. Move to infant's head and establish unresponsiveness while your partner moves to patient's side to be ready to deliver chest compressions. If patient is unresponsive, then simultaneously check for breathing and palpate for a brachial pulse; take no more than 10 seconds to do this. If patient has no pulse and is either not breathing or only gasping, then apply an AED if available.

Step 2 Place infant on a firm surface, using one hand to keep head in an open airway position. You can also use a pad or wedge under shoulders and upper body to keep head from tilting forward.

Step 3 Imagine a line drawn between nipples. Place two fingers in middle of sternum, about 0.5 in. (1 cm) below level of imaginary line (one finger width). Using two fingers, compress sternum at least one-third anterior-posterior diameter of chest (approximately 1.5 in. [4 cm] in most infants). Compress chest at a rate of 100 to 120/min. After each compression, allow sternum to return briefly to its normal position. Allow equal time for compression and relaxation of chest. Do not remove your fingers from sternum, and avoid jerky movements.

Step 4 Coordinate compressions and ventilations in a 30:2 ratio for one rescuer and 15:2 for two rescuers, making sure chest rises with each ventilation. At end of each cycle, pause for two ventilations. Continue cycles of compressions and ventilations until an AED becomes available or infant shows signs of spontaneous breathing. If infant resumes effective breathing, place him or her in a position that allows for frequent reassessment of airway and vital signs during transport.

Chapter 42

Skill Drill 42-1 Intubating a Newborn

Step 1 Pre-oxygenate newborn by bag-mask ventilation to an oxygen saturation greater than 95%. Administering 100% oxygen is not needed and can have deleterious effects in preterm infants.

Step 2 Suction oropharynx if there are copious secretions that prevent adequate ventilation. This can be a vagal stimulus, so pay close attention to pulse rate, and avoid repeated or vigorous suctioning. Provide bag-mask ventilation if bradycardia results.

Step 3 Place laryngoscope blade in oropharynx. Visualize vocal cords. Avoid applying torque to blade because it increases risk of trauma. Place ET tube between vocal cords until black line on ET tube is at level of cords. For full-term newborns, ET tube is usually advanced until it is at 9 cm at lip. For a premature newborn, you may need to advance ET tube to only 6.5 to 7 cm at lip. Limit intubation attempt to 20 seconds, and initiate bag-mask ventilation if it is unsuccessful or if significant bradycardia develops.

Step 4 Confirm ET tube placement. Observe chest rise, auscultate laterally in epigastric region and high on chest, note mist in ET tube (seen when patient exhales through tube from condensation of humidified air leaving lungs), note equal breath sounds on both sides, and observe for clinical improvement. Monitor $ETCO_2$ via waveform capnography, and consider using pulse oximetry. This is often earliest indicator of return of spontaneous circulation (ROSC). Pulse oximetry monitoring provides peripheral oxygen saturation and reflects response to adequate oxygenation and ventilation.

Step 5 Tape ET tube in place on face to minimize risk of tube dislodging. Monitor newborn closely for complications such as tube dislodgement, tube occlusion by mucous plug or meconium, or pneumothorax.

Skill Drill 42-2 Inserting an Orogastric Tube in the Newborn

Step 1 Measure for correct depth. Use an 8F feeding tube, and measure length from bottom of earlobe to tip of nose to halfway between xiphoid process (lower tip of sternum) and umbilicus.

Step 2 Insert tube through mouth to appropriate depth. Leave nose open to allow for ventilation.

Step 3 Attach a 10-mL syringe and suction stomach contents. Tape tube to newborn's cheek. Remove syringe from feeding tube to allow venting of air from stomach. Intermittently suction feeding tube.

Chapter 43

Skill Drill 43-1 Inserting an Oropharyngeal Airway in a Pediatric Patient

Step 1 Determine appropriately sized airway by measuring from corner of mouth to angle of jaw or by using a length-based resuscitation tape to measure patient. Place airway next to face, with flange at level of central incisors and bite block segment parallel to hard palate. The tip of airway should reach angle of jaw.

Step 2 Position patient's airway. For medical patients, use head tilt–chin lift maneuver, avoiding hyperextension. If patient has a traumatic injury, use jaw-thrust maneuver and provide in-line spinal stabilization.

Step 3 Open mouth by applying pressure on chin with your thumb. Insert airway by depressing tongue with a tongue blade on base of tongue and inserting airway directly over tongue blade. If a tongue blade is not available, point airway tip toward roof of mouth to depress tongue. Gently rotate airway into position as it passes through mouth toward curve of tongue. Insert airway until flange rests against lips. Reassess airway after insertion.

Skill Drill 43-2 Inserting a Nasopharyngeal Airway in a Pediatric Patient

Step 1 Determine appropriately sized airway. External diameter of airway should not be larger than diameter of naris, and there should be no blanching (turning white) of naris after insertion. Place airway next to patient's face to make sure length is correct. Airway should extend from tip of nose to tragus of ear (ie, small cartilaginous projection in front of opening of ear). Position patient's airway, using techniques described for oropharyngeal airway (OPA).

Step 2 Lubricate airway with a water-soluble lubricant. Insert tip into right naris with bevel pointing toward septum.

Step 3 Carefully move tip forward, following curvature of nose, until flange rests against outside of nostril. If you are inserting airway on left side, insert tip into left naris upside down, with bevel pointing toward septum. Move airway forward slowly until you feel a slight resistance, and then rotate airway 180°. Reassess airway after insertion.

Skill Drill 43-3 Performing One-Person Bag-Mask Ventilation on a Pediatric Patient

Step 1 Open airway and insert appropriate airway adjunct.

Step 2 Hold mask on patient's face by using one-handed head tilt–chin lift technique (E-C grip) method. To use E-C method, form a C with your thumb and index finger along mask while your other three fingers form an E along mandible. With infants and toddlers, support jaw with only your third finger. Do not compress area under chin because you may push tongue into back of mouth and block airway. Keep your fingers on mandible. Ensure mask forms an airtight seal on face. Maintain seal while checking that airway is open.

Step 3 Squeeze bag, using correct ventilation rate: 12 to 20 breaths/min for infants and children (1 breath every 3 to 5 seconds). Allow 1 second per ventilation, providing adequate time for exhalation.

Step 4 Assess effectiveness of ventilation by watching bilateral rise and fall of chest.

Skill Drill 43-4 Performing Pediatric Endotracheal Intubation

Step 1 Take standard precautions (gloves and face shield).

Step 2 Check, prepare, and assemble your equipment.

Step 3 Measure length of child using a length-based resuscitation tape to aid in determining needed equipment sizes.

Step 4 Manually open child's airway.

Step 5 Measure for proper size, and then insert oropharyngeal airway (OPA) or nasopharyngeal airway (NPA).

Step 6 Ventilate patient with a bag-mask device at a rate of 12 to 20 breaths/min with sufficient volume to produce visible chest rise. Attach pulse oximeter, and note child's oxygen saturation level. Preoxygenate child for at least 2 to 3 minutes with 100% oxygen.

Step 7 Place patient's head in a neutral or sniffing position; add padding as needed to achieve proper positioning. Remove airway adjunct, then insert laryngoscope into right side of mouth, and sweep tongue to left. Lift tongue with firm, gentle pressure. Avoid using teeth or gums as a fulcrum.

Step 8 Identify vocal cords. If cords are not yet visible, instruct your partner to perform BURP maneuver (also called external laryngeal manipulation) if possible.

Step 9 Introduce ET tube in right corner of child's mouth.

Step 10 Pass ET tube through vocal cords to approximately 2 to 3 cm below vocal cords. Remove laryngoscope from patient's mouth. Inflate cuff to proper pressure, and immediately remove syringe if a cuffed tube is used.

Step 11 Attach an end-tidal carbon dioxide detector (waveform capnography preferred). Attach bag-mask device, and auscultate for equal breath sounds over each lateral chest wall high in axillae. Ensure absence of breath sounds over epigastrium. Assess for hypoxia during intubation attempt.

Step 12 Secure ET tube with a commercial device or tape, noting placement of distance marker at child's teeth or gums. Ventilate patient at proper rate and volume while monitoring capnography and pulse oximetry.

Skill Drill 43-5 Performing Pediatric IO Infusion

Step 1 Check selected IV fluid for proper fluid, clarity, and expiration date. Look for any discoloration or particles floating in fluid. If any are found, discard fluid and choose another bag of fluid. Select appropriate equipment, including an intraosseous (IO) needle, syringe, saline, and extension set. A three-way stopcock may also be used to facilitate easier fluid administration.

Step 2 Select proper administration set. Connect administration set to bag. Prepare administration set. Fill drip chamber, and flush tubing. Ensure no air bubbles remain in tubing. Prepare syringe and extension tubing.

Step 3 At any time before IO puncture, cut or tear tape and prepare bulky dressings. Before IO puncture, take standard precautions. Identify proper anatomic site for IO puncture. To miss epiphyseal (growth) plate, you should measure two fingerbreadths below knee on medial side of leg.

Step 4 Cleanse site using aseptic technique (ie, in a circular manner from inside out). Stabilize tibia. Place a folded towel under knee, and hold it so that you keep your fingers away from puncture site. Insert needle at a 90° angle to leg. Advance needle with a twisting motion until you feel a "pop."

Step 5 Unscrew cap, and remove stylet from needle.

Step 6 Remove stylet from catheter. Attach syringe and extension set to IO needle. Pull back on syringe to aspirate blood and particles of bone marrow to ensure placement. If you are not able to aspirate marrow but IO flushes easily, with no signs of infiltration (swelling around insertion site), then continue to flush. Slowly inject saline to ensure proper placement of needle. Watch for infiltration, and stop infusion immediately if any is noted. It is possible to fracture bone during insertion of IO needle; if this happens, you should remove IO needle and switch to other leg. Connect administration set, and adjust flow rate as appropriate. Fluid does not flow well through an IO needle, and boluses are given by administering fluid using syringe and three-way stopcock.

Step 7 Secure needle with tape, and support it with a bulky dressing. Be careful not to tape around entire circumference of leg because doing so could impair circulation and create compartment syndrome. Dispose of needle in proper container.

Skill Drill 43-6 Immobilizing a Child

Step 1 Use a towel under shoulders of a child to maintain head in a neutral position.

Step 2 Apply an appropriately sized cervical collar.

Step 3 Carefully log roll child onto immobilization device.

Step 4 Secure child's torso to immobilization device first.

Step 5 Secure child's head to immobilization device.

Step 6 Complete immobilization by ensuring that child is strapped in properly.

Skill Drill 43-7 Immobilizing an Infant

Step 1 Carefully stabilize infant's head in a neutral position, and lay seat down into a reclined position on a hard surface.

Step 2 Position a pediatric board or a similar device between infant and surface on which infant is resting.

Step 3 Slide infant onto board.

Step 4 Make sure infant's head is in a neutral position by placing a towel under infant's shoulders.

Step 5 Secure torso first, and place padding to fill any voids.

Step 6 Secure infant's head to backboard.

Chapter 45

Skill Drill 45-1 Cleaning a Tracheostomy Tube

Step 1 Wash your hands and apply a mask, goggles, and clean nonlatex gloves. Suctioning a home care patient is a clean procedure, not a sterile one. Open supplies may be used. For cost reasons, home care patients often reuse their suction catheters. If catheters do not have visible contamination and have been stored in a clean manner, they are acceptable for use. Remove inner cannula, and check with your patient's caregiver, if available, regarding appropriate solution for soaking device, then place device to soak in recommended solution. If caregiver is not available, use a mixture of hydrogen peroxide and water. Placing cannula in plain water is acceptable in short-term situations. With one-piece tracheostomy tubes, this step is unnecessary. If patient is dependent on a ventilator, have a replacement cannula immediately available.

Step 2 Attach catheter to negative pressure. Check suction and clear catheter by drawing up a small amount of saline.

Step 3 Have patient take a deep breath, or preoxygenate patient using ventilator.

Step 4 Insert catheter into trachea without suction. Apply intermittent suction while removing catheter. Repeat as necessary. Keep patient well oxygenated during procedure.

Step 5 Clean inner cannula with tracheostomy brush, rinse, and replace and lock into place. Omit this step for a one-piece tracheostomy tube. Remove your gloves and wash your hands. Document procedure and assessment on PCR.

Skill Drill 45-2 Replacing an Ostomy Device

Step 1 Help position patient in a comfortable area in which to change appliance and easily dispose of contaminated articles. Wash your hands and apply a mask, goggles, and clean nonlatex gloves. Open supplies. Ostomy equipment includes a skin barrier called a wafer and one of several styles of drainage bags. Some bags can be opened along bottom and emptied at regular intervals; others are sealed around a system similar to a urine drainage bag. Empty/remove current appliance, and dispose of it appropriately.

Step 2 Wash area around stoma with soap and water. Cleanse stoma with water only, being careful not to rub or irritate area.

Step 3 Place a clean gauze pad over stoma to prevent contamination of clean skin with stool or urine.

Step 4 Cut wafer to correct size using patient's measurement or tracing. Home care patients usually have stoma already sized or have a tracing to cut a hole in wafer large enough for stoma but keeping exposed skin to a minimum.

Step 5 Attach appliance to wafer. Be sure distal end is closed.

Step 6 Remove gauze.

Step 7 Remove paper backing from wafer.

Step 8 Apply appliance with stoma centered in wafer cutout. Remove your gloves and wash your hands. Document procedure and assessment on PCR.

Skill Drill 45-3 Catheterizing an Adult Male Patient

Step 1 Help position patient supine with legs slightly spread apart. Maintain privacy as much as possible. Wash your hands and apply a mask, goggles, and sterile nonlatex gloves.

Open supplies, including urinary catheter and placement kit. Home care patients may reuse their catheters provided that they have been stored in a clean manner. Place necessary supplies onto a clean area within reach. If placing an indwelling catheter, use sterile technique throughout. Do not allow catheter that will be inserted to come into contact with anything that is not also sterile. If you are inserting an indwelling catheter, connect a syringe filled with saline to balloon port. Also, connect indwelling catheter to drainage system. There are no connecting ports for either a balloon or a drainage bag on a straight catheter.

Wash penis with solution included in kit. Make sure foreskin has been retracted. Use great caution throughout to avoid breaks in sterile technique.

Coat end of catheter with a water-soluble gel. Hold penis at a 90° angle to body and insert catheter.

Step 2 When urine is evident in tubing, insert catheter until Y between drainage port and balloon port is at tip of penis. For a straight catheter, insert approximately 1 inch (2.5 cm) more.

Inflate balloon, and gently pull back on catheter until you feel resistance, which indicates that balloon is snug against neck of bladder. This step is unnecessary for a straight catheter. Never inflate balloon if you do not see any urine in tubing or if you meet resistance to inflation, as doing so may indicate that balloon is in urethra instead of bladder, and inflation would therefore cause urethral injury.

Step 3 Allow urine to drain. Note amount and color.

To remove a catheter, remove saline in balloon port and pull back gently until catheter is free of tip of penis. Never remove an indwelling catheter without using a syringe to remove saline from balloon because it may damage urinary sphincter. For a straight catheter, simply pull back gently to remove catheter. Wash according to home care instructions. Remove your gloves and wash your hands, following standard precautions. If catheter is to remain in place, secure it to patient's leg according to home care instructions. Document procedure and assessment on PCR.

Skill Drill 45-4 Catheterizing an Adult Female Patient

Step 1 Help position patient supine with legs spread apart or side lying with top knee flexed. Maintain privacy as much as possible. Wash your hands and apply nonlatex gloves.

Open supplies including urinary catheter and placement kit. Home care patients may reuse their catheters provided that they have been stored in a clean manner. Place necessary supplies onto a clean area within reach. If placing an indwelling catheter, use sterile technique throughout. Do not allow catheter that will be inserted to come into contact with anything that is not also sterile. If you are inserting an indwelling catheter, connect a syringe filled with saline to balloon port. Also, connect indwelling catheter to drainage system. There are no connecting ports for either a balloon or a drainage bag on a straight catheter.

Wash perineal area with solution included in kit. First cleanse outer area of perineum, and then spread labia minora and thoroughly wash mucosa surrounding vagina and urinary meatus. Dry with a clean towel. Coat end of catheter with a water-soluble gel. Locate urinary meatus anterior to vagina and insert catheter. Depending on age of patient, integrity of her pelvic musculature, and other factors, locating urinary meatus can be difficult.

Step 2 When urine is evident in tubing, insert catheter another 1 to 3 inches (2.5 to 8 cm).

Step 3 Inflate balloon and gently pull back on catheter until you feel resistance, which indicates that balloon is snug against neck of bladder. This step is unnecessary for a straight catheter. Allow urine to drain. Note amount and color.

To remove a catheter, remove saline in balloon port and pull back gently until catheter is free of tip of meatus. Never remove an indwelling catheter without using a syringe to remove saline from balloon because it may damage urinary sphincter. For a straight catheter, simply pull back gently to remove catheter. If catheter is to be reused, it should be cleaned. Remove your gloves and wash your hands.

If catheter is to remain in place, secure it to patient's leg or abdomen according to patient's needs. Document procedure and assessment on PCR.

Chapter 48

Skill Drill 48-1 Breaking Tempered Glass Using a Spring-Loaded Center Punch

Step 1 Take standard precautions and don appropriate PPE. Ensure that scene is safe and vehicle is stable. Using window farthest from patient, place palm of your hand facedown against lower corner of window and frame, with your index finger and thumb facing upward. Position and rest body of spring-loaded center punch in ridge section of your palm (V-section of your hand) between your index finger and thumb.

Step 2 Ensure that patient is protected from flying glass. Warn personnel verbally, "Breaking glass!" With point of tool directly on glass, apply pressure until spring is activated and glass breaks.

Step 3 Use a piece of cribbing to remove remaining fragments of tempered glass from around window frame.

Skill Drill 48-2 Stabilizing a Suspected Spinal Injury in the Water

Step 1 Turn patient supine by rotating entire upper half of patient's body as a single unit. Twisting only head, for example, may aggravate any injury to cervical spine. Two rescuers are usually required to turn patient safely, although one may suffice.

Step 2 As soon as patient is turned, have other rescuer support head and trunk as a unit while you open airway and begin artificial ventilation using mouth-to-mouth method or a pocket mask. Immediate ventilation is primary treatment of all submersion patients as soon as patient is faceup in water.

Step 3 Float a buoyant backboard under patient as you continue ventilation.

Step 4 Secure trunk and head of patient to backboard to eliminate motion of cervical spine. Do not remove patient from water until this is done.

Step 5 Remove patient from water, on backboard.

Step 6 Remove patient's wet clothes and cover him or her with a blanket. Administer supplemental oxygen if patient is breathing adequately; give positive-pressure ventilation if he or she is apneic or breathing inadequately. Begin CPR if breathing and pulse are absent.

Chapter 49

Skill Drill 49-1 Using the *ERG* to Research Materials

Step 1 Identify chemical name and/or chemical ID number for suspect material.

Step 2 Look up material name in appropriate section. Use yellow section to obtain information based on chemical ID number. Use blue section to obtain information based on alphabetical chemical name. *Note any listing that has been highlighted because this should lead you to evacuation distance section of* ERG.

Step 3 Determine correct emergency action guide to use for chemical identified.

Step 4 Identify potential fire and explosion and/or health hazards of chemical identified.

Step 5 Identify isolation distance and protective actions required for chemical identified.

Step 6 Identify emergency response actions for chemical identified.

Answer Key

Section 1: Preparatory

Chapter 1: EMS Systems

Matching

1. C (page 27)
2. D (page 27)
3. A (page 27)
4. F (page 24)
5. G (page 9)
6. B (page 10)
7. J (page 27)
8. H (page 29)
9. E (pages 29–30)
10. I (page 21)

Multiple Choice

1. A (page 6)
2. C (page 8)
3. D (page 12)
4. B (page 21)
5. B (page 26)
6. D (pages 17–18)
7. C (page 23)
8. B (page 6)
9. C (page 11)
10. C (page 13)
11. C (pages 10–11)
12. D (pages 10–11)
13. B (page 11)

Fill in the Blank

1. mobile intensive care units (page 6)
2. dispatcher (page 11)
3. reciprocity (page 10)
4. empathy (page 18)
5. first priority (page 19)
6. continuous quality improvement (CQI) (page 22)
7. Prospective (page 26)

Ambulance Calls

1. a. When your spouse is calling for the ambulance, she should give the name and the location of the theater and possibly the theater number if it is a large multiplex. Always give the patient's chief complaint and the current status of the patient (eg, alert and oriented), and tell whether the patient is breathing. Your spouse should also tell the dispatcher that there is a paramedic on the scene.
   b. Any patient who experiences syncope needs to be seen by a physician in the emergency department (ED). Syncopal episodes can be caused by problems involving the heart (eg, life-threatening dysrhythmia), problems involving the brain (eg, a stroke or transient ischemic attack [TIA]), shock (eg, orthostatic hypotension, vasovagal syncope, dehydration, or blood loss), or a number of other problems. In this scenario, the patient could have also hurt herself when she fell.
2. a. You should always ensure scene safety for yourself, your crew, bystanders, and the patient. This is your number-one priority. Make sure the driver has moved the vehicle far enough away from the patient so that care can be given. You should also make sure the vehicle is in park, the engine is turned off, and the parking brake is set. You can also control the scene by having bystanders block traffic to the area until law enforcement arrives.
   b. You should begin treatment by having the EMT hold cervical spine immobilization on this patient. You should start with your primary survey (ABCDEs) and move to the secondary assessment. After completing the trauma exam, if you determine that the patient has a broken femur, you should apply manual traction to the leg to help stabilize it, and control the pain and bleeding until the ambulance arrives.

True/False

1. F (page 5)
2. F (page 6)
3. T (page 12)
4. F (page 13)
5. F (page 13)
6. F (page 19)
7. T (page 22)
8. T (page 26)
9. F (page 20)
10. T (page 18)

Short Answer

1. a. Integrity—Be open, honest, and truthful with patients. (page 17)
   b. Empathy—Understand and identify the feelings of patients and their families. (page 18)
   c. Self-motivation—Be driven to keep yourself competent in your skills and your professional manners. (page 18)
   d. Confidence—Instill confidence in your patients and colleagues by showing that you are confident in your abilities and skills. (page 18)
   e. Communications—Express and exchange your ideas, thoughts, and findings on the scene. (page 18)
   f. Teamwork and respect—All involved must work together to achieve a common goal to provide the best possible prehospital care to ensure the overall well-being of the patient. (page 18)
   g. Patient advocacy—Always act in the best interest of your patient. (page 18)
   h. Injury prevention—Help on the scene by pointing out dangerous situations for the patient in his or her home or surroundings. (page 18)
   i. Careful delivery of service—Follow protocols and procedures, and continuously evaluate your performance. (page 18)
   j. Time management—Use your time wisely; for example, prioritize your patient's needs. (page 18)
   k. Administration—Document each call thoroughly and professionally, and consider additional administrative roles as your career evolves. (page 18)
2. a. Preparation—Physical; mental; emotional; knowledge, skills, and abilities; equipment that is appropriate and in working order. (page 19)
   b. Response—Timely and safe. (page 19)
   c. Scene management—Safety of yourself and your team, safety of the patient and bystanders, assessing the situation, use of personal protective equipment (PPE). (pages 19–20)
   d. Patient assessment and care—Appropriate, organized assessment; recognize and prioritize patient's needs. (page 20)
   e. Management and disposition—Follow protocols or radio medical director; know capabilities of receiving facilities. (page 20)
   f. Patient transfer and report—Give brief, concise handoff report; protect the patient's privacy. (page 20)
   g. Documentation—Fill out PCR. (page 20)
   h. Return to service—Restock and prepare unit. (page 20)
3. Medical control is set up by law as a supervisor for the paramedic. The roles of the medical director are as follows: educating and training personnel (ensuring their competency in the field), participating in selection of new personnel, helping with equipment selection for the field, developing clinical protocols, ensuring a continuous quality improvement (CQI) program is in place, providing input on patient care, interfacing with the EMS systems and other health care agencies, acting as an EMS advocate in the community, and serving as the "medical conscience" of the EMS system. (pages 21–22)
4. a. Online medical control—Allows the paramedic immediate patient care resources. It allows the paramedic to transfer data immediately to the receiving facility for better patient care. (page 21)
   b. Protocols—Treatment plans for a specific illness or injury (eg, the patient with chest pain usually gets oxygen, acetylsalicylic acid [ASA], nitroglycerin, and sometimes morphine and metoprolol [Lopressor]). (page 21)
   c. Standing orders—Protocols that are written and signed by the medical director and outline specific directions, permissions, and sometimes publications (eg, the basic life support [BLS] care given to a patient with an allergic reaction, such as oxygen and epinephrine). (pages 21–22)

Chapter 2: Workforce Safety and Wellness

Matching

Part I

1. A (page 53)
2. B (page 53)
3. B (page 53)
4. A (page 53)
5. B (page 53)
6. A (page 53)
7. B (page 53)

Part II

1. B (page 56)
2. C (page 56)
3. A (page 56)

Part III

1. D (page 57)
2. F (page 46)
3. H (page 46)
4. J (page 63)
5. A (page 56)
6. C (page 56)
7. G (page 46)
8. I (page 46)
9. E (page 47)
10. B (page 46)

Multiple Choice

1. C (page 56)
2. D (page 57)
3. A (page 59)
4. C (page 51)
5. B (page 47)
6. D (page 56)
7. D (pages 55–56)
8. D (page 55)
9. A (page 56)
10. B (pages 58–59)

Fill in the Blank

1. a. projection (page 56)
   b. denial (page 56)
   c. conversion hysteria (page 57)
   d. displacement (page 56)
2. a. Take care of your own health. Get enough rest. Eat a balanced diet. Get regular physical exercise. Treat your body with respect (stop cigarettes and drugs). (page 60)
   b. Give yourself some "me" time every day.
   c. Learn how to relax.
   d. Do not make unreasonable demands on yourself.
   e. Do not make unreasonable demands on others.
   f. Stay in touch with your feelings.
   g. Learn techniques for managing stress while on duty.
   h. Debrief after tough calls.

Identify

1. Pertinent negatives (pages 58–60)
   a. Not sleeping
   b. Too much caffeine
   c. Not exercising
   d. Smoking
   e. Eating too much of the wrong foods
   f. Projecting his negative attitude
2. Stress reactions (page 56)
   a. Projection
   b. Anger

Ambulance Calls

1. a. This is a critical incident for all members of the team. This death of a child is particularly hard on John because he also has an infant boy. He is probably feeling that he is a bad paramedic because the child died, even though every effort was made during the resuscitation. This also might affect his feelings about being a father. (page 59)
   b. Paramedics are often under a lot of stress at their job. They can do several things to reduce stress and avoid burnout, such as get enough sleep, eat a balanced diet, and perform 30 minutes of aerobic activity three to four times a week. Avoid caffeine, smoking, and recreational drugs. Limit alcohol intake. Make sure you can devote some time during

each day to yourself, and learn to relax with hobbies and social activities. Don't make unreasonable demands on yourself or others. Share your stress by talking or crying. Always debrief after a tough call. (page 60)

2. a. You never want to just blurt out that you think the patient isn't going to make it. Tell the patient that his condition is serious but that you and the hospital team are going to do everything you can for him. Let him talk, and be sympathetic to anything he says. Remember, you might be the last to speak to him, so if he has dying words for his family, make sure to write them down. Make sure the doctor at the hospital has these words to give to the family when he breaks the news that their loved one has died. (pages 61–62)

b. Not all dying people will experience all five stages. They may not experience them "in order," either. Encourage the patient to talk about these feelings if possible. (page 61)

(1) Denial. The patient might say things like, "This can't happen to me."

(2) Anger. Anger might appear as blaming the paramedic, family, or even God. Anger can come in the form of yelling or physical outbursts.

(3) Bargaining. This can be a patient's way of praying: "Please just let me live long enough to see my family again." Patients may bargain with you, the doctor, and God.

(4) Depression. This is characterized by quiet time by the patient, crying, or perhaps physical contact with anyone close to the person, including you.

(5) Acceptance. The patient may leave the sorrow behind and reflect on his or her life. The patient might want to leave words for his or her family and to let them know that things will be okay. Usually, this is the hardest time for the family. The patient doesn't appear to be fighting for life, and that sometimes angers family members. Once again, anger is a stage of grief, and the family members will exhibit these feelings also.

True/False

1. F (page 39)
2. T (page 43)
3. F (page 44)
4. T (page 46)
5. T (page 50)
6. F (page 56)
7. F (page 57)
8. T (page 58)
9. T (page 61)
10. T (page 48)
11. F (page 47)
12. T (page 49)
13. F (page 42)
14. T (page 56)

Short Answer

1. a. Cold sweat
b. Pounding heart
c. Dry mouth
d. Feeling "energized" (page 55)

2. a. Let the family see the body.
b. Use the word *dead* instead of euphemisms for death (eg, "expired" or "passed away").
c. Let the family see your resuscitation efforts.
d. Give the family some time with the body.
e. Try to arrange for further support (eg, neighbors, clergy).
f. Accept the family's right to experience a variety of feelings. (page 62)

3. a. Anxiety
b. Blind panic
c. Depression
d. Overreaction
e. Conversion hysteria (page 57)

Problem Solving

1. a. 76
b. 220 – 46 = 174
c. 174 – 76 = 98 × 0.7 = 69
d. 69 + 76 = 145 (page 42)

Chapter 3: Public Health

Matching

Part I

1. P (page 74)
2. O (page 72)
3. N (page 83)
4. M (page 83)
5. L (page 81)
6. F (page 83)
7. E (page 83)
8. D (page 77)
9. C (page 72)
10. B (page 87)
11. A (page 83)
12. K (page 72)
13. J (page 72)
14. I (page 87)
15. H (page 81)
16. G (page 79)

Part II

(pages 77–79)

1. C
2. A
3. D
4. D
5. A
6. B
7. C
8. A
9. B
10. D

Multiple Choice

1. B (page 72)
2. B (page 72)
3. C (page 88)
4. A (pages 75–77)
5. C (page 81)
6. D (page 87)
7. C (page 74)
8. B (page 81)
9. C (page 81)
10. D (page 73)

Fill in the Blank

1. intervention (page 77)
2. intentional (page 72)
3. education; enforcement; engineering/environment; economic incentives (pages 77–79)
4. passive intervention (page 79)
5. heart disease, cancer, chronic lower airway disease, unintentional injuries, stroke (page 72)
6. process objective (page 87)
7. teachable moment (page 75)

Identify

1. Pertinent negatives: (page 78)
   a. Bathwater still standing
   b. Boiling water on stove
   c. Trampoline with no safety net
   d. Knitting needles and scissors left out

Ambulance Calls

1. a. Whenever you are entering a home with unknown scene factors, it is wise to call for law enforcement. As a result of not being able to gain entry, the officer has probable cause for breaking the window. This covers the paramedic for unlawful entry. This could also be a potential crime scene, so law enforcement is a must.
   b. When entering a home, you should always carry a radio to contact your team on the outside. A flashlight is also important because finding a light switch in the dark can be difficult. Pay attention to the broken glass from the window to prevent an injury to the person entering the home. An old blanket or tarp should be laid inside the window to prevent being cut by broken glass.
   c. The teachable moment here occurs after they determine the patient is okay and does not need to be transported. While waiting for the neighbor, Mary and Jake could talk to the patient about how and where to hide an outside key to the home and give the location to the lifeline personnel. Lifeline services could then let dispatch know where the key is hidden. Also, they could construct a list of neighbors with the key to the home. Finally, they could talk to the patient about always taking the cordless phone or cell phone with him into the bathroom or anytime he is away from a wall phone. (pages 75–77)

2. **a.** S: Simple. This display needs to be simple for the children to understand it.
   M: Measurable. They need to have a play cell phone for the children to practice calling. That way, they can see if their demonstration has helped the children understand.
   A: Accurate. All of the information given during the demonstration and during the practice session should be clear and accurate.
   R: Reportable. During the next year, the dispatch center will keep records on the children who use the 9-1-1 system. This allows the following years' programs to change if there is a need.
   T: Trackable. After the call, it is evident that the video helped Ryan. Once again, this should be reported, and the case should be kept on file. (page 88)
   b. This video took the scariness away for Ryan. He was able to realize that his mother would not wake up. When he was unable to rouse her, he remembered the 9-1-1 number to call for help. Good job, Larry and Courtney! Part of your job as a paramedic is to help members of the community help themselves.

True/False

1. F (page 81)
2. T (page 73)
3. T (page 84)
4. T (page 83)
5. F (page 72)
6. T (page 88)
7. T (pages 86–88)
8. F (page 88)
9. T (page 88)
10. F (pages 75–77)

Short Answer

1. *Primary injury prevention* is defined as keeping an injury from ever occurring. Example: Removal of small choking hazards, such as removal of buttons from a stuffed animal

   Secondary injury prevention is defined as reducing the effects of an injury that has already happened. Example: Airbags reduce the impact from the steering wheel during a motor vehicle crash. (page 81)
2. *Students should list three of the following:*
   a. EMS providers are widely distributed in a population.
   b. EMS providers reflect the composition of the community.
   c. In rural communities, EMS providers are sometimes the highest medically trained persons.
   d. EMS providers can reduce overall injuries as a result of intervention.
   e. EMS providers are high-profile role models.
   f. EMS providers are perceived as champions of their patients.
   g. EMS providers are welcomed by schools and organizations for their role in preventive programs.
   h. EMS providers are perceived as authorities on injuries and illness. (page 81)
3. **a.** Education: Education for the public to reduce injuries and illness (page 77)
   b. Enforcement: Laws to help curb destructive behaviors (page 79)
   c. Engineering/Environment: Changing the design of products or spaces to reduce injuries (page 79)
   d. Economic incentives: Monetary incentives to reinforce safe behavior (page 79)
4. **a.** Host: Child who drowns (page 84)
   b. Agent: Drowning (page 84)
   c. Environment: The swimming pool (page 84)

Fill in the Table

The Five Steps to Developing a Prevention Program (pages 86-88)
1. Conduct a community assessment.
2. Define the problem.
3. Set goals and objectives.
4. Plan and test interventions.
5. Implement and evaluate interventions.

Chapter 4: Medical, Legal, and Ethical Issues

Matching

Part I

1. A (page 109)
2. A (page 109)
3. B (page 109)
4. A (page 109)
5. A (page 109)
6. B (page 109)
7. B (pages 101–102)
8. C (pages 101–102)
9. A (pages 101–102)
10. D (pages 101–102)
11. M (pages 96–99)
12. E (pages 96–99)
13. UE (pages 96–99)
14. E (pages 96–99)
15. UE (pages 96–99)
16. M (pages 96–99)
17. UE (pages 96–99)
18. UE (pages 96–99)
19. M (pages 96–99)
20. UE (pages 96–99)

Part II

1. J (page 114)
2. H (page 112)
3. I (page 108)
4. G (page 104)
5. E (page 121)
6. C (page 103)
7. A (page 116)
8. D (page 100)
9. B (page 117)
10. F (pages 101–102)

Multiple Choice

1. B (page 101)
2. C (page 102)
3. D (pages 104–106)
4. A (pages 114–116)
5. D (page 116)
6. B (page 112)
7. C (page 100)
8. A (page 102)
9. C (page 112)
10. A (page 102)
11. B (page 97)
12. C (pages 119–120)
13. C (page 118)
14. A (page 117)
15. D (page 98)

Fill in the Blank

1. a. informed (page 109)
   b. custodial parent; legal guardian (page 112)
2. plaintiff; defendant (page 100)
3. scope of practice (page 104)
4. advance directive (page 117)
5. emancipated (page 112)
6. ethical; legal; falsification (page 99)

Identify

1. Chief complaints: Low blood glucose and unconsciousness. Blood glucose levels should be between 80 and 120 mg/dL. This patient's level was 42 mg/dL. He became unresponsive at the scene, which gives implied consent to treat him.
2. Vital signs: Oxygen saturation, 97%; respiration, 20 breaths/min; blood glucose, 42 mg/dL; blood pressure, 132/70 mm Hg; pulse, 96 beats/min; lung sounds, clear; skin, cool; pupils, sluggish. After IV and D_{50}, the scenario says vital signs were within normal limits, and blood glucose returned to a level of 118 mg/dL.
3. Pertinent negatives: What is *not* wrong with the patient? Look for why the patient became unresponsive. He did not choke, he is not hypoxic, and the medic cannot see any obvious trauma to his head. He has a strong pulse, so he is not in cardiac arrest. He also wakes up as soon as D_{50} is administered. This suggests that the most likely problem was the blood glucose levels. However, in calls involving a patient who becomes unresponsive, the medic should always complete a SAMPLE history before ending care and letting the patient sign off.

Ambulance Calls

1. a. Actions to take: The boy's injury is not life threatening, and it is not likely to be appreciably aggravated by waiting another hour or so. Tell the school authorities to keep trying to reach the boy's parents and call you back when they have gotten permission to have the boy treated.
   b. Provide treatment: This is a classic case of implied consent.
   c. Actions to take: Some people would argue that any person who attempts suicide is, by definition, not mentally competent and not able to give informed consent (or informed refusal). But you cannot depend on that argument to protect you from a charge of technical assault and battery if you touch the patient or false imprisonment if you take her to the hospital against her will. Ask the boyfriend if the patient is under psychiatric care; if so, perhaps her psychiatrist can be enlisted to help. In states where suicide is a felony, you can call the police for help. In any event, contact medical command for advice.

   d. Actions to take: The best thing to do in this situation is to call for police backup. In all probability, this patient will have to be forcibly restrained, and the police are the only people permitted to authorize that action.
   e. Provide treatment: This is a classic case of implied consent.
   f. Actions to take: This patient is probably having a heart attack and definitely needs to be in the hospital—but the only legal way to get him there is through patient, sympathetic persuasion. You will need to spend time talking with him, trying to understand his fears, and explaining to him the possible consequence of ignoring his symptoms. If he still refuses treatment and transport despite your best efforts at persuasion, you may not transport him against his will. Be sure to "leave the door open" so that he feels free to call you back later if he should change his mind. (pages 109–111)

2. Students should list three of the following:
   a. Oriented to person, place, and day
   b. Responds to questions appropriately
   c. Absence of signs of mental impairment from alcohol, drugs, head injury, and so on
   d. Evidence that the patient understands the nature of his condition
   e. Evidence that the patient can describe a reasonable plan for follow-up care
   f. Oxygen saturation levels within normal levels
   g. Blood glucose levels within normal limits (page 110)

True/False

1. F (page 102)
2. T (page 102)
3. T (page 103)
4. T (page 104)
5. F (page 121)
6. T (page 113)
7. F (page 118)
8. T (page 109)
9. F (page 112)
10. T (page 97)
11. F (page 96)
12. T (page 98)
13. T (page 98)
14. F (page 116)
15. T (page 119)
16. F (page 117)
17. T (page 118)
18. F (pages 119–120)
19. T (page 99)
20. F (page 120)

Short Answer

1. Students should list three of the following: (page 108)
   a. Obvious or suspected homicide
   b. Obvious or suspected suicide
   c. Any other violent or sudden, unexpected death
   d. Death of a prison inmate

2. Good Samaritan laws were written to provide immunity from liability to anyone who stops to help at the scene of an emergency. The care provided is free of charge. Paramedics have a legal duty to act, which is not covered by the Good Samaritan laws. (page 121)

3. a. That harm resulted (page 113)
   b. That the paramedic had a duty to act (page 113)
   c. That there was a breach of that duty (page 113)
   d. That the failure to act appropriately was the proximate cause of the plaintiff's injury (page 113)

4. Students should list four of the following: (page 108)
   a. Child abuse
   b. Elder abuse
   c. Injury sustained during commission of a felony
   d. Drug-related injuries
   e. Childbirth occurring outside a medical facility
   f. Rape
   g. Animal bites
   h. Certain communicable diseases
   i. Domestic violence

5. a. MOLST stands for Medical Orders for Life-Sustaining Treatment. Although similar to a DNR, the MOLST is more expansive and designed for both prehospital providers and health care providers. (page 120)
   b. Check with your instructor or medical director to see whether MOLST is used in your state.

6. Each person will have a private code of right and wrong. The paramedic's guiding principle, however it is worded, should be based on overriding concern for the welfare of the patient. (pages 97–99)

7. This is a very hard situation to handle. The first thing that should be done is to speak directly to the senior paramedic about how offensive his or her remarks are. If the remarks continue, it would be necessary to address this issue with the chain of command. (page 99)
8. When responding to code and presented with a DNR order, you must begin to verify the order quickly. Your local protocols will tell you everything you should look for. Things that should appear on every order include the name of the patient (confirm with the person's ID that this is the right patient), the original signatures of the patient and the doctor, and dates. Your online medical director will also be able to help you with any questions. (page 119)

Chapter 5: Communications

Matching

Part I

(page 152)

1. O
2. C
3. C
4. C
5. O
6. C
7. C
8. O
9. C
10. C

Part II

1. H (page 139)
2. G (page 140)
3. K (page 135)
4. L (page 140)
5. I (page 141)
6. M (pages 143–144)
7. J (page 140)
8. N (page 141)
9. A (page 139)
10. C (page 137)
11. F (page 140)
12. E (page 157)
13. B (page 143)
14. D (page 136)

Part III

1. (page 148)
   (1) F: The patient is a 60-year-old woman who collapsed in the bathroom while sitting on the toilet.
   (2) J: She was apparently well until this morning.
   (3) D: Her daughter says that the patient complained of a severe headache before she collapsed.
   (4) B: The patient has a history of high blood pressure. (In fact, this is really part of the history of the present illness, if you know what the patient's problem is! She seems to have had a hemorrhagic stroke, so her high blood pressure is one of the predisposing factors.)
   (5) L: She was hospitalized 6 years ago for an AMI.
   (6) H: The patient's medications include nitroglycerin and Aldomet (methyldopa).
   (7) E: The patient was still responsive when we arrived, but she rapidly became unresponsive.
   (8) A: Pulse is 50 beats/min and regular, respirations are 36 breaths/min and deep, blood pressure is 180/126 mm Hg, and Spo_2 is 94%.
   (9) I: Her left pupil is larger than the right and does not react to light.
   (10) K: Her neck is somewhat stiff.
   (11) C: The deep tendon reflexes are hyperactive.
   (12) G: We are administering oxygen at 4 L/min by nasal cannula.

Multiple Choice

1. C (pages 145–146)
2. C (pages 137–138)
3. D (page 144)
4. C (page 140)
5. D (page 135)
6. A (page 151)
7. C (page 151)
8. B (page 154)
9. D (page 151)
10. C (page 153)
11. A (page 151)
12. B (page 152)
13. D (pages 157–158)
14. B (pages 157–158)

Fill in the Blank

The order of answers given will vary for 1–5.

1. person calling for help; the dispatcher; landline (telephone) (pages 135–137)
2. dispatcher; the paramedics or other rescuers; a two-way radio (although a pager will suffice for dispatch) (page 137)
3. dispatcher; other agencies, such as police, fire, utility companies, and civil defense; landline (telephone) (page 137)
4. paramedic; medical command; radio or cellular telephone (page 148)
5. paramedic; the receiving hospital; radio or cellular telephone (page 139)
6. communication (page 134)
7. calm (page 151)
8. open-ended question (page 152)
9. neutral (page 154)
10. police (page 155)

11. toys (page 156)
12. cultural competence (page 157)

Identify

1. Chief complaint: Chest pain
2. History of the present illness: The pain was "squeezing" in character, 6 out of 10 in severity, radiated to the left shoulder and jaw, and had been present for 2 hours. The pain was accompanied by increasing difficulty in breathing.
3. Other medical history: He is known to have heart disease.
4. General appearance: The patient was sitting bolt upright; he appeared alert and apprehensive and was in moderate respiratory distress, breathing shallowly at 30 breaths/min.
5. Vital signs: Respiratory rate, 30 breaths/min; pulse, 130 beats/min, weak and regular; BP, 200/90 mm Hg; and Spo_2, 94%.
6. Physical exam: His neck veins were distended to the angle of the jaw at 45°. Wet crackles were heard at both lung bases, and auscultation of the heart revealed a gallop rhythm. The abdomen was not distended. There was a 1+ presacral and ankle edema.
7. Treatment given: The patient was given oxygen by non-rebreathing mask at 12 L /min, had a 12-lead ECG taken, had an IV of normal saline, and was transported to the regional cardiac care center in semi-Fowler position.
8. Pertinent negatives: The abdomen was not distended; the patient denied nausea, vomiting, sweating, or palpitations.

Ambulance Calls

Part I

1. Just about everything was wrong with the transmission quoted!
   a. The unit being called should be mentioned first. So, it should have been, "County Hospital, Medic 12."
   b. It was unnecessarily wordy, wasting a lot of time (eg, "Be advised that . . ."; "Please 10-9 your message").
   c. The patient's name was mentioned on the air, along with an abbreviation that a layperson could easily misunderstand. To compound the offense, the paramedic spelled out the initials of the chief complaint using a nonstandard phonetic alphabet, using insulting words to do so.
   d. The paramedic was apparently trying to be funny. He may have thought the whole thing was a laugh a minute, but Maggie Jones might be forgiven if she didn't think so. Making insulting references to the patient ("well endowed with adipose tissue") or to the other party on the radio ("Are you deaf or something?") is highly unprofessional and simply reflects on the immaturity of the speaker.
   e. The report of the patient's findings was not given in any sort of standard format. As a result, the people at County Hospital had to waste a lot of time trying to drag the important information out of the paramedics.
   f. Words that are poorly heard by radio, such as "yes," were used.
   g. The paramedic did not repeat back the medication orders to make sure he had received them correctly.
   h. The radio was used for nonmedical communications ("Pop a few doughnuts into the microwave").
2. The best way to find out just how difficult the dispatcher's job can be is to step into that job for a few hours. The information you need to try to obtain from the hysterical caller reporting a crash is as follows:
   - What is the exact location of the incident?
   - What is the telephone number from which the caller is phoning?
   - At this point, dispatch the (first) ambulance. ("Unspecified accident at such-and-such address. Details will follow.")
   - What is the nature of the incident (eg, explosion, road crash, train derailment, building collapse)?
   - How many victims are there?
   - Are there any hazards at the scene, specifically:
     (a) Traffic hazards
     (b) Fire
     (c) Spills
     (d) Downed electrical wires
   - If it is a *transport* collision (motor vehicles, train):
     (a) How many vehicles are involved?
     (b) Is it possible to determine what cargoes the vehicles are carrying?

     Contact the responding vehicle with additional information. Dispatch additional vehicles and contact other agencies as needed.

Part II

1. There is no single correct answer to the dilemma posed in this question: How do you reply to a patient when he asks, "Am I going to die?" However, there are some general guidelines:
   - Do not try to minimize the seriousness of the patient's situation. Most patients who are near death *know* at least that they are in serious condition. If you are merrily chirping, "There, there, everything is going to be fine," the patient will simply assume that (a) you don't understand the situation, or (b) it is forbidden for him to speak to you honestly about his fears. Those are *not* the messages you want to convey!
   - Do not, however, take away all hope. As long as the patient is alive, there is hope for him.
   - In the situation described, you might say something like this: "Sir, your situation is very serious, but we have an excellent rescue team here, with the best medical backup, and we're going to do everything we can to save your life." Also let the patient know that you are willing to listen to what he has to say, to transmit any messages he has for other people, and so forth.
2. In the case of a patient with diabetes, you have to remember that the patient can become violent. You should begin to talk calmly to the patient. Tell her your name, and reassure her that you are there to help her. Take a nonaggressive stance, but be wary of the patient. Explain to the patient that you want to test her blood glucose level, start an IV, and give her glucose through the IV. If the patient is fighting you, you may need to use law enforcement to subdue the patient. As soon as you get the patient's glucose levels to normal, she will calm down and thank you.
3. **a.** You should have asked if anyone able to translate for the patient and the family was available in the area.
   b. Explain to the translator why the candles must be blown out before using the oxygen. You may ask for permission first; if it is not granted, move the woman before applying the oxygen.
   c. The student's "rock out" sign has made her feel that the devil has just arrived in her bedroom, and because you used the red pen to write her name, she now feels you are both associated with the devil.
   d. Your translator can help keep the woman and her family calm and make your transition to her caregiver much easier. You should have the translator explain *everything* that you are doing *before* you do it. Most important is to take the translator to the hospital with you to continue care and keep the patient calm on the way to the hospital. (pages 157–160)

True/False

1. T (pages 139, 141)
2. T (page 143)
3. F (page 139)
4. T (page 135)
5. F (page 146)
6. T (page 149)
7. F (page 136)
8. T (page 153)
9. T (page 153)
10. F (page 154)
11. F (page 151)
12. T (page 151)
13. T (page 155)
14. F (page 154)
15. T (page 157)

Short Answer

1. Most radio communications systems require a basic minimum of components. (pages 137–138)

Component	Function
Base station	Dispatch and coordination area
Mobile transceiver	Communications with ambulances
Portable transceiver	Communications with paramedics when they are out of their vehicle
Repeater	To extend the range of low-power transceivers
Remote consoles in hospitals	To allow communications with receiving hospitals
Landline/cellular backup	To extend the user network

2. The job of the dispatcher (EMD) includes the following duties. *Students should list four of the following:* (pages 136–138)
   a. Extracting information from panicky callers
   b. Directing the right emergency vehicle to the right address
   c. Giving advice and first-aid instructions by telephone to distraught people
   d. Coordinating the response of different agencies to an emergency
   e. Monitoring field communications to determine if help is needed
   f. Keeping written records of data such as response times.

3. An EMS communications system has to provide for at least the following linkages (*students will draw a diagram*): (pages 135–138)
   a. Citizen to dispatch center
   b. Dispatch center to ambulances
   c. Dispatch center to hospitals
   d. Dispatch center to medical control
   e. Dispatch center to other services
   f. Ambulance to hospitals
   g. Paramedic to medical control
4. Telemetry dispatcher: Go ahead, Medic 785, you are clear to transmit with MD 802 from Saint Peter's Hospital on Med channel 2.

   Medic 785: MD 802, this is Medic 785 on Med 2. How do you read?

   MD 802: Medic 785, this is MD 802. You are loud and clear; proceed with your transmission.

   Medic 785: I am treating a 58-year-old man who is in moderate distress with a chief complaint of chest pain. He states it came on suddenly while shoveling snow. He describes the pain as crushing under his breastbone and radiating down his left arm. The pain is a 10 on 10, and he has had the pain for about 15 minutes. The patient states he has no prior history and denies any shortness of breath. He has an allergy to Novocain and takes three aspirins daily as well as 10 mg of Lipitor. He states he has a history of hypertension and high cholesterol with CAD in his family. His last oral intake was lunch 3 hours ago and the 162 mg of chewable aspirin the dispatcher advised him to take prior to our arrival. The events leading up to the incident involved shoveling heavy snow.

   Physical exam reveals some crackles at the bases of both lungs, not JVD or pedal edema. His vital signs are respirations of 20 breaths/min and regular; pulse of 110 beats/min, strong and regular; and a BP of 146/82 mm Hg. His oxygen saturation is 96% on a non-rebreathing mask, and his ECG is sinus tachycardia with no ectopy, but the 12-lead shows ST-segment elevation in V_3 and V_4 (possible anterior wall MI).

   We are treating him as a rule-out MI and have administered morphine and oxygen. Nitroglycerin and aspirin were self-administered. We are currently transporting, and our plan is to continue monitoring him and go through the rest of the fibrinolytic checklist. What's your pleasure on 5 mg of metoprolol?

   MD 802: Medic 785, go ahead with the metoprolol, and I will alert the cath lab staff right away.

   Medic 785: Received. Our ETA is 20 minutes.

Fill in the Table

(page 145)

A	Alpha	J	Juliette	S	Sierra
B	Bravo	K	Kilo	T	Tango
C	Charlie	L	Lima	U	Uniform
D	Delta	M	Mike	V	Victor
E	Echo	N	November	W	Whiskey
F	Foxtrot	O	Oscar	X	X-ray
G	Golf	P	Papa	Y	Yankee
H	Hotel	Q	Quebec	Z	Zebra
I	India	R	Romeo		

Chapter 6: Documentation

Matching

Part I

(pages 179–181)

1. F
2. C
3. B
4. E
5. G
6. A
7. F
8. D
9. H
10. B
11. E
12. F
13. F
14. C
15. B
16. F
17. E
18. D
19. C
20. D
21. B
22. G
23. B
24. H
25. B
26. F

27. In rearranging the sentences into the correct sequence for presentation, there may be some variation in the order of sentences within a given category (eg, the sentences that make up the "history of the present illness," which you labeled B). All sentences from category B should precede those from category C, which should precede those from category D, and so forth. (pages 179–181)

HISTORY

A. Chief Complaint
(1) 6: The patient is a 51-year-old man with chest pain.

B. History of the Present Illness
(2) 3: The pain came on while he was watching television.
(3) 25: He describes the pain as squeezing.
(4) 23: The pain radiates down his left arm.
(5) 10: Nothing seemed to make the pain better or worse.
(6) 15: He also felt nauseated.
(7) 21: He denies any shortness of breath.

C. Other Medical History
(8) 19: He is under the care of Dr. Tums for an ulcer.
(9) 14: The patient takes alumina/magnesia (Maalox) and cimetidine (Tagamet) regularly.
(10) 2: The patient is allergic to penicillin.

PHYSICAL ASSESSMENT

D. General Appearance
(11) 18: He was sitting in a chair and appeared to be frightened.
(12) 20: He was alert and oriented to person, place, and day.
(13) 8: His skin was pale, cold, and sweaty (diaphoretic).

E. Vital Signs
(14) 11: The pulse was 52 beats/min and full, with an occasional premature beat.
(15) 17: His respirations were 20 breaths/min and unlabored.
(16) 4: The blood pressure was 190/110 mm Hg.

F. Physical Examination
(17) 13: There was no cyanosis of the lips.
(18) 12: The neck veins were not distended.
(19) 7: The chest was clear.
(20) 26: Lung sounds were clear bilaterally.
(21) 16: His abdomen was soft and nontender.
(22) 1: There was no pedal edema.

MANAGEMENT
(23) 5: He was given supplemental oxygen by non-rebreathing mask at 12 L /min.
(24) 2: An 18-gauge IV was started with normal saline at TKO rate.

CONDITION DURING TRANSPORT
(25) 9: The patient was transported in semi-Fowler position.
(26) 24: The blood pressure came down to 170/90 mm Hg during transport.

Part II

(pages 179–181)

1. F
2. E
3. B
4. C, B
5. F
6. D
7. G
8. A
9. E
10. D
11. G
12. B
13. F
14. G
15. F
16. H
17. F
18. F
19. F

20. The following shows the sentences rearranged into the correct sequence for documentation on the PCR:

HISTORY

A. Chief Complaint
(1) 35: The patient is a middle-aged man who was struck by a car while crossing the street.

B. History of the Present Illness
(2) 39: He apparently staggered into the street without looking, as if he were drunk.
(3) 30: Bystanders state, "The car that hit him was traveling very fast."
(4) 31: His medical ID that says he is a diabetic.

C. Other Medical History
(Apparently, none is available; the medical ID bracelet could be listed here.)

PHYSICAL ASSESSMENT

D. General Appearance
(5) 37: The patient was unconscious and did not withdraw from painful stimuli.
(6) 33: His skin is pale, cool, and moist.

E. Vital Signs
(7) 29: The pulse was 92 beats/min, somewhat weak, and regular.
(8) 36: Respirations were 30 breaths/min, deep, and noisy; blood pressure was 160/110 mm Hg.

F. Physical Examination
(9) 32: There is a bruise on the left forehead.
(10) 44: There was no blood or fluid draining from his nose or ears.
(11) 42: The pupils were equal, midposition, and reactive to light.
(12) 40: Chest wall was stable, and breath sounds were equal bilaterally.
(13) 45: His abdomen was soft.
(14) 28: The right leg was severely angulated at the midfemur.
(15) 46: The dorsalis pedis pulses were equal.

G. Management
(16) 38: An OPA was inserted, and supplemental oxygen was given by non-rebreathing mask at 12 L /min.
(17) 41: We put the right leg in a traction splint.
(18) 34: He was secured to a scoop stretcher.

H. Condition During Transport
(19) 43: There was no change in his condition during transport.

Part III

1. In taking a history and carrying out a physical examination, you go to a lot of trouble to obtain important information about the patient. It would be a shame if that information were lost because you could not document it in an order that other health care providers could easily process. (pages 179–181)

AGE, SEX, AND CHIEF COMPLAINT
(1) F: The patient is a 60-year-old woman who collapsed in the bathroom while sitting on the toilet.

A. History of the Present Illness
(2) J: She was apparently well until this morning.
(3) D: Her daughter says the patient complained of a severe headache before she collapsed.

B. Past Medical History
(4) B: The patient has a history of high blood pressure. (In fact, this is really part of the history of the present illness, if you know what the patient's problem is! She seems to have had a hemorrhagic stroke, so her high blood pressure is one of the predisposing factors.)
(5) L: She was hospitalized 6 years ago for an AMI.
(6) H: The patient's medications include nitroglycerin and methyldopa (Aldomet).

PHYSICAL ASSESSMENT

C. State of Consciousness

(7) E: The patient was still conscious when we arrived, but she rapidly lost consciousness.

D. Vital Signs

(8) A: Pulse is 50 beats/min and regular, respirations are 36 breaths/min and deep, and blood pressure is 180/126 mm Hg.

E. Physical Exam

(9) I: Her left pupil is larger than the right and does not react to light.

(10) K: Her neck is somewhat stiff.

(11) C: The deep tendon reflexes are hyperactive.

MANAGEMENT SO FAR

(12) G: We are administering oxygen at 12 L/min by non-rebreathing mask.

Multiple Choice

1. C (page 171)
2. B (page 173)
3. A (page 178)
4. C (pages 178–179)
5. B (page 179)
6. B (page 170)
7. A (pages 171–172)
8. C (page 179)
9. C (pages 174–175)
10. C (page 184)

Fill in the Blank

How to Write a Narrative

(pages 179–181)

Topic	Items to Include
1. Standard precautions	State which precautions you used and why.
2. Scene safety	Did you have to make your scene safe? If so, then state what you did and why you did it. Did this step create a delay of patient care?
3. MOI/NOI	Simply state. For example, "motor vehicle crash" or "difficulty breathing."
4. Number of patients	Record only when more than one patient is present. For example, "This is patient 2 of 3."
5. Additional resources	Did you call for help? If so, then state why, at what time, and at what time the help arrived. Was transport delayed?
6. Cervical spine	State whether you applied manual stabilization or full spinal immobilization. You may want to include the reason why. For example, "Because of the significant MOI. . ."
7. Initial general impression	Simply state, if not already documented on the PCR.
8. LOC	Report LOC, any changes in LOC, and at what time changes occurred.
9. Chief complaint	Note and quote pertinent statements made by the patient and/or bystanders, including any pertinent negatives. For example, "Patient denies chest pain. . ."
10. Life threats	List all interventions and how the patient responded. For example, "Assisted ventilations with oxygen (15 L/min) at 20 breaths/min, with no change in LOC."
11. ABCDE	Document what you found and any interventions performed.
12. Oxygen	Record whether you administered oxygen, how you applied it, and how much you administered.
13. Primary survey, patient history, secondary assessment, or reassessment	State the type of assessment you used and any pertinent findings. For example, "Secondary assessment revealed unequal pupils, crepitus to right ribs, and an apparent closed fracture of the left tibia." Note the time each assessment was made and the findings.
14. SAMPLE/OPQRST	Note and quote any pertinent answers.
15. Vital signs	Record the times when you took the patient's vital signs and the findings. (Your service may want you to record vital signs in the narrative portion, as well as other places on the PCR.)
16. Medical direction	Quote any orders to you by medical control, and state who gave them.
17. Management of secondary injuries/treat for shock	Report all interventions, at what time they were completed, and how the patient responded.

Identify

1. Chief complaint: Chest pain
2. History of the present illness: The pain was described as "pressure in the center of the chest with left arm numbness" and had been present for 30 minutes. The pain was accompanied by difficulty in breathing.
3. Other medical history: She is known to have a history of angina and asthma.
4. General appearance: The patient was sitting bolt upright; she appeared alert and apprehensive and was in moderate respiratory distress, breathing shallowly at 26 breaths/min.
5. Vital signs: Respiratory rate, 26 breaths/min; pulse, 136 beats/min, weak and regular; blood pressure, 180/80 mm Hg; and Spo_2, 95%.
6. Physical exam: Her neck veins were distended to the angle of the jaw at 45°. Rales were heard at both lung bases, and auscultation of the heart revealed a gallop rhythm. The abdomen was not distended.
7. Management: The patient was given oxygen by non-rebreathing mask at 12 L /min; a 12-lead ECG was acquired and transmitted and shows a STEMI; an IV of normal saline was started at TKO rate; and 5 mg of morphine, 324 mg of ASA, and nitroglycerin have been administered. She was transported to St. Joseph's Hospital cath lab in semi-Fowler position.
8. Pertinent negatives: The abdomen was not distended; the patient denied vomiting.

True/False

1. F (page 186)
2. F (page 185)
3. T (page 172)
4. T (page 182)
5. T (page 185)
6. F (page 172)
7. T (page 186)
8. T (page 179)
9. T (page 170)
10. F (page 185)

Short Answer

1. a. Besides the standard information regarding the patient's medical history and physical findings, the trip sheet (PCR) should contain a record of the times (time the call was received, time the ambulance departed, time the ambulance reached the scene, and so on). (page 173)
   b. Such a record is important to enable evaluation of such things as response times or how much time is being spent at the scene. (pages 171–172)
2. Two reasons for making sure that your PCRs are accurate and complete are as follows:
   a. For the benefit of the patient, whose subsequent care may depend on the information that you have (or have not) provided.
   b. For your own benefit, if the case should ever become a subject of court proceedings. The trip sheet reflects on the person who wrote it. If your PCR is sloppy and incomplete, a court would not be unjustified in wondering whether the care you gave the patient was also sloppy and incomplete. (pages 183–184)
3. a. Number of patients: Record only when more than one patient is present (eg, "This is patient 2 of 3").
   b. Standard precautions: Were standard precautions initiated? If so, state which precautions you used and why.
   c. MOI/NOI: Simply state. For example, "motor vehicle crash" or "difficulty breathing."
   d. Oxygen: Record if oxygen was used, how it was applied, and how much was administered. (page 180)

Complete the Patient Care Report (PCR)

Show your completed PCR to your paramedic instructor, and ask for feedback on how well you recorded the case you were given.

Chapter 7: Medical Terminology

Matching

Part I

1. S (page 203)
2. Q (page 203)
3. O (page 202)
4. M (page 199)
5. K (page 198)
6. I (page 196)
7. T (page 204)
8. R (page 193)
9. N (page 199)
10. P (page 202)
11. L (page 204)
12. J (page 196)
13. H (page 204)
14. F (page 193)
15. D (page 203)
16. B (page 203)
17. G (page 203)
18. E (page 199)
19. C (page 198)
20. A (page 203)

Part II

1. S (page 204)
2. Q (page 203)
3. O (page 203)
4. T (page 206)
5. R (page 194)
6. P (page 203)
7. N (page 199)
8. L (page 199)
9. J (page 201)
10. H (page 204)
11. F (page 204)
12. D (page 199)
13. B (page 206)
14. A (page 203)
15. C (page 193)
16. E (page 204)
17. G (page 201)
18. I (page 204)
19. K (page 199)
20. M (page 201)

Multiple Choice

1. C (page 192)
2. B (page 193)
3. C (page 194)
4. B (page 194)
5. D (page 196)
6. B (page 196)
7. C (page 197)
8. B (page 199)
9. D (page 200)
10. C (page 200)
11. B (page 200)
12. A (page 201)
13. D (page 202)
14. B (page 201)
15. B (page 208)

Fill in the Blank

1. sac; pericardium (page 206)
2. transvaginal; across (page 206)
3. infrathoracic; bottom (page 206)
4. uterus; ectopic (page 206)
5. woman; first (page 196)
6. five; five (page 196)
7. cirrhosis; skin (page 197)
8. red; oxygen; erythrocyte (page 197)
9. plane; transverse (page 199)
10. muscle; shoulder (page 200)

True/False

1. T (page 200)
2. T (page 200)
3. F (page 200)
4. F (page 200)
5. T (page 200)
6. T (page 200)
7. F (page 201)
8. T (page 201)
9. F (page 201)
10. T (page 201)
11. T (page 203)
12. T (page 198)
13. F (page 203)
14. F (page 204)
15. T (page 204)

Section 2: The Human Body and Human Systems

Chapter 8: Anatomy and Physiology

Matching

Part I

1. G (page 240)
2. F (page 239)
3. D (page 284)
4. E (page 290)
5. A (page 337)
6. B (page 356)
7. C (page 320)
8. T (page 239)
9. S (page 360)
10. H (page 281)
11. I (page 290)
12. L (page 329)
13. K (page 316)
14. J (page 249)
15. R (page 388)
16. Q (page 240)
17. O (page 342)
18. P (page 330)
19. N (page 247)
20. M (page 310)

Part II

1. P (page 317)
2. Q (page 335)
3. O (page 294)
4. L (page 388)
5. N (page 278)
6. M (page 266)
7. T (page 294)
8. S (page 258)
9. R (page 297)
10. K (page 343)
11. J (page 343)
12. B (page 324)
13. A (page 280)
14. F (page 319)
15. E (page 266)
16. D (page 339)
17. C (page 281)
18. I (page 278)
19. H (page 320)
20. G (page 359)

Part III

1. O (page 258)
2. M (page 335)
3. L (page 233)
4. N (page 338)
5. K (page 253)
6. I (page 239)
7. H (page 296)
8. J (page 338)
9. T (page 253)
10. S (page 359)
11. R (page 287)
12. Q (page 322)
13. P (page 268)
14. A (page 290)
15. B (page 306)
16. F (page 300)
17. G (page 249)
18. D (page 267)
19. C (page 280)
20. E (page 340)

Part IV

(pages 253–254)

1. H
2. D
3. I
4. G
5. B
6. C
7. E
8. A
9. F

Multiple Choice

1. D (page 243)
2. B (page 250)
3. C (page 270)
4. C (page 384)
5. B (page 281)
6. D (page 290)
7. C (page 288)
8. A (page 288)
9. C (page 339)
10. D (page 334)
11. B (page 345)
12. A (page 351)
13. D (page 333)
14. B (page 334)
15. B (page 299)
16. D (page 300)
17. D (page 309)
18. B (page 309)
19. B (page 309)
20. B (page 321)

Fill in the Blank

1. liver; gallbladder; bile (pages 380–381)
2. small intestine; large intestine; colon (pages 379–380)
3. endocrine; hormones; endocrine; exocrine (page 323)
4. growth; thyroid; luteinizing; oxytocin; contract (page 327)
5. ovaries; fallopian tubes; placenta; vagina; labia majora; labia minora; vestibule (page 397)

Labeling

1. **Bones of the skull** (page 274, Figure 8-31)
   - **A.** Frontal bone
   - **B.** Orbit
   - **C.** Nasal bone
   - **D.** Zygoma
   - **E.** Maxilla
   - **F.** Mandible
   - **G.** Parietal bone

- **H.** Temporal bone
- **I.** External auditory meatus
- **J.** Mastoid process
- **K.** Temporomandibular joint
- **L.** Cervical vertebrae

2. Lower extremity (page 284, Figure 8-46)

- **A.** Pelvis
- **B.** Femoral head
- **C.** Greater trochanter
- **D.** Lesser trochanter
- **E.** Femur
- **F.** Patella
- **G.** Fibula
- **H.** Tibia
- **I.** Tarsals
- **J.** Metatarsals
- **K.** Phalanges

3. Respiratory system (page 356, Figure 8-106)

- **A.** Nasal air passage
- **B.** Mouth
- **C.** Nasopharynx
- **D.** Oropharynx
- **E.** Pharynx
- **F.** Epiglottis
- **G.** Larynx
- **H.** Apex of the lung
- **I.** Trachea
- **J.** Bronchioles
- **K.** Main bronchus
- **L.** Base of the lung
- **M.** Diaphragm
- **N.** Carina

True/False

1. T (page 314)
2. T (page 314)
3. T (page 314)
4. F (page 314)
5. F (page 314)
6. F (page 314)
7. F (page 314)
8. T (page 314)
9. T (page 314)
10. F (page 314)
11. T (page 282)
12. F (page 282)
13. T (pages 282–283)
14. T (page 289)
15. F (page 302)

Chapter 9: Pathophysiology

Matching

Part I

1. Q (page 446)
2. R (page 451)
3. S (page 457)
4. T (page 456)
5. I (page 437)
6. J (pages 450–451)
7. K (page 441)
8. L (page 441)
9. M (page 433)
10. N (page 457)
11. P (page 420)
12. O (page 457)
13. A (page 426)
14. E (page 428)
15. D (page 448)
16. C (page 448)
17. B (page 441)
18. F (page 426)
19. G (page 437)
20. H (page 451)

Part II

1. G (page 447)
2. F (page 447)
3. E (page 448)
4. D (page 440)
5. C (page 435)
6. T (page 460)
7. S (page 443)
8. R (page 442)
9. Q (page 431)
10. L (page 447)
11. K (page 421)
12. J (page 420)
13. I (page 437)
14. H (page 448)
15. P (page 431)
16. O (page 466)
17. N (page 429)
18. M (page 447)
19. A (page 427)
20. B (page 445)

Part III

1. H (page 454)
2. G (page 439)
3. F (page 439)
4. E (page 437)
5. D (page 467)
6. T (page 432)
7. S (page 428)
8. R (page 447)
9. Q (page 428)
10. P (page 428)
11. O (page 451)
12. A (page 422)
13. B (page 434)
14. C (page 424)
15. I (page 442)
16. J (page 444)
17. K (page 456)
18. N (page 448)
19. M (page 450)
20. L (page 446)

Multiple Choice

1. B (page 427)
2. A (page 420)
3. C (page 422)
4. B (page 456)
5. B (page 425)
6. D (page 458)
7. D (page 460)
8. B (page 426)
9. C (page 435)
10. C (page 433)
11. D (page 462)
12. C (page 430)
13. B (page 428)
14. A (page 423)
15. C (page 421)

Fill in the Blank

1. oxygen; nutrients; removal; tissues; circulatory (page 434)
2. shock; heart; blood; oxygen (page 435)
3. shock; flow; blocked (page 435)
4. hypovolemic; exogenous; fluid (page 437)
5. vasodilator; released; allergen (page 437)
6. Hyperkalemia (page 423)
7. buffers (page 426)
8. apoptosis (page 433)
9. Multiple organ dysfunction syndrome (page 438)
10. Endotoxins (page 431)

Labeling

1. **Type I allergic reaction** (page 452, Figure 9-18)
   - **A.** Allergen
   - **B.** Plasma
   - **C.** Antibodies
   - **D.** Mast cells
   - **E.** IgE
   - **F.** Histamine
   - **G.** Dilation
   - **H.** Mucus
   - **I.** Contraction
   - **J.** Smooth

Identify

1. Chief complaint: Can't breathe
2. Vital signs: Respirations are 28 breaths/min and shallow. Pulse is 90 beats/min, with occasional irregular beats. BP is 160/90 mm Hg. Oxygen saturation is 90%, and skin is warm and moist.
3. Pertinent patient history: COPD, fever, coughing with bloody sputum
4. Presumptive diagnosis: Acute exacerbation of COPD

Ambulance Calls

1. a. Based on the ACE inhibitor and the peaked T wave, this patient is likely hyperkalemic, having an elevated potassium level.
   b. The immediate treatment is to contact medical control to discuss administering calcium chloride.
2. a. Crohn disease affects the gastrointestinal system. It is a chronic inflammatory condition that affects the colon and/or the terminal part of the small intestine.
   b. Symptoms include diarrhea, abdominal pain, nausea, fever, weakness, and weight loss. (page 463)
3. Patients with Alzheimer disease might have memory loss and be disoriented to time and day in the early stages. In later stages, they may exhibit restlessness and agitation. In the final stages of the disease, they may be unable to communicate, may experience urinary and fecal incontinence, and possibly may have seizures. (page 464)

True/False

1. T (page 440)
2. F (page 440)
3. F (page 441)
4. F (page 441)
5. T (page 445)
6. F (page 456)
7. F (page 437)
8. T (page 441)
9. T (page 453)
10. T (page 439)
11. F (page 453)
12. T (page 461)
13. T (page 461)
14. F (page 458)
15. T (page 462)

Short Answer

1. a. Inhalants
   b. Food
   c. Drugs
   d. Infectious agents
   e. Contactants
   f. Physical agents (page 453)
2. *Students should provide five of the following:*
   a. Hypoxic injury
   b. Ischemia
   c. Chemical injury
   d. Infectious injury
   e. Immunologic injury
   f. Physical damage
   g. Inflammatory injury (page 429)
3. a. Emphysema
   b. Chronic bronchitis
   c. Acute bronchitis
   d. Sinusitis
   e. Laryngitis
   f. Pneumonia
   g. Asthma (page 457)
4. a. Exercise-induced syncope
   b. Syncope associated with chest pain
   c. History of syncope in a close family member (ie, parent, sibling, child)
   d. Syncope associated with startle, such as the response to a loud noise (pages 460–461)

5. a. Margination
   b. Activation
   c. Adhesion
   d. Transmigration (diapedesis)
   e. Chemotaxis (pages 447–448)
6. a. Alarm
   b. Resistance
   c. Exhaustion (pages 466–467)

Fill in the Table

(page 435)

Signs and Symptoms of Compensated and Decompensated Hypoperfusion	
Compensated	**Decompensated**
Agitation, anxiety, restlessness	Altered mental status (verbal to unresponsive)
Sense of impending doom	**Hypotension**
Weak, rapid (thready) pulse	**Labored or irregular breathing**
Clammy (cool, moist) skin	Thready or absent peripheral pulses
Pallor with cyanotic lips	Ashen, mottled, or cyanotic skin
Shortness of breath	**Dilated pupils**
Nausea, vomiting	**Diminished urine output (oliguria)**
Delayed capillary refill time in infants and children	Impending cardiac arrest
Thirst	
Normal BP	

Chapter 10: Life Span Development

Matching

Part I

1. O (page 477)
2. P (page 488)
3. Q (page 488)
4. T (page 487)
5. S (page 487)
6. R (page 486)
7. F (page 484)
8. G (page 479)
9. H (page 480)
10. N (page 490)
11. M (page 479)
12. L (page 479)
13. A (page 485)
14. B (page 488)
15. C (pages 480–481)
16. J (page 481)
17. I (page 485)
18. K (page 487)
19. E (page 484)
20. D (page 488)

Part II

1. J (page 481)
2. K (page 484)
3. L (page 480)
4. M (page 485)
5. D (page 484)
6. E (page 485)
7. F (page 485)
8. G (page 482)
9. T (page 481)
10. S (page 481)
11. R (page 482)
12. Q (page 491)
13. C (page 479)
14. B (page 490)
15. A (page 479)
16. I (page 479)
17. H (page 481)
18. O (page 481)
19. N (page 485)
20. P (page 479)

Multiple Choice

1. D (page 479)
2. B (page 478)
3. D (page 479)
4. B (page 481)
5. C (page 490)
6. D (page 490)
7. A (page 491)
8. A (pages 489–490)
9. B (page 488)
10. C (page 485)

Fill in the-Blank

1. 7.5; 5; 10; fluid (page 478)
2. palmar grasp (page 479)
3. fontanelles (page 479)
4. Growth plates (page 479)
5. Bonding (page 480)
6. Trust; mistrust (page 482)
7. aneurysm (page 488)
8. mesentery (page 490)
9. terminal drop hypothesis (page 491)
10. increases; decreases (page 489)

Labeling

(page 480, Figure 10-4)

A. Anterior
B. Posterior
C. Mastoid
D. Sphenoidal

Identify

1. Chief complaint: Fell and hip hurts a great deal
2. Vital signs: Pulse 90 beats/min and thready; respirations 24 breaths/min and shallow; and blood pressure 100/70 mm Hg
3. SAMPLE history:

   Signs/symptoms: Externally rotated foot, discoloration, and a great deal of pain

   Allergies: None

   Medications: Medications for heart failure

   Pertinent medical history: Heart failure, past smoker, and heart attack last year

   Last oral intake: Ate breakfast a few hours ago

   Event: Tripped and fell

Ambulance Calls

1. (page 479)

Reflex	How to Test	Appropriate Response
Moro reflex	Startle the infant (clap your hands once near the child).	Infant opens arms wide and spreads fingers; seems to grab at things.
Palmar grasp	Place an object–a finger–in the infant's palm.	The infant should grasp your finger.
Rooting reflex	Touch the infant's cheek.	The infant should turn his or her head toward the touch.
Sucking reflex	Stroke the infant's lips.	The infant should respond as if preparing to feed.

2. a. The patient is considered a late adult. It is not uncommon to have visual issues that make it difficult for her to get around and that may also contribute to trauma such as a low fall. She may not be able to read small print such as that found on a prescription medical container, and she may not be focusing well.

   In addition, she may have some hearing loss that makes it difficult for her to hold a conversation and be understood, potentially leading to confusion and inaccurate responses to questions. (pages 488–492)

   b. While going through body systems, be concerned about cardiac-related issues and aneurysms when addressing cardiovascular issues. The patient may have a cardiac history and diminished cardiac output as a result of her age. Her body may not be able to compensate with rapid blood pressure changes, so vital signs are important, and you must consider asking if she gets dizzy when she sits up or stands. A cardiac event is always a consideration even if there are no overt signs present. When considering respiratory issues, be aware of an elderly person's diminished ability to clear secretions and the fact that she may have diminished lung capacity, which can mean low air exchange. Ask yourself whether there are any signs of respiratory distress in this patient. Because stagnant air can remain in the lungs, hypercarbia is a concern. When considering renal and gastric issues, ask about pain and discomfort as well as bowel and urinary habits. The renal and gastrointestinal systems become less efficient with age, causing an inability to process fluids, nutrients, and electrolytes properly. The nervous system should be addressed. Elderly people have slower motor and sensory responses, which can place them at risk for injury.

   Slow bleeds into the brain may initially appear with subtle signs. If there is a concern, perform a stroke assessment. (pages 491–492)

3. a. Privacy is an issue among adolescents. Therefore, with both her mother and girlfriend in the room, asking if she is pregnant is inappropriate. Your partner should have waited until no family or friends were present before asking this question. If the opportunity doesn't present itself before reaching the ED, let the staff know.

   b. Palpation of the abdomen must be done in a way that respects the patient's privacy and, if possible, by a paramedic of the same gender as the patient. It may have been appropriate to wait until the patient was loaded into the ambulance to perform this assessment. (page 486)

True/False

1. T (page 479)
2. F (page 479)
3. F (page 479)
4. T (pages 480–481)
5. F (page 485)
6. T (page 488)
7. T (pages 489–490)
8. F (page 491)
9. T (page 490)
10. F (page 490)

Short Answer

1. a. Moro reflex
   b. Palmar grasp
   c. Rooting reflex
   d. Sucking reflex (page 479)
2. a. Cholesterol
   b. Calcium (page 488)
3. a. Decreased ability to clear secretions
   b. Decreased cough reflex
   c. Decreased gag reflex

d. Diminished cilia with age
e. Decreased innervation of airway structures, resulting in decreased sensation (page 489)

4. a. Diminished visual acuity
b. Visual distortions
c. Harder for the eye to focus
d. Narrower peripheral field
e. Greater sensitivity to glare
f. Hearing loss
g. Loss of taste bud sensation (page 491)

5. a. Gastrointestinal distress
b. Upper respiratory tract infection (page 482)

6. a. Control
b. Following rules
c. Competitiveness (page 483)

7. a. Loss of respiratory muscle mass
b. Increased stiffness of the thoracic cage
c. Decreased surface area available for air exchange (page 489)

Fill in the Table

1. (pages 485–486)

Male Characteristics	Female Characteristics
External organs enlarge.	Breasts and thighs increase in size.
Pubic and ancillary hair begins to appear.	Menstruation begins (can begin younger than teenage years).
Voice changes.	Acne occurs.
Acne occurs.	Follicle-stimulating hormone and luteinizing hormone (both of which increase estrogen and progesterone production) are released.

2. (page 481, Table 10-1)
A. Tracks objects with the eyes
B. Smiles and frowns
C. Recognizes family from strangers
D. Sits upright in a chair; speaks one-syllable words
E. Has mood swings
F. Places objects in mouth to explore them
G. Starts to walk without help; frustrated with restrictions

Section 3: Patient Assessment

Chapter 11: Patient Assessment

Matching

Part I

1. L (page 507)
2. M (page 537)
3. N (page 555)
4. K (page 541)
5. U (page 569)
6. T (page 555)
7. S (page 581)
8. J (page 565)
9. I (page 547)
10. A (page 558)
11. B (page 588)
12. D (page 560)
13. C (page 571)
14. R (page 568)
15. Q (page 510)
16. P (page 531)
17. O (page 573)
18. Y (page 581)
19. X (page 584)
20. W (page 586)
21. V (page 510)
22. H (page 569)
23. G (page 563)
24. F (page 594)
25. E (page 560)

Part II

1. I
2. J, M
3. D, O, U
4. A, G, V
5. T
6. J, L
7. N, C
8. K, L
9. B
10. S
11. O
12. C
13. R
14. F
15. Q
16. H
17. E
18. P

Part III

(page 503)

1. S
2. NS
3. S
4. NS
5. NS
6. S
7. S
8. NS

Multiple Choice

1. B (page 520)
2. C (page 523)
3. A (page 523)
4. D (page 524)
5. B (page 522)
6. D (page 527)
7. C (page 528)
8. B (page 529)
9. A (page 528)
10. C (pages 525–526)
11. D (page 510)
12. B (page 547)
13. A (page 547)
14. C (page 512)
15. C (page 556)
16. A (page 575)
17. B (page 581)
18. C (page 569)
19. D (page 585)
20. C (page 555)
21. A (page 502)
22. C (page 502)
23. D (page 509)
24. A (page 507)
25. A (page 503)
26. C (pages 510–511)
27. D (page 535)
28. D (page 541)
29. C (pages 549, 552)
30. A (page 512)

Labeling

(page 570, Figure 11-36)

A. Right hypochondrial region
B. Epigastric region
C. Left hypochondrial region
D. Right lumbar region
E. Umbilical region
F. Left lumbar region
G. Right iliac region
H. Hypogastric region
I. Left iliac region

Fill in the Blank

1. field impression (page 503)
2. introduce yourself (page 520)
3. present illness (page 532)
4. jargon (page 522)

5. face-to-face (page 529)
6. Empathy (page 521)
7. reflection (page 523)
8. HIPAA (page 525)
9. medical history (page 526)
10. age; education (page 519)

Ambulance Calls

1. Accident scenes like the one pictured in this question are fairly characteristic of those you will encounter in your work. You can learn a lot from the scene and the people there if you know what to look for and what to ask.
   a. The potential sources of information about what happened to the patient at the scene are as follows:
      (1) The scene itself
      (2) The patient
      (3) The bystanders at the bus stop and perhaps in the diner
      (4) Any medical identification devices the patient might be carrying
   b. From observing the scene, you can tell the following:
      (1) The driver was driving somewhat erratically.
      (2) Something caused him to swerve off the road (perhaps he saw something in the road or thought he saw something).
      (3) The driver was conscious when he went off the road (he was able to apply the brakes).
      (4) Massive forces were involved in the accident (enough to break the telephone pole).
      (5) The driver struck his head against the windshield.
   c. It is necessary to take a history for the following reasons:
      (1) To find out what happened. Why did he swerve off the road? Did something cross his path? Did he suddenly feel ill?
      (2) To find out what hurts—that is, to start searching for his most serious injuries.
      (3) To find out whether he has any underlying medical problems that might complicate his care. If, for example, he is taking anticoagulant medications after a previous heart attack, he could lose a great deal of blood from what might otherwise be a fairly minor wound.
      (4) To gather information that might otherwise be unavailable to the hospital staff, such as data on the MOI.
   d. Before you start taking the history, you need to do the following:
      (1) Clear your mind of any preconceived ideas about the patient (eg, "He must have been drunk").
      (2) Introduce yourself, and explain your role.
      (3) Find out the patient's name.
      (4) Try to position yourself at the patient's level; to do so, lean over or crouch down near the car window.
      (5) Initiate some physical contact; for example, put a hand on the patient's shoulder and instruct him not to move until you have examined him.

True/False

1. T (page 539)
2. F (page 524)
3. F (page 523)
4. T (page 522)
5. T (page 528)
6. T (page 552)
7. T (page 504)
8. F (page 539)
9. F (page 521)
10. T (page 523)
11. F (page 555)
12. T (page 507)
13. T (page 588)
14. F (page 584)
15. T (page 569)
16. F (page 579)
17. F (page 577)
18. T (pages 574–575)
19. T (page 569)
20. F (pages 547–549)

Short Answer

1. a. In eliciting the history of the present illness from a patient whose chief complaint is "pain in my gut," one would want to know at least the following:
      (1) Did anything in particular provoke the pain? What brought it on? Does anything make it worse? Does anything make it better?
      (2) What is the quality of the pain? What is it like?
      (3) Does the pain radiate anywhere? Where is it precisely?
      (4) How severe is the pain?
      (5) What was the timing of the pain; that is, when did it come on? Has it been there constantly since, or does it come and go?
      (6) Are there any associated symptoms, such as nausea, vomiting, diarrhea, or constipation? (pages 532–533)

b. In inquiring about the patient's other medical history, you need to find out the following:
   (1) Does he have any major underlying medical problems? One way to find out is to ask, "Are you presently under a doctor's care for any condition?"
   (2) Does he take any medications regularly?
   (3) Does he have any allergies?
   (4) Does he have a family doctor, or does he regularly go to a particular hospital? (page 534)

2. In taking the history of a patient, excellent communications skills are needed. The following are communications techniques used by paramedics in the field:
   a. Facilitation
   b. Reflection
   c. Clarification
   d. Confrontation
   e. Interpretation (page 523)
3. The four questions you need to answer in making your survey of the scene are the following:
   a. Is it safe for me to approach the victim(s)?
   b. Is there any hazard to the patient?
   c. Will I need any help?
   d. Do I need any special equipment to reach the patient?

   If you do not ask and answer those questions at every incident scene, your career as a paramedic may be very short indeed, for you will not notice the downed high-tension line draped over the car, or the little trail of fire creeping toward the vehicle, or the bus about to plow into the disabled vehicle that is still in the middle of the road. (pages 505–508)
4. Possible sources of information about what happened to the patient include the following:
   a. The patient himself or herself (the most important source if the patient is conscious)
   b. Bystanders or family
   c. The scene (MOI)
   d. Medical identification devices

Fill in the Table

1. (page 585)

Tests for Disability in Cranial Nerves

Cranial Nerve	Test
I	**Check smell**
II	**Check visual acuity**
III	**Check pupil size, shape, symmetry, response to light, eye movements**
IV	**Check eye movements**
V	**Check jaw clench; touch both sides of face at forehead, cheeks, and jaw**
VI	**Check eye movements**
VII	**Check facial symmetry; look for abnormal movements; raise eyebrows, grin broadly, frown, shut eyes tightly, puff out cheeks; note any asymmetry**
VIII	**Check hearing and balance**
IX, X	**Check swallowing; perform general physical exam**
XI	**Check shoulder shrug; turn head from left to right and back**
XII	**Check swallowing; turn head from left to right and back**

2. When you assess an injured patient from head to toe, it helps to know what you are looking for. (pages 556–583)

Body Region	What I Will Be Looking for in Particular
Head	**Deformity, lacerations, cerebrospinal fluid (CSF) leak, Battle sign, maxillofacial injury**
Neck	**Open wounds, subcutaneous emphysema, tracheal deviation, jugular distention, bruises over cervical spine**
Chest	**Bruises, open wounds, instability, inequality of breath sounds, dullness or hyperresonance**
Abdomen	**Contusions, open wounds, evisceration, distention, rigidity, cough rebound**
Extremities	**Deformity, swelling, ecchymosis, pulses, movement, sensation**
Back/buttocks	**Just soft-tissue injuries**

Chapter 12: Critical Thinking and Clinical Decision Making

Matching

Part I

(pages 605–606)

1. A
2. B
3. A
4. A
5. B
6. B
7. A
8. B
9. A
10. B

Part II

1. E (page 611)
2. D (page 603)
3. A (page 608)
4. B (page 604)
5. F (page 609)
6. C (page 608)

Multiple Choice

1. C (page 604)
2. B (page 608)
3. D (page 608)
4. A (pages 609–610)
5. B (pages 611–614)
6. D (pages 611–614)
7. C (page 611)
8. B (page 604)
9. A (page 607)
10. C (page 606)

Fill in the Blank

1. gathering (page 603)
2. protocols (page 605)
3. think; work (page 606)
4. concept formation (page 608)
5. life threats (page 607)
6. working diagnosis (page 608)
7. reading (page 611)
8. trends (page 612)

Identify

1. Chief complaint: General malaise.
2. Vital signs: Blood glucose is 110 mg /dL; blood pressure (BP) is 160/100 mm Hg. The ECG is normal sinus rhythm with some slight ST-segment depression, with a pulse of 92 beats/min and regular. Spo_2 is 97%, lungs are clear, and respirations are 18 breaths/min. Skin is warm and dry, and she is PERRLA and alert.
3. Pertinent negatives: After the intervention of the IV at TKO and the nitroglycerin paste, the BP drops to 120/70 mm Hg.

Ambulance Call

1. a. The child in this scenario is unable to tell you her name or where she is. This tells you that she is only a V (verbal response) using the AVPU scale. She will respond but is not oriented to person, place, or day. She is classified as having an altered mental status and is a priority patient from the start.
   b. You can treat this child under implied consent. Because she has a severe life threat, you can assume the parents would want life-saving treatment to be provided for their daughter.
   c. The vital signs suggest that the intracranial pressure is rising. BP is high for this child's age, and the pulse and respirations are dropping. This tells the paramedics they should begin moving toward a regional trauma center as fast and as safely as they can.
   d. The major concern here is to keep a patent airway and provide supplemental oxygen for this patient. Because the patient is breathing at a rate less than 8 breaths/min and her oxygen saturation is 88%, you know that she is hypoxic. She needs an advanced airway to be inserted as soon as possible, and she may be a candidate for rapid-sequence intubation (RSI) if she continues to have a gag reflex.

2. a. Use the highest point, or even stand on a car hood (not the one that crashed), and have someone honk the horn until you get the attention of the people around you. Identify yourself and ask the crowd if anyone has medical training. Then, identify a bystander for crowd control. Also designate someone to go down the line of cars, instructing them to move to the road's shoulder so that emergency vehicles can get through.
   b. Everything the local responders have is needed! Use a cell phone to communicate with dispatch. Identify yourself and the fact that you are incident command until someone arrives to take over for you. Jaws of Life will be needed, as well as any medical helicopters and nearby advanced life support (ALS) units. Try to get the number of injured patients to the dispatcher as soon as possible. When using the Jaws of Life, a fire truck should be present, so try to get the area cleared of vehicles that were not involved in the collision.
   c. You will start to triage the occupants of the two vehicles. That way, when help arrives, you can direct them to the most critical of patients. Always remember that your safety and the bystanders' safety come first.

True/False

1. T (page 603)
2. T (page 604)
3. F (page 605)
4. F (page 607)
5. F (page 608)
6. T (page 609)
7. F (page 611)
8. T (page 611)

Short Answer

1. a. Read the scene: As a paramedic, you must ensure your safety and the safety of your crew, patient, and bystanders. Scene safety is first! You will also use your scene size-up to give you clues to the patient's condition. Weather and MOI are also something to look for when reading the scene. (pages 611–612)
   b. Read the patient: In this phase, you decide if the patient is sick or not sick. You will observe, talk to, and touch your patient in this phase. You will also look for any life threats and take baseline vital signs. (page 612)
   c. React: Always address any life threats first, and handle them as they come up in your assessment. At this time, you will begin to think about your working diagnosis. (page 613)
   d. Reevaluate: Always check your interventions to make sure they are helping the patient. You will also check that you have gathered all the information on your patient at this time and will watch for any other problems to pop up. (page 614)
   e. Revise the plan: Once you have begun your treatment, you may realize that a "drunken" patient is really a patient who is having a diabetic emergency. So your treatment plan will have to be revised at this time to treat the patient correctly. (page 614)
   f. Review your performance: After your call is over, you should do an informal review to see where you can improve your patient care. Sometimes this can be a formal process. It always helps to talk to your team members about each call and learn something from every call you run. (page 614)
2. When gathering information, start by asking all the questions you are taught to ask. Begin with the chief complaint, SAMPLE history, OPQRST, and all the mnemonics you have been taught to use. The good paramedic will be able to use open- and closed-ended questions. Frequently, there will be circumstances that will make it hard to gather a good history. Perhaps the patient is unconscious, with no family members present to answer questions. There may be a language barrier, or the patient may be unable to speak clearly or hear your questions clearly. You will need to look at the surrounding scene to help gather information about the patient. You will often need to look at the patient's body position or facial expression. These clues will help you quickly gather information about the patient.

   When evaluating the information that you have gathered, you must begin to ask whether your information is pertinent to the patient's current condition. This is the point where you begin to formulate and enact your treatment plan for the patient. Remember, you must constantly reevaluate the patient and your treatments.

   Synthesizing your information goes hand in hand with the evaluation process. This process takes you a little deeper into understanding the disease process or which organ systems have been affected by trauma. This helps you prepare for any upcoming problems the patient may face. A thinking paramedic will be able to put all the information together and treat the patient in the best way possible. (pages 603–605)

Section 4: Pharmacology

Chapter 13: Principles of Pharmacology

Matching

Part I

(page 623)

1. III
2. V
3. I
4. II
5. IV
6. IV
7. I
8. II
9. II
10. III

Part II

1. U (page 631)
2. T (page 650)
3. S (page 650)
4. R (pages 628, 646)
5. Y (page 658)
6. X (page 631)
7. W (page 625)
8. V (page 663)
9. Q (page 641)
10. P (page 650)
11. O (page 631)
12. N (page 631)
13. A (page 661)
14. B (page 628)
15. C (page 664)
16. D (page 646)
17. M (page 631)
18. L (page 629)
19. K (page 644)
20. J (page 638)
21. E (page 645)
22. F (page 626)
23. G (page 630)
24. I (page 629)
25. H (page 629)

Part III

1. U (page 645)
2. V (page 647)
3. W (page 642)
4. X (page 639)
5. Y (page 647)
6. A (page 639)
7. B (page 661)
8. C (page 639)
9. D (page 665)
10. E (page 628)
11. T (page 658)
12. S (page 645)
13. R (page 663)
14. Q (page 629)
15. P (page 628)
16. F (page 631)
17. G (page 630)
18. H (page 627)
19. I (page 638)
20. J (page 622)
21. O (page 628)
22. N (page 630)
23. M (page 660)
24. K (page 626)
25. L (page 674)

Multiple Choice

1. B (page 625)
2. C (page 622)
3. A (page 623)
4. C (page 640)
5. B (page 644)
6. D (page 624)
7. B (page 624)
8. D (page 630)
9. C (page 638)
10. A (page 645)
11. C (page 628)
12. C (page 628)
13. D (page 634)
14. B (page 669)

Fill in the Blank

1. indications (page 626)
2. neutralization (page 640)
3. antagonist (page 673)
4. potentiation (page 640)
5. alpha-1 (page 630)
6. beta-2 (page 630)
7. Diuretic (page 631)
8. beta-blocking (page 655)
9. Cardiac glycosides (page 655)
10. corticosteroids (page 655)

Identify

1. Chief complaint: Heart palpitations
2. Vital signs: Pulse is 60 beats/min, regular, and weak; respirations are slightly labored at 22 breaths/min; BP is 90/60 mm Hg; Spo_2 is 97%; and skin is pale.
3. Pertinent negatives: No pain (she may be having a "silent MI," which is a myocardial infarction [MI] without pain or discomfort), no nausea, and relatively good health.

   Note: The fact that the patient started a new medication might be a significant finding because she may be having an adverse effect.

Ambulance Calls

1. **a.** Right patient: Does this patient meet the criteria based on the assessment, vital signs, and SAMPLE history?
   b. Right medication: Is morphine the correct medication for this patient?
   c. Right dose: Based on the patient's weight and your protocols, are you giving the right amount?
   d. Right route: Is the drug being given in the optimal way?
   e. Right time: Is this drug being given when it should be, and has the patient already taken or been given any other drugs that could interact with it?
   f. Right documentation and reporting: At what time was the medication administered, exactly what amount was administered, and by which route was it administered? Because this is a controlled substance, are there any other legal requirements for documentation?
   g. Right assessment: Confirm indications and contraindications.
   h. Right to refuse: Respect patient autonomy.
   i. Right evaluation: Continually monitor your patient.
   j. Right patient education: Inform the patient of any pertinent risks and benefits as soon as possible, prior to medication administration. (pages 648–649)
2. **a.** An inactive substance can become active, capable of producing desired or unwanted clinical effects (active metabolite).
   b. An active medication can be changed into another active medication (active metabolite).
   c. An active medication can be completely or partially inactivated (inactive metabolite).
   d. A medication can be transformed into a substance (active or inactive metabolite) that is easier for the body to eliminate. (page 646)
3. **a.** Age
   b. Weight (the doses for many drugs administered are calculated based on the weight of the patient)
   c. Environment
   d. Genetic factors
   e. Pregnancy
   f. Psychosocial factors (pages 632–635)

True/False

1. F (page 625)
2. F (page 623)
3. T (page 632)
4. T (page 647)
5. T (page 632)
6. F (page 633)
7. T (pages 660–661)
8. T (page 637)
9. F (page 639)
10. F (pages 654, 674)
11. T (page 628)
12. T (page 668)
13. T (page 634)

Short Answer

1. **a.** Chemical name
   b. Generic name
   c. Trade or brand name (page 625)
2. **a.** Medication names
   b. Category or class of medication
   c. Uses/indications
   d. Mechanism of action (pharmacodynamics)
   e. Pregnancy risk factor
   f. Contraindications
   g. Available forms
   h. Dosages (often differentiated based on age indication)
   i. Administration and monitoring considerations
   j. Potential incompatibility
   k. Adverse effects
   l. Pharmacokinetics (page 626)
3. **a.** No trailing zero after decimal point; for example, 4.0 mg can be interpreted as 40 mg, so do not include the decimal point and zero: 4 mg.
   b. No leading zero before decimal point; for example,.8 mg can be interpreted as 8 mg, so use a zero before the decimal point: 0.8 mg.
   c. MSO can be misinterpreted as magnesium sulfate, so write out *morphine sulfate*.

d. $MgSO_4$ can be misinterpreted as morphine sulfate, so write out *magnesium sulfate*.
e. SC may be interpreted as SL, so write out *subcutaneous*.
f. IN can be interpreted as IV or IM, so write out *intranasal*. (page 650)

4. *Students should provide eight of these common adverse effects:*
a. Nausea
b. Vomiting
c. Sedation
d. Palpitations
e. Hypotension
f. Hypertension
g. Bradycardia
h. Tachycardia
i. Respiratory depression
j. Endocrine abnormalities
k. Dizziness (page 637)

5. a. Antiemetics
b. Antidiarrheals
c. Antibiotics
d. Antacids
e. Antihistamines
f. Beta-blocking agents
g. Benzodiazepines
h. Corticosteroids
i. Fibrinolytics
j. Hormone replacement drugs
k. Narcotic analgesics
l. Sympathomimetics (pages 654–657)

Fill in the Table

1. (page 643)

Veins Used During Intraosseous (IO) Infusion	
Intraosseous Site	**Vein**
Proximal tibia	**Popliteal vein**
Femur	**Femoral vein**
Distal tibia (medial malleolus)	Great saphenous vein
Proximal humerus	Axillary vein
Manubrium (sternum)	**Internal mammary and azygos veins**

2. (page 641)

Gastrointestinal Medication Absorption	
Factor	Medication Absorption
GI motility	Ability of medication to pass through the GI tract into the bloodstream
GI pH	Perfusion of the GI system (may be decreased during systemic trauma or shock)
Presence of food, liquids, or chemicals in the stomach	Injury or bleeding in the GI system (both can alter GI motility, decreasing the time that oral medications can be absorbed)

3. (page 624)

Sources of Medication	
Source	**Examples**
Plants	Atropine, aspirin, digoxin, morphine
Animals	Heparin, antivenom, thyroid preparations, insulin
Microorganisms	Streptokinase, numerous antibiotics
Minerals	Iron, magnesium sulfate, lithium, phosphorus, calcium

Chapter 14: Medication Administration

Matching

Part I

(page 762)

1. D
2. C
3. B
4. A
5. C
6. B
7. A

Part II

1. L (page 725)
2. K (page 693)
3. E (page 689)
4. F (page 753)
5. D (page 699)
6. C (page 733)
7. B (page 695)
8. A (page 695)
9. J (page 711)
10. T (page 693)
11. S (page 699)
12. N (page 696)
13. M (page 734)
14. O (page 734)
15. P (page 729)
16. Q (page 706)
17. R (page 701)
18. I (page 751)
19. H (page 716)
20. G (page 687)

Part III

1. L (page 753)
2. R (page 701)
3. M (page 755)
4. S (page 711)
5. N (page 693)
6. O (page 709)
7. P (page 693)
8. T (page 712)
9. Q (page 699)
10. A (page 693)
11. C (page 709)
12. B (page 759)
13. D (page 746)
14. F (page 737)
15. E (page 753)
16. K (page 693)
17. J (page 692)
18. I (page 694)
19. H (page 713)
20. G (page 753)

Multiple Choice

1. C (page 716)
2. C (page 757)
3. D (page 692)
4. B (page 696)
5. B (page 700)
6. C (page 702)
7. A (page 710)
8. B (page 716)
9. B (page 712)
10. B (page 689)
11. D (page 740)
12. B (page 733)
13. C (page 738)
14. C (page 753)
15. B (page 731)
16. C (page 688)
17. A (page 688)
18. C (page 729)
19. D (page 751)
20. C (page 710)

Fill in the Blank

1. colloid (page 693)
2. crystalloid; saline (page 692)
3. hypertonic; hypotonic; isotonic; hypertonic; isotonic; hypotonic (page 693)
4. lower; higher; osmosis (page 693)
5. dyspnea; hypertension (page 711)

Labeling

Common sites for intramuscular injections

(page 740, Figure 14-56)

A. Deltoid
B. Gluteus maximus
C. Vastus lateralis
D. Rectus femoris muscle

Ambulance Calls

Intravenous lines are supposed to help save lives, but they may cause problems (most of which can be prevented!).

1. **a.** You are the patient's problem! You weren't keeping an eye on the IV. The 59-year-old man who is suddenly short of breath has most probably developed circulatory overload because his to-keep-open (TKO) IV became a "runaway IV" and poured an extra liter of fluid into his vascular space in a very short period of time.

   b. You need to slow the IV to TKO rate, sit the patient up with his legs dangling, and radio the physician for further instructions. (page 711)

2. a. The frail old woman probably has very frail veins, and your IV has apparently ruptured the wall of one of those veins and infiltrated.

b. You need to discontinue the IV and start a new one at another site, if she really needs it. If not, wait until you reach the emergency department (ED), where a new IV can be inserted under more controlled conditions.

c. Other problems that might cause an IV to slow down include tightening of the clamp, a kink in the tubing, the tip of the catheter resting against the wall of the vein, flexion at a joint causing the vein to kink, and the IV bag hung too low. (page 709)

3. a. When bright red blood comes spurting back in your face, it is a good indication that you have accidentally cannulated an artery.

b. You need to immediately withdraw the catheter and hold firm pressure over the puncture site for at least 5 minutes. (page 710)

4. a. A painful, red, swollen venipuncture site is a sign of thrombophlebitis.

b. The treatment is to discontinue the IV and put a warm compress (hot pack) over the puncture site.

c. The following can minimize the likelihood of thrombophlebitis:

(1) Adequately disinfecting the skin before venipuncture
(2) Wearing sterile gloves to start an IV
(3) Covering the puncture site with a sterile dressing
(4) Securing the catheter firmly so that it cannot wobble around inside the vein (page 710)

5. a. Yes, this patient is probably seriously injured. The reason for that conclusion is the signs of shock already evident: restlessness; cold, clammy skin; and the thirst itself.

b. You decide to start an IV with lactated Ringer solution, which is a **crystalloid** solution. To calculate the IV rate, you need to recall the equation:

$$\frac{\text{Volume to be infused} \times \text{gtt/mL}}{\text{Time of infusion (in minutes)}} = \frac{200 \text{ mL} \times 10 \text{ gtt /mL}}{60 \text{ min}}$$

2,000 gtt ÷ 60 min = 33.3 gtt/min

For practical purposes, that is 30 gtt/min. (page 727)

c. The steps in troubleshooting an IV are as follows:

(1) Check the IV fluid.
(2) Check the administration set.
(3) Check the height of the IV bag.
(4) Check the type of catheter used.
(5) Check the constricting band. (page 708)

True/False

1. T (page 757)
2. T (pages 693–694)
3. F (page 693)
4. T (page 757)
5. T (page 751)
6. F (page 749)
7. F (page 691)
8. T (page 693)
9. F (page 693)
10. T (page 696)
11. F (page 698)
12. F (page 699)
13. F (page 700)
14. F (pages 702, 705)
15. T (page 709)
16. T (page 710)
17. F (page 711)
18. T (page 712)
19. F (page 720)
20. F (page 720)
21. T (page 721)
22. F (page 726)
23. T (page 725)
24. T (page 728)
25. T (page 690)

Short Answer

1. a. Allow the arm to hang off the stretcher.

b. Pat or rub the area.

c. Apply chemical heat packs for at least 60 seconds (page 702)

2. a. The gauge of the needle

b. The IV attempts versus successes

c. The site (eg, left forearm, left external jugular)

d. The type of fluid that you are administering

e. The rate at which the fluid is running (page 702)

3. *Students should list three of the following:*

a. Infiltration: Signs and symptoms are local edema around the site, continued IV flow after occlusion of the vein above the insertion site, and patient complaints of tightness and pain around the IV site. (page 709)

b. Occlusion: Signs and symptoms are decreasing drip rate or the presence of blood in the tubing or a positional IV. Also, if the bag of fluid is empty, it can cause an occlusion by clotting around the site of the IV. (page 709)
c. Vein irritation: Signs and symptoms include the solution tingling, stinging, itching, or burning. If redness develops at the IV site, discontinue the IV, and start a new IV with all new equipment and fluids. (page 709)
d. Thrombophlebitis: Signs and symptoms are tenderness and pain along the vein, as well as redness and edema at the site of the venipuncture. (page 710)
e. Hematoma: Signs and symptoms are rapid blood pooling below the skin around the IV site, leading to tenderness and pain. Use direct pressure to stop the hematoma. Evaluate the site to see if the IV is good and can be used. If not, pull out the IV, and apply direct pressure. (page 710)
f. Nerve, tendon, or ligament damage: Signs and symptoms are numbness, tingling, and sudden, shooting pain. Remove the IV and select a different site. (page 710)
g. Arterial puncture: Signs and symptoms are bright red spurting blood with a much faster flow. Discontinue the site and apply direct pressure to the IV site until the bleeding stops. (page 710)

4. a. Name of the drug
b. The dose of the drug
c. Time you administered the drug
d. Route of administration (eg, IV, IM)
e. Name of the paramedic who administered the drug
f. The patient's response to the medication, whether positive or negative (page 688)

Fill in the Table

Route of Administration	Where in the Body the Medication Goes
Enteral	1. **Gastrointestinal tract** (page 729)
Oral	2. **By the mouth** (page 729)
Intradermal	3. **Injection into the dermis** (page 737)
Percutaneous	4. **Through the skin and mucous membranes** (page 749)
Sublingual	5. **Under the tongue** (page 71)
Endotracheal	6. **Bagged in through the ET tube** (pages 755, 757)
Buccal	7. **Between the cheek and gums** (page 751)
Transdermal	8. **Applied topically** (page 749)
Intramuscular	9. **Injection into the muscl**e (page 739)
Rectal	10. **Into the rectal mucosa** (page 730)
Parenteral	11. **Any route other than the gastrointestinal tract** (page 732)
Subcutaneous	12. **Injection between dermis and muscle** (page 737)
Intravenous	13. **Directly into a vein** (page 694)
Ocular	14. **Drop or ointment into the eye** (pages 751-752)
Aural	15. **Into the ear canal** (page 753)
Inhalation	16. **Inhaled into the lungs** (page 753)
Intranasal	17. **Within the nose** (page 753)

Problem Solving

1. To give the baker 200 mL/h with a macrodrip set (page 727):

$$\frac{\text{Volume to be infused} \times \text{gtt/mL of administration set}}{\text{Total time of infusion in minutes}} = \text{gtt/min}$$

$$\frac{200 \text{ mL/h} \times 10 \text{ gtt/mL}}{60 \text{ min}} = \text{approximately } 33.3 \text{ gtt/min}$$

2. For the patient who needs only a keep-open line (page 727):

$$\frac{30 \text{ mL} \times 60 \text{ gtt/mL}}{60 \text{ min}} = 30 \text{ gtt/min}$$

3. This problem, which involves calculating concentrations and flow rates, is not merely a theoretical exercise; it is typical of the calculations you will be making every day in your work as a paramedic, and a slip of the decimal point could kill someone!

a. Your vial of lidocaine contains 50 mL of 4% lidocaine, so by definition, it contains (pages 727–728):

$$\frac{4 \text{ g of lidocaine}}{100 \text{ mL}} = \frac{2 \text{ g of lidocaine}}{50 \text{ mL}}$$

b. When you add that 2 g of lidocaine to a volume of 500 mL:

$$\frac{2 \text{ g}}{500 \text{ mL}} = \frac{2{,}000 \text{ mg}}{500 \text{ mL}} = 4 \text{ mg/mL} = 0.0004$$

(Ignore the volume in which the lidocaine was suspended.)

c. If the patient is to receive 2 mg/min, he must receive:

$$\frac{2 \text{ mg/min}}{4 \text{ mg/mL}} = 0.5 \text{ mL/min}$$

d. Thus, the number of drops per minute at which you have to set the infusion is 0.5 mL/min × 60 gtt/mL = 30 gtt/min.

4. 12 g × 1,000 mg/g = 12,000 mg (page 722)

5. $$\frac{156 \text{ lb}}{2.2 \text{ lb/kg}} = 70.9 \text{ kg}$$

Round up to 71 kg (page 724)

6. Step 1: 135 ÷ 2 = 67.5

Step 2: 67.5 × 0.10 = 6.75

Round 6.75 to 7.

Step 3: 67.5 – 7 = 60.5

Round up to 61.

Patient's weight in kilograms for field purposes is 61 kg. (page 724)

7. $$\frac{6 \text{ mg}}{10 \text{ mg/mL}} = 0.6 \text{ mL}$$

(page 725)

8. Concentration on hand (pages 725–726):

$$\frac{20 \text{ mg}}{10 \text{ mL}} = 2 \text{ mg/mL}$$

Volume you will give:

$$\frac{2 \text{ mg}}{2 \text{ mg/mL}} = 1 \text{ mL}$$

9. (pages 728–729)

a. 10 mcg/kg/min × 80 kg = 800 mcg/min (desired dose)

b. $$\frac{800 \text{ mg (or 800,000 mcg)}}{500 \text{ mL}} = 1.6 \text{ mg/mL}$$

c. 1.6 mg/mL × 1,000 mcg/mg = 1,600 mcg/mL

d. $$\frac{800 \text{ mcg/min}}{1{,}600 \text{ mcg/mL}} = 0.5 \text{ mL/min}$$

e. 0.5 mL/min × 60 gtt/mL = 30 gtt/min

10. (page 722)

Microgram (mcg)	Milligram (mg)	Gram (g)	Kilogram (kg)
500.0	0.5	0.0005	0.0000005
1,000,000.0	**1,000.0**	1.0	**0.001**
1,000,000,000.0	**1,000,000.0**	**1,000**	1.0
1,000.0	1.0	**0.001**	**0.000001**
1.0	**0.001**	**0.000001**	**0.000000001**
800,000.0	800.0	**0.8**	**0.0008**
15.0	**0.015**	**0.000015**	**0.000000015**

Milliliter (mL)	Deciliter (dL)	Liter (L)
5,000.0	50.0	5.0
1.0	**0.01**	**0.001**
10.0	**0.1**	**0.01**
1,000.0	**10.0**	1.0
250.0	**2.5**	0.25

11. (page 724)

Patient's Weight (lb)	Patient's Weight (lb) ÷ 2	Weight (lb) ÷ 2 10%	Subtract Your 10% from the Weight ÷ 2	Patient's Weight in Kilograms (kg)	Patient's Weight in lb ÷ 2.2 = Patient's Weight in Kilograms (kg)
60	60 ÷ 2 = 30	30 × 10% = 3	30 - 3 = 27	27	27.27
16	**8**	**0.8 (≈ 1)**	**8 - 1 = 7**	**7**	**7.27**
138	**69**	**6.9 (≈ 7)**	**69 - 7 = 62**	**62**	**62.72**
8	**4**	**0.4 (≈ 0.5)**	**4 - 0.5 = 3.5**	**3.5**	**3.64**
250	**125**	**12.5**	**125 - 12.5 = 112.5**	**112.5**	**113.64**
36	**18**	**1.8 (≈ 2)**	**18 - 2 = 16**	**16**	**16.36**
82	**41**	**4.1 (≈ 4)**	**41 - 4 = 37**	**37**	**37.27**
180	**90**	**9.0**	**90 - 9 = 81**	**81**	**81.82**
330	**165**	**16.5 (≈ 17)**	**165 - 17 = 148**	**148**	**150**

12. (page 723)

1,000 mL NS	500 mL NS	250 mL NS	100 mL NS	50 mL NS
100 g	50 g	25 g	10 g	5 g
1,600 g	800 g	**400 g**	**160 g**	**80 g**
1,000 g	**500 g**	250 g	**100 g**	**50 g**
40 g	**20 g**	**10 g**	4 g	**2 g**
100 g	50 g	**25 g**	**10 g**	**5 g**

13. (page 727)

a. 120 ÷ 60 = 2 mL/min
b. 120 ÷ 15 = 8 mL/min
c. 120 ÷ 30 = 4 mL/min

14. (page 725)

Temperature in °F	°F - 32	(°F - 32) × 0.555	Temperature in °C
32	**0**	**0**	**0**
95.0	**95 − 32 = 63**	**63 × 0.555 = 34.97**	**34.97 (approximately 35)**
98.6	98.6 − 32 = 66.6	66.6 × 0.555 = 36.96	36.96 (approximately 37)
101.0	**101 − 32 = 69**	**69 × 0.555 = 38.3**	**38.3 (approximately 38)**
104.0	**104 − 32 = 72**	**72 × 0.555 = 39.96**	**39.96 (approximately 40)**

15. (pages 726–727)

Desired Dose	Patient's Weight in Pounds (lb)	Patient's Weight in Kilograms (kg)	Medication Administered
1 mg/kg lidocaine	90	90 ÷ 2.2 = 40.9 kg (≈ 41 kg)	41 kg × 1 mg lidocaine = 41 mg lidocaine to administer
0.2 mg/kg atropine	30	**30 ÷ 2.2 = 13.6**	**13.6 kg × 0.2 mg atropine = 2.72 mg atropine to administer**
0.05 mg/kg lorazepam	180	**180 ÷ 2.2 = 81.8**	**81.8 kg × 0.5 mg = 4.09 mg lorazepam to administer**
30 mg/kg methylprednisolone	220	**220 ÷ 2.2 = 100**	**100 kg × 30 mg = 3,000 mg = 3 g methylprednisolone to administer**
15 mg/kg phenobarbital	12	**12 ÷ 2.2 = 5.5**	**5.5 kg × 15 mg = 82.5 mg phenobarbital to administer**

16. (pages 728–729)

Patient's Weight in Pounds (lb)	Patient's Weight in Kilograms: Weight in lb ÷ 2.2 = Weight in kg (or Use the "10% Trick")	Volume to be Infused with First Bolus at 20 mL/kg
60	**60 lb ÷ 2.2 = 27 kg**	**27 kg × 20 mL/kg = 540 mL**
80	**80 lb ÷ 2.2 = 36 kg**	**36 kg × 20 mL/kg = 720 mL**
100	**100 lb ÷ 2.2 = 45 kg**	**45 kg × 20 mL/kg = 900 mL**
125	**125 lb ÷ 2.2 = 57 kg**	**57 kg × 20 mL/kg = 1,140 mL**
150	**150 lb ÷ 2.2 = 68 kg**	**68 kg × 20 mL/kg = 1,360 mL**
175	**175 lb ÷ 2.2 = 80 kg**	**80 kg × 20 mL/kg = 1,600 mL**
190	**190 lb ÷ 2.2 = 86 kg**	**86 kg × 20 mL/kg = 1,720 mL**
20	**220 lb ÷ 2.2 = 100 kg**	**100 kg × 20 mL/kg = 2,000 mL (= 2 L)**
300	**300 lb ÷ 2.2 = 136 kg**	**136 kg × 20 mL/kg = 2,720 mL**

17. (pages 726–727)

a. 100 mg/10 mL lidocaine = 10 mg/1 mL lidocaine
b. 1 mg/10 mL epinephrine = 0.1 mg/1 mL epinephrine
c. 40 mg/14 mL furosemide = 2.9 mg/1 mL furosemide
d. 6 mg/2 mL adenosine = 3 mg/1 mL adenosine
e. 20 mg/5 mL diazepam = 4 mg/1 mL diazepam
f. 10 mg/5 mL naloxone = 2 mg/1 mL naloxone
g. 2 mg/5 mL albuterol = 0.4 mg/1 mL albuterol
h. 150 mg/3 mL amiodarone = 50 mg/1 mL amiodarone
i. 25 g/125 mL activated charcoal = 0.2 g/1 mL activated charcoal = 200 mg/1 mL activated charcoal

18. (pages 725–726)

- **a.** 1% xylocaine = 1 g/100 mL = 0.01 /1 mL (or 10 mg/mL)
- **b.** 10% dextrose = 10 g/100 mL = 0.1 g/1 mL (or 100 mg/mL)
- **c.** 0.5% albuterol = 0.5 g/100 mL = 0.005 g/1 mL (or 5 mg/mL)
- **d.** 10% calcium chloride = 10 g/100 mL = 0.1 g/1 mL (or 100 mg/mL)
- **e.** 50% magnesium sulfate = 50 g/100 mL = 0.5 g/1 mL (or 500 mg/mL)
- **f.** 5% alupent = 5 g/100 mL = 0.05 g/1 mL (or 50 mg/mL)
- **g.** 0.9% sodium chloride = 0.9 g/100 mL = 0.009 g/1 mL (or 9 mg/mL)

19. (pages 726–727)

- **a.** 800 mg/500 mL = 1.6 mg/1 mL = 1,600 mcg/1 mL
- **b.** 800 mg/250 mL = 3.2 mg/1 mL = 3,200 mcg/mL
- **c.** 800 mg/1,000 mL = 0.8 mg/1 mL = 800 mcg/mL
- **d.** 800 mg/100 mL = 8.0 mg/1 mL = 8,000 mcg/mL

20. (pages 726–727)

- **a.** Desired dose = 15 mg labetalol
  Concentration = 100 mg/20 mL = 5 mg/1 mL
  15 mg ÷ 5 mg/mL = 3 mL of medication will be administered
- **b.** Desired dose = 3 mg haloperidol
  Concentration = 5 mg haloperidol/1 mL
  3 mg ÷ 5 mg/mL = 0.6 mL of haloperidol will be administered
- **c.** Desired dose = 750 mg calcium chloride
  Concentration = 1,000 mg calcium chloride/10 mL = 100 mg calcium chloride/1 mL
  750 mg ÷ 100 mg/mL = 7.5 mL of calcium chloride will be administered

Section 5: Airway Management

Chapter 15: Airway Management

Matching

Part I

1. J (page 785)
2. I (page 838)
3. H (page 785)
4. F (page 785)
5. E (page 866)
6. D (page 783)
7. L (pages 861–862)
8. N (page 783)
9. M (page 777)
10. K (page 787)
11. P (page 823)
12. O (page 783)
13. T (page 789)
14. S (page 862)
15. V (page 787)
16. U (page 781)
17. X (page 823)
18. W (page 787)
19. Q (page 831)
20. R (page 783)
21. D (page 783)
22. C (page 785)
23. A (page 804)
24. B (page 784)

Part II

1. T (pages 831–832)
2. C (page 878)
3. T (pages 831–832)
4. N (page 847)
5. N (page 847)
6. T (pages 831–832)
7. T (pages 831–832)
8. C (page 878)

Part III

1. E, F (pages 816–818)
2. B (pages 808–809)
3. C (page 813)
4. A (page 809)
5. D, E (pages 814–817)
6. B (pages 808–809)
7. C, D (pages 813–816)
8. B (pages 808–809)

Multiple Choice

1. C (page 777)
2. A (page 779)
3. D (page 809)
4. B (page 831)
5. B (page 876)
6. D (page 863)
7. A (page 883)
8. C (page 829)
9. C (page 784)
10. D (page 785)
11. C (page 876)
12. D (page 876)
13. C (page 876)
14. A (page 869)
15. C (page 830)
16. B (page 867)
17. C (page 866)
18. D (pages 863–864)
19. B (page 862)
20. D (page 858)

Fill in the Blank

1. hypoxia; preoxygenation (page 834)
2. sniffing (page 835)
3. 30 (page 838)
4. i-gel; bite block; channel; gastric; support (page 871)
5. stroke (pages 802)
6. French; whistle-tip; tonsil-tip (page 797)
7. camera; distal; airway; clouded (page 846)
8. preoxygenate (page 834)
9. intact gag reflex; caustic (page 867)
10. partially exposed; Mallampati (page 830)

Labeling

1. Parts of the larynx (page 777, Figure 15-2)
   - A. Hyoid bone
   - B. Thyrohyoid ligament
   - C. Laryngeal prominence (Adam's apple)
   - D. Cricothyroid membrane
   - E. Trachea
   - F. Corniculate cartilage (behind larynx)
   - G. Thyroid cartilage
   - H. Arytenoid cartilage (behind larynx)
   - I. Cricoid cartilage

Identify

1. Chief complaint: Choking.
2. Vital signs: Respirations are 28 breaths/min and shallow. Decreased right-side lung sounds. Pulse is 98 beats/min and regular. Blood pressure is 128/86 mm Hg. Skin is cyanotic and cool. Spo_2 is 90%, and the patient is confused.
3. Pertinent negatives: The patient has clear lung sounds on the left, which suggests that the cap has gone down the right mainstem. Because there are sounds on the right, you know that only a portion of the right lung has been blocked, and the cap must be stuck in the bronchial tree.

   There is nothing other than oxygen and a fast but safe ride that you can give this patient! He needs to get to surgery as soon as possible.

Complete the Patient Care Report (PCR)

Show your completed PCR to your paramedic instructor, and ask for feedback on how well you recorded the case you were given.

Ambulance Calls

1. a. The patient described in this question is showing classic signs of choking. He gives the universal distress sign for choking (clutches his neck), staggers, and falls—all without making a sound. The reason he is not making a sound is because no air is moving past his vocal cords, which means his upper airway is completely obstructed—and that means he is going to die if you do not act immediately. (page 804)
   b. The most urgent priority is to try to expel the foreign body from his airway, which means giving the patient manual thrusts. There is no reason to pump his stomach (answer 1) because his problem is what *did not* make it into his stomach, not what *did*. Clearly, he is not in any shape to gargle with saltwater (answer 3), nor would it help him if he could. At the moment, he does not need epinephrine (answer 4), although he may need it very soon if his airway obstruction is not relieved and he suffers cardiac arrest as a consequence. He certainly doesn't need a sedative such as diazepam (Valium) (answer 5); he is already sedated quite enough by his hypoxemia. (What's hypoxemia? Check the glossary if you don't remember.) Both this question and the one preceding illustrate why it is not a good idea to try to grab a quick dinner while you are on duty. The Law of Dining on Duty states: If you are going to get called to a cardiac arrest during your shift, the call will come at the precise moment that the pizza you ordered comes out of the oven. (pages 804–805)
2. a. When your friend starts to choke on his hot dog, as evidenced by his paroxysm of violent coughing, the first thing you should do is encourage him to keep coughing (answer 5). A cough generates airflows of gale-force velocity—far more powerful than anything you could generate artificially by, for example, using manual thrusts (answer 3). Sticking your finger in the mouth of a panicky, choking person (answer 2) is a good way to lose a finger; reaching blindly into the throat with any instrument, let alone barbecue tongs (answer 4), is as likely to produce a rather messy tonsillectomy as it is to snare a wayward hot dog. There is no point in trying to ventilate your friend artificially (answer 1); he still has some air exchange by his own efforts, and blowing into his mouth may just force the hot dog farther down his airway. (page 804)
   b. When coughing fails to expel the foreign object and the person's airway becomes completely obstructed (as evidenced by your friend's aphonia), that is the time to give the Heimlich maneuver (abdominal thrust) (answer 3). Your friend is still conscious, so the finger sweep (answer 2) and head tilt (answer 1) are still inappropriate. The barbecue tongs (answer 4) are always inappropriate. There is no point now in encouraging your friend to keep coughing (answer 5); if he could cough, he would. (page 804)
   c. When the Heimlich maneuver (abdominal thrust) does not work and your friend becomes unconscious, your next steps should be as follows:
      (1) Carefully position him on the ground.
      (2) Begin 30 chest compressions.
      (3) Open the airway and look in the mouth. Attempt to remove the foreign body only if you actually see it, and then attempt to ventilate the patient.
      (4) If you cannot force air past the obstruction, give chest compressions until the foreign body is expelled from the victim's airway. (page 804)
   d. When the paramedics arrive with all their gear, you finally have the means to take definitive action. At that point, you should take the following steps:
      (1) With the patient's head in the sniffing position, open the patient's mouth and insert the laryngoscope blade.
      (2) Visualize the obstruction.

(3) Remove the object with the Magill forceps.
(4) Attempt to ventilate the patient. (pages 805–806)

3. Probably this male bodybuilder has a short, very muscular neck, which is a classic situation for a difficult intubation.
a. When the cords will not come into view, ask your partner to apply the **BURP maneuver**, which is **backward, upward, rightward** pressure on the larynx. (page 838)
b. gum elastic bougie (page 837)
c. When you finally have the tube in and have confirmed its position, you need to secure it. Be sure to document the following on the PCR:
(1) You visualized it going through the vocal cords.
(2) You auscultated both lungs and the stomach.
(3) The end-tidal waveform capnography reading
(4) The depth of the tube as noted by the centimeter marking at the teeth (page 841)

4. Nasotracheal intubation does not always go smoothly, and you need to be prepared to spend a little time getting it right.
a. You can tell that the tip is moving toward the glottis by:
(1) Putting your ear over the tube and hearing and feeling the movement of air through the tube. This can also be done using a stethoscope. (page 848)
(2) Seeing misting inside the tube (from condensation of the patient's breath). (page 850)
(3) Using a Beck Airway Airflow Monitor device and listening for the sounds of breathing. (pages 848, 850)
b. When the beeps from the monitor start getting further and further apart, it means that the patient's heart is slowing down (ie, she is developing bradycardia).
c. You must immediately:
(1) Stop advancing the tube.
(2) Attach the tube to an oxygen source and consider ventilating.
(3) Consider using a basic life support (BLS) airway until the patient is no longer hypoxic.

5. a. 33 minutes
b. The oxygen will run out before you get back.

$$\text{Duration of flow} = \frac{(\text{Tank pressure in psi} - 200\text{ psi}) \times \text{Cylinder constant}}{\text{Flow rate in L/min}}$$

$$\frac{(800\text{ psi} - 200\text{ psi}) \times 0.28}{5\text{ L/min}} = 33.6$$

Only if you let the cylinder run down all the way to zero will you manage to squeeze 40 minutes' worth of oxygen out of it, but you will have to make sure you keep up your pace as you trudge through the woods carrying the stretcher. If you are starting to drag, you would be better advised to decrease the flow rate to the nasal cannula to about 4 L/min. And next time, make sure you take a full oxygen cylinder with you. (pages 806–807)

6. (1) Seeing the patient's chest rise and fall with each breath you give
(2) Feeling the compliance of the patient's lungs in your own lungs
(3) Hearing and feeling air escape through the patient's mouth during passive exhalation (page 814)

7. a. To minimize gastric distention during artificial ventilation, you need to:
(1) Reposition and reassess the airway to keep it fully open.
(2) Observe the chest for adequate rise and fall, avoiding excessive ventilation volumes. Blow in only that volume of air needed to obtain visible chest rise.
(3) Limit ventilation times to 1 second. (page 820)
b. If the patient's gastric distention begins to interfere seriously with your ability to get any air into his lungs, you will have to attempt to decompress the stomach. It will not be a pleasant job. Follow the steps for insertion of an orogastric tube or nasogastric tube.

If you answered either of those "What should you do?" questions with the phrase, "Call an ambulance!" give yourself an extra point. Unless you want to spend the night doing CPR all by yourself in the movie theater, you should send someone for help at the very outset. (pages 820–823)

8. The advantages of the pocket mask over other devices for giving artificial ventilation include:
(1) Its immediate availability (assuming you remember to carry it in your pocket).
(2) Its adaptability; it can be deployed with or without supplemental oxygen.

(3) Its potential to be used as a simple face mask if the patient resumes breathing.

(4) Its effectiveness; it is much easier to maintain a good seal with a pocket mask (and therefore deliver good volumes) than it is with a bag-mask device as a single rescuer. (page 813)

9. The patient in heart failure has fluid in his alveoli, and for that reason, a portion of his cardiac output is not picking up any oxygen as it passes through the lungs (a situation called shunting). It is not surprising, therefore, that his oxygen saturation is reduced.

- **a.** The Spo_2 reading of 86% is abnormally low. A normal reading would be greater than 95% on room air. There is no reason to suspect an artifact (erroneous reading) because the reading is consistent with the patient's clinical presentation. (pages 787–788)
- **b.** The measure you need to take immediately when you see a reading like that (or, even without a pulse oximeter, when you see a patient in respiratory distress) is to administer oxygen. (What would be the best device for administering supplemental oxygen to this patient?) (page 788)
- **c.** Possible sources of an erroneous reading in this patient include the following. *Students should list three of the following:*
  - (1) Bright ambient light may be interfering with the reading. Cover the sensor with a towel or aluminum foil if you suspect that is the problem.
  - (2) Check whether the patient is moving. The oximeter may confuse patient motion for a pulse.
  - (3) If it is cold in the ambulance, causing the patient's peripheral blood vessels to constrict as a consequence, the resulting poor perfusion of the extremities may lead to false oximetry readings.
  - (4) Nail polish will prevent the sensor from working properly.
  - (5) The sensor may be picking up venous pulsations. Move it to a different finger or to the earlobe and recheck.
  - (6) Abnormal hemoglobin may produce a false-normal reading. (page 789)

10. Probably the primary indication for using an end-tidal carbon dioxide monitor is to confirm and monitor the placement of an endotracheal tube.

- **a.** In the case described, you can conclude that the tracheal tube is in the esophagus. If the tube were in the trachea, as it is supposed to be, the carbon dioxide concentration of the exhaled gas ought to be at least 2%, translating into a tan or yellow color on the sensor. (page 790)
- **b.** The action you should take right away is to deflate the cuff and remove the tracheal tube. Preoxygenate the patient before you make another attempt to intubate. (pages 848–852)

11. a. The situation is much more serious than it might seem from a 33% reduction in minute volume. A person whose tidal volume is so small is doing little more than moving his dead space back and forth (do you remember what dead space is?), so there is little true alveolar ventilation and, therefore, little carbon dioxide removal.
Because carbon dioxide will not be removed efficiently, the level of carbon dioxide in the blood will rise, and the arterial Pco_2 will rise—by definition, a situation of hypoventilation. (page 792)

- **b.** As a result, the patient's pH will **fall**, reflecting the increased acidity of his blood. (pages 781–782)
- **c.** The resulting derangement in his acid–base balance is called a **respiratory acidosis**—"acidosis" because the pH is lower than normal, "respiratory" because the source of the problem is in the respiratory system (the failure to breathe deeply enough). (pages 781–782)
- **d.** The treatment required in the acute situation is to assist the patient's ventilations to improve the tidal volume and flush out some of that excess carbon dioxide. (pages 781–782)

12. The next time you have to walk up four flights of steps, you will probably remember to take a full E cylinder, not a half-empty D cylinder.

$$\text{Duration of flow} = \frac{(\text{Tank pressure} - 200\text{ psi}) \times C}{\text{Flow rate}}$$

$$\frac{(900\text{ psi} - 200\text{ psi}) \times 0.16\text{ L/psi}}{10\text{ L/min}} = \text{about 11 (11.2) minutes (page 807)}$$

13. In this question about a head-injured patient, you had to review both some respiratory physiology and the pathophysiology of head injury.

- **a.** You can conclude that the patient's arterial Pco_2 will tend to **increase**, so his pH will **decrease**. The net effect will be an acid–base disorder called a **respiratory acidosis**. The way you can help correct that abnormality is to **assist the patient's ventilations. This will increase the patient's minute volume (which will blow off more carbon dioxide).** (pages 781–782)

14. a. *Students will list five of the following conditions that can cause respiratory distress and inadequate ventilation:*
(1) Severe infection
(2) Trauma
(3) Brainstem insult
(4) A noxious or oxygen-poor environment
(5) Upper or lower airway obstruction
(6) Respiratory muscle impairment (eg, spinal injury)
(7) A central nervous system impairment (eg, head trauma) (page 783)

b. The treatment for hypoxia/hypoxemia is to give supplemental oxygen. That may sound obvious, but it is truly remarkable how many hypoxemic patients arrive at the emergency room by ambulance without oxygen being administered. Don't be stingy with oxygen. (page 783)

True/False

One of the most important things to remember about suctioning is that suctioning removes air as well as liquids.

1. T (pages 797–799)
2. T (pages 797–799)
3. F (page 824)
4. T (page 787)
5. T (page 874)
6. F (page 777)
7. F (page 777)
8. T (page 779)
9. F (page 829–830)
10. F (page 873)

Short Answer

1. *Students should list four of the following:*
a. The tongue
b. A foreign body*
c. Swelling (edema)
d. Trauma to the face or neck
e. Aspirated vomitus (page 802)

2. a. Provides a secure airway
b. Protects the airway from aspiration
c. Enables delivery of aerosolized drugs directly into the lung for rapid absorption into the bloodstream (page 831)

3. *Students should list three of the following:*
a. Airway control needed as a result of coma, respiratory arrest, and/or cardiac arrest
b. Ventilatory support before impending respiratory failure
c. Prolonged ventilator support required
d. Absence of a gag reflex
e. Traumatic brain injury
f. Unresponsiveness
g. Impending airway compromise (as in burns or trauma)
h. Medication administration (as a last resort) (page 833)

4. a. Accidental intubation of the esophagus (page 838)
b. This complication can be avoided by:
(1) Positioning the patient correctly for intubation
(2) Seeing the tube pass through the vocal cords
(3) Checking for breath sounds over both lungs after intubation and epigastrium
(4) Always using end-tidal waveform capnography to confirm and monitor the tube (page 839)

c. If it does occur, intubation of the esophagus can be detected by:
(1) Gurgling noises over the epigastrium during ventilation
(2) Absence of breath sounds over the lungs during ventilation
(3) Failure of the patient to "pink up" on ventilation

Once detected, accidental intubation of the esophagus can be corrected by immediately withdrawing the tracheal tube and ventilating the patient with a bag-mask device. No further attempt to intubate the patient should be made until the patient has been reoxygenated for at least 3 minutes. (page 839)

d. Accidental intubation of a bronchus (usually the right main bronchus) (page 839)
e. Can be avoided by stopping as soon as the cuff passes the vocal cords (page 839)
f. If it does occur, bronchial intubation can be detected by the absence of breath sounds over one lung (usually the left). Once detected, bronchial intubation can be corrected by deflating the cuff, and then slowly drawing the tube back until breath sounds become audible in both lungs. Then, reinflate the cuff and mark the tube at the teeth. (page 839)

5. The principal hazard of using a neuromuscular blocker is that it converts a breathing patient with some sort of airway into a nonbreathing patient without any airway; therefore, if you are unable to intubate within 30 seconds and you have trouble maintaining an airway manually, the patient will need a surgical airway urgently. (page 862)
6. *Students should list five of the following:*
   a. Pulmonary edema
   b. Pneumonia
   c. Submersion (drowning)
   d. Chest trauma
   e. Airway obstruction
   f. Pneumothorax
   g. Inhalation of smoke or toxic fumes
   h. Respiratory arrest (page 806)
7. *Students should list four of the following:*
   a. Tachypnea (rapid breathing)
   b. Hyperpnea (abnormally deep breathing)
   c. Use of accessory muscles to breathe
   d. Nasal flaring
   e. Cyanosis (bluish tinge to the lips and nail beds)
   f. If you mentioned dyspnea—a feeling of shortness of breath—that's acceptable, but technically speaking, dyspnea is a symptom, not a sign. (pages 783–784)
8. *Students should list six of the following:*
   a. No smoking!
   b. No grease.
   c. Keep out of extreme heat.
   d. Use the right valve.
   e. Keep all valves closed when not in use.
   f. Keep cylinders firmly secured.
   g. Keep your face and body to the side of the cylinder.
   h. Have the cylinder tested every 10 years. (pages 806–807)
9. a. Observe the chest to see if it rises and falls. For a respiratory complaint, make a visual observation.
   b. Listen over the nose and mouth for the sound of airflow. For a respiratory complaint, listen to (auscultate) the lungs for air movement.
   c. Feel with your cheek over the nose and mouth for the movement of air. For a respiratory complaint, palpate the chest for equal movement. (pages 783–787)
10. A person who has suffered respiratory arrest will need **artificial** ventilation. (page 811)
11. In artificial ventilation, the rescuer has to breathe for the patient. In assisted ventilation, by contrast, the patient is breathing spontaneously, and the rescuer simply boosts the tidal volume. (pages 811–814)
12. With any form of artificial ventilation, the primary objective is to normalize the PCO_2 by moving air in and out of the lungs. Controlled ventilation also aims to supply oxygen to the alveoli. (pages 811–814)
13. In general, with any patient whose state of oxygenation may be in jeopardy, the pulse oximeter can help you keep tabs on things. *Students should list three situations.* (page 788)
    a. A patient with trauma to the chest, in whom pneumothorax or hemothorax (or both) may interfere with oxygenation
    b. A patient in pulmonary edema, who has a large shunt because of fluid in his or her alveoli
    c. A patient undergoing tracheal intubation
    d. A patient undergoing suctioning
    e. A patient having a severe asthma attack or deterioration of chronic lung disease
    f. A submersion (drowning) victim
14. The spine-injured patient with weakness or partial paralysis of the respiratory muscles does not have the strength to inhale deeply. Thus, his tidal volume will be smaller than normal, so his minute volume will also **decrease**, leading to an **increase** in his arterial PCO_2. (page 779)

Fill in the Table

1. Knowing when to deploy a piece of equipment is just as important as knowing how to deploy it. (pages 779–801)

	Oropharyngeal Airway	Nasopharyngeal Airway
Use for:	Deeply unconscious patient who has no gag reflex, especially if being ventilated by bag-mask device Bite block for intubated patient	Patient with an altered mental status
Do not use for:	Patient with intact gag reflex	Patient with trauma to the nose Suspected basilar skull fracture (blood or clear fluid draining from nose)

2. Oxygen-delivery devices (page 809)

Device	Flow Rate (L/min)	Oxygen Delivered (%)
Nasal cannula	1-6	24-44
Nonrebreathing mask	15	90-100
Bag-mask device with reservoir	15 flush	Nearly 100

3. Every piece of equipment in the ambulance has its indications and sometimes contraindications. You need to be aware of both. (pages 799–800, 831–841, 868–871, 875–877)

Adjunct	Indicated for:	Do Not Use in:
Oropharyngeal airway	Airway maintenance in deeply unconscious, breathing patient To improve effectiveness of bag-mask ventilation	Patient who is not deeply unconscious Severe trauma in the mouth Any patient with intact gag reflex
Combitube	Cardiac arrest when it is not feasible to intubate the trachea Patient who has swallowed corrosives	Patient who is not deeply unconscious
LMA	Cardiac arrest when it is not feasible to intubate the trachea	Patient who has food in his stomach and may aspirate
Endotracheal intubation	Cardiac arrest Deep coma Absent gag reflex Imminent danger of upper airway obstruction (eg, respiratory burns)	Patients with intact gag reflex or likelihood of laryngospasm

Section 6: Medical

Chapter 16: Respiratory Emergencies

Matching

Part I

1. Q (page 923)
2. P (page 912)
3. O (page 909)
4. N (page 936)
5. M (page 916)
6. A(page 915)
7. B (page 905)
8. C (page 937)
9. D (page 945)
10. E (page 922)
11. T (page 907)
12. S (page 909)
13. R (page 949)
14. I (page 905)
15. H (page 949)
16. G (page 911)
17. L (page 907)
18. K (page 912)
19. J (page 910)
20. F (page 909)

Part II

1. P (page 946)
2. O (page 911)
3. N (page 907)
4. M (page 928)
5. L (page 916)
6. E (page 907)
7. D (page 909)
8. C (page 928)
9. B (page 924)
10. A (page 946)
11. T (page 918)
12. S (page 938)
13. R (page 916)
14. Q (page 907)
15. K (page 946)
16. J (page 915)
17. I (page 936)
18. H (page 910)
19. G (pages 923–924)
20. F (page 943)

Multiple Choice

1. B (page 905)
2. C (page 948)
3. D (page 923)
4. C (page 945)
5. A (page 918)
6. C (page 917)
7. C (page 918)
8. B (page 909)
9. D (pages 939–940)
10. A (page 910)

Fill in the Blank

1. atelectasis (page 945)
2. Paroxysmal nocturnal; left-sided (page 911)
3. polycythemia (page 907)
4. flail chest (page 908)
5. orthopnea (page 928); cyanosis (page 920)
6. paroxysmal nocturnal dyspnea (page 911)
7. Tactile fremitus (page 925)
8. three; two (page 905)
9. thyroid; upward (page 914)
10. pursed-lip breathing (page 939)

Labeling

1. Respiratory patterns (page 920, Figure 16-12)
   - **A.** Cheyne-Stokes breathing
   - **B.** Central neurogenic hyperventilation
   - **C.** Apneustic respiration
   - **D.** Biot respiration
   - **E.** Ataxic respiration
   - **F.** Agonal gasps

Identify

1. Chief complaint: Unresponsive, not breathing
2. Vital signs: Heart rate 46 beats/min; oxygen saturation 64%
3. Pertinent negatives: No chest rise and fall

   Tommy was unconscious and not breathing. He had no chest rise and fall upon trying to ventilate him. He did have a faint brachial pulse, which identified that compressions were not needed yet because his airway had not been blocked for very long. Oxygen saturation was 64%, heart rate was 46 beats/min, and there were no spontaneous respirations. BP was unattainable. After the airway was opened, Tommy quickly returned to normal with 100% supplemental oxygen.

Ambulance Calls

1. **a.** Although it is possible for a 22-year-old to suffer a heart attack, it is not very likely; thus, when you are confronted with a patient of this age complaining of chest pain, you need to think about other possibilities—such as a pulmonary embolism, a spontaneous pneumothorax, or, as this case turns out to be, hyperventilation syndrome. The tip-offs are the paresthesia around the mouth, the carpopedal spasm, and, incidentally, the increased respiratory rate. That last is significant because, strangely enough, often tachypnea and hyperpnea are not the most prominent features of hyperventilation syndrome, and, as in this case, other signs or symptoms may predominate. (page 910)

   b. The steps in management are:
   (1) Calm and reassure the patient.
   (2) Help her to take conscious control of her breathing by telling her to breathe as you slowly count (about one number every 5 seconds).
   (3) If the acute episode does not pass, the patient needs to be evaluated in the ED. (pages 910–911)

   c. This woman's arterial P_{CO_2} is probably *lower* than normal because her minute ventilation is increased; that is, she is blowing off more carbon dioxide than usual. (page 910)

2. Later during the history, you learn that Mr. Smith has been smoking three packs a day for 48 years. The 1,051,200 cigarettes (give or take a few) that Mr. Smith has smoked over this time frame seem to be catching up with him. You can do the arithmetic yourself: 3 packs/day × 20 cigarettes/pack × 365 days/year × 48 years.

   a. Now you find him in respiratory distress. Signs of respiratory distress (increased work of breathing) include the following:
   (1) Bony retractions
   (2) Soft-tissue retractions
   (3) Nasal flaring
   (4) Tracheal tugging
   (5) Paradoxical respiratory movement
   (6) Pulsus paradoxus
   (7) Pursed-lip breathing
   (8) Grunting (page 914)

   b. What needs to be done immediately on encountering a patient in this condition is to administer supplemental oxygen before you ask any more questions or proceed any further with your examination. It is also a good idea to attach the patient to a cardiac monitor and to obtain a 12-lead electrocardiogram (ECG) at this stage because a hypoxic patient is a patient who is very likely to develop serious, possibly life-threatening cardiac dysrhythmias—and you would like to have some warning that they are coming. (page 928)

   c. In taking the history, the following are the pieces of information you would like to know (pages 921–923):

   Regarding the dyspnea, the OPQRST questions are, in order:
   (1) O: Onset—When it did start?
   (2) P: We already have a general idea of what provoked the symptoms (probably it was being in the recumbent position for several hours), but it would be useful to know what palliates them. Is there a position in which the patient is more comfortable? Has he taken anything to try to relieve his symptoms? If so, did it help?
   (3) Q: What is the quality of the dyspnea? Is it the same as his usual shortness of breath or qualitatively different?
   (4) R: Radiates—Does pain go anywhere else?
   (5) S: How severe is the dyspnea? Ask the patient to rate it on a 1 to 10 scale, with 1 being nothing and 10 being the worst, against his usual dyspnea, in terms of ability to do specific things (eg, walk up a flight of stairs).
   (6) T: What was the timing of this particular attack? When specifically did it come on? Which symptom came first, and what came next?
   (7) Take a SAMPLE history.

   d. In conducting the secondary assessment, you are looking for some very specific signs. (pages 923–927)

Part of the Body	What I Am Looking for in Particular
General appearance	**Position; level of consciousness (to indicate cerebral oxygenation); degree of distress; skin–sweating cyanosis**
Vital signs	**Tachycardia; abnormal respiratory rate, depth, or pattern; noisy breathing**
Head	**Cyanosis of mucous membranes; nasal flaring**
Neck	**Tracheal tugging or deviation; use of neck muscles to breathe; distended neck veins**
Chest	**Barred chest; abnormal or unequal breath sounds; inadequate air exchange**
Abdomen	**Paradoxical respiratory movement; painful, palpable liver in right upper quadrant**
Extremities	**Cigarette stains; clubbing of the fingers; pedal edema**

e. (1) Answer: (b) Chronic obstructive pulmonary disease (COPD). This patient is most likely suffering from an acute decompensation of COPD. (page 943)
(2) The steps of management should include the following: (pages 943–944)
- Administer supplemental oxygen. (You should have done that already.)
- Keep the patient sitting up. (He probably won't allow you to do otherwise).
- Start IV fluids at to-keep-open (TKO) rate.
- Monitor ECG.

If you chose to withhold oxygen from this patient, or even to give it in a stingy fashion, you flunk—because the patient may die. Go back and reread the section in your textbook on COPD. No, oxygen should not be withheld from this patient, nor should it be given in very low flows. The treatment of choice for COPD in decompensation is oxygen, oxygen, oxygen. That is one of the few medications that can save the patient's life.

The doctor has ordered a breathing treatment for the patient as well. You will see in a moment whether that was a judicious choice, but meanwhile, it gives you an opportunity to review the pharmacology of albuterol (Proventil, Ventolin). (page 931)

3. a. Answer: (1) Pulmonary embolism. The 56-year-old man with the sudden onset of dyspnea and pleuritic chest pain has most probably experienced a pulmonary embolism, to which his chronic heart disease predisposed him. (page 949)
b. Prehospital management of the case includes the following steps:
(1) Administer 100% supplemental oxygen.
(2) Start a large-bore IV line with fluid to keep a vein open.
(3) Monitor ECG.
(4) Transport without delay. (page 949)

True/False

1. T (page 907)
2. T (page 915)
3. T (page 905)
4. T (page 919)
5. F (page 928)
6. T (page 917)
7. T (page 912)
8. T (page 924)
9. T (page 925)
10. T (page 926)
11. T (page 919)
12. F (page 947)
13. F (pages 943–944)
14. T (page 940)
15. T (page 932)
16. F (page 930)
17. F (page 930)
18. F (page 933)
19. F (page 933)
20. F (pages 933–935)

Short Answer

1. Four things that can cause a pulmonary embolism (page 949):
a. Fat embolism from a broken bone
b. Amniotic fluid leakage
c. Air embolism from trauma or IV line
d. Blood clot caused by heart rhythms or lifestyle

2. Diagnosis of a pulmonary embolism is cyanosis that does not resolve with the administration of supplemental oxygen. A good history, finding out about such events as a recent surgery or broken bone, also helps with the diagnosis. Cardiac history and the patient's current heart rhythm are helpful as well. The patient may have a history of deep vein thrombus. Also, the patient may present with an acute pain centered in the chest that does not radiate. Lung sounds are generally good with perhaps a small area of diminished sounds. (page 949)

3. There are no contraindications to oxygen in the prehospital setting as long as the patient's clinical picture warrants its use (ie, respiratory distress/failure and Spo_2 less than 95%). (page 928)

4. Not everything that wheezes is an acute asthmatic attack. Other causes of wheezing include the following:
   a. Left-sided heart failure (page 942)
   b. Smoke inhalation or inhalation of toxic fumes
   c. Chronic bronchitis (page 942)
   d. Foreign body obstruction of a major airway (eg, the patient who has a peanut lodged in a bronchus or a tumor compressing a bronchus) (page 942)
5. Signs that should alert you to the seriousness of an asthmatic attack in a child include the following (pages 939–941):
   a. Sleepiness
   b. Pulsus paradoxus
   c. Cyanosis
   d. Hyperinflation of the chest
   e. A silent chest

Fill in the Table

1. Breathing patterns (page 919, Table 16-5)

Pattern	Comments
Agonal	**Irregular gasps** that are widely spaced; usually represent **stray neurologic impulses** in a dying patient; occasional agonal gasps are not unusual in patients with no pulse; not actually considered a form of breathing
Apneustic	Characterized by a **prolonged inspiratory hold** (sometimes called "**fish** breathing"); follows damage to the **pneumotaxic center** in the brain; an ominous sign of severe **brain injury**
Ataxic	Chaotically irregular respirations that indicate **severe** brain injury or **brainstem herniation**
Biot respirations	Irregular pattern, **rate**, and depth of respirations, characterized by intermittent patterns of **apnea**; indicates severe brain injury or **brainstem** herniation
Bradypnea	Unusually **slow** respirations
Central neurogenic hyperventilation	Tachypneic **hyperpnea**; rapid and deep respirations caused by **increased intracranial pressure** or direct **brain injury**; drives **carbon dioxide** level down and **pH** up, resulting in respiratory **alkalosis**
Cheyne-Stokes respirations	**Crescendo-decrescendo** breathing with a period of **apnea** between cycles; not considered ominous unless grossly **exaggerated** or occurs in a patient with brain **trauma**
Cough	Forced exhalation against a closed **glottis**; an airway-clearing maneuver; also seen when **foreign substances** irritate the airways; controlled by the cough center in the brain (**Antitussive** medications work on the cough center to reduce this sometimes annoying physiologic response.)
Eupnea	**Normal** breathing
Hiccup	Spasmodic contraction of the **diaphragm**, causing short **exhalations** with a characteristic sound; sometimes seen in cases of diaphragmatic (or **phrenic**) nerve irritation from **acute myocardial infarction**, ulcer disease, or **endotracheal intubation**
Hyperpnea	Abnormally **increased** rate and depth of breathing; seen in various **neurologic** or chemical disorders, including overdose with certain drugs
Hypopnea	Abnormally **decreased** rate and depth of breathing
Kussmaul respirations	The same pattern as in **central neurogenic hyperventilation**, but caused by the body's response to metabolic **acidosis**, attempting to rid itself of blood **acetone** via the lungs; seen in diabetic **ketoacidosis**; accompanied by a **fruity** (acetone) breath odor and, usually, **cracked** and dry mouth and lips
Sighing	Periodically taking a very deep breath of about **twice** the normal volume; forces open **alveoli** that routinely close from time to time
Tachypnea	Unusually **rapid** breathing; does not reflect **depth** of respiration and does not mean a patient is **hyperventilating** (breathing too rapidly and deeply, resulting in a lowered **carbon dioxide** level); often involves moving only small volumes of air, or **hypoventilation** (much like a panting dog)
Yawning	Seems beneficial in the same manner as **sighing**

Complete the Patient Care Report (PCR)

Show your completed PCR to your paramedic instructor, and ask for feedback on how you recorded the case you were given.

Chapter 17: Cardiovascular Emergencies

Part 1: Cardiac Function

Matching

Part I

1. F (page 965)
2. G (page 1039)
3. E (page 964)
4. L (page 971)
5. K (page 1039)
6. J (page 1039)
7. O (page 1005)
8. N (page 1056)
9. M (page 1026)
10. R (page 1027)
11. Q (page 995)
12. P (page 978)
13. A (page 1027)
14. B (page 970)
15. C (page 964)
16. D (page 1005)
17. H (page 976)
18. I (page 995)
19. Y (page 964)
20. X (page 963)
21. W (page 979)
22. S (page 972)
23. T (page 967)
24. U (page 1064)
25. V (page 1028)

Part II

1. M (page 979)
2. L (page 1005)
3. K (page 1049)
4. G (page 1060)
5. F (page 988)
6. A (page 1004)
7. B (page 972)
8. C (page 968)
9. D (page 965)
10. E (page 961)
11. Y (page 965)
12. X (page 982)
13. T (page 1006)
14. U (page 1004)
15. W (page 1041)
16. P (page 981)
17. O (page 964)
18. N (page 971)
19. S (page 1038)
20. R (page 1029)
21. Q (page 963)
22. H (page 1027)
23. I (page 1045)
24. J (page 1020)
25. V (page 1061)

Multiple Choice

1. B (page 1060)
2. B (page 970)
3. D (page 971)
4. B (page 969)
5. C (page 967)
6. C (page 975)
7. D (page 1039)
8. C (page 967)
9. A (pages 1042–1043)
10. B (page 1045)

Fill in the Blank

1. collateral circulation (page 1064)
2. aortic (page 1062)
3. Contiguous (page 979)
4. pulmonary circulation (page 963)
5. rapid; anaphylaxis (page 1017)
6. first-degree; rhythm; P; QRS (page 1020)
7. AV junction (page 971)
8. ventricular; enlarged (page 1029)
9. absolute refractory period (page 970)
10. T wave (page 970)

Labeling

1. Coronary arteries (pages 962–963, Figures 17-1B and 17-1C)
   - **A.** Superior vena cava
   - **B.** Right atrium
   - **C.** Right coronary artery in coronary sulcus
   - **D.** Inferior vena cava
   - **E.** Aorta
   - **F.** Pulmonary artery
   - **G.** Left coronary artery
   - **H.** Left atrium
   - **I.** Circumflex branch of left coronary artery
   - **J.** Anterior descending branch of left coronary artery
   - **K.** Coronary vein

L. Aorta
M. Left pulmonary artery
N. Pulmonary veins
O. Left atrium
P. Coronary sinus
Q. Left ventricle
R. Superior vena cava
S. Right pulmonary artery
T. Pulmonary veins
U. Right atrium
V. Inferior vena cava
W. Right ventricle
X. Posterior descending coronary artery in posterior interventricular groove

2. Location of precordial leads (page 980, Figure 17-13)
A. Left ventricle
B. Left atrium
C. Right atrium
D. Interventricular septum
E. Right ventricle
F. Sternum

True/False

1. T (pages 966, 1059)
2. F (pages 1063–1064)
3. F (page 1056)
4. T (page 1054)
5. F (page 1054)
6. T (pages 1045–1047)
7. F (page 1047)
8. F (page 1042)
9. T (page 1042)
10. T (page 1041)

Fill in the Table

1. Role of electrolytes in cardiac function (page 970, Table 17-1)

Electrolyte	Role in Cardiac Function
Sodium (Na+)	Flows into the cell to initiate depolarization
Potassium (K+)	Flows out of the cell to initiate **repolarization** Decreased or increased levels of potassium result in the following: • ***Hypokalemia*** → increased myocardial irritability • ***Hyperkalemia*** → decreased automaticity/conduction
Calcium (Ca^{+2})	Has a major role in the depolarization of **pacemaker** cells (maintains depolarization) and in myocardial contractility (involved in contraction of heart muscle tissue) Decreased or increased levels of calcium result in the following: • ***Hypocalcemia*** → decreased contractility and increased myocardial irritability • ***Hypercalcemia*** → increased contractility
Magnesium (Mg^{+2})	Stabilizes the cell membrane; acts in concert with **potassium**, and opposes the actions of calcium Decreased or increased levels of magnesium result in the following: • ***Hypomagnesemia*** → decreased conduction • ***Hypermagnesemia*** → increased myocardial irritability

Part 2: Heart Rhythms and the ECG

Matching

Part I

1. G (page 978)
2. C (page 978)
3. I (page 984)
4. D (page 985)
5. B (pages 987–988)
6. F (page 991)
7. E (page 999)
8. A (page 1020)
9. J (page 1005)
10. H (page 997)

Part II

1. J (page 1062)
2. K (page 1029)
3. L (page 963)
4. M (page 967)
5. I (page 965)
6. H (page 970)
7. G (page 994)
8. F (page 1032)
9. Y (page 997)
10. X (page 1041)
11. W (page 1041)
12. V (page 984)
13. Q (pages 961, 963)
14. P (page 1062)
15. O (page 985)
16. N (page 1029)
17. D (page 1026)
18. C (page 972)
19. B (page 1014)
20. A (page 1034)
21. U (page 991)
22. T (page 992)
23. S (page 988)
24. R (page 987)
25. E (page 983)

Multiple Choice

1. B (page 985)
2. D (page 978)
3. C (page 1031)
4. A (page 979)
5. B (page 1014)
6. C (page 993)
7. C (page 1008)
8. A (page 1007)
9. B (page 1037)
10. A (page 982)

Fill in the Blank

1. Sinus arrest (page 992)
2. supraventricular tachycardia (page 993)
3. accelerated junctional rhythm (page 1002)
4. third-degree (page 1021)
5. Ventricular fibrillation (page 1007)
6. bigeminy; trigeminy (page 1005)
7. Asystole (page 1014)
8. delta wave (page 997)
9. unifocal; multifocal (page 1004)
10. sinus bradycardia (page 988)

True/False

1. T (page 976)
2. F (page 1003)
3. F (page 986)
4. T (page 991)
5. F (page 1001)
6. F (page 999)
7. T (page 1020)
8. F (page 972)
9. T (page 1006)
10. F (page 1005)

Short Answer

1. Shave the patient's body hair to prevent movement and facilitate skin contact. Wipe the chest area with an alcohol swab to remove oil and dead tissue. Wait for the alcohol to dry before application. Always attach electrodes to the cable before applying them to the chest area. Confirm the proper placement of all electrodes. (page 976)
2. The P wave is the depolarization of the SA node. The PR interval occurs while the impulse is delayed at the AV node. This delay allows the ventricles to fill fully. The QRS complex is the depolarization of both ventricles. The T wave represents the repolarization of both ventricles. (pages 982–984)
3. A 12-lead ECG "looks" at the heart as a whole. It gives views of the heart different from the standard three leads. It helps in localizing the site of injury in the heart. (page 1023)
4. Always start with scene safety and standard precautions. Check for responsiveness, open the airway, and assess breathing; if the patient is not breathing, give two breaths. Check pulse and start compressions if needed. Ready the defibrillator and check the patient's rhythm. After the rhythm is established, follow the advanced cardiac life support and/or your local protocol. (pages 1014–1019)
5. You and the medical director should practice different scenarios in preparation for having to deliver any bad news. You should role-play and discuss the correct way to break the news of the patient's death to the family. You must feel comfortable and develop strategies in advance for dealing with these situations. (pages 1018–1019)

Part 3: Putting It All Together and Practice ECG Strips

Matching

(page 966)

1. I
2. B
3. E
4. F
5. A
6. C
7. H
8. D
9. J
10. G

Labeling

1. Electrical conduction system (page 971)
   A. Sinoatrial (SA) node (pacemaker)
   B. Atrioventricular (AV) node
   C. Conduction myofibers (Purkinje fibers)
   D. Atrioventricular bundle
   E. Purkinje fibers
   F. Interventricular septum
   G. Right and left branches of AV bundle

Fill in the Table

1. Components of the ECG (page 985, Table 17-4)

ECG Representation	Cardiac Event
P wave	Depolarization of the **atria**
PRI	Depolarization of the atria and delay at the **AV** junction
QRS complex	Depolarization of the **ventricles**
ST segment	Period between ventricular depolarization and beginning of **repolarization**
T wave	Ventricular **repolarization**
R-R interval	Time between two **successive** ventricular depolarizations

Ambulance Calls

1. a. Chief complaint: Severe chest pain

Vital signs: Skin is pale and cool, pulse is 82 beats/min and thready, respirations are 32 breaths/min and shallow, BP is 90/62 mm Hg, and oxygen saturation is 91% on room air.

b. (1) Apply high-flow supplemental oxygen.
(2) Listen to lung sounds.
(3) Apply the heart monitor.
(4) Start an IV medication line.

The patient is not a candidate for nitroglycerin at this point, but having him chew 325 mg of aspirin would be appropriate. (page 1045)

c. (1) Yes
(2) About 135 beats/min
(3) Hidden in QRS; some are seen as inverted after QRS
(4) Not present
(5) Not present
(6) 0.12 seconds
(7) Present and upright
(8) Junctional tachycardia (page 1003)

d. Without a 12-lead ECG, you cannot confirm an AMI. However, because the patient has chest pain, the AMI and chest pain protocols should be followed. (pages 1042–1048)
e. Treatment should consist of advanced cardiac life support (ACLS) guidelines. Nitrates would not be good for this patient because of the low BP. (page 1044)

2. a. Chief complaint: Severe dyspnea

Vital signs: Skin is cyanotic, pulse is 102 beats/min and irregular, respirations are 60 breaths/min and labored, BP is 170/94 mm Hg, lungs have crackles, and oxygen saturation is 86%.

b. (1) Provide high-flow supplemental oxygen.
(2) Monitor the ECG.
(3) Obtain a 12-lead ECG if possible.
(4) Start an IV line. Keep the patient sitting up. (pages 1054–1055)
c. Right-sided heart failure (page 1051)
d. Provide oxygen to help bring up the oxygen saturation. Follow ACLS guidelines for pulmonary edema, and give a nitrate to decrease the patient's BP after an IV line has been started. (pages 1054–1055)

3. a. Chief complaint: Syncope/low heart rate.

Vital signs: Skin is cool, pulse is 44 beats/min and regular, respirations are 22 breaths/min, BP is 82/40 mm Hg, and oxygen saturation is 94%. Chest pain is not measurable. Lungs are clear. (page 965)

b. (1) Decreased cerebral perfusion
(2) Dysrhythmias
(3) Increased vagal tones
(4) Heart lesions (page 965)
c. (1) Provide high-flow oxygen.
(2) Start an IV line. Atropine 0.5 mg can be used to increase the heart rate. An epinephrine drip or a bolus of epinephrine can also be used. Consult your protocols. (pages 988–989)
d. Transcutaneous pacing (TCP) (pages 989–991)

4. a. Chief complaint: Feeling poorly

Vital signs: Skin is cool, pulse is 76 beats/min and irregular, BP is 110/74 mm Hg, and oxygen saturation is 97%. Lungs are clear.

b. (1) No (irregular)
(2) 76 beats/min (approx.)
(3) Absent
(4) Not present
(5) n/a (P waves not present)
(6) None
(7) QRS complex is normal.
(8) Atrial fibrillation
(9) Treatment is supportive. Monitor the patient. Do not convert atrial fibrillation in the field unless absolutely necessary. (page 999)

5. a. Accelerated idioventricular rhythm (page 1006)
b. Sinus dysrhythmia (page 992)
c. Atrial flutter (pages 999–1000)
d. Second-degree heart block, Mobitz type II (pages 1020–1021)
e. Polymorphic ventricular tachycardia (pages 1006–1007)
f. Third-degree heart block (pages 1021–1022)
g. Accelerated junctional rhythm (pages 1002–1003)
h. Junctional escape rhythm (page 1002)
i. Idioventricular rhythm (pages 1005–1006)
j. Sinus arrest (page 992)
k. Multifocal atrial tachycardia (page 1001)
l. Second-degree heart block, Mobitz type I (pages 1020–1021)
m. Monomorphic ventricular tachycardia (page 1006)
n. First-degree AV block (page 1020)
o. Wandering atrial pacemaker (pages 1000–1001)
p. Supraventricular tachycardia (pages 993–994)
q. Sinus bradycardia (page 988)
r. Ventricular fibrillation (pages 1007–1008)

6. a. Premature junctional complexes (pages 1001–1002)
   b. Premature ventricular complex (pages 1003–1004)
   c. Premature atrial complex (page 993)

Short Answer

1. 0.04 seconds (page 982)
2. 5 (page 982)
3. a. Altered level of consciousness (LOC) and mental status
   b. Chest pain
   c. Hypotension
   d. Other signs of shock
   e. Heart rate greater than 150 beats/min (pages 995–996)
4. Adenosine (page 995)
5. Amiodarone (page 996)
6. Begin transcutaneous pacing (TCP) (if the patient is conscious, consider administering an analgesic if that can be accomplished rapidly) (page 989)
7. a. Epinephrine 1 mg (page 1009)
   b. Epinephrine 2–10 mcg/kg/min (page 989)
   c. Adenosine 6 mg (page 996)
   d. Amiodarone 150 mg/10 min (page 996)
8. a. Hypovolemia
   b. Hypoxemia
   c. Hypothermia
   d. Hypokalemia
   e. Hyperkalemia
   f. Hydrogen ion (acidosis)
   g. Tension pneumothorax
   h. Tamponade, cardiac
   i. Toxins
   j. Thrombosis (coronary or pulmonary) (page 1017)

Problem Solving

1. 75 mL /min × 72 mL = 5,400 mL/min (page 1049)
2. 100 beats/min × 90 mL = 9,000 mL/min (page 1049)
3. a. L
   b. R
   c. R
   d. L
   e. R
   f. R
   g. L (pages 1049–1054)
4. MAP = DBP + 1/3 (SBP – DBP) (page 1059)
   a. 116 (approximately)
   b. 151 (approximately)
   c. 105 (approximately)

Practice ECG Strips

1. Rate: 75

   Rhythm: Regular

   Significant findings: Anteroseptal AMI with elevated ST and flat ST segments in V_1 to V_4

2. Rate: 75

   Rhythm: Regular

   Significant findings: Anteroseptal AMI with elevated ST in V_1 to V_4 and Q waves in V_2 to V_4

3. Rate: 70

   Rhythm: Regular

   Significant findings: Anteroseptal AMI with lateral extension and ST changes in V_1 to V_5 and I and aVL

4. Rate: 150

   Rhythm: Regular

   Significant findings: Anteroseptal AMI with lateral extension and elevated ST in V_1 to V_5, I, and aVL and reciprocal changes in the inferior leads

5. Rate: 60

   Rhythm: Regular

   Significant findings: High lateral AMI with flat ST segments and elevation in I and aVL and reciprocal changes in the inferior leads

6. Rate: 60 to 70

   Rhythm: Regular

   Significant findings: Inferolateral AMI with ST elevation in II, III, and aVF; reciprocal changes of ST depression in I and aVL; and ST elevation in V_3 to V_6

7. Rate: 120 to 130

   Rhythm: Regular

   Significant findings: Inferolateral AMI with ST segment elevations in II, III, aVF, and V_3 to V_6 and reciprocal changes in I and aVL

8. Rate: 150

   Rhythm: Regular

   Significant findings: Inferolateral (apical) AMI with ST elevation in I, II, III, aVF, and V_2 to V_6

9. Rate: 100

   Rhythm: Regular

   Significant findings: Inferolateral (apical) AMI with ST segment elevation in I, II, III, aVF, and V_2 to V_6 and Q waves in the inferior leads

10. Rate: 75 to 100

    Rhythm: Irregular with aberrantly conducted APCs and/or JPCs

    Significant findings: Oh my! Take it piece by piece. Rule out wandering pacemaker and multifocal atrial tachycardia and notice the ST elevation in I, II, aVL, aVF, and V_2 to V_6

11. Rate: 90

    Rhythm: Regular

    Significant findings: Inferior wall AMI with ST elevations and Q waves in II, III, and aVF; reciprocal changes in I and aVL; and ST elevation in V_1 to V_3

12. Rate: 80

    Rhythm: Regular

    Significant findings: Inferior wall AMI with right ventricular involvement and ST elevation in II, III, and aVF; reciprocal changes in the inferior leads; and ST elevation in lead III

13. Rate: 60 or less

    Rhythm: Irregular

    Significant findings: Inferoposterior AMI with lateral extension and ST elevation in II, III, and aVF; reciprocal ST depression in aVL; and ST elevation in V_5 and V_6

14. Rate: 120

Rhythm: Regular

Significant findings: Inferior posterior lateral AMI with ST elevations in II, III, aVF, and V_4 to V_6: reciprocal ST depression in aVL; and ST depression in V_1 and V_2

15. Rate: 75

Rhythm: Regular

Significant findings: Inferior right ventricular posterior AMI with elevations in limb leads and reciprocal changes in lateral, ST elevation in III that are taller than II, and positive ST elevation in V_4R

16. Rate: 60 to 75

Rhythm: Irregular

Significant findings: Inferior right ventricular posterior AMI with lateral extension and ST elevation in II, III, and aVF and reciprocal changes in I, V_1, V_2, V_3, and V_4

17. Rate: 100

Rhythm: Regular

Significant findings: Hyperkalemia, massive peaked T waves in leads V_2 to V_4 and tall T waves in III and aVF

18. Rate: 75

Rhythm: Regular

Significant findings: Hyperkalemia, very tall symmetrical T waves in leads I, II, III, aVF, and V_2 to V_6

19. Rate: 60

Rhythm: Regular

Significant findings: Wide ventricular complex with no P waves and hyperkalemia with peaked T waves

20. Rate: Not for long

Rhythm: Irregular

Significant findings: Oh no! Start CPR and hope the defibrillator is handy. Get an IV or IO line started, and administer epinephrine and magnesium. This patient has a long QT with frequent aberrant beats leading to torsades de pointes and then to VF. With high-quality CPR and quick actions, you may be able to return the patient to a normal sinus rhythm.

Chapter 18: Neurologic Emergencies

Matching

Part I

1. H (page 1090)
2. G (page 1096)
3. F (page 1095)
4. E (page 1089)
5. Y (page 1095)
6. X (page 1095)
7. W (page 1091)
8. V (page 1122)
9. Q (page 1119)
10. P (page 1091)
11. O (page 1087)
12. N (page 1087)
13. A (page 1114)
14. B (page 1119)
15. C (page 1123)
16. D (page 1096)
17. M (page 1092)
18. L (page 1091)
19. K (page 1091)
20. J (page 1096)
21. U (page 1095)
22. I (page 1123)
23. S (page 1127)
24. T (page 1127)
25. R (page 1095)

Part II

1. K (page 1119)
2. J (page 1095)
3. I (page 1093)
4. H (page 1121)
5. G (page 1121)
6. Y (page 1095)
7. X (page 1090)
8. W (page 1091)
9. V (page 1087)
10. U (page 1118)
11. O (page 1129)
12. N (page 1123)
13. M (page 1096)
14. L (page 1114)
15. F (page 1083)
16. E (page 1115)
17. D (page 1101)
18. C (page 1095)
19. B (page 1114)
20. A (page 1101)
21. T (page 1086)
22. S (page 1095)
23. R (page 1129)
24. P (page 1129)
25. Q (page 1114)

Multiple Choice

1. D (page 1083)
2. C (page 1083)
3. A (page 1121)
4. A (page 1089)
5. C (page 1087)
6. C (pages 1092)
7. A (page 1114)
8. C (page 1083)
9. D (page 1121)
10. B (page 1090)

Labeling

1. Pupil responses (page 1093, Figure 18-8)
    1. C. Dilated
    2. A. Normal
    3. D. Unequal
    4. B. Constricted (pinpoint)

Fill in the Blank

1. synapse; neuron (page 1084)
2. Cheyne-Stokes; increases; apnea (page 1088)
3. endotoxin (page 1127)
4. brain; blood; cerebrospinal fluid (page 1101)
5. decrease; increase (page 1088)
6. extreme; hyperpnea (page 1088)
7. Tonic; body (page 1096)
8. Glucose; 60–120 (pages 1092–1093)
9. ischemic; hemorrhagic (page 1101)
10. tonic-clonic; absence (page 1114)

Identify

1. Chief complaint: General weakness, visual disturbance
2. Vital signs: BP is 128/76 mm Hg, pulse is 84 beats/min, oxygen saturation is 95%, blood glucose is 112 mg/dL
3. Pertinent negatives: No pain, vital signs in normal ranges, no facial droop, no trauma, normal temperature, no history of illness

    Vital signs are all pretty normal, BP is 128/76 mm Hg, pulse is 84 beats/min and regular, and oxygen saturation is 95%. The patient is alert and has a patent airway. He is breathing regularly. His blood glucose level is 112 mg/dL. The vital signs are telling you that nothing is wrong, but the negatives are telling you more. The patient has no signs of trauma, infection, or illness. He is not in any pain. His symptoms and signs are very vague, and only supportive care and transport are required.

Complete the Patient Care Report (PCR)

Show your completed PCR to your paramedic instructor, and ask for feedback on how you recorded the case you were given.

Ambulance Calls

1. This is a case of status epilepticus.
   a. When you get around to doing a rapid medical assessment, you will want to be particularly alert for the following causes of seizures (pages 1113–1114). *Students should list 10 of the following:*
      (1) abscess
      (2) alcohol
      (3) birth anomaly
      (4) brain infections (meningitis, encephalitis)
      (5) brain trauma
      (6) diabetes mellitus
      (7) febrile
      (8) idiopathic (no known cause)
      (9) inappropriate medication dosage
      (10) organic brain syndromes
      (11) recreational drug use
      (12) stroke or TIA
      (13) systemic infection
      (14) tumor
      (15) uremia (kidney failure)
   b. The steps in treating a patient in status epilepticus are (page 1097):
      (1) Protect the patient from injury.
      (2) Ensure an open airway, which may mean inserting an endotracheal (ET) tube the first chance you get once the seizure activity subsides. It will be difficult to impossible during the actual seizure. After the tube is in, insert an oropharyngeal airway (OPA) as well to prevent the patient from biting down on the ET tube, and secure them both in place. (Patients having seizures have been known to bite an ET in half!)
      (3) Administer supplemental oxygen. Remember: Deaths from seizures are hypoxic deaths.
      (4) Start an IV line with a large-bore catheter and secure it very well.
   c. The medication most commonly used in the field for status epilepticus is diazepam (Valium) (page 1117).
      (1) The contraindications to giving diazepam are in patients who are pregnant and those who have already taken other sedative drugs or alcohol.
      (2) The correct dosage is 5.0 mg slowly via IV line given after you have measured a baseline BP. Then, wait a few minutes and recheck the BP. You may repeat diazepam every 10 to 15 minutes with 5.0 mg (total dosage should not exceed 30 mg). You may also use lorazepam 0.05 mg/kg (maximum dose at one time is 4 mg). Repeat the lorazepam in 10 to 15 minutes with a maximum dose of 8 mg in a 12-hour period. (pages 1502–1503)
      (3) The possible side effects of IV diazepam include hypotension and even respiratory or cardiac arrest (those more serious complications are more likely to occur in elderly patients). (You may need to refer to the Medication Formulary appendix, pages 1502–1503, for more details on the drug.)
2. The person calling 9-1-1 got it right: The woman with a "possible stroke" has almost certainly had a stroke.
   a. She is most likely right-handed. Remember that the left side of the brain controls the right side of the body and vice versa. You know that the stroke involves the left side of her brain because the right side of her body is paralyzed. You suspect that the left side of her brain is the dominant side because the stroke has robbed her of speech. Most right-handed people are "left-dominant"; that is, the left side of the brain is the dominant side in terms of speech and several other functions. (page 1095)
   b. The steps in treating this woman are as follows (pages 1102–1103):
      (1) Protect her airway because she cannot (she has no gag reflex). Suction secretions as needed, and keep her in the stable side position.
      (2) Administer supplemental oxygen.
      (3) Monitor cardiac rhythm, and be prepared to deal with dysrhythmias.
      (4) Start an IV line with a microdrip infusion set, and hang normal saline at a to-keep-open rate.
      (5) Protect the paralyzed extremities. The patient should be lying on her nonparalyzed (left) side so that she can feel if she is putting too much pressure on an arm or leg.
      (6) Maintain a running conversation with the patient, and provide honest reassurance.

3. Here you have a patient in a coma of unknown cause.
   a. The easiest way to remember the possible causes of coma is through the mnemonic AEIOU-TIPS (pages 1110–1111):
      (1) A Alcohol/acidosis
      (2) E Epilepsy/endocrine/electrolyte imbalance
      (3) I Insulin
      (4) O Opiates/other drugs
      (5) U Uremia
      (6) T Trauma/temperature
      (7) I Infection
      (8) P Poisoning/psychogenic causes
      (9) S Shock/stroke/syncope/space-occupying lesion/subarachnoid hemorrhage
   b. (1) Establish an airway (consider holding off intubation, though, until you can assess the results of dextrose and naloxone).
      (2) Administer supplemental oxygen.
      (3) Establish an IV line in a large vein.
      (4) Give thiamine, 100 mg slowly IV (if still carried in your emergency medical services [EMS] system).
      (5) Give 50% dextrose, 50 mL slowly IV, preferably after checking the blood glucose level.
      (6) If the patient does not wake in response to dextrose and there is reason to suspect narcotic overdose (eg, pinpoint pupils), give naloxone, 0.4 to 2 mg slowly IV; if there is no response after 2 to 3 minutes, repeat the dose.
      (7) If there is no response to two doses of naloxone, intubate the trachea.
      (8) Monitor cardiac rhythm.

   Other steps include: Keep a flow sheet of neurologic and vital signs; protect the patient's eyes (tape them shut); and transport the patient to the hospital (pages 1109–1112).

True/False

1. T (page 1081)
2. T (page 1099)
3. F (page 1088)
4. T (page 1119)
5. T (page 1088)
6. F (page 1102)
7. T (page 1087)
8. T (page 1107)
9. F (page 1102)
10. T (page 1117)
11. F (page 1099)
12. F (page 1107)
13. T (page 1109)
14. F (page 1115)

Short Answer

1. Vocabulary
   Hemiparesis: Weakness of one side (half) of the body (*hemi-* + *-paresis*) (page 1095)
   Pseudoseizures: Psychogenic nonepileptic seizures; a type of generalized neurologic event (page 1114)
2. a. Seizure disorders (page 1090)
   b. Diabetes (page 1090)

Fill in the Table

1. Types of dystonias (page 1126, Table 18-20)

Type	Presentation
Cervical dystonia (torticollis)	Most common form of focal dystonia; intermittent, patterned, repetitive, spasmodic motion of the head in a twisting, flexing, extending, or tilting manner; can involve more than one motion type
Oculogyric crisis	Deviation of the eyes in any direction, usually with eyes strained toward the top of the head
Oromandibular	Forceful contractions of the face, which can involve the tongue darting in and out of the mouth
Blepharospasm	Eyelid spasms or uncontrollable blinking
Athetosis	Slow, writhing motions commonly involving the face and distal extremities
Upper limb dystonia	Cramping of the hands, elbows, and arms (eg, graphospasm [writer's cramp])
Choreiform movements	Quick, jerky, irregular, and unpredictable movements; often found in the face, arms, and hands
Spasmodic dysphonia	Involuntary contraction of the vocal cords, interrupting speech

2. Common causes of seizures (page 1114, Table 18-12)

Common causes of seizures
Abscess
Alcohol
Birth anomaly
Brain infections (meningitis, encephalitis)
Brain trauma
Diabetes mellitus
Fever (rapid rate of rise)
Hypertension during pregnancy (eclampsia)
Idiopathic (of no known cause)
Inappropriate medication dosage
Organic brain syndromes
Recreational drug use (cocaine)
Stroke or TIA
Systematic infection
Tumor
Uremia (kidney failure)

3. Cranial nerves (page 1094, Table 18-5)

Cranial Nerve	Function
I. Olfactory	Smell
II. Optic	Vision
III. Oculomotor	Movement of the eye, pupil, and eyelid
IV. Trochlear	Movement of the eye
V. Trigeminal	Chewing Pain Temperature Touch of the mouth and face
VI. Abducens	Movement of the eye
VII. Facial	Movement of the face Tears Salivation and taste
VIII. Auditory	Hearing and balance
IX. Glossopharyngeal	Swallowing, taste, and sensation in the mouth and pharynx
X. Vagus	Sensation and movement of the pharynx, larynx, thorax, and GI system
XI. Accessory	Movement of the head and shoulders
XII. Hypoglossal	Movement of the tongue

Problem Solving

1. Cincinnati Prehospital Stroke Scale (page 1107)
   a. Smile is not equal.
   b. She has difficulty saying, "You can't teach an old dog new tricks."
   c. When she closes her eyes, her right arm drifts down.
2. Los Angeles Prehospital Stroke Screen (page 1107)
   a. Age is greater than 45.
   b. Smile is unequal.
   c. Blood glucose is normal.
   d. Her grip strength is not equal.
   e. Right arm drifts.
   f. Patient is not bedridden.
   g. Symptom onset is less than 24 hours.
   h. She has no history of seizures or epilepsy.

Chapter 19: Diseases of the Eyes, Ears, Nose, and Throat

Matching

1. S (page 1161)
2. R (page 1152)
3. Q (page 1147)
4. P (page 1146)
5. O (page 1140)
6. Y (page 1160)
7. X (page 1141)
8. W (page 1144)
9. V (page 1140)
10. U (page 1152)
11. A (page 1143)
12. B (page 1150)
13. C (page 1147)
14. D (page 1155)
15. E (page 1150)
16. T (page 1161)
17. J (page 1140)
18. K (page 1142)
19. L (page 1157)
20. M (page 1158)
21. N (page 1154)
22. I (page 1158)
23. H (page 1159)
24. G (page 1142)
25. F (page 1146)

Multiple Choice

1. B (pages 1140–1141)
2. B (page 1147)
3. C (page 1142)
4. D (page 1142)
5. C (page 1147)
6. B (page 1142)
7. C (page 1149)
8. D (page 1152)
9. A (page 1166)
10. B (page 1163)
11. C (pages 1151–1152)
12. D (page 1156)

Labeling

1. Structures of the eye (page 1141, Figure 19-1)
   A. Iris
   B. Cornea
   C. Pupil
   D. Lens
   E. Optic nerve
   F. Retina
   G. Choroid
   H. Sclera
2. Structures of the ear (page 1149, Figure 19-9)
   A. Auricle (pinna)
   B. External auditory canal
   C. Tympanic membrane
   D. Semicircular canals
   E. Cochlea
   F. Eustachian (auditory) tube
   G. Stapes
   H. Incus
   I. Malleus
3. Structure of a tooth (page 1157, Figure 19-14B)
   A. Crown
   B. Enamel
   C. Dentin
   D. Root
   E. Root canal

Fill in the Blank

1. eyelids; swelling (page 1142)
2. contact lenses; remove (page 1143)
3. ophthalmoscope; eye (page 1144)
4. conjunctivitis; conjunctiva (page 1144)
5. chalazion; painless; pustule (page 1146)
6. open-angle; slowly (page 1147)

Identify

1. a. Chief complaint: Dizziness
   b. Vital signs: Respiratory rate of 20 breaths/min and regular, pulse of 118 beats/min and regular, BP of 98/P mm Hg, and Spo_2 of 89%
   c. Pertinent negatives: Denies LOC; denies pain to head, chest, or abdomen
2. a. Chief complaint: Nosebleed and headache
   b. Vital signs: Respiratory rate of 20 breaths/min and regular, pulse of 108 beats/min and irregular, BP of 170/102 mm Hg, and Spo_2 of 95%
   c. Pertinent negatives: No LOC, no trauma

Ambulance Calls

1. a. Very serious, potentially vision-threatening injury. Corneal abrasion is commonly caused by direct trauma, foreign bodies, contact lenses, or exposure to UV radiation. The signs and symptoms of corneal abrasion include pain with extraocular movement, redness, excessive tearing, sensation of foreign object in the eye, blurred or loss of vision, photophobia, and/or headache. (page 1142)
   b. Rule out life threats, lightly cover the eye, apply cold to the swelling of the orbit bone, and transport to the most appropriate emergency department (ED).
2. a. Flush with plenty of saline or sterile water, flowing away from the injured eye and not into the uninjured eye. Transport the patient as soon as possible to the most appropriate ED.

True/False

1. F (page 1155)
2. T (page 1155)
3. T (page 1156)
4. T (page 1157)
5. T (page 1152)
6. T (page 1158)
7. T (page 1159)
8. T (page 1160)
9. F (page 1160)
10. F (page 1161)

Chapter 20: Abdominal and Gastrointestinal Emergencies

Matching

Part I

1. R (page 1190)
2. Q (page 1192)
3. P (page 1171)
4. O (page 1171)
5. Y (page 1185)
6. X (page 1188)
7. W (page 1200)
8. V (page 1183)
9. I (page 1178)
10. H (page 1184)
11. G (page 1190)
12. F (page 1190)
13. B (page 1171)
14. A (page 1197)
15. N (page 1174)
16. M (page 1197)
17. U (page 1187)
18. T (page 1172)
19. S (page 1184)
20. C (page 1196)
21. D (page 1187)
22. E (page 1189)
23. L (page 1182)
24. K (page 1190)
25. J (page 1190)

Part II

1. R (page 1183)
2. Q (page 1184)
3. P (page 1186)
4. O (page 1195)
5. Y (page 1183)
6. X (page 1185)
7. W (page 1185)
8. V (page 1179)
9. A (page 1171)
10. B (page 1184)
11. C (page 1183)
12. D (page 1198)
13. E (page 1189)
14. N (page 1199)
15. M (page 1194)
16. U (page 1193)
17. T (page 1203)
18. S (page 1202)
19. L (page 1201)
20. K (page 1201)
21. J (page 1197)
22. F (page 1200)
23. G (page 1186)
24. H (page 1178)
25. I (page 1178)

Multiple Choice

1. A (page 1185)
2. C (page 1190)
3. B (pages 1192–1193)
4. C (page 1195)
5. A (page 1179)
6. D (page 1184)
7. C (page 1184)
8. B (page 1179)
9. D (page 1191)
10. B (pages 1198–1199)

Fill in the Blank

1. liver disease; longer (page 1197)
2. alcohol; smoking; mucosal (page 1171)
3. portal; venous; absorbed (page 1174)
4. non-narcotic; hypotension (page 1180)
5. immunocompromised; food-borne (page 1196)
6. *Helicobacter pylori*; nonsteroidal (page 1185)
7. Biliary tract disorders (page 1190)
8. colitis (page 1194)
9. Ulcerative colitis; hereditary (page 1194)
10. early; ripe; rupture (page 1191)

Labeling

1. Normal versus hiatal hernia (page 1186, Figure 20-5)

Normal:

A. Esophagus
B. Diaphragm
C. Stomach

Hiatal hernia:

A. Esophagus
B. Weak diaphragm
C. Stomach

2. Common locations of abdominal hernias (page 1201, Figure 20-11)

A. Xiphoid process
B. Epigastric
C. Umbilical
D. Inguinal
E. Femoral

Identify

1. a. Chief complaint: GI bleed, hypovolemic shock, and near syncope
b. Vital signs: Skin is diaphoretic, ashen, cool; BP is 88/P mm Hg by palpation; heart rate is 118 beats/min; oxygen saturation is 89%
c. Pertinent negatives: None indicated for this call

2. a. Chief complaint: Per law enforcement, "man down"; per the patient, abdominal pain
b. Vital signs: Skin is jaundiced, cool, dry; capillary refill is delayed; ECG shows sinus tachycardia; oxygen saturation is 94%; BP is 142/86 mm Hg; blood glucose level is 110 mg/dL
c. Pertinent negatives: Patient denies any injuries or falls

3. a. Chief complaint: Severe abdominal pain
b. Vital signs: ECG shows sinus rhythm; bilateral radial pulses are equal; capillary refill is normal; pulse is 92 beats/min, strong and regular; oxygen saturation is 99%; skin color is normal, and skin is warm and diaphoretic
c. Pertinent negatives: No recent injury or trauma

Ambulance Calls

1. a. The patient in this ambulance call has a classical presentation of appendicitis. (page 1191)
b. (1) Oxygen
(2) IV access
(3) Volume resuscitation as necessary
(4) Dopamine for septicemia, if authorized in your EMS system
(5) Pain management
(6) Nausea management (page 1192)
b. (1) Ondansetron (Zofran): This medication should be administered slowly over at least 2 minutes.
(2) Diphenhydramine (Benadryl): Be cautious when using this medication because it can cause drowsiness and a drop in BP.
(3) Hydroxyzine (Vistaril): Be cautious when administering this medication to patients who have taken any medication that has central nervous system (CNS) depressive effects. Hydroxyzine (Vistaril) increases the CNS depressive effects of other medications.
(4) Promethazine (Phenergan): Be cautious when administering this medication to patients who have taken any medication that has CNS effects. Like hydroxyzine, promethazine increases the CNS depressive effects of other medications. Also, this medication tends to cause a marked burning sensation during injection. Administer slowly. (page 1181)

2. a. Aggressive management of ABCs, including positioning to facilitate drainage and suctioning
b. Rapid but safe immediate transport
c. Fluid resuscitation
d. Pharmacologic management of nausea and vomiting (page 1184)

3. a. Standard precautions.
b. Effective positioning of the patient to ensure adequate drainage of material out of the mouth.
c. Oxygen.
d. Listen to lung sounds.
e. Administer hypotonic solution.
f. Consider pain management.
g. Consider medications that may be administered for management of nausea. (pages 1175–1176)

True/False

1. T (page 1181)
2. F (pages 1194)
3. T (page 1197)
4. T (page 1185)
5. F (pages 1178–1179)
6. F (page 1178)
7. T (page 1176)
8. T (page 1178)
9. T (page 1175)
10. F (page 1185)

Short Answer

1. a. Borborygmi: A bowel sound characterized by increased activity within the bowel. (page 1177–1178)
   b. Cholecystitis: Inflammation of the gallbladder. (page 1182)
   c Scaphoid: A concave shape of the abdomen. This can be caused by evisceration. (page 1177)
   d. Mallory-Weiss syndrome: A condition in which the junction between the esophagus and the stomach tears. (page 1184)
2. a. Somatic (page 1179)
   b. Appendicitis (page 1191)
   c. Irritation or injury to tissue, causing activation of peripheral nerve tracts (page 1179)
3. a. Somatic (page 1179)
   b. Usually occurs after an initial visceral, parietal, or somatic pain; similar nerve tracts cause "pain" in distant locations. (page 1179)

Fill in the Table

1. The patient's symptoms and signs can tell you a lot.

Finding	What the Finding Tells Me
Coffee-ground vomitus	**The patient is bleeding into his stomach, and the blood has been there for some time.**
Melena	**The patient is bleeding somewhere in the GI tract.**
Tenting of the skin	**The patient is severely dehydrated.**
Patient very still	**The patient probably has peritonitis.**

Chapter 21: Genitourinary and Renal Emergencies

Matching

Part I

1. N (page 1214)
2. M (page 1229)
3. L (page 1227)
4. K (page 1229)
5. J (page 1225)
6. T (page 1214)
7. S (page 1221)
8. R (page 1214)
9. Q (page 1223)
10. P (page 1223)
11. O (page 1222)
12. I (page 1214)
13. H (page 1229)
14. G (page 1225)
15. F (page 1230)
16. A (page 1223)
17. B (page 1229)
18. C (page 1223)
19. D (page 1227)
20. E (page 1225)

Part II

1. Q (page 1214)
2. R (page 1214)
3. S (page 1214)
4. T (page 1221)
5. M (page 1227)
6. N (page 1230)
7. O (page 1217)
8. P (page 1225)
9. L (page 1227)
10. K (page 1220)
11. J (page 1214)
12. I (page 1230)
13. D (page 1229)
14. C (page 1229)
15. B (page 1223)
16. A (page 1214)
17. E (page 1229)
18. F (page 1224)
19. G (page 1223)
20. H (page 1229)

Multiple Choice

1. C (page 1214)
2. C (page 1217)
3. B (page 1220)
4. C (page 1223)
5. A (page 1222)
6. B (page 1222)
7. C (page 1223)
8. A (page 1233)
9. B (page 1229)
10. A (page 1222)

Labeling

1. The urinary system (page 1214, Figure 21-1A)
   - **A.** Kidneys
   - **B.** Ureters
   - **C.** Urinary bladder
   - **D.** Urethra
2. The four-quadrant system (page 1219, Figure 21-4A)
   - **A.** Liver
   - **B.** Gallbladder
   - **C.** Iliac crest
   - **D.** Appendix
   - **E.** Costal arch
   - **F.** Spleen
   - **G.** Small intestine
   - **H.** Rectum
3. The nine-section system(page 1219, Figure 21-4B)
   - **A.** Right hypochondriac region
   - **B.** Right lumbar region
   - **C.** Right iliac region
   - **D.** Left hypochondriac region
   - **E.** Left lumbar region
   - **F.** Left iliac region

Fill in the Blank

1. comfort; support (pages 1222–1223)
2. cortex; medulla; pelvis (page 1214)
3. Acute kidney injury (page 1223)
4. hemodialysis (page 1227)
5. Disequilibrium syndrome (page 1229)
6. priapism (page 1229)
7. Visceral (page 1218)

8. cardiovascular (page 1226)
9. pain relief (page 1222)
10. lower (page 1220)

Identify

1. Chief complaint: Kidney stone, abdominal pain.
2. Vital signs: Patient is alert; oxygen saturation is 98%; respirations are 18 breaths/min; lungs are clear; pulse is 96 beats/min; ECG shows sinus tachycardia; BP is 148/94 mm Hg; blood glucose is 96 mg/dL; skin is warm and dry; temperature is 98.6°F. Pain is 10/10.
3. Pertinent negatives: History of salty food and drink with no water consumption.

Ambulance Calls

1. The first patient with abdominal pain you had to deal with is a 42-year-old man.
   a. Poorly localized, crampy pain associated with other autonomic symptoms such as nausea is called visceral pain. (page 1218)
   b. Visceral pain usually comes about because of obstruction of a hollow organ that causes distention and stretching of the organ wall.
   c. Visceral pain is characteristic of conditions such as bowel obstruction, urethral stone, or a stone in the bile duct. (page 1218)
2. E. The patient is in obvious pain and is probably bleeding internally as a result of the trauma to the kidneys. Remember that kidneys are solid organs that filter the blood, and they hold a lot of blood. Rapid assessment of this patient with IV support should be established quickly, and then he should be transported to the regional trauma center.
3. With more and more patients being maintained on chronic renal dialysis, paramedics will find themselves dealing more often with the problems to which dialysis patients are prone.
   a. (1) The patient who feels too weak to move and has peaked T waves on his ECG is most likely suffering from hyperkalemia. (page 1224)
      (2) The steps to take are as follows:
         (a) Continue to monitor his cardiac rhythm carefully.
         (b) Give atropine, 0.5 mg rapidly IV.
         (c) Contact medical control to consider giving 10 mL of a 10% solution of calcium chloride IV.
         (d) Make sure the calcium chloride has infused. Then contact medical control to consider giving 50 mEq of sodium bicarbonate IV.
         (e) Transport without delay, and be prepared to deal with a cardiac arrest en route. (page 1225)
   b. (1) The patient with paroxysmal nocturnal dyspnea has classic signs of heart failure.

True/False

1. F (page 1223)
2. F (page 1233)
3. T (page 1223)
4. T (page 1214)
5. T (page 1225)
6. F (page 1227)
7. T (page 1228)
8. T (page 1214)
9. F (page 1214)
10. T (page 1223)

Short Answer

1. We scarcely ever think about our kidneys and how much they do for us. It is only when the kidneys are not working that we can begin to appreciate all the things they do when they are functioning. And when they aren't working, a whole lot of other things start going wrong as well. Thus, patients with chronic kidney disease, who have dialysis treatments, are much more vulnerable to the following conditions (page 1226):
   a. Heart failure
   b. Hypertension
   c. Myocardial infarction
   d. Pericardial tamponade
   e. Uremic pericarditis

Fill in the Table

(page 1223)

Signs and Symptoms of Acute Kidney Injury	
Type of Acute Kidney Injury	**Signs and Symptoms**
Prerenal	**Hypotension** **Tachycardia** **Dizziness** **Thirst**
Intrarenal	**Flank pain** **Joint pain** **Oliguria** **Hypertension** **Headache** **Confusion** **Seizure**
Postrenal	**Pain in lower flank, abdomen, groin, and genitalia** **Oliguria** **Distended bladder** **Hematuria** **Peripheral edema**

Chapter 22: Gynecologic Emergencies

Matching

Part I

1. G (page 1246)
2. F (page 1245)
3. E (page 1243)
4. D (page 1239)
5. T (page 1244)
6. S (page 1238)
7. R (page 1238)
8. Q (page 1239)
9. K (page 1238)
10. J (page 1245)
11. I (page 1245)
12. H (page 1238)
13. C (page 1238)
14. B (page 1243)
15. A (page 1239)
16. P (page 1239)
17. O (page 1239)
18. N (pages 1238–1239)
19. M (page 1239)
20. L (page 1238)

Part II

1. K (page 1238)
2. J (page 1245)
3. O (page 1243)
4. N (page 1243)
5. M (page 1243)
6. I (page 1248)
7. H (page 1244)
8. G (page 1248)
9. F (page 1243)
10. L (page 1238)
11. E (page 1238)
12. D (page 1242)
13. C (page 1239)
14. B (page 1238)
15. A (page 1244)

Multiple Choice

1. C (page 1239)
2. D (page 1239)
3. B (page 1246)
4. B (page 1239)
5. B (page 1247)
6. A (pages 1243–1248)
7. C (page 1248)
8. D (page 1246)
9. B (pages 1248–1249)
10. C (page 1245)

Labeling

1. Anatomy of the female genital tract and pelvis (page 1238, Figure 22-1)
   - **A.** Ovary
   - **B.** Uterine (fallopian) tube
   - **C.** Uterus
   - **D.** Cervix
   - **E.** Vagina
2. Reproductive system with an ectopic pregnancy (page 1246, Figure 22-5)
   - **A.** Fallopian tube
   - **B.** Fertilized oocyte
   - **C.** Uterus
   - **D.** Ovary

Fill in the Blank

1. vagina (page 1238)
2. imperforate hymen (page 1239)
3. amenorrhea (page 1239)
4. Menopause (page 1239)
5. endometriosis (page 1245)
6. ectopic; after (page 1247)
7. Scene safety (page 1240)
8. modesty (page 1241)
9. Cullen; Grey Turner (page 1241)
10. Cystitis; bacteria; perineum (page 1243)

Identify

1. Chief complaint: Severe abdominal pain.
2. Vital signs: Patient is alert, pain is 10 out of 10, pulse is 120 beats/min, blood pressure (BP) is 140/92 mm Hg, ECG shows sinus tachycardia, oxygen saturation is 94%, respirations are 20 breaths/min, the temperature is 102°F, pupils are PERRLA, and lungs are clear.

3. Pertinent negatives: No illness, no trauma, and no sexual activity yet.

   What is wrong? She has a ruptured ovarian cyst. The lack of sexual activity eliminates the possibility of ectopic pregnancy. She is running a fever with no other signs of illness. The rebound tenderness, abdominal distention, and vomiting tell you that this patient is very ill; her vital signs indicates that she is in septic shock. Rapid transport is indicated. (page 1244)

Ambulance Calls

1. **a.** The 25-year-old woman with fever and abdominal pain that began not long after her menstrual period most likely has pelvic inflammatory disease (answer E).
   b. (1) The prehospital management is gentle transport.
   (2) In view of the woman's tachycardia, fever, and history of vomiting, she is probably dehydrated, so it is a good idea to start an IV line with crystalloid and run in fluids en route to the ED. (pages 1242-1243)
2. **a.** The 24-year-old woman who thinks she has appendicitis more likely has an embryo developing in her right fallopian tube—that is, an ectopic pregnancy (answer D). Crampy, unilateral abdominal pain followed by spotting and signs of early shock are good enough evidence to start treatment.
   b. Treatment is as follows:
   (1) Administer supplemental oxygen.
   (2) Keep the patient recumbent.
   (3) Start a large-bore IV line and run it wide open (or per local protocol).
   (4) Allow nothing by mouth.
   (5) Keep the patient warm.
   (6) Monitor ECG rhythm and vital signs.
   (7) Notify the receiving hospital.
   (8) Transport without delay. (pages 1246-1248)

True/False

1. F (page 1248)
2. F (page 1243)
3. T (page 1249)
4. F (page 1248)
5. T (page 1243)
6. T (page 1243)
7. T (page 1239)
8. F (page 1245)
9. F (page 1239)
10. T (page 1239)

Short Answer

1. In evaluating a woman of childbearing age whose chief complaint is abdominal pain, you will want to know more about the pain, about associated symptoms, and about her obstetric and gynecologic history. (pages 1240–1241)
   a. Among the questions you should ask in taking the history are the following. (*Students should list 10.*)
   (1) What provoked the pain? Does anything make it better or worse?
   (2) What is the pain like? Sharp? Dull? Crampy?
   (3) Where is the pain? Does it radiate anywhere else?
   (4) How severe is the pain? Compare it to prior experience, or rate it on a scale of 1 to 10.
   (5) When did the pain start? What is the temporal relationship between the pain and other symptoms?
   (6) Which other symptoms has the patient noticed? Has she had vaginal bleeding? Has she felt dizzy or faint?
   (7) When was her last normal menstrual period?
   (8) Has she noticed any breast tenderness, urinary frequency, or nausea in the mornings?
   (9) Which, if any, type of contraception does the woman use?
   (10) Has she had any vaginal discharge?
   (11) How many previous pregnancies has she had? How many deliveries?
   (12) Which gynecologic problems has she had in the past?
   (13) Does she have any serious underlying illnesses?
   b. On physical examination, what you want to look for in particular are the following:
   (1) Signs of hypovolemia, such as anxiety, restlessness, cold and clammy skin, tachycardia, and postural changes in vital signs
   (2) Signs of peritoneal irritation, such as abdominal rigidity or pain on movement (page 1241)
2. Risk factors for ectopic pregnancy include the following. (*Students should list two.*)
   a. Previous pelvic inflammatory disease
   b. Previous ectopic pregnancy
   c. Using an IUD for contraception
   d. Previous pelvic surgery (page 1246)

3. The classic triad of findings in ectopic pregnancy is:
   a. Abdominal pain
   b. Amenorrhea
   c. Vaginal bleeding (page 1247)

Fill in the Table

1. (page 1240, Table 22-1)

Elements of the Gynecologic History
Current symptoms: Vaginal bleeding? Amount? Any tissue passed?
Current symptoms: Abdominal pain? Onset, duration, character, location, radiation, severity?
Current symptoms: Vaginal discharge? Color, amount, odor, itching?
Currently pregnant?
Current sexual activity? Birth control?
Last menstrual period (LMP)
Prior pregnancies (gravidity)
Prior births (parity)
Prior pregnancy complications or losses?
Prior cesarean sections or other abdominal surgery?
Other past medical history, medications, allergies
Prior or current sexually transmitted diseases

Chapter 23: Endocrine Emergencies

Matching

Part I

1. T (page 1260)
2. S (page 1264)
3. R (page 1261)
4. Q (page 1260)
5. P (page 1260)
6. F (page 1259)
7. E (page 1259)
8. D (page 1260)
9. C (page 1260)
10. B (page 1259)
11. Y (page 1261)
12. X (page 1282)
13. W (page 1261)
14. V (page 1282)
15. U (page 1265)
16. A (page 1280)
17. O (page 1265)
18. N (page 1265)
19. M (page 1263)
20. L (page 1264)
21. J (page 1261)
22. I (page 1261)
23. H (page 1259)
24. G (page 1280)
25. K (page 1284)

Part II

1. U (page 1282)
2. T (pages 1266–1267)
3. S (page 1265)
4. R (page 1265)
5. Q (page 1265)
6. Y (page 1261)
7. X (page 1260)
8. W (page 1260)
9. V (page 1279)
10. O (page 1259)
11. N (page 1261)
12. M (page 1260)
13. L (page 1260)
14. K (page 1261)
15. J (page 1266)
16. A (page 1274)
17. B (page 1277)
18. C (page 1261)
19. D (page 1260)
20. E (page 1268)
21. I (page 1259)
22. H (page 1265)
23. G (page 1275)
24. F (page 1260)
25. P (page 1281)

Multiple Choice

1. D (page 1259)
2. C (page 1259)
3. B (page 1260)
4. A (page 1259)
5. B (page 1259)
6. B (page 1260)
7. B (page 1260)
8. B (page 1266)
9. C (page 1268)
10. A (page 1275)
11. D (page 1277)
12. A (page 1280)
13. D (page 1281)
14. A (pages 1282–1283)
15. D (page 1283)

Labeling

1. Diabetic emergencies (page 1274, Figure 23-5)
   - A. DKA, HHS, or symptomatic hyperglycemia
   - B. Hyperglycemia
   - C. Normal
   - D. Hypoglycemia
   - E. Hypoglycemic crisis

Fill in the Blank

1. Myxedema (page 1283)
2. thyroid-stimulating hormone (page 1259)
3. sodium; potassium (page 1260)
4. rehydration; electrolyte (page 1276)
5. 12 to 48; deteriorating (page 1275)
6. fatigue; seizure (pages 1268–1269)
7. type 1; type 2 (page 1266)
8. islets of Langerhans; glucagon; insulin (page 1260)
9. endocrine (page 1259)
10. hyperosmolar; hyperosmolar; coma (page 1277)

Identify

1. a. Chief complaint: Altered level of consciousness
   b. Vital signs: Respirations are shallow and the patient is diaphoretic. Her pulse is 118 beats/min, and her BP is 104/88 mm Hg.
   c. Pertinent negatives: Her blood glucose is 48 mg/dL.
   d. Nature of the endocrine disorder: Type 1 diabetes

This patient is likely suffering from hypoglycemia. Hypoglycemia in the patient with insulin-dependent diabetes is often the result of having taken too much insulin, too little food, or both. Her vital signs include a mental status of being unresponsive, a tachycardia of 118 beats/min, and a blood pressure (BP) of 104/88 mm Hg. Her skin indicates diaphoresis as well as blood glucose of 48 mg/dL. (pages 1270–1274)

2. a. Chief complaint: Shortness of breath
   b. Vital signs: Rapid breathing. He is tachycardic with a BP of 108/82 mm Hg.
   c. Pertinent negatives: Fruity, acetone breath. He has poor skin turgor, and skin tenting is present.
   d. Nature of the endocrine disorder: Diabetes

   This patient is likely suffering from diabetic ketoacidosis. His vital signs include tachycardia, an elevated blood glucose level, and BP of 108/82 mm Hg. Oxygen saturation is 95%. (pages 1274–1277)

3. a. Chief complaint: Altered mental status
   b. Vital signs: Bradycardic and hypotensive
   c. Pertinent negatives: Cannot get a pulse oximeter reading. The patient is acting confused and psychotic.
   d. Nature of the endocrine disorder: Myxedema coma

   This patient is most likely suffering from myxedema coma. Myxedema coma is associated with elderly females, behavioral/mental status changes, and hypothermia. (pages 1282–1283)

Ambulance Calls

1. The patient is showing characteristic signs of diabetic ketoacidosis (DKA). The steps of prehospital management are aimed primarily at stabilizing vital functions and restoring fluid. The goals of prehospital treatment are as follows:
   a. Begin rehydration and correct the patient's electrolyte and acid–base abnormalities.
   b. Follow the procedure for any comatose patient with regard to airway maintenance and supplemental oxygen. Be particularly alert for vomiting, and have suction ready.
   c. Start an IV line and infuse up to 1 L of normal saline over the first half hour or at the rate suggested by protocol or online medical control.
   d. Monitor cardiac rhythm. Changes in serum potassium caused by DKA can lead to marked myocardial instability. (pages 1274–1277)
2. a. Probable underlying illness(es): Hypoglycemia (pages 1270–1274)
   b. Probable underlying illness(es): Diabetes
   c. The patient has an insulin pump. Consider the possibility of a malfunctioning pump, the patient not loading the insulin into the pump, or, regardless of the pump, the patient disregarding proper dietary control. Any of these scenarios could cause a hypoglycemic emergency. (pages 1270–1274)
   d. Do not let a known diagnosis of diabetes prevent you from considering other causes of coma. Patients with diabetes are not immune to—for example—head injury, stroke, seizures, meningitis, and other traumatic injuries or conditions. Keep an open mind, and assess the patient thoroughly. (page 1272)

Complete the Patient Care Report (PCR)

Show your completed PCR to your paramedic instructor, and ask for feedback on how well you recorded the case you were given.

True/False

1. T (page 1263)
2. F (page 1260)
3. T (page 1282)
4. T (page 1259)
5. F (page 1280)
6. T (page 1275)
7. F (page 1270)
8. T (page 1268)
9. T (pages 1268–1269)
10. F (page 1266)
11. T (page 1265)
12. T (page 1260)
13. F (page 1260)
14. T (page 1259)
15. F (page 1281)

Short Answer

1. Vocabulary:
   a. Hypoglycemia: Hypoglycemia in the patient with insulin-dependent diabetes is often the result of having taken too much insulin, too little food, or both. Unlike other tissues, which can usually metabolize fat or protein in addition to sugar, the tissues of the central nervous system (including the brain) depend entirely on glucose as their source of energy. If the level of glucose in the blood drops dramatically, the brain is literally starved. (pages 1270–1271)
   b. Diabetic ketoacidosis (DKA): A life-threatening condition, DKA occurs when certain acids accumulate in the body because insulin is not available. Patients who develop this condition tend to be young—teenagers and young adults. In DKA, the deficiency of insulin prevents cells from taking up the extra sugar. (pages 1274–1275)

   c. Thyrotoxicosis: A toxic condition caused by excessive levels of circulating thyroid hormone. Although hyperthyroidism can cause thyrotoxicosis in some patients, the two conditions are not identical. Thyrotoxicosis may also be caused by goiters, autoimmune disease (Graves disease—the most common cause of hyperthyroidism), and thyroid cancer. Graves disease, which has an incidence of 1.4 cases per 1,000 persons, has a chronic course with remissions and relapses. If left untreated, it may be fatal. (page 1283)
   d. Insulin: A hormone produced by the pancreas that is vital to the control of the body's metabolism and blood glucose level. Insulin causes sugar, fatty acids, and amino acids to be taken up and metabolized by cells. (page 1260)
   e. Cushing syndrome: A condition caused by an excess of cortisol production by the adrenal glands or by excessive use of cortisol or other similar steroid (glucocorticoid) hormones. (page 1281)
2. Treatment:
   a. Myxedema coma: Administer supplemental oxygen therapy to correct hypoxia. Intubation and ventilation are indicated for patients with diminished respiratory drive or those who are unable to protect their airway; these measures help prevent respiratory failure. Monitor the patient's cardiac status. Hypotension may respond to crystalloid therapy, and a vasopressive agent, such as dopamine (Intropin), may be necessary. Administer 25 to 50 g of D_{50} (or D_{10} if your system has switched to that concentration) if glucose levels are less than 60 mg/dL. Treat hypothermia with passive rewarming methods—aggressive rewarming may lead to vasodilation and hypotension. Hemodynamically unstable patients with profound hypothermia, however, require active rewarming. Avoid sedatives, narcotics, and anesthetics because of the delayed metabolism. (pages 1282–1283)
   b. Adrenal insufficiency: The treatment for adrenal insufficiency is based on the clinical presentation and findings and is geared toward maintaining the airway, breathing, and circulation until arrival at the emergency department (ED). Other goals of prehospital treatment are to begin rehydration of the patient and to correct the electrolyte and acid–base abnormalities. Follow the procedure for a patient with altered mental status or comatose patient with regard to airway maintenance and supplemental oxygen. Be alert for vomiting, and have suction ready. Start an IV line and infuse up to 1 L of 0.9% normal saline. If the patient is hypotensive, administer a normal saline bolus at 20 mL/kg. Remember, a patient in adrenal insufficiency may be severely dehydrated, often to the point of shock, and needs volume. Check the patient's glucose level. Administer 25 to 50 g of D_{50} (or D_{10} if your system has switched to that concentration) to correct the hypoglycemia. D_5NS is the preferred IV fluid, but a second IV line administering D_5W can be used to maintain the patient's blood glucose level. Monitor cardiac rhythm because changes in serum electrolytes can lead to marked myocardial instability. (pages 1279–1280)
   c. Hyperosmolar nonketotic coma: The treatment of hyperosmolar nonketotic coma (HONK)/hyperosmolar hyperglycemic syndrome (HHS) in the prehospital setting follows the pathway for dehydration and altered mental status. Airway management is the top priority. The comatose patient is often unable to maintain and protect his or her airway. For this reason, endotracheal intubation may be indicated and should be completed as early as possible. Cervical spine immobilization should be used for all unresponsive patients found in a down position, unless witnesses can validate that no fall occurred. Large-bore IV access should be gained as soon as possible, but do not delay transfer while initiating the IV. If necessary, obtain IV access during the transport to the ED. Also obtain a blood glucose level as soon as possible. After you have initiated the IV line, a bolus of 500 mL 0.9% normal saline is appropriate for nearly all adults who are clinically dehydrated. In patients with a history of congestive heart failure or renal insufficiency, a 250-mL bolus may be a more appropriate starting point. Fluid deficits in HONK/HHNC patients may amount to 10 L or more. These patients may receive 1 to 2 L in the first hour. If the glucose level is less than 60 to 80 mg/dL, then (depending on your local protocols) administer 25 g of D_{50} as soon as possible. (pages 1277–1278)

Fill in the Table

1. (page 1269, Table 23-1)

Oral Agents Used to Treat Type 2 Diabetes Mellitus		
Medication Class	**Function**	**Examples**
Sulfonylureas	**Stimulate beta cells to produce more insulin**	Chlorpropamide (Diabinese) Glipizide (Glucotrol) Glyburide (Micronase, Glynase, DiaBeta) Glimepiride (Amaryl)
Meglitinides	Stimulate beta cells to produce more insulin	Repaglinide (Prandin) Nateglinide (Starlix)
Biguanides	**Decrease the amount of glucose produced by the liver**	Metformin (Glucophage)
Thiazolidinediones	Increase insulin effectiveness in the muscle and decrease liver glucose production	Rosiglitazone (Avandia) Pioglitazone (ACTOS)
Alpha-glucosidase inhibitors	**Prevent the breakdown of starches**	Acarbose (Precose) Miglitol (Glyset)
DPP-4 inhibitors	Inhibit the breakdown of GLP-1, a naturally occurring compound in the body that reduces blood glucose levels	Sitagliptin (Januvia) Saxagliptin (Onglyza)

Chapter 24: Hematologic Emergencies

Matching

Part I

1. T (page 1303)
2. S (page 1294)
3. R (page 1297)
4. Q (page 1299)
5. P (page 1294)
6. K (page 1294)
7. J (page 1294)
8. I (page 1294)
9. H (page 1306)
10. G (page 1297)
11. O (page 1301)
12. N (page 1294)
13. M (page 1294)
14. L (page 1294)
15. F (page 1298)
16. A (page 1302)
17. B (page 1302)
18. C (page 1301)
19. D (page 1301)
20. Y (page 1304)
21. X (page 1303)
22. W (page 1301)
23. V (page 1294)
24. E (page 1297)
25. U (page 1304)

Part II

1. O (page 1297)
2. N (page 1297)
3. G (page 1296)
4. M (page 1294)
5. L (page 1303)
6. R (page 1301)
7. Q (page 1308)
8. P (page 1307)
9. F (page 1299)
10. A (page 1304)
11. B (page 1305)
12. C (page 1307)
13. K (page 1294)
14. J (page 1302)
15. I (page 1299)
16. E (page 1294)
17. D (page 1296)
18. H (page 1299)

Multiple Choice

1. D (page 1299)
2. D (page 1300)
3. D (page 1307)
4. A (page 1298)
5. C (page 1295)
6. C (page 1308)
7. C (pages 1304–1305)
8. A (page 1306)
9. B (page 1307)
10. D (page 1294)

Labeling

1. Major organs for producing and regulating the blood (page 1298, Figure 24-4)
   - A. Liver
   - B. Bone marrow
   - C. Spleen

Fill in the Blank

1. connective (page 1294)
2. hematopoietic (page 1294)
3. blood cells; blood cells; platelets (thrombocytes) (page 1294)
4. stem cells (page 1294)
5. RBC count; hemoglobin level; hematocrit (page 1294)
6. Platelets (page 1297)
7. Hodgkin lymphoma (page 1305)
8. sickle cell disease (page 1301)
9. fatigue; headaches; dyspnea (pages 1304–1305)
10. pain (page 1305)
11. von Willebrand disease (page 1297-1298)
12. Bohr effect (page 1294)

Identify

1. a. Chief complaint: Extreme weakness, fatigue, and dyspnea
   b. Vital signs: Pulse is 86 beats/min, slightly irregular, and difficult to palpate; BP is 92/P. Skin is pale, warm, and dry. PERRLA. Oxygen saturation is 91% on ambient air.
   c. Pertinent negatives: Denies chest pain or shortness of breath
2. a. Chief complaint: Altered mental status and possible syncope
   b. Vital signs: His radial pulses are equal bilaterally and regular at 86 beats/min. Skin is jaundiced but cool and dry. PERRLA. Oxygen saturation is 98% on a nonrebreathing face mask.
   c. Pertinent negatives: Not sure if the patient lost consciousness

3. a. Chief complaint: Acute sickle cell crisis, pain
   b. Vital signs: Pulse is 112 beats/min, regular; pulse oximetry is 91%; BP is 148/96 mm Hg. Skin is warm/moist. PERRLA.
   c. Pertinent negatives: None

Ambulance Calls

1. a. The patient who develops back pain, diaphoresis, cyanosis, and other symptoms during a blood transfusion is showing signs of a hemolytic reaction to the blood transfusion. (pages 1308–1309)
   b. To deal with this situation, you need to do the following:
      (1) Stop the transfusion! Disconnect the blood bag, and save it for testing.
      (2) Keep the IV line open with D_5W (if signs of shock develop, switch to normal saline or lactated Ringer's solution).
      (3) Draw a blood sample (red-top tube) from a site other than the IV line.
      (4) Notify the physician and request orders.
2. a. Polycythemia is characterized by an overabundance or overproduction of RBCs. The increased RBC production can be caused by a rare disorder. It can arise in persons who live in high-altitude areas for long periods. The disease causes hyperviscosity of the circulatory system. (pages 1305–1306)
   b. Prehospital care largely consists of supportive care and transporting the patient to an appropriate facility. Administer oxygen as needed. Establish IV access for possible pharmacologic interventions for pain or pulse rate control as appropriate. (page 1306)

True/False

1. F (pages 1294–1296)
2. F (page 1294)
3. T (page 1298)
4. F (page 1308)
5. T (page 1305)
6. F (page 1307)
7. T (page 1307)
8. T (page 1299)
9. F (page 1299)
10. T (pages 1298–1299)

Short Answer

1. Blood disorders present differently from other typical injuries and diseases encountered by paramedics. Students should provide some of the following common findings: (page 1300)
   a. Level of consciousness: Alterations in level of consciousness, ranging from excitability, agitation, and combativeness, to complete unresponsiveness
   b. Skin: Uncontrolled bleeding, unexplained or chronic bruising, itching, pallor, or jaundice (yellow appearance usually indicates liver problems)
   c. Visual disturbances: Visual disturbances, including blurred vision, decreased vision, and seeing black or gray spots
   d. Gastrointestinal system: Epistaxis (bloody nose), bleeding or infected gums, ulcers, melena (blood in the stool), and liver failure (causes jaundice)
   e. Skeletal system: Chronic joint or bone pain or rigidity
   f. Cardiovascular system: Dyspnea, tachycardia, chest pain, hemoptysis (coughing up blood)
   g. Genitourinary system: Hematuria, menorrhagia, chronic or recurring infections
2. a. Leukemia (pages 1304–1305)
      (1) Depends on stage.
      (2) Patient complains of fatigue, headaches, or dyspnea.
      (3) Fever, bone pain, and diaphoresis may be present.
      (4) Vital signs may indicate shock.
      (5) Treatment includes ABCs, IV access, and pain medications.
   b. Hemophilia (page 1307)
      (1) Acute and chronic bleeding may occur at any time.
      (2) Spontaneous intracranial bleeding may be common.
      (3) Be supportive of patients and families.
      (4) Treatment includes ABCs and IV access; treat all bleeding as potentially life threatening.
   c. Polycythemia (pages 1305–1306)
      (1) Characterized by an overabundance of RBCs.
      (2) Can be caused by a rare disorder or congestive heart failure.
      (3) Can lead to strokes, transient ischemic attacks (TIAs), headaches, and abdominal pain.

(4) Found more frequently in adults older than 50 years.
(5) Clinical treatment includes phlebotomy.
(6) Support ABCs.

3. Provide definitions for the following terms:
   a. Leukopenia: A reduction in the number of white blood cells (WBCs) (page 1303)
   b. Polycythemia: An overabundance or overproduction of RBCs, WBCs, and platelets (page 1305)
   c. Reticuloendothelial system: The system in the body that is primarily used to defend against infection (page 1312)
   d. Pruritus: Unspecified itching (page 1306)
   e. Hematocrit: The proportion of RBCs in total blood volume (page 1294)
   f. Melena: Blood in the stool (page 1307)

Fill in the Table

1. (page 1308, Table 24-4)

ABO Rh Type and Preferred and Alternative Donor Types		
Recipient Blood Type	**Preferred Donor Type**	**Additional Permissible Types**
A+	A+	A–, O+, O–
A–	**A–**	**O–**
AB+	AB+	AB–, A+, A–, B+, B–, O+, O–
AB–	**AB–**	**A–, B–, O–**
B+	B+	B–, O+, O–
B–	**B–**	**O–**
O+	O+	O–
O–	**O–**	**None**

Chapter 25: Immunologic Emergencies

Matching

Part I

1. K (page 1331)
2. L (page 1321)
3. M (page 1317)
4. H (page 1320)
5. I (page 1317)
6. J (page 1320)
7. N (page 1317)
8. O (page 1317)
9. A (page 1317)
10. B (page 1317)
11. C (page 1316)
12. G (page 1317)
13. F (page 1317)
14. E (page 1316)
15. D (page 1317)

Part II

1. I (page 1320)
2. H (page 1320)
3. G (page 1332)
4. L (page 1318)
5. K (page 1317)
6. J (page 1331)
7. F (page 1323)
8. E (page 1317)
9. D (page 1320)
10. A (page 1317)
11. B (page 1317)
12. C (page 1320)

Multiple Choice

1. D (page 1327)
2. D (page 1329)
3. B (page 1330)
4. D (page 1330)
5. D (page 1329)
6. D (page 1330)
7. C (page 1317)
8. A (pages 1328–1331)
9. C (pages 1317–1318)
10. C (page 1321)
11. B (page 1333)
12. D (page 1334)

Labeling

(page 1322, Figure 25-2)

1. Antigen introduced into the body
2. Mast cells
3. Bronchospasm, vasoconstriction
4. Decreased cardiac output, decreased coronary flow
5. Vasodilation, leakiness
6. Pruritus, urticaria, edema

Fill in the Blank

1. primary; sensitivity (page 1320)
2. secondary; reexposure (page 1320)
3. antibody (page 1317)
4. Mast (page 1326)
5. Histamine (page 1326)
6. noisy upper (page 1323)
7. systemic; multiple (page 1317)
8. Hypersensitivity; immune; exaggerated (page 1317)
9. Collagen; autoimmune (page 1331)
10. oxygen (page 1330)

Identify

1. **a.** Chief complaint: This patient is probably having a localized reaction at the sting site.
   b. Vital signs: She is conscious and alert. Her skin color is normal, warm, and dry. Capillary refill is normal. Her oxygen saturation is 99%, and her BP is 112/68 mm Hg. PERRLA.
   c. Pertinent negatives: No history and no medications
2. **a.** Chief complaint: This call isn't all that unusual, especially given the recent concerns about Lyme disease. This patient does not appear to be suffering from an allergic reaction.
   b. Vital signs: He is conscious and alert. His pulse is 110 beats/min and regular. BP is 142/84 mm Hg. PERRLA. Skin is warm and moist.
   c. Pertinent negatives: No previous medical history, no allergies, and no known drug allergies

3. a. Chief complaint: This call seems as though it is a true medical emergency. Many schools and classrooms are "peanut-free." In fact, many restaurants and bakeries have signs posted regarding their ingredients and the use of products that may cause allergic reaction. The patient presents as being in noticeable distress with a well-documented allergy history.
   b. Vital signs: Pulse is 124 beats/min, oxygen saturation is 90%, and BP is 90/62 mm Hg.
   c. Pertinent negatives: None indicated
4. a. Chief complaint: It's not uncommon to respond to a reported allergic reaction only to find the patient in minor distress. What is not really clear is the time the patient had dinner. If several hours have gone by, it is less likely that the cause is an allergic reaction. A number of ailments can cause GI upset, including bacterial and viral infections.
   b. Vital signs: Pulse is 124 beats/min, oxygen saturation is 90%, and BP is 112/62 mm Hg.
   c. Pertinent negatives: None
5. a. Chief complaint: Once again, this is a true life-threatening emergency. It's hard to predict how babies and small children may present after receiving routine inoculations. The vast majority of small patients suffer only from minor systemic complications, such as pain and fever. But occasionally, you may encounter a child who has had serious side effects. Remember to maintain ABCs aggressively, contact medical control immediately, and follow pediatric advanced life support as well as local protocols.
   b. Vital signs: Apical pulse is 190 beats/min. Capillary refill is delayed, and skin is mottled.
   c. Pertinent negatives: None

Ambulance Calls

1. This 58-year-old man who was stung by a bee is also suffering an anaphylactic reaction, but because of his age, you have to be a little more careful in giving epinephrine.
   a. The treatment is as follows:
      (1) Ensure that his airway stays patent.
      (2) Administer high-flow oxygen by nonrebreathing mask.
      (3) Monitor the electrocardiogram (ECG) throughout (keep the beep tone on).
      (4) Start a large-bore IV, and run in normal saline (according to your protocols).
      (5) Administer epinephrine per your protocols.
      (6) Remove the stinger from the patient's skin, taking care not to squeeze it. If the site is on an extremity, put a constricting band (venous tourniquet) proximal to the sting site.
      (7) Consult medical command regarding any other pharmacotherapy (eg, Benadryl or corticosteroid).
      (8) Transport without delay. (pages 1328–1331)
   b. Adverse reactions to or side effects of epinephrine include:
      (1) Nervousness
      (2) Restlessness
      (3) Headache
      (4) Tremor
      (5) Pulmonary edema
      (6) Dysrhythmias
      (7) Chest pain
      (8) Hypertension
      (9) Tachycardia
      (10) Nausea
      (11) Vomiting (page 1330, and page 1506 of the Volume 1 Appendix, *Emergency Medications*)
2. If you want to stay out of trouble on your night off, stay out of restaurants! The lady at the next table is suffering an anaphylactic reaction, apparently to something she ate. The sensation of a lump in the throat along with her squeaky voice indicates that she is in a lot of trouble. The steps in management are as follows:
   a. Administer epinephrine per your protocols.
   b. Administer supplemental oxygen by nasal cannula.
   c. Start transport.
   d. Start an IV line with a large-bore cannula.
   e. Consider a corticosteroid per your protocols. (pages 1329–1330)

3. a. Patient A is showing classic signs of choking, and a shot of epinephrine will not help him a bit (except during resuscitation from the cardiac arrest he will surely suffer if you failed to diagnose his choking and act immediately).
   b. Patient B is simply experiencing a very common untoward side effect of erythromycin, about which he should have been warned by the doctor who prescribed the drug.
   c. Patient C is having an anaphylactic reaction.
4. Use the following steps to manage patient C:
   a. Ensure that his airway stays open. It is already in jeopardy, judging from his hoarse voice.
   b. Monitor the ECG; cardiac dysrhythmias are likely.
   c. Administer epinephrine per your protocol.
   d. Start at least one large-bore IV line, and run it wide open.
   e. Consider the use of a corticosteroid per your protocols. (pages 1328–1331)
5. The contraindications to diphenhydramine (Benadryl) are the following:
   a. Hypersensitivity to antihistamines
   b. Newborns or premature infants
   c. Breastfeeding
   d. Use with caution in infants, children, older adults, patients with asthma or narrow-angle glaucoma, and patients taking monoamine oxidase inhibitors (MAOIs). (page 1504 of the Volume 1 Appendix, *Emergency Medications*)
6. The dosage in this case would be 25 to 50 mg slowly IV. (page 1504 of the Volume 1 Appendix, *Emergency Medications*)

Complete the PCR

Show the completed PCR to your instructor to obtain feedback on your completion of the form.

True/False

1. F (page 1328)
2. T (page 1335)
3. T (page 1330)
4. F (page 1329)
5. F (page 1329)
6. T (page 1318)
7. T (pages 1317–1320)
8. F (page 1316)
9. T (page 1330)
10. T (page 1330)

Short Answer

1. Effects produced by chemical mediator histamine include the following:
   a. Systemic vasodilation
   b. Increased permeability of blood vessels
   c. Decreased cardiac contractility
   d. Decreased coronary blood flow
   e. Dysrhythmias
   f. Bronchoconstriction
   g. Pulmonary vasoconstriction (page 1321)
2. *Students should provide four of the following main categories:*
   Foods
   Medications
   Latex
   Blood transfusions (mismatched)
   Hymenoptera stings: bees, yellow jackets, hornets, wasps, fire ants
   Animals
   Seminal fluid
   Allergen-specific subcutaneous immunotherapy
   Chlorhexidine (antiseptic)
   Anti-cancer drugs
   Radio contrast media (pages 1318–1319)

Fill in the Table

(pages 1318–1319)

Causes of Anaphylactic Reactions	
Antigen, General Category	**Comments**
Foods	**Peanuts, shellfish, cow's milk, wheat, soy, eggs**
Medications	**Penicillin, antibiotics, muscle relaxants, opioids, salicylates, nonsteroidal anti-inflammatory drugs (NSAIDs)**
Latex	**Gloves, supplies, or materials containing latex**
Blood transfusions	**Mismatched blood**
Hymenoptera stings	**Bees, yellow jackets, hornets, wasps, fire ants**
Animals	**Dander (long-haired animals), animal serum products (horse serum, gamma globulins)**

Chapter 26: Infectious Diseases

Matching

Part I

1. M (page 1366)
2. N (page 1382)
3. O (page 1345)
4. L (page 1377)
5. K (page 1368)
6. Y (page 1345)
7. X (page 1374)
8. W (page 1347)
9. V (page 1348)
10. U (page 1350)
11. F (page 1368)
12. E (page 1347)
13. D (page 1385)
14. C (page 1347)
15. B (page 1347)
16. T (page 1377)
17. S (page 1354)
18. R (page 1347)
19. Q (page 1348)
20. P (page 1356)
21. A (page 1373)
22. J (page 1366)
23. I (page 1354)
24. H (page 1368)
25. G (page 1345)

Part II

1. V (page 1363)
2. U (page 1378)
3. T (page 1367)
4. S (page 1370)
5. Y (page 1380)
6. X (page 1358)
7. W (page 1357)
8. O (page 1356)
9. N (page 1353)
10. M (page 1370)
11. L (page 1368)
12. K (page 1372)
13. E (page 1375)
14. D (page 1347)
15. C (page 1347)
16. B (page 1383)
17. A (page 1345)
18. G (page 1365)
19. F (page 1368)
20. H (page 1379)
21. I (page 1345)
22. J (page 1355)
23. R (page 1359)
24. Q (page 1375)
25. P (page 1345)

Multiple Choice

1. D (page 1345)
2. D (pages 1346–1347)
3. B (page 1355)
4. B (page 1345)
5. D (page 1349)
6. A (page 1350)
7. C (page 1357)
8. A (page 1347–1348)
9. C (pages 1357–1364)
10. D (page 1367)

Fill in the Blank

1. Standard precautions (page 1347)
2. handwashing (page 1349)
3. postexposure medical follow-up (page 1350)
4. Pathogenic organisms (page 1355)
5. Epstein-Barr; oral (page 1364)
6. Lyme disease (page 1378)
7. sexually transmitted diseases (page 1365–1368)
8. viral hepatitis (page 1370)
9. patient; patient; unwashed (page 1382)
10. mammals; birds (page 1384)

Identify

1. a. Chief complaint: Flu-like symptoms that include fever, chills, dry cough
   b. Vital signs: Respiratory rate is 20 breaths/min, oxygen saturation on ambient air is 95%, pulse is 106 beats/min and regular, and BP is 128/68 mm Hg. Skin is warm and dry. Victim is conscious and alert.
   c. Pertinent negatives: He denies medication, allergies to medication, international travel, and other previous medical history.
2. a. Chief complaint: Infestation of lice; patient is contaminated.
   b. Vital signs: Pulse is 88 beats/min and irregular, BP is 98/72 mm Hg, oxygen saturation is 88%. He is tachypneic, and there is obvious skin tenting and delayed capillary refill.
   c. Pertinent negatives: He believes he just put on the "new clothing" this morning and rarely "needs" to take any pills.
3. a. Chief complaint: ALS interfacility transport.
   b. Vital signs: BP as noted on the noninvasive monitor is 98/54 mm Hg with a heart rate of 62 beats/min.
   c. Pertinent negatives: Patient is "stable" for transport.

Ambulance Calls

1. a. The college student with fever, headache, stiff neck, vomiting, and an altered state of consciousness is showing typical signs of meningitis, perhaps meningococcal.
   b. The paramedic can minimize the risk of catching meningitis from a patient by wearing a mask and washing his or her hands after the call. (page 1358)
2. a. The 54-year-old man with hemoptysis, night sweats, and weight loss most probably has tuberculosis.
   b. The paramedic can minimize the risk of contracting the infection by wearing a mask and washing his or her hands after the call. It is also a good idea to check, about 2 months later, for evidence of new tuberculosis infection by having a tuberculin test. (page1362)
3. a. The IV drug user with yellow eyes, dark urine, anorexia, and distaste for cigarettes has classic symptoms of hepatitis B virus.
   b. To minimize the risk of contracting hepatitis from a patient, the paramedic should employ standard precautions, including gloves when handling blood or body fluids and extreme caution with needles and IV equipment. And, as always, wash your hands after the call. (pages 1370–1371)
4. a. The 8-year-old with fever, loss of appetite, and swelling of the salivary glands under the ears most likely has mumps.
   b. The paramedic's best protection against mumps is immunization, either by mumps vaccine or by having had the illness as a child. The paramedic who is not immunized should wear a mask and guard against droplets. Whether immune or not, wash your hands after the call. (page 1360)
5. a. The young woman with fever, conjunctivitis, and the blotchy red rash has measles.
   b. Prevention is by vaccination. If you haven't had measles or immunization against measles, you can try wearing a mask, but in all likelihood, you will soon have measles, too—just wait about 10 days. Be sure to wash your hands after the call, though, to minimize the risk to the next patients you treat. (page 1363–1364)

Complete the PCR

Show the completed PCR to your instructor to obtain feedback on your completion of the form.

True/False

1. T (page 1374)
2. T (page 1373)
3. F (page 1373)
4. F (page 1373)
5. T (page 1372)
6. F (page 1373)
7. F (page 1373)
8. T (page 1366)
9. F (page 1365)
10. F (page 1366)

Short Answer

1. a. Students will check the illnesses they had as a child or up to this point.
   b. What did your personal immunization survey turn up? Are you completely covered, or do you have some deficits to make up?
   c. If your last tetanus booster was more than 10 years ago, or if you never had an immunization against hepatitis B, make sure you remedy those and any other immunization deficits before you take your first call. And be sure to wash your hands.
2. There is no need to be panicky about AIDS or any other communicable disease if you know something about it.
   a. There are only three ways in which HIV can be transmitted from one person to another:
      (1) Through sexual contact
      (2) Through contaminated blood or blood products (eg, being stuck by a needle used on an HIV-positive person)
      (3) From mother to fetus (pages 1372–1373)
   b. To minimize the risk of acquiring HIV from a patient, follow standard precautions. *Students should provide three of the following:*
      (1) Wear disposable gloves for any contact with blood or other potentially infectious materials (OPIM).
      (2) Use needle-safe or needleless devices.
      (3) Use good handwashing technique.
      (4) Perform routine cleaning of the vehicle after transport. (page 1373)

Fill in the Table

1. (page 1348, Table 26-1)

Recommended Personal Protective Equipment for Preventing Transmission of Human Immunodeficiency Virus and Hepatitis B Virus in the Prehospital Setting				
Task or Activity	**Disposable Gloves**	**Gown**	**Mask**	**Protective Eyewear**
Bleeding control with spurting blood	Yes	**Yes**	Yes	**Yes**
Bleeding control with minimal bleeding	Yes	**No**	No	**No**
Emergency childbirth	Yes	**Yes**	Yes, if spatter is likely	**Yes, if spatter is likely**
Drawing blood samples	Yes	**No**	No	**No**
Inserting an IV line	Yes	**No**	No	**No**
Advanced airway insertion (eg, endotracheal intubation, laryngeal mask airway, Combitube)	Yes	**No**	No, unless spatter is likely[a]	**No, unless spatter is likely[a]**
Oral/nasal suctioning, manually cleaning airway	Yes	**No**	No, unless spatter is likely[a]	**No, unless spatter is likely[a]**
Handling and cleaning instruments with microbial contamination	Yes	**No, unless soiling is likely**	No	**No**
Measuring blood pressure	No	**No**	No	**No**
Measuring temperature	No	**No**	No	**No**
Giving an injection	No	**No**	No	**No**
[a]Spatter is often likely, so use personal protective equipment accordingly.				

Data from Centers for Disease Control and Prevention (CDC): Guidelines for prevention of transmission of human immunodeficiency virus and hepatitis B virus to health-care and public-safety workers: A response to P.L. 100-607 The Health Omnibus Programs Extention Act of 1988. MMWR. 1989;38(S-6):Table 4, (d)(3)(ix)(A)-(C). Available at: http://wonder.cdc.gov/wonder/prevguid/p0000114/p0000114.asp. Accessed November 10, 2011; and Ask the expert: gloves for injections. HCPro OSHA Heathcare Advisor website. http://blogs.hcpro.com/osha/2012/01/ask-the-expert-gloves-for-injections/; and Standard interpretations. United States Department of Labor, OSHA website. https://www.osha.gov/pls/oshaweb/owadisp.show_document?p_table=INTERPRETATIONS&p_id=20819

2. (pages 1348–1385)

Disease	Mode(s) of Transmission	Protective Measures
AIDS	**Sexual contact; injection of contaminated blood products; from mother to fetus**	**Gloves, mask; extreme caution with needles and sharp objects; handwashing**
HAV	**Fecal-oral; from ingesting contaminated water, shellfish, etc**	**Handwashing**
HBV	**Sexual contact; injection of contaminated blood products**	**Immunization; gloves, mask; extreme caution with needles and sharp objects; handwashing**
Meningitis	**Droplet spread**	**Mask; handwashing**
Mumps	**Saliva; droplet spread**	**Immunization; mask; handwashing**
Syphilis	**Sexual contact; infected saliva; semen, vaginal discharge**	**Gloves; handwashing**
Tuberculosis	**Droplet spread**	**Mask; handwashing**
MERS	**Spread of material from infected wound**	**Handwashing; gloves; excellent cleaning routines, airborne precautions**
SARS	**Direct contact with respiratory secretions or body fluids**	**Handwashing; mask that has been fit-tested (ie, N95 or P100)**

Chapter 27: Toxicology

Matching

Part I

1. O (page 1404)
2. N (page 1398)
3. M (page 1441)
4. L (page 1412)
5. Y (page 1415)
6. X (page 1436)
7. W (page 1398)
8. V (page 1442)
9. J (page 1401)
10. I (page 1428)
11. H (page 1442)
12. G (page 1442)
13. U (page 1398)
14. T (page 1432)
15. S (page 1416)
16. R (page 1404)
17. F (page 1420)
18. E (page 1419)
19. D (page 1400)
20. C (page 1406)
21. Q (page 1442)
22. P (page 1404)
23. K (page 1413)
24. A (page 1409)
25. B (page 1414)

Part II

1. H (page 1404)
2. I (page 1398)
3. J (page 1406)
4. K (page 1404)
5. Y (page 1404)
6. X (page 1435)
7. W (page 1398)
8. V (page 1403)
9. A (page 1414)
10. B (page 1435)
11. C (page 1421)
12. D (page 1421)
13. U (page 1398)
14. T (page 1399)
15. S (page 1404)
16. R (page 1406)
17. E (page 1421)
18. F (page 1424)
19. G (page 1398)
20. L (page 1415)
21. M (page 1437)
22. N (page 1419)
23. O (page 1436)
24. P (page 1436)
25. Q (page 1448)

Multiple Choice

1. C (page 1400)
2. D (page 1400)
3. B (page 1409)
4. D (page 1411)
5. D (page 1412)
6. D (page 1408)
7. B (page 1400)
8. B (page 1404)
9. C (page 1415)
10. D (pages 1422–1424)
11. D (page 1404)
12. C (page 1427)
13. A (page 1435)
14. C (pages 1437)
15. C (page 1442)

Fill in the Blank

1. poison; drug (page 1398)
2. Toxicologic emergencies; intentional; unintentional (page 1399)
3. ingestion; inhalation; injection; absorption (page 1400)
4. Toxidromes; clinical umbrella (page 1403)
5. toxic; liver; complications; GI (page 1411)
6. Stimulants; abuse; crack; prescription; stimulants (page 1412)
7. heroin; lucid (page 1421)
8. unintentional (page 1422)
9. poisoning; oxygen; hemoglobin (page 1426)
10. water-soluble; alkalis; alkalis (page 1429)
11. MDMA (page 1430)
12. rubber cement; vomiting (page 1433)
13. gastric irritation; pain; toxicity (page 1433)
14. prolonged; tachycardia; QT (page 1435)
15. mercury; accumulates; liver (page 1439)

Identify

1. **a.** Sedative and hypnotic
   b. *Students should provide two of the following:*
   (1) Phenobarbital
   (2) Secobarbital
   (3) Diazepam (Valium)
   (4) Thiopental
   (5) Midazolam
   (6) Lorazepam
   (7) Propofol

(8) Ethanol
(9) Flunitrazepam
(10 Zolpidem tartrate (page 1404)

2. a. Stimulant
b. *Students should provide two of the following:*
(1) Cocaine
(2) Amphetamine
(3) Methamphetamine
(4) Diet aids
(5) Nasal decongestants (pages 1412–1414)

3. The odor of alcohol (ETOH) along with nausea and vomiting may indicate ingestion and poisoning as a result of alcohol. (page 1405)

4. A seizing patient could be consistent with amphetamines, camphor, cocaine, strychnine, arsenic, carbon monoxide (CO), or petroleum poisoning. Depressed respirations could be indicative of narcotic, alcohol, propoxyphene, CO, or barbiturate poisoning. The type of poisoning common to both symptoms might lead you to be suspicious of a narcotic overdose. CO does not seem likely because family members are able to give you some information, and there is no indication that they are suffering any of the same symptoms. (page 1405)

Ambulance Calls

1. a. Questions to ask the patient's neighbors include the following:
(1) When was the patient last seen?
(2) Do you have any idea of what happened to him?
(3) Is he known to suffer any chronic illnesses (eg, diabetes, epilepsy)?
(4) Has he been injured recently?
(5) Did he complain of any symptoms when last seen?
(6) Is he a known abuser of drugs or alcohol?
b. Besides the neighbors, the scene itself may provide valuable information about what may have caused the patient's coma. Check out:
(1) The bathroom and bedroom for medicine bottles or drug paraphernalia
(2) The kitchen for insulin in the refrigerator or other medications on the counter
(3) The living room and the kitchen trash for empty liquor bottles
c. The patient's physical findings can also help narrow down the possible causes of his coma:

Finding	Possible Diagnostic Significance
Cold, dry skin	**Overdose of alcohol or sedative drugs**
Pulse = 110 beats/min, thready	**Hypovolemia, hypoglycemia, overdose of barbiturates**
BP = 90/60 mm Hg	**Hypovolemia**
Respirations = 12 breaths/min and shallow	**Overdose with sedative drugs**
Pupils dilated and not reactive to light	**Cerebral anoxia, barbiturate overdose, certain eye drops**
Breath smells of alcohol (ETOH)	**Patient ingested alcohol**

(page 1405)

d. The patient is best described as comatose, answer (3).
e. The steps in managing this patient are as follows:
(1) Ensure that the scene is safe for access and egress.
(2) Maintain the airway. (Check whether the patient accepts an oropharyngeal airway [OPA].)
(3) Ensure that breathing is adequate. (Assist ventilations as needed.)
(4) Ensure that circulation is not compromised (eg, by hypoperfusion or dysrhythmia).
(5) Administer high-concentration supplemental oxygen to maintain saturation levels of 94% or higher.
(6) Establish vascular access. (Check blood glucose and administer dextrose IV if hypoglycemic.)
(7) Consider administration of an antidote or mitigating medication, if available.
(8) Be prepared to manage shock, coma, seizures, and dysrhythmias. (Consider administering naloxone [Narcan] per local protocol and/or medical control.)

(9) Transport the patient as soon as possible. To reduce the risk of aspiration, place the patient in the left lateral recumbent position if there is any risk of vomiting.

(10) Other considerations specific to this patient: intubation, 12-lead ECG, frequently rechecking vitals and neurologic function (and noting any trends), splinting the patient's left arm in a position of function. (page 1412)

2. When Junior, or anyone else for that matter, swallows something he shouldn't have swallowed, it is important to obtain details of the ingestion.

a. What was swallowed? (Bring the container to the hospital with the patient if possible.)

b. When was it swallowed?

c. How much was swallowed? (Check to see how much is left in the container if there is any uncertainty; doing so will give you an upper limit of the amount that could have been ingested.)

d. What else was swallowed? Did Junior perhaps sample some washing powder as an hors d'oeuvre or maybe a bit of furniture polish as a chaser?

e. Did he vomit? (pages 1407–1408)

3. When a person is found unconscious and there is reason to suspect a toxic cause, the physical assessment should focus not only on the evaluation of the level of consciousness but also on parameters that might provide clues to a specific toxic agent. *Students should provide five of the following:*

a. Unusual odors on the breath

b. A precise assessment of the mental status, charted on a patient care report (PCR)

c. The condition of the skin (CTC: color, temperature, condition)

d. The respirations, for signs of respiratory depression or metabolic acidosis

e. Abnormalities of the pulse and BP

f. Abnormalities of the pupils (very dilated or very constricted) (page 1405)

4. When the teenager swallows his father's tricyclic antidepressant medications:

a. Activated charcoal is given, by some EMS systems, to absorb poisonous compounds to its surface and thereby effectively remove them from the body. (pages 1401, 1435)

b. Activated charcoal is not effective with poisoning from certain substances, such as alcohols. It is not recommended for acid or alkali ingestions. (pages 1401, 1430)

c. The steps in treatment for this teenager are as follows:

(1) Maintain the airway. If mental status suddenly deteriorates, insert an advanced airway.

(2) Administer high-flow supplemental oxygen to maintain blood saturation levels of greater than 94%.

(3) Establish vascular access.

(4) Provide continuous ECG monitoring.

(5) Administer activated charcoal per medical control orders.

(6) Consult with medical control to consider sodium bicarbonate administration.

(7) Manage hypotension with sequential boluses of normal saline.

(8) Assess blood glucose levels. Administer IV dextrose if the patient is hypoglycemic.

(9) Be alert for agitation or violence. Provide reassurance and administer benzodiazepines, if needed.

(10) Do not give flumazenil (Romazicon; may cause seizures) or physostigmine (Eserine, Antilirium).

(11) Treat seizures with benzodiazepines.

(12) Provide rapid transport to the appropriate facility. (page 1435)

5. The gentleman who swallowed crystalline Drano ingested a very strong alkali that will continue burning holes in everything it touches until it is removed from the body.

a. From a management perspective, advanced life support care for a toxicologic emergency builds on the following basics:

(1) Ensure the scene is safe for access and egress.

(2) Maintain the airway.

(3) Ensure breathing is adequate.

(4) Ensure circulation is not compromised (ie, either by hypoperfusion or a dysrhythmia).

(5) Administer high-concentration supplemental oxygen to maintain saturation levels of 94% or higher.

(6) Establish vascular access.

(7) Consider administration of antidote or mitigating medication, if available.

(8) Prepare to manage shock, coma, seizures, and dysrhythmias.

(9) Transport the patient as soon as possible. If any risk of vomiting exists, then place the patient in the left lateral recumbent position to reduce the risk of aspiration. (page 1409)

6. Down by the railway, some of the community's homeless population have congregated to console themselves with whatever they can find to drink. Sometimes, the substances chosen as cheap substitutes for ethanol can have disastrous consequences when ingested.

a. The first patient is showing classic signs of ethylene glycol toxicity. The pleasant taste of the substance, the gastrointestinal symptoms some hours later, and the severe respiratory distress about 24 hours later are all characteristic. (page 1432)

b. The steps of management are the same as that of methanol, which are as follows:
(1) Establish and manage the airway. (Consider advanced airway placement as needed.)
(2) Establish vascular access.
(3) Assess the blood glucose level, and administer glucose if the patient has hypoglycemia.
(4) Consult with medical control for consideration of sodium bicarbonate and/or 10% calcium gluconate.
(5) Provide immediate transport to an appropriate facility. (page 1432)

c. The second patient, who appears drunk, is most likely suffering from methyl alcohol poisoning. (pages 1431–1432)

d. The care plan for a patient with suspected methanol poisoning is the same as for ethylene glycol poisoning, with the exception of possibly getting an order from medical control to administer 10 mL of 10% calcium gluconate via slow IV push, which is appropriate for the ethylene glycol but not the methanol.
(1) Establish and manage the airway (consider advanced airway placement as needed).
(2) Establish vascular access.
(3) Assess the blood glucose level and administer glucose if the patient has hypoglycemia.
(4) Consult with medical control for consideration of sodium bicarbonate.
(5) Provide immediate transport to an appropriate facility. (page 1430)

7. There's something called too much of a good thing, and too much insulation of a cabin heated by a wood stove is definitely in the too-much-of-a-good-thing category!

a. In the case in question, everyone inside the cabin is showing signs of carbon monoxide poisoning. (pages 1425–1426)

b. The steps to take are as follows:
(1) Remove the patient from the exposure. Bundle up in warm clothes, and open all the windows of the cabin.
(2) Establish and maintain the airway, inserting an advanced airway as needed.
(3) Administer high-flow supplemental oxygen by a tight-fitting nonrebreathing mask.
(4) Establish vascular access.
(5) Keep the patients quiet and at rest to minimize oxygen demand.
(6) Monitor the ECG rhythm and level of consciousness.
(7) Transport to the appropriate facility. If the patient is unresponsive or has signs of serious CO poisoning, direct transport to a facility capable of providing hyperbaric medicine is preferred. (page 1426)

8. a. The patient stricken with a "possible heart attack" while sitting out on the lawn is in fact the victim of his next-door neighbor's insecticide spray. Although you must take very seriously the possibility of acute myocardial infarction in any middle-aged man who complains of weakness, nausea, and a tight feeling in his chest, the hypersalivation combined with constricted pupils and severe bradycardia all point to organophosphate poisoning. And, indeed, your partner returns from his discussion with Mr. Greenthumb carrying the offending bottle of parathion. (page 1425)

b. The drug used to treat organophosphate poisoning is the parasympathetic blocking agent atropine. (page 1425)

c. Massive doses of atropine are often required to counteract the effects of organophosphates. Paramedics administer 1 mg IV. Thereafter, atropine is administered 1 mg IV every 3 to 5 minutes until the patient is atropinized. (page 1425)

d. (1) The first component of patient assessment and management is decontamination, which is likely performed by a hazmat crew according to local protocol. The patient care includes the following measures:
(2) Establish and maintain the airway. Consider an advanced airway as needed.
(3) Suction as needed.
(4) Administer high-flow oxygen to maintain saturation levels of greater than 94%.
(5) Establish vascular access (IV or IO), without delay if possible.
(6) Administer 1.0 mg atropine IV/IO push or by auto-injector, and repeat the dose every 3 to 5 minutes until easing of ventilation and reduction of secretions (atropinization) occur.
(7) Administer up to three pralidoxime (2-PAM) auto-injectors (600 mg/each) in the first hour. Multiple doses may be required for patients with severe exposure.
(8) Apply the ECG monitor, pulse oximeter, and capnometer.
(9) Notify the receiving hospital early, and transport to the appropriate facility. (page 1425)

9. The boy who suffered a seizure after inhaling typewriter correction fluid should be treated as any other postictal patient:
   a. Ensure the patient with contaminated skin or clothing has been decontaminated prior to treatment because the vapors can be harmful to others.
   b. Establish and maintain the airway, and ensure adequate ventilation.
   c. Administer high-flow supplemental oxygen to maintain blood saturation levels of greater than 94%.
   d. Establish vascular access.
   e. Continuously monitor the ECG rhythm; consider running a 12-lead ECG.
   f. Administer sequential bolus infusions of normal saline to treat hypotension.
   g. Transport the patient to the most appropriate facility. (page 1434)

Complete the PCR

Show the completed PCR to your instructor to obtain feedback on your completion of the form.

True/False

1. T (page 1400)
2. F (page 1426)
3. T (page 1401)
4. T (page 1404)
5. T (pages 1409–1411)
6. T (page 1410)
7. T (page 1411)
8. F (page 1407)
9. F (page 1413)
10. T (page 1437)
11. T (page 1429)
12. T (page 1433)
13. T (page 1414)
14. F (page 1438)

Short Answer

1. The patient whom you are tempted to write off as "just another drunk" is in fact much more vulnerable to a host of injuries and medical problems than the more sober John Q. Citizen. The conditions to which alcoholics are particularly susceptible include the following (*students should list 10 of the following*):
   a. Subdural hematoma
   b. Gastrointestinal bleeding
   c. Pancreatitis
   d. Hypoglycemia
   e. Pneumonia
   f. Burns
   g. Hypothermia
   h. Seizures
   i. Dysrhythmias
   j. Cancer
   k. Esophageal varices (page 1411)

Fill in the Table

1. You don't have to look very far to find commonly ingested poisons. Just check your own home. (pages 1428, 1429, 1431–1434, and 1441–1442)

Type of Poison	Examples
Strong acid	**Toilet bowl cleaner, battery acid, bleach disinfectant**
Strong alkali	**Drain buildup remover (Drano), Clinitest tabs, chlorine bleach, dishwasher detergent**
Hydrocarbons	**Benzene industrial solvents, toluene spray paints and lacquer thinner, gasoline for power tools**
Toxic plants	**Lantana, dieffenbachia, caladium, castor bean**

2. (Page 1438, Table 27-7)

Signs and Symptoms of Acetaminophen Toxicity		
Stage	**Time Frame**	**Signs and Symptoms**
I	< **24 h**	Nausea, vomiting, loss of appetite, pallor, malaise
II	**24-72 h**	Right upper quadrant abdominal pain; abdomen tender to palpation
III	**72-96 h**	Metabolic acidosis, renal failure, coagulopathies, recurring GI symptoms
IV	**4-14 d (or longer)**	Recovery slowly begins, or liver failure progresses, and the patient dies

Chapter 28: Psychiatric Emergencies

Matching

Part I

1. U (page 1452)
2. V (page 1470)
3. W (page 1453)
4. X (page 1467)
5. Y (page 1467)
6. A (page 1452)
7. B (page 1480)
8. C (page 1455)
9. D (page 1469)
10. E (page 1475)
11. O (page 1464)
12. N (page 1458)
13. M (page 1476)
14. L (page 1460)
15. K (page 1472)
16. T (page 1452)
17. S (page 1461)
18. R (page 1456)
19. Q (page 1456)
20. P (page 1456)
21. F (page 1476)
22. G (page 1474)
23. H (page 1480)
24. I (page 1452)
25. J (page 1452)

Part II

1. R (page 1454)
2. Q (page 1474)
3. F (page 1452)
4. P (page 1456)
5. O (page 1472)
6. Y (page 1455)
7. X (page 1474)
8. W (page 1456)
9. V (page 1477)
10. U (page 1456)
11. A (page 1456)
12. B (page 1476)
13. C (page 1456)
14. D (page 1456)
15. E (page 1474)
16. S (page 1452)
17. T (page 1475)
18. L (page 1472)
19. M (page 1480)
20. N (page 1459)
21. K (page 1472)
22. J (page 1469)
23. I (page 1459)
24. H (page 1456)
25. G (page 1477)

Part III

(page 1454)

1. P
2. P
3. O
4. B
5. P
6. O
7. O
8. B
9. O
10. P

Part IV

(page 1456, Table 28-3)

1. F
2. B
3. E
4. D
5. H
6. G
7. A
8. C
9. D
10. B
11. E
12. H

Multiple Choice

1. A (page 1454)
2. D (page 1456)
3. C (pages 1457–1459)
4. D (page 1459)
5. A (pages 1473–1474)
6. D (pages 1471–1472)
7. A (page 1463)
8. D (page 1452)
9. B (page 1454)
10. A (page 1474)
11. B (page 1462)
12. C (page 1468)

Fill in the Blank

1. biologic; organic; environment; illness; injury; substance-related (page 1454)
2. clearly; confused; delusional; frequent (page 1457)
3. fear; dread; autonomic (page 1475)
4. bulimia nervosa; anorexia nervosa (page 1476)
5. *Students should list three of the following*: amoxapine (Asendin), desipramine (Norpramin, Pertofrane), doxepin (Adapin, Sinequan), imipramine (Imavate, Janimine, Pramine, Presamine, Tofranil), amitriptyline (Amitril, Endep, Elavil), and nortriptyline (Aventyl, Pamelor) (page 1478)
6. orthostatic hypotension; supportive (page 1479)
7. Suicide (page 1470)
8. 100; schizophrenia (page 1474)

Identify

1. Fluoxetine (Prozac) and diazepam (Valium) (pages 1478–1479)
2. Phenelzine (Nardil) and bupropion (Wellbutrin) (pages 1478–1479)
3. Aripiprazole (Abilify) (page 1480)

Ambulance Calls

1. The shortest answer to this question is that the paramedic did just about everything wrong! Furthermore, he or she was inexcusably rude.
   a. The paramedic never identified himself (assume it was a male paramedic).
   b. The paramedic used a demeaning term to address the patient ("dearie") instead of asking her name and addressing her with respect as Miss, Ms., or Mrs. So-and-so.
   c. The paramedic stood in front of the patient, towering over her and also blocking her escape—a very threatening stance. He should have crouched down to be at the same level as the patient and positioned himself somewhat to the side so that she wasn't trapped in the corner.
   d. The paramedic passed judgment on the patient's feelings ("Big girls don't cry"). Furthermore, he belittled the patient's problem without even waiting to find out what the problem was! ("You're making a mountain out of a molehill.")
   e. The paramedic gave inappropriate and premature reassurance, telling the patient in essence that everything will be all right by tomorrow without even knowing what's wrong today.
   f. The paramedic tried to forestall the patient's expressions of feeling, urging her to stop crying.
   g. The paramedic never gave the patient a chance to talk.
   h. The paramedic then turned his back on the patient and asked if someone else could tell him what was going on, implying that the patient's version of things was of no importance. (page 1462)
2. The fact that Mr. Crosby has admitted you into his apartment, even reluctantly, is a hopeful sign.
   a. You might start the interview something like this: "Your neighbors have been worried about you; that's why they called us. They thought there might be some kind of problem here. Is there any way we can help?" If the patient then says something to the effect that there's nothing anyone can do to help, you might comment on his statement: "You seem really discouraged." The objective is to indicate that you are a "sympathetic ear," prepared to listen to his troubles. (page 1462)
   b. The symptoms of depression that this patient is showing include the following:
      (1) A sense of worthlessness
      (2) Decreased appetite
      (3) No apparent interest in anything
      (4) Lack of energy (pages 1473–1474)
   c. Other symptoms and signs of depression include:
      (1) Sleep disturbances
      (2) Difficulty concentrating
      (3) Psychomotor abnormalities (retardation or agitation)
      (4) Suicidal thoughts (pages 1473–1474)
   d. The risk factors for suicide in this patient's history include:
      (1) Male, although he does not fit the < 55 age group since he is 62
      (2) Widower
      (3) Social isolation
      (4) Depression
      (5) Possible alcohol problem (empty bottles lying around) (page 1470)
   e. Other risk factors for suicide include the following. *Students should provide six of the following:*
      (1) Depression or sudden improvement in depression
      (2) Male sex, age <55 years
      (3) Single, widowed, or divorced
      (4) Alcohol or other drug abuse
      (5) Recent loss of spouse or significant relationship
      (6) Chronic, debilitating illness
      (7) Schizophrenia
      (8) Expresses suicidal thought and concrete plans for carrying them out
      (9) Caucasian
      (10) Social isolation
      (11) Previous suicide attempt(s)
      (12) Financial setback or job loss
      (13) Family history of suicide (page 1470)

f. Among the questions to ask in evaluating this patient's suicide risk are the following: (*Student should list three of the following five*)
   (1) Did you ever feel that you would be better off dead?
   (2) Have you ever thought of harming yourself? Do you feel that way now?
   (3) Do you have a plan for going about it? Do you have the things you need to carry out the plan?
   (4) Has anyone in your family ever died by suicide?
   (5) Have you ever tried to kill yourself before? (page 1470)

3. The young woman with a "possible heart attack" is unlikely to be suffering a heart attack (although it's not completely out of the question).
   a. Her problem is most likely a panic attack. (page 1475)
   b. The symptoms and signs that suggest that diagnosis include the following:
      (1) Dyspnea
      (2) Chest tightness
      (3) Feeling faint
      (4) Her feelings of unreality and impending death
      (5) Tachycardia
      (6) Sweating
      (7) Trembling (page 1475)
   c. Yes, there certainly are other possibilities that must be taken into account, including:
      (1) Pulmonary embolism, which is highest on the list of possibilities
      (2) Cardiac dysrhythmia
      (3) A reaction to a drug
      (4) An anaphylactic reaction
      (5) An acute myocardial infarction (AMI), which is seen much more frequently among young people these days because of the widespread use of cocaine
   d. To manage this patient, therefore:
      (1) Separate her from all the panicky bystanders.
      (2) Create a calm environment.
      (3) Tolerate the patient's disability.
      (4) Reassure the patient that he or she is safe.
      (5) Give the patient's symptoms a name.
      (6) Help the patient regain control. (pages 1475–1476)

4. The police officer who summoned you to the bar was on the right track, even if "psycho case" is not a very specific diagnosis.
   a. The patient is probably in the manic phase of a bipolar mood disorder. (page 1472)
   b. The evidence to suggest this diagnosis includes the following:
      (1) His pressure of speech
      (2) His grandiose ideas (big business deals, big spender)
      (3) His apparently euphoric mood that is, nonetheless, very brittle (His good cheer easily turns to a less pleasant affect when he is challenged by the bartender or the police officer.)
      (4) His hyperactivity, pacing up and down (pages 1472–1473)
   c. In managing this patient, you will have to try to persuade him to go voluntarily to the hospital. If he will not be persuaded, and probably he will not, coercion will be necessary. Consult your medical director first. (page 1473)

5. The strangely dressed man found wandering down the middle of the street is a good example of disorganized behavior. Because walking in traffic is not a healthy activity, the patient must be assumed to be unable to care for himself and probably needs institutional care. From the description, it does not sound as if you will be able to obtain a useful history. You should simply tell the patient gently but firmly that you are going to take him to the hospital for care. He will probably go along without much fuss if you are nonthreatening about it. (page 1469)

6. The karate expert is seriously ill and probably dangerous.
   a. He is showing signs of psychosis (answer 2)—hallucinations, persecutory delusions, loosening of associations. (pages 1467–1469)
   b. Yes, there are indications that he might become violent.
   c. Indications. *Students should provide four of the following:*
      (1) His body language—sitting there like a coiled spring, gripping the armrests of the chair
      (2) The fact that he is easily startled
      (3) His avoidance of eye contact

(4) The fact that he views the paramedics as adversaries (He thinks you're the FBI!)
(5) His hearing of voices that tell him to put up a fight

d. In managing this situation:
(1) Observe your surroundings. Keep yourself between the patient and the door to his room. Make note of any potential weapons. Maintain a safe distance, at least two arm lengths (which will keep you out of range of his foot).
(3) Identify yourself again as a paramedic. Explain in plain language what you are doing and what the patient's role is.
(4) Explain to the patient the need to be seen by a physician, and that you will take the patient to the medical facility to get help.
(5) If the patient is experiencing disorientation, keep orientating the patient to time, place, and the people in the environment.
(6) Reassure the patient, and point out landmarks to help orient the patient.
(7) When a patient's behavior becomes so excited that it threatens his or her well-being or the safety of others, you must take more aggressive steps to prevent injury. (page 1469)

True/False

1. T (page 1462)
2. F (pages 1460–1462)
3. F (page 1461)
4. F (page 1462)
5. T (page 1462)
6. T (page 1463)

Short Answer

1. The paramedic needs to develop a "nose for danger" and be able to predict which situations present a high risk for violence.
a. Situations where alcohol or illicit drugs are being consumed (eg, tavern, party)
b. Incidents involving large crowds
c. Incidents in which violence has already occurred (eg, shooting, stabbing, domestic disturbances) (page 1471)

2. a. Patients intoxicated with drugs or alcohol
b. Patients withdrawing from drugs or alcohol
c. Psychotic patients
d. Patients with delirium (page 1471)

Fill in the Table

(page 1454, Table 28-2)

Selected Disease States That May Produce Psychotic Symptoms	
Disease State	**Psychotic Symptoms**
Toxic and deficiency states	Drug-induced psychoses, especially from: Digitalis • Steroids • Disulfiram • Amphetamines • LSD, PCP, and other psychedelics Nutrition disorders: • Alcohol abuse • Vitamin deficiencies Poisoning with bromide or other heavy metals Kidney failure Liver failure
Infections	Syphilis Parasites Viral encephalitis (eg, after measles) Brain abscess
Neurologic disease	Seizure disorders (especially temporal lobe seizures) Primary and metastatic tumors of the brain Dementia Stroke Closed head injury
Cardiovascular disorders	Low cardiac output (eg, in heart failure)
Endocrine disorders	Thyroid hyperfunction (thyrotoxicosis) Adrenal hyperfunction (Cushing syndrome)
Metabolic disorders	Electrolyte imbalances (eg, after severe diarrhea) Hypoglycemia Diabetic ketoacidosis

Section 7: Trauma

Chapter 29: Trauma Systems and Mechanism of Injury

Matching

Part I

1. C (page 1547)
2. B (page 1547)
3. D (pages 1555–1556)
4. A (page 1547)
5. B (page 1547)
6. A–D (pages 1547, 1555–1556)
7. A (page 1547)
8. A (page 1547)
9. B (page 1547)
10. A, B (page 1547)

Part II

1. J (page 1562)
2. I (page 1543)
3. H (page 1562)
4. G (page 1543)
5. F (page 1543)
6. Y (page 1559)
7. X (page 1543)
8. W (page 1542)
9. V (page 1545)
10. U (page 1543)
11. A (page 1544)
12. B (page 1545)
13. C (page 1563)
14. D (page 1548)
15. E (page 1558)
16. N (page 1543)
17. O (page 1559)
18. P (page 1559)
19. Q (page 1544)
20. R (page 1559)
21. K (page 1559)
22. L (page 1543)
23. M (page 1545)
24. S (page 1544)
25. T (page 1542)

Part III

1. P (page 1568)
2. O (page 1569)
3. N (page 1542)
4. M (page 1543)
5. L (page 1548)
6. G (page 1559)
7. F (page 1557)
8. E (page 1559)
9. D (page 1545)
10. C (page 1545)
11. T (page 1550)
12. S (page 1556)
13. R (page 1544)
14. Q (page 1563)
15. B (page 1562)
16. A (page 1545)
17. K (page 1568)
18. J (page 1563)
19. I (pages 1542–1543)
20. H (page 1562)

Multiple Choice

1. A (page 1571)
2. C (page 1566)
3. D (page 1572)
4. B (page 1556)
5. A (page 1560)
6. D (page 1561)
7. D (pages 1558–1559)
8. A (page 1542)
9. D (page 1571)
10. A (page 1551)

Labeling

(page 1561)

A. Primary blast injury (injuries due to the blast wave itself)
B. Secondary blast injury (injuries due to missiles being propelled by blast force)
C. Tertiary blast injury (injuries due to impact with another object)
D. Quaternary blast injury (collateral injuries such as burns, crush injuries, toxic inhalation)
E. Quinary blast injury (long-term damage from biologic, chemical, or radioactive contaminants added to explosive device)

Fill in the Blank

1. **a.** The size of the explosive charge
   b. The nature of the surrounding medium
   c. The distance from the explosion
   d. The presence or absence of reflecting surfaces (page 1563)
2. anatomic; penetration (page 1558)
3. Arterial air embolism (page 1563)
4. **a.** Height
   b. Position
   c. Surface
   d. Physical condition
   e. Area (pages 1556–1557)
5. cervical; neck (page 1553)

Identify

1. **a.** Mechanism of injury: Rollover motor vehicle crash
   b. Chief complaint: Pain to radius/ulna, neck pain
   c. Vital signs: Pulse 110 beats/min and regular, respiration 16 breaths/min and unlabored, blood pressure (BP) 106/96 mm Hg, Spo_2 98%, and ashen-colored skin
   d. Pertinent negatives: Denies LOC
2. **a.** Mechanism of injury: High-speed motorcycle-versus-guardrail crash
   b. Chief complaint: Hurts all over
   c. Vital signs: Conscious and alert, skin ashen and diaphoretic, no palpable BP, >2-second capillary refill, respiration 28 breaths/min, and Spo_2 92%
   d. Pertinent negatives: None
3. **a.** Mechanism of injury: Possible fall, TIA, cardiac
   b. Chief complaint: Per patient, none; staff states she fell and has pain to hip.
   c. Vital signs: Pulse 58 beats/min and irregular; BP 158/110 mm Hg; Spo_2 95%; skin cool and dry; normal capillary refill
   d. Pertinent negatives: Denies chest pain, shortness of breath, neck or back pain

Complete the Patient Care Report

Show the completed PCR to your instructor to obtain feedback on your completion of the form.

Ambulance Calls

1. Evaluate the mechanism of injury, and examine the trauma scene for evidence of high-energy trauma.
   a. Speed
   b. Restrained versus airbag deployment
   c. Loss of consciousness
   d. Physical damage to pole and vehicle, and any intrusion into the vehicle
   e. Patient's chief complaint
   f. Secondary assessment (physical exam) (pages 1545, 1547, 1552–1553)
2. **a.** Height: The distance that he jumped. This will determine the speed at which he fell and, therefore, the force of impact with which he hit the ground.

   Position: How he landed. This will tell you which part(s) of the body absorbed the greatest amount of kinetic energy.

   Area: The area over which the impact is distributed—the larger the area of contact at the time of the impact, the greater dissipation of the force and the lesser the peak pressures generated.

   Surface: Which kind of surface he landed on. A pile of hay has a lot more give than a concrete sidewalk. The more the surface can "give," the less the falling body will have to deform.

   Physical condition: The physical condition of the patient before the fall. Does he have any underlying physical problems—such as an ulcer or an enlarged spleen—that might predispose him to certain injuries?

   b. Spine, legs, pelvis (pages 1556–1557)
3. Children tend to fall head-first, so head injuries are common in children, as are injuries to the wrists and upper extremities when the child attempts to break the fall. The surface on which the child falls is very important. (page 1557)
4. **a.** Call the police.
   b. (1) The type of weapon that was used (handgun, rifle, or shotgun; type and caliber)
   (2) At which range was it fired?
   (3) Which kind of bullet was used?
   (4) Look for powder residue around the wound.
   (5) Look for entrance and exit wounds. (page 1560)
5. Explosions produce several different mechanisms of injury, and one needs to anticipate each type; otherwise, it is easy to miss the less obvious injuries.
   a. Primary blast injury: Body damage caused by the explosion
   b. Secondary blast injury: Damage from being struck by flying debris
   c. Tertiary blast injury: Patient being hurled against a stationary object
   d. Quaternary blast injury: Collateral injuries such as burns, crush injuries, and toxic inhalation (page 1561)

6. (page 1563)

Tissues at Risk	Evidence
1. Tympanic membrane	Blood in the ear
2. Pulmonary blast injury	Tight feeling in chest
3. Arterial air embolism	Blurry vision

True/False

1. T (page 1563)
2. F (page 1572)
3. F (page 1573)
4. T (page 1546)
5. T (page 1551)
6. F (page 1554)
7. T (page 1570)
8. F (page 1570)

Short Answer

1. In this question, you are asked to consider the forces involved when a 2,000-lb automobile traveling at 20 mph strikes a pedestrian. (pages 1544–1545)
   a. Some of the kinetic energy of the vehicle will remain energy of motion, assuming the vehicle keeps moving. (If the driver hits the brakes, the friction of the brakes will transform that kinetic energy into heat.) Some energy will be absorbed by the vehicle in the deformation of the bumper or hood, and the remainder will be absorbed by the pedestrian who has been struck by the vehicle.
   b. Had the vehicle weighed 6,000 lb instead of 2,000 lb—that is, had its weight (mass) been tripled—its kinetic energy at any given speed would also have tripled, according to the kinetic energy equation: $KE = m/2 \times V^2$.
   c. Had the vehicle been traveling at 60 mph instead of 20 mph—that is, had its velocity been tripled—its kinetic energy would have increased nine times because kinetic energy increases as the *square* of the velocity. That is why it is nearly impossible for a pedestrian to survive an impact with a vehicle, even a relatively small vehicle, going faster than about 40 mph—the kinetic energies become overwhelming.

2. When a car traveling at a speed of 50 mph slams into a concrete wall, the effects of progressive deceleration occur in five phases. The first three distinct collisions that take place are as follows:
   a. Collision 1 is between the *automobile* and the concrete wall. Because the automobile is both more mobile and more deformable than the concrete wall, the majority of the kinetic energy is absorbed by the automobile in its rebound off the wall and deformity of the front end.
   b. Collision 2 is between the *occupant* and the automobile. In that collision, some of the kinetic energy is absorbed by the automobile (eg, in denting the dashboard), but the larger proportion is absorbed by the occupant.
   c. Collision 3 is between the internal *organs* of the occupant and the restraining walls of the person's body (eg, the skull, the chest cage, the pelvic girdle). The majority of the kinetic energy in that collision is absorbed by the internal organs. (page 1546)

3. When you arrive at the crash scene, a close inspection of the scene and of the damaged vehicle(s) can provide extremely important information—information that will enable the physicians who take over the patient's care to detect and manage the patient's problems much more expeditiously. Indeed, what you observe (or fail to observe) about the crash scene could make the difference between life and death for the patient—so keep your eyes open, report what you have observed to the base physician, and record your findings on the patient's PCR. (page 1547)
   a. Deformed dashboard
      (1) Ruptured spleen, liver, bowel, diaphragm
      (2) Fractured patella
      (3) Dislocated knee
      (4) Femoral fracture
      (5) Dislocated hip
   b. Deformed steering column
      (1) Sternal or rib fracture
      (2) Flail chest
      (3) Myocardial contusion
      (4) Pericardial tamponade
      (5) Pneumothorax or hemothorax
      (6) Exsanguinations from aortic tear

c. Cracked windshield
   (1) Brain injury
   (2) Scalp, facial cuts
   (3) Cervical spine injury
   (4) Tracheal injury
d. Door smashed in
   (1) Fractured hip
   (2) Fractured iliac wing
   (3) Fractured clavicle or ribs

4. *Students should provide six of the following:*
   a. Facial injuries
   b. Soft-tissue neck trauma
   c. Larynx and tracheal trauma
   d. Fractured sternum
   e. Myocardial contusion
   f. Pericardial tamponade
   g. Pulmonary contusion
   h. Hemothorax, rib fracture
   i. Flail chest
   j. Ruptured aorta
   k. Intra-abdominal injuries (page 1551)

Fill in the Table

1. (Table 29-6, page 1572)

Key Elements for Trauma Centers		
Level	**Definition**	**Key Elements**
Level I	A comprehensive regional resource that is a tertiary care facility. Capable of providing total care for every aspect of injury—from prevention through rehabilitation.	**1. 24-hour in-house coverage by general surgeons** **2. Availability of care in specialties such as orthopedic surgery, neurosurgery, anesthesiology, emergency medicine, radiology, internal medicine, and critical care** **3. Should also include cardiac, hand, pediatric, and microvascular surgery and hemodialysis** **4. Provides leadership in prevention, public education, and continuing education of trauma team members** **5. Committed to continued improvement through a comprehensive quality assessment program and organized research to help direct new innovations in trauma care**
Level II	Able to initiate definitive care for all injured patients.	**1. 24-hour immediate coverage by general surgeons** **2. Availability of care in specialties such as orthopedic surgery, neurosurgery, anesthesiology, emergency medicine, radiology, and critical care** **3. Tertiary care needs such as cardiac surgery, hemodialysis, and microvascular surgery may be referred to a Level I trauma center** **4. Committed to trauma prevention and continuing education of trauma team members** **5. Provides continued improvement in trauma care through a comprehensive quality assessment program**

Key Elements for Trauma Centers		
Level	**Definition**	**Key Elements**
Level III	Able to provide prompt assessment, resuscitation, and stabilization of injured patients and emergency operations.	1. **24-hour immediate coverage by emergency medicine physicians and prompt availability of general surgeons and anesthesiologists** 2. **Program dedicated to continued improvement in trauma care through a comprehensive quality assessment program** 3. **Has developed transfer agreements for patients requiring more comprehensive care at a Level I or Level II trauma center** 4. **Committed to continuing education of nursing and allied health personnel or the trauma team** 5. **Must be involved with prevention and have an active outreach program for its referring communities**
Level IV	Able to provide ATLS before transfer of patients to a higher-level trauma center.	1. **Include basic emergency department (ED) facilities to implement ATLS protocols and 24-hour laboratory coverage** 2. **Transfer to higher-level trauma centers follows the guidelines outlined in formal transfer agreements** 3. **Committed to continued improvement of these trauma care activities through a formal quality assessment program** 4. **Involved in prevention, outreach, and education within its community**

2. (Table 29-3, page 1551)

"Ring" of Chest Injuries From Impact With the Steering Wheel or Dashboard
• **Facial injuries**
• Soft-tissue neck trauma
• Larynx and tracheal trauma
• **Fractured sternum**
• **Myocardial contusion**
• **Pericardial tamponade**
• Pulmonary contusion
• Hemothorax, rib fractures
• **Flail chest**
• **Ruptured aorta**
• Intra-abdominal injuries

Problem Solving

1. $KE = \frac{(200+120)}{2} \times 50^2 = 400{,}000$

(page 1486)

2. $KE = \frac{120}{2} \times 50^2 = 150{,}000$

(page 1486)

Chapter 30: Bleeding

Matching

1. K (page 1592)
2. L (page 1592)
3. J (page 1584)
4. I (page 1592)
5. H (page 1592)
6. Q (page 1587)
7. P (page 1587)
8. O (page 1585)
9. N (page 1592)
10. M (page 1587)
11. Y (page 1587)
12. X (page 1583)
13. W (page 1584)
14. V (page 1584)
15. U (page 1584)
16. A (page 1583)
17. B (page 1584)
18. C (page 1583)
19. D (page 1588)
20. E (page 1588)
21. G (page 1586)
22. F (page 1583)
23. T (page 1592)
24. S (page 1587)
25. R (page 1585)

Multiple Choice

1. B (page 1584)
2. C (page 1584)
3. A (page 1595)
4. D (page 1589)
5. D (page 1594)
6. A (page 1592)
7. C (page 1592)
8. B (page 1589)
9. C (page 1597)
10. B (page 1587)

Labeling

1. The circulatory system (page 1582, Figure 30-1)
   - **A.** Head, arm, and upper trunk
   - **B.** Arteriole
   - **C.** Artery
   - **D.** Aorta
   - **E.** Lung
   - **F.** Heart
   - **G.** Abdominal organs
   - **H.** Lower body and legs
   - **I.** Vein
   - **J.** Venule

Fill in the Blank

1. hemoglobin (page 1584)
2. perfusion (page 1584)
3. Hemostasis (page 1587)
4. melena (page 1592)
5. Epistaxis (page 1595)
6. Hypoperfusion (page 1585)
7. hematochezia (page 1592)
8. clotting; hemophilia (page 1587)
9. SVR; CO; worsening (page 1589)
10. heart; liver (page 1588)
11. compensated; decompensated; irreversible (page 1589)
12. normal saline; lactated Ringer's (page 1602)
13. mouth; vomit (page 1602)
14. crystalloids (page 1602)

Identify

1. Chief complaint: Abdominal GSW
2. Vitals signs: Sinus tachycardia rate of 120 beats/min, and equal lung sounds. Respirations are 24 breaths/min; BP is 80/56 mm Hg; skin is pale, diaphoretic, and clammy. Patient is alert with oxygen administration. An eye assessment shows PERRLA.
3. Pertinent negatives: No pulse at wrist, little external bleeding, no ectopy on ECG

Complete the Patient Care Report

Show the completed PCR to your instructor to obtain feedback on your completion of the form.

Ambulance Calls

1. In assessing the state of perfusion:
   a. You can judge *peripheral* perfusion by checking the radial pulse.
   b. The best indicator in the field of *perfusion of the brain* is the patient's state of consciousness. (page 1589)
2. You are called to a bar to attend a bleeding, unresponsive man. The place is full of noise and confusion—unruly customers, police, curiosity seekers. *This is the time to remember the priorities of the primary survey:* ABC or CAB.

   First, before you even enter that bar, make certain that the police have the situation under control. (If you did not include that step in your answer, you do not get *any* points for your answer and, furthermore, you are a very poor risk for life insurance!) Look first to your own safety, remember?
   a. Open the patient's airway. (*Note:* If you suspect this is a cardiac arrest, the approach is CAB, not ABC.)
   b. Check whether the patient is breathing. If not, start artificial ventilation.
   c. Check whether the patient has a pulse. If he does not have a pulse, start external chest compressions.
   d. Cut away the patient's trouser leg, and find the source of his bleeding. When you have found it, control the bleeding by applying direct pressure to the wound, preferably over a sterile dressing. Check quickly for other lower-extremity injuries.
   e. Transfer the patient to the vehicle (he should be on a scoop by now).
   f. Get under way to the hospital and start an IV infusion en route. Complete your rapid secondary assessment as time permits. (page 1594)
3. This patient earns his "load-and-go" status by virtue of uncontrollable bleeding from the femoral artery.
   a. Steps to be taken at the scene:
      (1) Seal the open wound of the neck.
      (2) Administer supplemental oxygen.
      (3) Try at least to slow the bleeding from the groin by using direct pressure, a pressure dressing, and pressure to the artery. If your system uses hemostatic dressings, they should be used on this patient. (page 1599)
      (4) Communicate with medical control or the receiving hospital.
   b. Steps to be taken en route:
      (1) Start two large-bore IV lines with rapid infusion of fluids.
      (2) Complete a secondary assessment and physical exam.
      (3) Recheck vital and neurologic signs every 5 minutes. (pages 1601–1602)
4. Abdominal evisceration is certainly an attention-getter, but it does *not* pose an immediate threat to life.
   a. Steps to be taken at the scene:
      (1) Administer supplemental oxygen.
      (2) Complete the secondary assessment and a physical exam.
      (3) Cover the eviscerated organs with sterile dressings soaked in sterile saline and an occlusive dressing.
   b. Steps to be taken en route:
      (1) Communicate with medical control or the receiving hospital.
      (2) Start a large-bore IV with normal saline or lactated Ringer's (depending on your regional protocols).
      (3) Recheck vital and neurologic signs every 5 minutes. (pages 1601–1602)

True/False

1. F (page 1589)
2. F (page 1589)
3. F (page 1602)
4. T (page 1588)
5. T (page 1583)
6. F (page 1584)
7. T (page 1586)
8. T (page 1586)
9. F (page 1598)
10. T (page 1591)

Short Answer

1. Three components are required for a functioning regulatory system:
   a. A functioning pump: the heart
   b. Adequate fluid volume: the blood and body fluids
   c. An intact system of tubing capable of reflex adjustments (constriction and dilation) in response to changes in pump output and fluid volume: the blood vessels (page 1582)

2. Causes of hypovolemic shock *(students should provide four of the following)*:
   a. External bleeding
   b. Blunt chest trauma
   c. Blunt abdominal trauma
   d. Fractures of the pelvis or femur
   e. Ruptured ectopic pregnancy
   f. Bleeding ulcer
   g. Burns
   h. Dehydration (page 1588)
3. Knowing the findings in hemorrhagic shock is important to a paramedic. Estimates for Class II fluid and blood loss would include (page 1589):

Findings in Class II Fluid and Blood Loss (Hemorrhagic Shock)	
Heart rate (beats/min)	**Increased**
Systolic blood pressure (mm Hg)	**Minimal to no change at this point**
Pulse pressure (mm Hg)	**Decreased (narrowing)**
Capillary refill	**Decreased (may be delayed)**
Respiratory rate (breaths/min)	**Increased**
Central nervous system/mental status	**Increased agitation (mildly anxious)**
Skin condition	**Cool and moist**
Urine output (mL/h)	**Flat (at this point)**

4. It is absolutely essential that a paramedic be able to recognize the signs of shock—that is why we keep coming back to them. Symptoms and signs of shock include *(students should provide six of the following)*:
   a. Restlessness and anxiety
   b. Thirst
   c. Nausea, sometimes with vomiting
   d. Cold, clammy, pale, or mottled skin
   e. Weak, rapid pulse
   f. Rapid, shallow breathing
   g. Changes in the state of consciousness/mental status
   h. Fall in blood pressure (pages 1589–1590)
5. The four steps in managing external hemorrhage:
   a. Take standard precautions. Apply direct, even pressure over the wound with a dry, sterile dressing.
   b. If bleeding stops, apply a pressure dressing and/or splint. Hold the pressure dressing in place using gauze (bandage).
   c. If direct pressure does not rapidly control bleeding on an extremity injury, apply a tourniquet above the level of the bleeding. *Note:* Some EMS systems also use hemostatic dressings at this point.
   d. Tighten the tourniquet until the bleeding stops. Position the patient supine unless contraindicated. Administer oxygen as necessary. Keep the patient warm, transport promptly, monitor the serial vital signs, and watch diligently for developing shock. (page 1594)

Fill in the Table

(Table 30-3, page 1589)

Compensated Versus Decompensated Shock	
Compensated	**Decompensated**
• **Agitation, anxiety, restlessness** • Sense of impending doom • **Weak, rapid (thready) pulse** • Clammy (cool, moist) skin • **Pallor with cyanotic lips** • Shortness of breath • **Nausea, vomiting** • Delayed capillary refill in infants and children • **Thirst** • Normal systolic blood pressure	• Altered mental status (verbal to unresponsive) • **Hypotension** • Labored or irregular breathing • **Thready or absent peripheral pulses** • Ashen, mottled, or cyanotic skin • **Dilated pupils** • Diminished urine output (oliguria) • **Impending cardiac arrest**

Chapter 31: Soft-Tissue Trauma

Matching

Part I

1. G (page 1614)
2. H (page 1612)
3. I (page 1615)
4. V (page 1634)
5. N (page 1627)
6. W (page 1612)
7. K (page 1612)
8. L (page 1618)
9. M (page 1612)
10. O (page 1612)
11. U (page 1614)
12. T (page 1630)
13. A (page 1623)
14. B (page 1626)
15. C (page 1625)
16. J (page 1612)
17. P (page 1614)
18. D (page 1618)
19. E (pages 1613–1614)
20. F (page 1612)
21. S (page 1630)
22. R (page 1630)
23. Q (page 1612)

Part II

1. I (page 1630)
2. H (page 1630)
3. E (page 1623)
4. F (page 1616)
5. R (page 1611)
6. G (page 1630)
7. S (page 1612)
8. Q (page 1612)
9. J (page 1614)
10. K (page 1612)
11. L (page 1630)
12. M (pages 1621–1622)
13. A (page 1614)
14. B (page 1623)
15. C (page 1611)
16. D (page 1614)
17. P (page 1627)
18. O (page 1624)
19. N (page 1614)

Multiple Choice

1. D (page 1628)
2. B (page 1618)
3. D (page 1625)
4. A (page 1628)
5. A (page 1617)
6. C (page 1626)
7. C (page 1630)
8. C (page 1617)
9. D (page 1622)
10. D (page 1614)

Labeling

1. The skin (page 1611, Figure 31-1)
   - **A.** Hair
   - **B.** Pore
   - **C.** Germinal layer of epidermis
   - **D.** Sebaceous gland
   - **E.** Erector pillae muscle
   - **F.** Nerve (sensory)
   - **G.** Sweat gland
   - **H.** Hair follicle
   - **I.** Blood vessel
   - **J.** Subcutaneous fat
   - **K.** Fascia
   - **L.** Muscle
2. Types of open wounds
   - **A.** Abrasion (page 1623, Figure 31-9A)
   - **B.** Laceration (page 1624, Figure 31-10A)
   - **C.** Avulsion (page 1625, Figure 31-13A)
   - **D.** Puncture wound/impaled object (page 1624, Figure 31-11A)
   - **E.** Amputation (page 1626, Figure 31-14)

Fill in the Blank

1. Degloving; debridement (page 1615)
2. erythema; pus; warmth; edema; local discomfort (page 1616)
3. toxin; contractions (page 1630)
4. Gangrene; blood (page 1630)
5. Paronychia (page 1630)
6. collagen (page 1614)
7. superficial (page 1619)

Identify

1. The injury described appears to be a laceration with moderately uncontrolled bleeding. Even though this appears to be an isolated injury, a thorough primary survey is warranted. Treatment would generally include bleeding control. Usually, this can be completed with direct pressure. Sometimes, in extreme cases, a tourniquet may be needed. Perhaps splinting the extremity to minimize movement and applying a sterile dressing and roller gauze are appropriate. Do not forget to check distal capillary refill and motor neurologic function (PMS) before and after bandaging. (page 1617)
2. This sounds like a classic amputation. Of immediate concern is stopping the bleeding. Doing so will require the paramedic to don personal protective equipment (PPE), which at the very least includes gloves and may include a disposable gown and blankets. Paramedics must very quickly prepare bulky trauma dressings and be prepared for the potential of uncontrolled bleeding. Bleeding control is often self-limiting in this type of situation. However, if it is not controlled, methods such as direct pressure, elevation, and use of an arterial tourniquet may be required. It may be necessary to maintain these steps all the way to the hospital. If necessary, request additional resources. Once bleeding is controlled, begin treating the patient for shock with high-flow oxygen and IV fluid replacement. It is also beneficial as soon as practical to have the patient lie down with his feet elevated. Doing so on your cot enables you to initiate transport immediately. If the patient has adequate vital signs, pain medication may also be in order. Above all, do not forget about the amputated fingers. Follow local protocols regarding wet or dry dressings and placing the parts on ice. (page 1626)
3. This patient has incurred some type of puncture or stab wound. In her combative state, she might not realize how serious the injury could be. As a paramedic, you realize that she might have suffered a hemothorax or pneumothorax. You rapidly treat the obvious wound with an occlusive dressing and immediately prepare for transportation with high-flow oxygen. You also prepare IV lines en route. In a worst-case situation, this patient may require ventilatory assistance and intubation. (page 1619)

Ambulance Calls

1. a. To control the bleeding from Bugsy's left calf, you have several methods available:
      (1) Directing manual pressure over the bleeding site (likely to be the most effective)
      (2) Splinting the left leg
      (3) As a last resort, applying a tourniquet (pages 1620–1621)
   b. If Bugsy's wound had been on the forearm rather than on the leg, the brachial artery would most likely have been the cause of severe bleeding.
2. When Frank accidentally amputates two of his fingers, you have two problems: (1) treating the patient and (2) preserving the amputated parts in optimal condition.
   a. To treat the injury, the first priority is to stop the bleeding. Probably direct pressure will be sufficient because amputations ordinarily do not bleed profusely. Apply lots of fluffed gauze to the stumps of the fingers and bandage the whole hand in a position of function (fingers slightly flexed). The patient will doubtless require a lot of calming down; if you can remain calm, it will help a great deal.
   b. Once you have taken care of the patient, you can turn your attention to the amputated parts. Rinse the two fingers free of contaminants with cool, sterile saline. Wrap them loosely in saline-moistened sterile gauze. Then, place them in a plastic bag, seal the bag, and place it in a cool container for transport. Do *not* place the amputated part in water or directly on ice! (page 1626)
3. Bugsy's Butcher Shop is definitely not a healthy workplace. Now poor Hercules has become a casualty—not only of the meat grinder that mangled his hand but also of a Good Samaritan who was trying to help. The mistakes made in caring for Hercules include the following:
   a. No attempt was made to stop the bleeding by other means, such as direct pressure alone or in combination with elevation, splinting, and so on. *A tourniquet is a last resort*, not a first choice!
   b. A rope should not be used as a tourniquet, nor should any other narrow materials that can damage underlying tissues.
   c. The tourniquet was twisted too tightly. It is almost never necessary to twist a tourniquet as tight as it will go; the objective is to slow the bleeding sufficiently that it can be controlled by direct pressure.
   d. A tourniquet should never be covered, lest it escape attention. The Good Samaritan covered the patient's whole arm in a butcher's apron, perhaps to spare the patient the sight of his mangled extremity. (page 1620)

4. It is rather rare to encounter a patient with an impaled object, but considerable attention is given to the problem in emergency medical technician (EMT) and paramedic courses because the consequences of mismanagement could be disastrous.
   a. When the impaled object is in the eye, the usual principle applies: Stabilize the impaled object in place. For the eye, the most efficient way to do so is usually with a stack of gauze pads that has a hole in the middle. The gauze pads are passed gently over the impaled object and bandaged in place. If the impaled object is an arrow, as in the present case, it will not be possible to cover it with a paper cup. Do not try to shorten the impaled object. Just protect it from being jarred, and be sure to patch the other eye as well to prevent the injured eye from moving every time the uninjured eye shifts its gaze. (pages 1624–1625)
   b. When an object is impaled in the cheek, you have to break the usual rule about not removing an impaled object because it will be impossible to control bleeding inside the mouth as long as the arrow is sticking through the cheek. Therefore, gently pull the arrow out of the cheek. Then, pack the inside of the cheek with sterile gauze, and apply counterpressure with a dressing secured firmly against the outside of the cheek. Keep the patient on his side so that he can more easily spit any blood out of his mouth (instruct him not to swallow blood because blood in the stomach is a stimulus to vomit).
5. For the man bitten by the Doberman pinscher, the treatment is as follows:
   a. Have him stop walking on the injured leg.
   b. Clean the wound with lots of soap and water, and then rinse the wound with alcohol (there goes the rest of your gin).
   c. Send someone back along the beach to find out details about the dog (eg, name and address of owner), which must be reported to the local health authorities.
   d. See that the patient is transported to the hospital for further evaluation of his wound. (page 1627)

True/False

1. T (page 1626)
2. T (page 1610)
3. F (page 1611)
4. F (page 1612)
5. T (page 1623)
6. T (page 1626)
7. F (page 1614)
8. T (page 1630)
9. T (page 1621)
10. T (page 1613)

Short Answer

1. a. It protects underlying tissue from injury.
   b. It plays a major role in temperature regulation.
   c. It prevents excessive loss of water from the body.
   d. It serves as a sense organ for temperature, touch, and pain. (page 1611)
2. a. Hemostasis
   b. Inflammation
   c. Epithelialization
   d. Neovascularization
   e. Collagen synthesis (pages 1613–1614)
3. a. Contusion
   b. Ecchymosis
   c. Hematoma (page 1612)

Chapter 32: Burns

Matching

Part I

1. (page 1650)
   (1) A
   (2) A
   (3) B
   (4) A
   (5) B
   (6) A
   (7) A
   (8) A
2. (1) D. Put out the fire.
   (2) C. Open the airway manually.
   (3) A. Administer supplemental oxygen.
   (4) H. Intubate the trachea (if a basic life support [BLS] airway is not adequate).
   (5) F. Pass a nasogastric tube into his stomach.
   (6) B. Start an IV line.
   (7) J. Obtain a set of baseline vital signs.
   (8) E. Remove the patient's clothing.
   (9) G. Determine the extent and depth of the burn.
   (10) I. Cover the burns with sterile dressings. (pages 1651–1655)

Part II

1. P (page 1639)
2. O (page 1639)
3. N (page 1639)
4. M (page 1644)
5. L (page 1642)
6. T (page 1639)
7. S (page 1648)
8. R (page 1655)
9. Q (page 1660)
10. A (page 1665)
11. F (page 1642)
12. E (page 1652)
13. D (page 1639)
14. C (page 1655)
15. B (page 1650)
16. K (page 1641)
17. J (page 1646)
18. I (page 1639)
19. G (page 1639)
20. H (page 1639)

Part III

1. J (page 1641)
2. I (page 1642)
3. H (page 1644)
4. G (page 1642)
5. F (page 1642)
6. M (pages 1642–1643)
7. L (page 1643)
8. K (page 1642)
9. A (page 1660)
10. B (page 1644)
11. C (page 1648)
12. D (page 1648)
13. E (page 1641)

Multiple Choice

1. D (page 1663)
2. B (page 1665)
3. A (page 1648)
4. C (page 1643)
5. B (page 1648)
6. C (page 1646)
7. D (pages 1652–1653)
8. A (page 1653)
9. B (page 1656)
10. C (page 1662)

Labeling

1. The layers of the skin
   (page 1640, Figure 32-3)
   A. Epidermis
   B. Dermis
   C. Subcutaneous tissue
2. Burn severity
   (page 1643, Figure 32-8)
   A. Partial-thickness burn
   B. Superficial burn
   C. Full-thickness burn

Fill in the Blank

1. epidermis (page 1639)
2. dermis (page 1640)
3. scald (page 1641)
4. acids; alkalis; bases (page 1655)
5. Oxidizing agents (page 1655)
6. scene is safe (page 1665)
7. alpha; beta; gamma (page 1665)
8. zone of coagulation (page 1642)
9. dry dressing (page 1655)
10. decontaminated (page 1665)

Identify

1. Chief complaint: Woman burned by oil from a hot fryer. Upon arrival, you find her with holes in her jeans on the top of both thighs. She is crying and immediately rates her pain as unbearable.
2. Vital signs: Respirations are 22 breaths/min, oxygen saturation is 97%, lungs are clear, blood pressure (BP) is 150/100 mm Hg, pulse is 114 beats/min with sinus tachycardia, skin is cool, pain is 10/10, patient is alert × 3.
3. Pertinent negatives: Airway is open; patient does not have any mental deficits; there are no burns other than on the top of her thighs.

Complete the Patient Care Report

Show the completed PCR to your instructor to obtain feedback on your completion of the form.

Ambulance Calls

1. The patient who jumped from his bedroom window to escape a fire is in grave jeopardy. He is unresponsive, so his airway is liable to be obstructed. He may have additional respiratory injury (note the burns to his face), along with head and neck injuries (note the mechanisms of injury). Finally, he almost certainly has at least one broken bone. The steps in treating him are as follows:
   a. Put out the fire in his pants!
   b. Open his airway with cervical spine precautions (ie, chin lift or jaw thrust only).
   c. Administer supplemental oxygen—the patient has been in a smoky environment.
   d. Intubate the trachea. This patient is unresponsive, so his airway is already in jeopardy. In addition, he has almost certainly sustained airway injury—note the singed beard and swollen lips—so do not wait until laryngeal edema closes off his airway altogether. Get the endotracheal (ET) tube in while it is still relatively easy to do so.
   e. Cut away the pants, and perform the secondary trauma assessment. In doing so, you should evaluate the extent, depth, and severity of the burn.
   f. Cover the burns with sterile dressings.
   g. Splint the left leg and any other fractures; immobilize the patient on a backboard. (He fell from 15 feet, so you have to assume until proved otherwise that he injured his spine.)
   h. Start an IV line (can be done en route to hospital). *Note:* The precise time at which you start the IV line will be determined by the patient's overall condition and the amount of help you have at the scene. If the patient is in shock, start the IV line as soon as you have managed the airway. (pages 1651–1654)
2. Among the questions you would like answered about the burned patient are the following:
   a. When precisely did the burn occur? (ie, when did the fire break out?)
   b. Was the patient in a closed space with smoke or other products of combustion?
   c. Does the patient have any significant underlying medical problems?
   d. Does the patient take any medications regularly? Had he taken any drugs or alcohol within the past few hours?
   e. Does the patient have any allergies?

   You already know the answers to most of the other questions you would usually ask. You can assume that the patient did not lose consciousness while still in the burning building because he managed to jump out the window. You know what he was burned with (flame). Also, you know that nothing was done until the ambulance arrived. It would be helpful to question the fire personnel regarding toxic products of combustion to which the patient might have been exposed.

3. **a.** The burn on the right arm is probably a **partial-thickness (second-degree)** burn. The severe pain virtually rules out a third-degree burn, and the mottling suggests it is more serious than a superficial (first-degree) burn. The appropriate treatment is to **cover the burn with cool, wet, sterile dressings**. If the application of cool dressings is not sufficient to relieve the patient's pain, it may be necessary to give him a small dose of morphine in addition.

b. The burn on the flank is probably a **superficial (first-degree)** burn, although it could also be a partial-thickness burn (it will be impossible to tell for sure until at least another few hours). **Treat it as you would treat a partial-thickness burn** because it might well be one.

c. The burn on the right leg is probably a **full-thickness (third-degree)** burn. The leathery appearance, thrombosed veins, and absence of sensation are all characteristic. **Cover the burn with a dry sterile dressing**. (pages 1654–1655)

4. Electric burns can be very deceptive because the extent of injury may not be at all apparent from the burn that is visible on the surface of the body.

a. The four types of *burns* that may occur from electricity:

(1) A contact burn, which usually produces a bull's-eye lesion at the point of entry and sometimes also at the point of exit
(2) A flash burn, an electrothermal injury caused by the arcing of electric current
(3) A flame burn, which occurs if the electricity ignites a person's clothing or surroundings
(4) A TASER effect produced by an electric weapon (page 1661)

b. Besides burns, electricity may cause a variety of other injuries or disorders of function, including the following:

(1) Respiratory arrest
(2) Cardiac arrest
(3) Neurologic disorders (seizures, coma, paralysis)
(4) Kidney damage
(5) Fractures and dislocations
(6) Cervical spine injuries (page 1662)

c. In dealing with this electrocuted patient lying beside a live cable, you need to take the following steps:

(1) Secure the scene. Keep all bystanders well back from the live wire. Do not get within reach of the wire if you are not fully trained and fully equipped to deal with power lines. Radio for help, and do not get within the range of the wire until it has been inactivated. If you have some creative idea for extricating the patient that does not require your coming within the range of the cable (eg, lassoing him and dragging him toward you), you may try such a method, but bear in mind that the patient may have a spinal injury.
(2) As soon as it is safe to approach the patient, ensure that he has an open airway, taking precautions not to hyperextend his neck.
(3) Provide artificial ventilation or cardiopulmonary resuscitation (CPR) as needed.
(4) Administer supplemental oxygen.
(5) If the patient remains unresponsive, intubate the trachea (if a BLS airway is not adequate).
(6) Start an IV line, and run in normal saline solution as fast as the IV line will flow.
(7) Consult the base physician for medication orders.
(8) Cover burns with a sterile dressing.
(9) Splint fractures.
(10) Immobilize the spine (per local protocol) on a backboard/scoop. (page 1665)

5. In this question, an unresponsive young man was rescued from a house fire.

a. Signs suggestive of respiratory injury (airway involvement) in a burned patient include the following:

(1) Hoarseness
(2) Cough
(3) Stridor
(4) Singed nasal or facial hairs
(5) Facial burns
(6) Carbon in the sputum
(7) History of burn in an enclosed space (page 1647)

b. The first step to take in managing this patient is to *put out the fire* in his clothing!

c. (1) To calculate the extent of his burns, you need to use a combination of the rule of nines and the rule of palms (pages 1648–1649):
Posterior surface of both legs: 18%
Whole left arm: 9%
Hand-sized patch of left flank: 1%
Total: **28%**

(2) Yes, the patient does have a critical burn on at least three counts:
(a) He has full-thickness burns over more than 10% of his body.
(b) He has burns of all depths or thicknesses over more than 25% of his body.
(c) He has burns involving the genitals.

d. The Consensus formula states that during the *first 8 hours* the patient should receive (page 1653):

$$\tfrac{1}{2} \times 4 \text{ mL/kg body weight} \times \% \text{ body surface burned}$$

For this patient, that means:

$$\tfrac{1}{2} \times 4 \text{ mL} \times 70 \text{ kg} \times 28 = 3{,}920 \text{ mL}$$

Therefore, during each hour, the patient needs to receive:

$$\text{mL/h} = \frac{3{,}920 \text{ mL}}{8 \text{ h}} = 490 \text{ mL/h}$$

$$\text{mL/h} = \frac{490 \text{ mL}}{60 \text{ min/h}} = 8 \text{ mL/min}$$

$$\text{gtt/min} = 8 \text{ mL/min} \times 10 \text{ gtt/mL} = \mathbf{80 \text{ gtt/min}}$$

e. (1) The dosage of morphine usually given to an adult in the field is **5 mg (may be as high as 10 to 20 mg)**. (Per the Volume 1 Appendix, *Emergency Medications.*)
(2) It is usually given **intravenously** because absorption after intramuscular administration may be erratic if the patient has any perfusion problems.
(3) Possible adverse side effects include the following (*students should provide three of the following*):
(a) Hypotension
(b) Bradycardia
(c) Respiratory depression
(d) Nausea and vomiting (per Volume 1 Appendix, *Emergency Medications*)

6. a. Percentage of the patient's body that is burned (page 1648):
Entire left leg: 18%
Posterior right leg: 9%
Left forearm: 4%
Total: **31%**

b. Yes, the patient has a critical burn, which we know for two reasons:
(1) The burn covers more than 25% of the body surface.
(2) The burn involves the genitals.

c. If the pedal pulses are absent in a burned leg, you have to assume that swelling from circumferential burns has cut off the circulation to the foot. If you do not act quickly in such a situation, the patient may lose his leg.

d. You need to cool the burned leg with towels that have been soaked in cold water and transport the patient immediately to the hospital.

True/False

The principles of treating chemical burns do not differ significantly from the principles of treating thermal burns. In both cases, the first priority is to put out the *fire*, but in a chemical burn, putting out the fire is a more difficult and time-consuming operation.

1. F (pages 1655–1656)
2. T (page 1656)
3. F (page 1656)
4. F (page 1657)
5. T (pages 1658–1659)
6. T (page 1654)
7. T (page 1638)
8. F (page 1646)
9. T (page 1661)
10. F (page 1647)

Short Answer

1. a. Rule 1: Never be the tallest object. Stay out of the middle of open fields or open areas. Don't use ladders, umbrellas, or anything else that makes you taller. Make yourself as small as possible.

b. Rule 2: Never stand under or near the tallest object that is a good conductor. Stay away from trees, metal umbrellas, or towers of any kind.

c. Rule 3: Take shelter in the most substantial structure in which you will be safe if it is hit by lighting. Try to get in an enclosed building if possible. A small metal shed probably would not be a good idea.

d. Rule 4: Avoid touching a good conductor during a lightning storm. This can apply to things inside your home, such as the TV, telephone, and computer. (page 1663)

2. Suspect that a victim of flame burns has suffered respiratory injury (airway involvement) if any of the following signs are present (page 1647):
   a. Hoarseness
   b. Cough
   c. Stridor
   d. Singed nasal or facial hair
   e. Facial burns
   f. Carbon in the sputum
   g. History of burn in an enclosed space
3. Injury from a high-voltage electric source or from lightning may produce many conditions. Students should list six of the following: (page 1662)
   a. Asphyxia to apnea
   b. Peripheral nerve deficits
   c. Cardiac arrest
   d. Fracture and/or spine injury if the patient has fallen
   e. Kidney damage
   f. Cataracts
   g. Exit wound
   h. Seizures
   i. Delirium, confusion, or coma
   j. Severe tetanic muscle spasms

Fill in the Table

(pages 1652–1653)

Consensus Formula Chart										
% Burn	10 kg	20 kg	30 kg	40 kg	50 kg	60 kg	70 kg	80 kg	90 kg	100 kg
10	25	**50**	**75**	100	125	150	175	**200**	225	250
20	50	**100**	**150**	200	250	300	350	**400**	450	500
30	75	**150**	**225**	300	375	450	525	**600**	675	750
40	100	**200**	**300**	400	500	600	700	**800**	900	1,000
50	125	**250**	**375**	500	625	750	875	**1,000**	1,125	1,250
60	150	**300**	**450**	600	750	900	1,050	**1,200**	1,350	1,500
70	175	**350**	**525**	700	875	1,050	1,225	**1,400**	1,575	1,750
80	200	**400**	**600**	800	1,000	1,200	1,400	**1,600**	1,800	2,000
90	225	**450**	**675**	900	1,125	1,350	1,575	**1,800**	2,025	2,250
20 mL/kg	200	**400**	**600**	800	1,000	1,200	1,400	**1,600**	1,800	2,000

Note: Values in this table are based on the high end of the 2- to 4-mL range in the formula.

Problem Solving

1. To calculate the patient's fluid needs, first you must assess the extent of his burns. Then, you can calculate the IV rate in the usual fashion.
   a. The percentage of the patient's body that has been burned is calculated as follows (page 1648):
      Whole right leg: 18%
      Anterior left leg: 9%
      Anterior trunk: 18%
      Whole right arm: 9%
      Total: 54%
   b. Now you have to calculate the patient's fluid needs. First, you must convert his weight from pounds to kilograms:

$$\frac{154 \text{ lb}}{2.2 \text{ lb/kg}} = \mathbf{70 \text{ kg}}$$

   Now, according to the Consensus formula, the patient's fluid needs over the first 8 hours will be: (page 1653)

$$\tfrac{1}{2} \times 4 \text{ mL/kg body weight} \times \% \text{ of body surface burned}$$

$$\tfrac{1}{2} \times 4 \text{ mL} \times 70 \text{ kg} \times 54 = 7{,}560 \text{ mL}$$

   So his fluid needs *per hour* will be:

$$\frac{7{,}560 \text{ mL}}{8 \text{ h}} = \mathbf{945 \text{ mL/h}}$$

   (Practically speaking, that figure can be regarded as equivalent to 1 liter per hour, but you should complete the calculations using the precise figures.)
   Thus, you will need to deliver:

$$\frac{945 \text{ mL/h}}{60 \text{ min/h}} = 15.8 \text{ mL/min (ie, } \mathbf{16 \text{ mL/min}}\text{)}$$

   c. If your infusion set delivers 10 gtt per milliliter, you therefore need to set the rate of the infusion at:

$$10 \text{ gtt/mL} \times 16 \text{ mL/min} = \mathbf{160 \text{ gtt/min}}$$

   We included this question to give you a little practice in computing IV infusion rates—just in case you were getting rusty. In this particular case, however, it is an academic exercise only because to deliver the kind of volumes we are talking about—nearly 1 liter per hour—you will have to run the IV line wide open, probably under pressure. Usually, when volumes of this sort are required, it makes more sense to start a second and even a third IV line.
   d. For a burned patient, give an IV fluid that will remain in the vascular space, such as normal saline solution.

Chapter 33: Face and Neck Trauma

Matching

Part I

1. G (page 1688)
2. F (page 1678)
3. E (page 1677)
4. P (page 1684)
5. O (page 1702)
6. N (pages 1692–1693)
7. Q (page 1678)
8. B (page 1679)
9. A (page 1691)
10. D (page 1689)
11. C (page 1684)
12. X (page 1678)
13. W (page 1679)
14. R (page 1677)
15. S (page 1684)
16. T (page 1702)
17. M (page 1685)
18. L (page 1679)
19. K (page 1679)
20. I (page 1684)
21. H (page 1678)
22. V (page 1689)
23. U (page 1702)
24. J (page 1679)

Part II

1. S (page 1702)
2. T (page 1697)
3. U (page 1688)
4. V (page 1704)
5. R (page 1684)
6. Q (page 1693)
7. P (page 1704)
8. O (page 1704)
9. N (page 1704)
10. M (page 1678)
11. A (page 1684)
12. B (page 1684)
13. C (page 1702)
14. K (page 1678)
15. J (page 1678)
16. I (page 1679)
17. E (page 1677)
18. D (page 1679)
19. H (page 1697)
20. G (page 1677)
21. F (page 1677)
22. L (page 1690)

Multiple Choice

1. D (page 1679)
2. B (page 1677)
3. A (page 1679)
4. B (page 1678)
5. D (pages 1679, 1707)
6. B (page 1677)
7. A (page 1684)
8. B (page 1693)
9. C (page 1684)
10. B (page 1686)
11. C (page 1690)
12. B (pages 1692–1693)
13. B (page 1682)
14. D (page 1696)
15. A (page 1702)

Labeling

1. Structures of the eye (page 1678, Figure 33-5)
   - A. Iris
   - B. Cornea
   - C. Pupil
   - D. Lens
   - E. Sclera
   - F. Retina
   - G. Optic nerve
2. Structures of the anterior neck (page 1679, Figure 33-8)
   - A. Thyroid cartilage
   - B. Cricoid cartilage
   - C. Cricothyroid membrane
   - D. Trachea
   - E. Sternocleidomastoid muscle
   - F. Carotid arteries
3. Arteries of the neck (page 1679, Figure 33-9)
   - A. Internal carotid
   - B. Carotid sinus
   - C. Vertebral
   - D. Subclavian
   - E. Facial
   - F. External carotid
   - G. Superior thyroid
   - H. Common carotid
   - I. Brachiocephalic

Fill in the Blank

1. whiplash (page 1704)
2. strain (page 1704)
3. blowout (page 1677)
4. drainage; bloody (page 1682)
5. lymph (page 1682)
6. horizontal; hard palate (page 1684)
7. nasal; cerebrospinal fluid (CSF) (page 1685)
8. inner ear (page 1708)
9. airway (page 1687)
10. hyphema (page 1689)
11. Chemicals; heat; light (page 1691)
12. 20 (page 1694)
13. chemical burn (page 1696)
14. 1 (page 1699)
15. occlusive (page 1701)
16. light; adnexa (page 1691)
17. blood (page 1698)
18. sympathetic eye movement (page 1693)
19. pressure (page 1694)
20. craniofacial disjunction (page 1684)

Identify

1. Chief complaint: A head injury and severe facial injuries caused by the rollover and the patient's ejection from the vehicle.
2. Vital signs: The patient presents with decerebrate posturing and unresponsiveness; Glasgow Coma Scale (GCS) score is 8; respirations are 34 breaths/min and deep; oxygen saturation is 95%; pupils are sluggish; blood pressure (BP) is 160/90 mm/Hg; pulse is 72 beats/min; and skin is cool.
3. Pertinent negatives: No outward bleeding aside from the face.
4. This patient has an obvious head injury. A trauma center will have a neurosurgeon on hand to treat her. A community hospital would only be able to try to stabilize her and then ship her to a trauma center. This patient does not have that much time. The Golden Hour rule states that this patient needs surgery within an hour of the incident.
5. The patient has severe facial fractures, and the blood in her airway can easily be vomited or aspirated. Thus, the airway must be positioned properly (jaw thrust) and suctioned to remain clear.
6. The rising BP; slowing heart rate; and deep, fast respirations are the elements of the classic Cushing triad, which indicates a rising intracranial pressure.

Ambulance Calls

1. If you are able to salvage this young woman's lost tooth, you will have made a friend for life.
   a. Locate the tooth.
   b. Handle the tooth by the crown only. Do not touch the root surface of the tooth.
   c. Rinse the tooth and the empty socket with sterile saline or water (do not allow it to dry).
   d. Carefully place the tooth back in the socket.
   e. Once the tooth is in place, have the patient gently bite down on a gauze roll to maintain pressure against the tooth. (pages 1698–1699)
2. A thorough examination of an injured eye includes assessment of:
   a. The orbital rim for ecchymosis, swelling, laceration, and tenderness
   b. The eyelids for ecchymosis, swelling, and lacerations
   c. The corneas for foreign bodies
   d. The conjunctivae for redness, foreign bodies, inflammation, and pus
   e. The globes for redness, abnormal pigmentation, and lacerations

f. The pupils for size, shape, equality, and reaction to light (PERRLA)
g. Eye movements in all directions, for evidence of paralysis of gaze or no coordination between the movements of the two eyes
h. Most important, visual acuity (pages 1692–1693)

3. a. The principal dangers associated with a laceration of the neck are massive hemorrhage from major blood vessel disruption, airway compromise secondary to soft-tissue swelling, or direct damage to the larynx or trachea. Fatal air embolism is also considered a special danger.
   b. Open neck wounds should be sealed with an occlusive dressing immediately. (pages 1699–1701)

True/False

1. F (page 1677)
2. T (page 1690)
3. F (page 1691)
4. T (page 1692)
5. F (page 1697)
6. T (page 1684)
7. F (page 1684)
8. T (page 1685)
9. F (page 1699)
10. T (page 1684)
11. F (page 1686)
12. T (page 1690)
13. F (page 1693)
14. T (page 1700)
15. T (page 1698)
16. T (page 1701)
17. F (page 1702)
18. T (page 1702)
19. T (page 1697)
20. F (page 1698)

Short Answer

1. a. Closed head injury
   b. Cervical spine injury (page 1683)
2. *Students should provide five of the following:*
   a. Swelling of the face
   b. Ecchymosis over the face
   c. Crepitus over a broken bone
   d. Pain to palpation
   e. Instability of the facial bones
   f. Impaired ocular movement
   g. Malocclusion in cases where the jaw is fractured
   h. Visual disturbances
   i. Obvious deformity of the face (eg, flattening of one side) (page 1684)

Fill in the Table

1. Summary of maxillofacial fractures (Table 33-1, page 1686)

Injury	Signs and Symptoms
Multiple facial bone fractures	• Massive facial swelling • **Dental malocclusion** • **Palpable deformities** • Anterior or **posterior** epistaxis
Zygomatic and orbital fractures	• Loss of sensation below the **orbit** • Flattening of the **patient's cheek** • **Paralysis** of upward gaze
Nasal fractures	• Crepitus and instability • Swelling, tenderness, **lateral displacement** • Anterior or **posterior** epistaxis
Maxillary (Le Fort) fractures	• Mobility of the **midface** • Dental **malocclusion** • Facial swelling
Mandibular fractures	• Dental malocclusion • **Mandibular** instability

2. Signs and symptoms of injuries to the anterior part of the neck (Table 33-4, page 1702)

Injury	Signs and Symptoms
Laryngeal fracture, tracheal transection	• Labored breathing or reduced **air movement** • Stridor • Hoarseness, voice changes • **Hemoptysis** (coughing up blood) • Subcutaneous emphysema • Swelling, edema • Structural irregularity
Vascular injury	• **Gross external** bleeding • Signs of shock • Hematoma, swelling, edema • **Pulse** deficits
Esophageal perforation	• **Dysphagia** (difficulty swallowing) • **Hematemesis** • **Hemoptysis** (suggests aspiration of blood)
Neurologic impairment	• Signs of a stroke (suggests air embolism or **cerebral infarct**) • **Paralysis** or paresthesia • **Cranial** nerve deficit • Signs of **neurogenic** shock

Chapter 34: Head and Spine Trauma

Matching

Part I

1. H (page 1714)
2. G (page 1730)
3. F (page 1742)
4. E (page 1737)
5. D (page 1773)
6. Y (page 1728)
7. X (page 1714)
8. W (page 1713)
9. V (page 1722)
10. U (page 1722)
11. C (page 1716)
12. B (page 1739)
13. A (page 1751)
14. K (page 1716)
15. J (page 1728)
16. I (page 1727)
17. T (page 1714)
18. S (page 1742)
19. R (page 1738)
20. Q (page 1716)
21. L (page 1751)
22. M (page 1718)
23. N (page 1751)
24. O (page 1751)
25. P (page 1728)

Part II

1. P (page 1742)
2. O (page 1748)
3. N (page 1748)
4. M (page 1742)
5. L (page 1716)
6. E (page 1738)
7. D (page 1737)
8. C (page 1713)
9. B (page 1714)
10. A (page 1750)
11. Z (page 1745)
12. Y (page 1751)
13. X (page 1746)
14. W (page 1750)
15. V (page 1730)
16. K (page 1738)
17. J (page 1742)
18. I (page 1726)
19. H (pages 1723, 1734)
20. G (page 1738)
21. U (pages 1722, 1738)
22. T (page 1713)
23. S (page 1713)
24. R (page 1749)
25. Q (page 1714)
26. F (page 1738)

Part III (pages 1742–1746)

1. C
2. A
3. B
4. D
5. C
6. C
7. A
8. B
9. E
10. F

Multiple Choice

1. D (page 1734)
2. C (page 1738)
3. B (page 1736)
4. B (page 1736)
5. D (page 1716)
6. C (page 1735)
7. D (page 1737)
8. B (page 1739)
9. B (page 1745)
10. C (pages 1724–1725)
11. D (page 1741)
12. A (page 1721)
13. B (page 1717)
14. C (page 1718)
15. A (page 1718)
16. B (page 1720)
17. A (page 1720)
18. C (page 1754)
19. D (pages 1759–1760)
20. A (page 1763)
21. B (pages 1771–1772)
22. D (page 1731)

Labeling

1. Structures of the cervical, thoracic, and lumbar spine (page 1719, Figure 34-8)
   - **A.** Cervical plexus (C1–C5): Innervates the diaphragm
   - **B.** Brachial plexus (C5–T1): Controls the upper extremities
   - **C.** Lumbar plexus (L1–L4): Supplies the skin and muscles of the abdominal wall, external genitalia, and part of the lower limbs
   - **D.** Sacral plexus (L4–S4): Supplies the buttocks, perineum, and most of the lower limbs
2. The meninges (page 1716, Figure 34-7)
   - **A.** Skin
   - **B.** Fascia
   - **C.** Muscle
   - **D.** Bone of skull
   - **E.** Dura mater
   - **F.** Arachnoid
   - **G.** Cerebrospinal fluid
   - **H.** Blood vessel
   - **I.** Pia mater

3. Major regions of the brain (page 1715, Figure 34-4)
   A. Hypothalamus
   B. Thalamus
   C. Meninges
   D. Corpus callosum
   E. Skull
   F. Spinal cord
   G. Medulla
   H. Pons
   I. Midbrain

Fill in the Blank

1. vertebral (page 1717)
2. lamina, pedicles (page 1717)
3. cerebrum (page 1714)
4. pons; medulla (page 1716)
5. arachnoid (page 1716)
6. coup-contrecoup (page 1714)
7. hypertension; Cushing triad (page 1738)
8. epidural (page 1742)
9. rapid sequence intubation (page 1721)
10. body temperature (page 1746)
11. lamina; pedicles (page 1717)
12. C1; C2 (page 1748)
13. brain; spinal cord (page 1712)
14. medulla; pons; midbrain (page 1716)
15. foramen magnum (page 1718)
16. peripheral (page 1717)
17. Complete (page 1750)
18. neurogenic shock (page 1752)
19. spinal; cauda (page 1718)
20. downward; upward (page 1730)

Identify

Part I

1. Chief complaint: A head injury caused by the rollover and striking the windshield of the vehicle.
2. Vital signs: Patient presents with decerebrate posturing and unresponsiveness; GCS score is 7; respirations are 34 breaths/min and deep; oxygen saturation is 98%; pupils are sluggish; blood pressure (BP) is 160/90 mm/Hg; pulse is 64 beats/min; and skin is cool.
3. Pertinent negatives: No major outward bleeding, just some minor head lacerations
4. This patient has an obvious head injury. A trauma center will have a neurosurgeon on hand to treat her. A community hospital would only be able to try to stabilize her and then ship her to a trauma center. She does not have that much time. The Golden Hour rule states that this patient needs surgery within an hour of the incident.
5. The patient shows decerebrate posturing, which indicates that she already has swelling or bleeding inside the brain. The pressure is already building on the middle brainstem.
6. The rising BP; slowing heart rate; and deep, fast respirations are components of the Cushing triad, which indicates a rising ICP.

Part II

1. Chief complaint: Multiple trauma
2. Vital signs: Patient is V on the AVPU scale, GCS score is 9, skin is cool, BP is 100/62 mm Hg, pulse is 124 beats/min with sinus tachycardia, oxygen saturation is 96%, respirations are 26 breaths/min.

3. Pertinent negatives: Lungs are clear; no feeling or response in lower extremities.

The chief complaint in this case study is multiple trauma caused by a rollover crash. The patient is responding to voice and can answer only what her name is. Thus, you can call her a V on the AVPU scale and assign a score close to 9 on the GCS because of the inability to move her legs. The patient is hypothermic by touch. BP is 100/62 mm Hg, and pulse is 124 beats/min with sinus tachycardia on the monitor. Oxygen saturation is 96% but comes up to 98% with 100% oxygen. The breathing rate is 26 breaths/min and shallow. Lungs are clear. The absence of a pulse in either foot could be caused by the hypothermia. The patient has no feeling or response in her lower extremities. BP comes up slightly with a warm fluid bolus, which also helps to warm her. The second BP measurement is 108/64 mm Hg. You did your job by stabilizing the patient and securing her neck and body to the backboard. The physician later tells you the break was very bad, and there was nothing else you could have done to help her.

Complete the Patient Care Report (PCR)

Show the completed PCR to your instructor to obtain feedback on your completion of the form.

Ambulance Calls

1. a. The bad guy probably has a severe injury to the larynx, such as a laryngeal "fracture," as evidenced by the bruise over his throat, his hoarseness, and his subcutaneous emphysema. Furthermore, given the MOI, one has to assume that he has a cervical spine injury as well.
   b. The steps of treatment are as follows:
      (1) Administer 100% oxygen, and instruct the patient to breathe slowly (rapid inhalation may cause an unstable trachea to collapse inward). It is preferable to avoid intubating the patient in the field, but if the airway becomes compromised further, you may have no choice.
      (2) Immobilize the spine by immobilizing the whole patient on a long backboard.
      (3) Transport the patient immediately, preferably to a major trauma center.
2. a. This patient has a sensory level around T8 and intact motor function at least from T1 upward. You can assume that his injury is no higher than T8.
   b. His hypotension could mean either neurogenic shock or hypovolemic shock. It is very difficult, if not impossible, to distinguish between the two under these circumstances because if the sympathetic nervous system has been disrupted by the spinal cord injury, you will not see the usual signs of shock, such as sweating and tachycardia. Furthermore, the patient's sensory deficit may mask pain from damage to intra-abdominal structures. When you encounter shock in such circumstances, you have to treat it as hypovolemic shock until proven otherwise.
3. In this question about a patient with a head injury, you had to review some respiratory physiology along with the pathophysiology of head injury.
   a. If the patient's respiratory rate is 8 breaths/min and his tidal volume is 500 mL, his minute volume is calculated as follows:

$$\begin{aligned}\text{Minute volume} &= \text{Tidal volume} \times \text{Respiratory rate}\\ &= 500 \text{ mL/breath} \times 8 \text{ breaths/min}\\ &= 4{,}000 \text{ mL/min (4 L/min)}\end{aligned}$$

   b. The minute volume is less than normal. (Normal is around 6 L/min.)
   c. Therefore, you can conclude that the patient's arterial P_{CO_2} will tend to **increase**, so his pH will **decrease**. The net effect will be an acid–base disorder called a **respiratory acidosis**. The way you can help correct that abnormality is to **assist the patient's ventilations and thereby increase his minute volume (which will blow off more carbon dioxide)**.
   d. The signs of increasing ICP include the following (*students should provide five of the following*):
      (1) Vomiting
      (2) Headache
      (3) Altered level of consciousness
      (4) Seizures
      (5) Hypertension with a widening pulse pressure
      (6) Bradycardia
      (7) Irregular respirations
      (8) Unequal and nonreactive pupil
      (9) Coma
      (10) Posturing (page 1728)

- **e.** (1) The patient's AVPU rating is P (responds only to painful stimuli).
  (2) His score on the GCS is 8 points. (pages 1724–1725)

4. It should be clear, after carrying out this exercise, that the GCS enables a much more precise description than does the AVPU rating of the patient's level of consciousness. (pages 1724–1725)

- **a.** AVPU: somewhere between V and P
  GCS: 10
- **b.** AVPU: V
  GCS: 13
- **c.** AVPU: somewhere between P and U
  GCS: 5
- **d.** AVPU: A
  GSC: 15

5. In treating the victim of the whiskey bottle, how well did you remember your priorities?

- **a.** Eliminate the safety hazard. So long as there are tables and chairs being launched into orbit, you and everyone else in the bar are in danger. Try to get all bystanders to leave the premises (call in police help if needed). The first priority is to ensure scene safety and then, from a safe distance, to see if you can calm the patient. Explain that you are paramedics and that you have come to help him. Such an explanation is often of particular importance in municipalities where paramedics wear uniforms that could be mistaken for police uniforms (a very dangerous practice!).
- **b.** When you are reasonably certain that it is safe to approach the patient, encourage him to sit down, and examine his scalp by palpating the scalp wound lightly with a gloved finger to make certain that the skull beneath the wound is not fractured.
- **c.** If there is no evidence of skull fracture, control scalp bleeding by direct manual pressure, and apply a pressure dressing.
- **d.** Complete the secondary assessment, and manage any other injuries detected thereby.

True/False

1. F (page 1713)
2. T (page 1722)
3. F (page 1716)
4. T (page 1722)
5. T (page 1714)
6. F (page 1719)
7. T (page 1780)
8. T (page 1720)
9. T (pages 1736–1737)
10. F (pages 1738–1739)
11. T (page 1745)
12. T (page 1716)
13. F (page 1718)
14. T (page 1719)
15. T (page 1748)
16. F (pages 1748–1749)
17. F (page 1751)
18. T (page 1718)
19. F (pages 1722–1723)
20. F (page 1729)
21. F (page 1758)
22. T (pages 1759–1762)
23. F (page 1763)
24. F (page 1721)

Short Answer

1. *Students should list eight of the following:*

- **a.** High-velocity crash (greater than 40 mph) with severe vehicle damage
- **b.** Unrestrained occupant of moderate- to high-speed motor vehicle crash
- **c.** Vehicular damage with compartmental intrusion (12 inches) into the patient's seating space
- **d.** Fall from three times the patient's height
- **e.** Penetrating trauma near the spine
- **f.** Ejection from a motor vehicle
- **g.** Motorcycle crash at greater than 20 mph with separation of driver from bike
- **h.** Diving injury
- **i.** Auto–pedestrian or auto–bicycle crash with impact greater than 5 mph
- **j.** Death of an occupant in the same passenger compartment
- **k.** Rollover crash (unrestrained) (page 1720)

Fill in the Table

1. Signs and symptoms of head trauma (Table 34-2, page 1720)

Lacerations, contusions, or **hematomas** to the scalp
Soft area or **depression** noted on palpation of the scalp
Visible skull **fractures** or **deformities**
Battle sign or **raccoon** eyes
CSF rhinorrhea or **otorrhea**
Traumatic Brain Injury
Pupillary abnormalities • **Unequal** pupil size • Sluggish or **nonreactive** pupils
A period of unresponsiveness
Confusion or disorientation
Repeatedly asks the same questions (perseveration)
Amnesia (**retrograde** and/or **anterograde**)
Combativeness or other abnormal behavior
Numbness or tingling in the **extremities**
Loss of sensation and/or motor function
Focal **neurologic** deficits
Seizures
Cushing triad: hypertension, **bradycardia**, and irregular or erratic respirations
Dizziness
Visual disturbances, blurred vision, or double vision (**diplopia**)
Seeing "stars" (flashes of light)
Nausea or vomiting
Posturing (**decorticate** and/or **decerebrate**)

2. Dermatomes (Table 34-6, page 1731)

Nerve Root	Anatomic Location	Nerve Root	Anatomic Location
C2	**Occipital protuberance**	T10	Umbilicus
C3	**Supraclavicular fossa**	L1	**Inguinal** line
C5	Lateral side of **antecubital fossa**	L2	Mid-anterior thigh
C6	Thumb and medial index finger (six-shooter)	L3	Medial aspect of the **knee**
C7	**Middle** finger	L5	**Dorsum of the foot**
C8	**Little** finger	S1–S3	Back of **leg**
T2	**Apex of axilla**	S4–S5	**Perianal** area
T4	**Nipple** line		

Chapter 35: Chest Trauma

Matching

Part I

1. K (page 1808)
2. J (page 1791)
3. I (page 1804)
4. H (page 1805)
5. G (page 1794)
6. A (page 1790)
7. B (page 1806)
8. C (page 1797)
9. D (page 1809)
10. E (page 1791)
11. X (page 1812)
12. Y (page 1809)
13. T (page 1813)
14. W (page 1788)
15. V (page 1800)
16. P (page 1807)
17. Q (page 1797)
18. R (page 1795)
19. F (page 1813)
20. U (page 1791)
21. O (page 1806)
22. N (page 1798)
23. M (page 1801)
24. L (page 1808)
25. S (page 1798)

Part II

1. D (page 1805)
2. C (page 1801)
3. A (pages 1797–1798)
4. B (pages 1798–1799)
5. E (pages 1805–1806)

Multiple Choice

1. A (pages 1794–1796)
2. C (page 1798)
3. B (page 1806)
4. C (page 1791)
5. D (page 1807)
6. A (page 1788)
7. B (page 1810)
8. C (page 1799)
9. B (page 1801)
10. D (page 1801)

Labeling

1. The thorax (page 1789, Figure 35-2)
   - **A.** Thoracic inlet
   - **B.** Clavicle
   - **C.** Pericardium
   - **D.** Suprasternal notch
   - **E.** Manubrium
   - **F.** Angle of Louis
   - **G.** Body of sternum
   - **H.** Xiphoid process
   - **I.** Heart
   - **J.** Lung
   - **K.** Pleura
   - **L.** Diaphragm
   - **M.** Scapula
   - **N.** Ribs
   - **O.** Intercostal space

Fill in the Table

1. The MOIs, or easily detected injuries, may give clues to the presence of injuries that are harder to find.

If you find:	The patient may have:
1. Steering wheel imprint on anterior chest	**Myocardial contusion** (page 1808) **Cardiac tamponade** (pages 1806–1807) **Aortic rupture** (page 1810) **Pneumothorax or hemothorax** (pages 1797–1805) **Tracheobronchial injury** (page 1812)
2. Caved-in door on driver's side	**Diaphragmatic tear** (page 1811)
3. Fall from a height	**Thoracic aortic dissection/transection** (1809-1810) **Pulmonary contusion** (pages 1805–1806)
4. Bullet entrance wound in fifth left intercostal space	**Cardiac tamponade** (pages 1806–1807) **Injury to liver, spleen, stomach, lungs (look for exit wound)**
5. Fracture of ribs 5 to 7 in a young man	**Pulmonary contusion** (pages 1805–1806) **Pneumothorax and/or hemothorax** (pages 1797–1805)
6. Fracture of first and second ribs	**Major vascular injury** (pages 1809–1810) **Hemothorax** (pages 1804–1805)

Identify

1. a. Chief complaint: Patient's chest hurts.
   b. Physical findings: Patient is verbal and has bruising on the lower chest, diaphoresis, cyanosis dyspnea, equal bilateral breath sounds, tachycardia, weak peripheral pulses, hypotension, and electrical alternans.
   c. Signs of Beck triad: Muffled heart tones, hypotension, and jugular vein distention
   d. The patient most likely has pericardial (cardiac) tamponade. (pages 1806–1807)
2. a. Physical findings: Crackles, vital signs are within normal limits, an ECG shows ischemic changes, and no other signs of hypovolemia.
   b. Spalding effect: You believe that the pressure waves generated by the blunt trauma disrupted the capillary–alveolar membrane.
   c. Inertial effects: The tissues accelerated and decelerated at different rates, causing a tear.
   d. Implosion: The pressure created by the trauma compressed the gases within the lung.
   e. Do not run the IV infusion wide open. If the MOI suggests pulmonary contusion, be stingy with IV fluids unless the patient shows signs of shock. (pages 1795–1796)

Ambulance Calls

1. In this case, the young woman suffered unspecified deceleration injuries serious enough to render her unresponsive. The damage to the car—a caved-in dashboard and smashed windshield—also hints at significant head and chest injury. (pages 1808–1810)
   a. The major threats to this woman's airway are the following:
      (1) Her tongue, which is liable to fall back against her posterior pharynx
      (2) Blood or broken teeth in her mouth
      (3) Vomitus
      (4) Possible injury to the airway (eg, ruptured larynx)
   b. In assessing the adequacy of her breathing, you must
      (1) LOOK for:
         (a) Signs of respiratory embarrassment (nasal flaring, intercostal or supraclavicular retractions)
         (b) Tracheal deviation
         (c) Obvious bruises or open wounds of the chest
         (d) Paradoxical movement of any part of the chest
      (2) LISTEN for:
         (a) Sucking chest wound
         (b) Inequality of breath sounds
         (c) Dullness or hyperresonance to percussion

(3) FEEL for:
(a) Tracheal deviation
(b) Subcutaneous emphysema
(c) Instability of the rib cage

c. The steps that need to be taken immediately to ensure adequate breathing are as follows:
(1) Suction out the mouth as needed.
(2) Administer 100% supplemental oxygen.

d. To evaluate and manage the circulation during the primary survey, you must do the following:
(1) Identify and control significant external bleeding.
(2) Check the pulse (quality, rate, regularity, presence of paradoxus).
(3) Note the skin CTC (ie, color, temperature, condition).
(4) Check capillary refill if this is pediatric patient.
(5) Assess neck veins for distention.

2. a. The patient who has a shotgun wound to the chest in a "friendly" encounter has an open pneumothorax (answer 3) —indeed, a quite significant one (a 2-inch hole would be hard not to notice!). The wound inflicted by a shotgun at close range is essentially a blast injury, so you would also expect to find a considerable amount of damage to the lung tissue beneath, probably accompanied by disruption of major blood vessels. (pages 1798–1799)

b. The steps in managing this patient are the following:
(1) Make certain that the "friend" with the shotgun has left the scene or has been "neutralized" by police.
(2) Seal the open chest wound with an occlusive dressing as quickly as possible. Tape the dressing on three sides only, so that air can escape from it during exhalation.
(3) Administer 100% supplemental oxygen, preferably by nonrebreathing mask. Try to avoid giving oxygen under positive pressure.
(4) Start transport.
(5) Start an IV line en route, with lactated Ringer solution.

3. The elderly woman struck by a car has very well-localized pain over the fifth right rib as well as diminished breath sounds and hyperresonance on that side of the chest. (pages 1796–1799)

a. This patient probably has a rib fracture together with a simple pneumothorax on the right.

b. The principal danger associated with rib fracture is the development of atelectasis because of the patient's reluctance to breathe deeply. Atelectasis, in turn, predisposes the patient to develop pneumonia.

c. The treatment necessary in the field is as follows:
(1) Administer 100% supplemental oxygen by nonrebreathing mask.
(2) Encourage the patient to take periodic deep breaths; have her splint the fractured rib against a pillow each time she does so.
(3) Given the MOI, it would be a good idea to immobilize the patient's spine.

d. (1) If a patient becomes suddenly shows signs of shock, while at the same time showing signs of increased venous pressure (neck veins distended), she has probably developed a tension pneumothorax. (pages 1800–1804)
(2) If you are more than 2 to 3 minutes from the hospital when that happens, stop the vehicle, and decompress the patient's chest with a needle.

4. The primary survey revealed to you that the man ejected from his convertible has a partially obstructed airway, is bleeding, and is in shock and therefore is critically injured. In fact, that is all you need to know to start appropriate treatment. Although the following steps of treatment are listed in sequence, you will, in practice, have to accomplish the first few steps almost simultaneously. (pages 1793–1794)

a. Open the patient's airway with the jaw-thrust maneuver. As soon as the equipment to do so is available, suction out the mouth and pharynx.

b. With the hand that is maintaining the jaw thrust, seal off the bleeding wound of the neck. Apply a pressure dressing as soon as possible. Then, apply a pressure dressing to the scalp wound.

c. Administer 100% supplemental oxygen as soon as it is available.

d. Immobilize the spine.

e. Start transport.

f. Start at least one large-bore IV line en route. Run it wide open.

g. Monitor cardiac rhythm.

5. The clues to this patient's tension pneumothorax are the signs of shock in the face (jugular vein distention) and decreased breath sounds on one side. (pages 1800–1804)
   a. Steps to take at the scene:
      (1) Administer supplemental oxygen.
      (2) Decompress the chest with a cannula in the second right intercostal space, midclavicular line.
      (3) Immobilize the patient on a long backboard.
      (4) Communicate with medical control or the receiving hospital.
   b. Steps to be taken en route:
      (1) Perform a detailed secondary assessment.
      (2) Start a large-bore IV line with fluids.
      (3) Recheck vital and neurologic signs every 5 minutes.
6. Assessment (pages 1801–1804)
   a. Mental status (AVPU)
   b. Airway while providing manual stabilization
      (1) Check for obstructions.
   c. Breathing
      (1) Look for abnormal respirations.
      (2) Palpate the chest (note evidence of instability, crepitus, or subcutaneous emphysema).
      (3) Look for jugular vein distention.
      (4) Auscultate lung sounds (note absent or decreased breath sounds).
      (5) Observe for signs and symptoms of hypoxia.
      (6) Check for signs of hypocapnia.
   d. Circulation
      (1) Examine for external bleeding.
      (2) Obtain a complete set of vital signs and oxygen saturation.
      (3) Look at and feel the skin.
   e. Disability
      (1) Check extremities for pulses.
   f. History taking and secondary assessment (depending on the severity of the patient)
      (1) SAMPLE history
   g. Detailed secondary assessment with head-to-toe exam

   Management (pages 1801–1804)
      a. Ensure the airway is maintained.
      b. Provide oxygen (consider the need for ventilatory assistance and endotracheal [ET] intubation).
      c. Consider the need for a needle decompression.
      d. Control any external bleeding.
      e. Take frequent vital signs.
      f. Attach the patient to a pulse oximeter and capnography if intubated.
      g. Monitor ECG.
      h. Complete cervical spine immobilization before beginning transport.
7. In working out the answers to this question, you may have noticed that the mechanisms and signs of various chest injuries are very similar to one another. If it is difficult to distinguish such injuries in the relative calm and quiet of your study, consider how difficult it will be at midnight in a ditch by the side of the interstate highway in the pouring rain—which is where you will inevitably be making such determinations.
   a. D. This patient's distended neck veins tell you that something is increasing pressure on the venae cavae. The two most likely possibilities are air in the pleural space or blood in the pericardium. Because the breath sounds are equal, the best bet is cardiac tamponade, and the apparent pulsus paradoxus supports that diagnosis. Under ideal conditions, you might also be able to appreciate that the heart sounds are muffled, but conditions in the field are seldom ideal, and even evaluating breath sounds is usually quite challenging. Steps of management:
      (1) Provide oxygen.
      (2) Start transport.
      (3) Monitor cardiac rhythm.
      (4) Start an IV line with lactated Ringer solution or normal saline en route. (page 1807)

b. E. This is the classic picture of traumatic asphyxia, the so-called bloated frog appearance, and it bespeaks massive, often-fatal chest injury. Steps of management:
  (1) Provide cervical spine precautions.
  (2) Establish an airway. Don't take time at the scene to perform endotracheal intubation unless absolutely necessary.
  (3) Administer 100% supplemental oxygen.
  (4) Start transport.
  (5) Start at least one IV line en route. (pages 1812–1813)

c. C. If a patient has three ribs broken in two places, it's a good bet he's got a flail chest. You may not actually be able to see the paradoxical movement of the chest, especially if the patient is conscious and splinting the injured part of the chest (which he will do automatically, to reduce the pain that breathing causes). Even so, the nature of the injury tells you that there probably is a flail, and the asymmetry of chest movements supports this hypothesis. Steps of management:
  (1) Administer 100% supplemental oxygen by nonrebreathing mask. Be prepared to intubate and provide positive pressure ventilation.
  (2) Splint the flail segment by having the patient hold a pillow against it or by taping the unstable segment to the adjacent stable segment.
  (3) Encourage the patient to take deep breaths. If he is unable to do so, assist ventilations gently with a bag-mask device. Be alert for pneumothorax.
  (4) Start transport.
  (5) Monitor cardiac rhythm.
  (6) Start an IV lifeline en route, at a keep-open rate. (pages 1794–1796)

d. A. Here again, distended neck veins point to a process that is increasing intrathoracic pressure or otherwise preventing venous return to the heart. The decrease in breath sounds on the right side tells you that the problem is in the right chest, and the hyperresonance argues for a tension pneumothorax there. Steps of management:
  (1) Administer 100% supplemental oxygen by nonrebreathing mask.
  (2) Obtain orders from medical control as required by protocols.
  (3) Identify the second right intercostal space in the midclavicular line.
  (4) Prep the point you have identified (with povidone-iodine).
  (5) Use a 14-gauge long (3.25 inches if possible, for an adult) angiocatheter, or whatever other 14-gauge needle is at hand, to pop through into the pleural space and vent the pneumothorax. Secure the catheter or needle in place. Use a flutter valve if possible.
  (6) Immobilize the spine.
  (7) Start transport.
  (8) Start an IV line en route. (pages 1800–1804)

e. B. Like the patients with cardiac tamponade and tension pneumothorax, this patient with massive hemothorax is showing signs of shock (cold, sweaty skin; rapid, weak pulse). In contrast to those patients, however, his venous pressure is low (neck veins not distended), which should make you suspect hypovolemia. The decreased breath sounds in the left chest indicate that something is going on there, and the dullness to percussion suggests that fluid (blood) has taken the place of air in that side of the chest. It all adds up to massive bleeding within the chest. (Given the location of the stab wound, it is not unreasonable to consider the possibility of myocardial trauma and pericardial tamponade as well.) Steps of management:
  (1) Administer 100% supplemental oxygen.
  (2) Start transport.
  (3) Start two large-bore IV lines en route. (pages 1804–1805)

True/False

1. T (page 1788)
2. T (page 1812)
3. F (page 1806)
4. T (page 1809)
5. T (page 1790)
6. T (page 1811)
7. F (page 1812)
8. F (page 1801)
9. T (page 1801)
10. T (page 1801)

Short Answer

What you need to remember to answer this question correctly is that any injury below the nipples is both an abdominal injury and a chest injury. The bullet apparently took a straight line through the right upper quadrant (RUQ), and it could be expected to have hit the liver, kidney, and perhaps part of the lung. (pages 1788–1790)

Chapter 36: Abdominal and Genitourinary Trauma

Matching

Part I

1. L (page 1831)
2. J (page 1821)
3. K (page 1831)
4. A (page 1830)
5. B (pages 1830–1831)
6. C (page 1829)
7. D (page 1833)
8. E (page 1830)
9. I (page 1821)
10. H (page 1824)
11. F (page 1821)
12. G (page 1824)

Part II

1. C (page 1833)
2. B (page 1833)
3. B (page 1833)
4. D (pages 1835–1836)
5. D (pages 1835–1836)
6. F (page 1830)
7. G (page 1832)
8. B (page 1833)
9. A (page 1833)
10. B (page 1833)

Multiple Choice

1. D (pages 1829–1831)
2. D (page 1835)
3. C (page 1821)
4. C (page 1824)
5. D (page 1833)
6. C (page 1832)
7. D (page 1834)
8. D (pages 1824–1825)
9. A (page 1829)
10. D (pages 1828–1829)

Labeling

1. Organs in the peritoneum (page 1822, Figure 36-2A)
   - A. Liver
   - B. Peritoneum
   - C. Ascending colon
   - D. Diaphragm
   - E. Stomach
   - F. Spleen
   - G. Transverse colon
2. Organs in the retroperitoneal space (page 1822, Figure 36-2B)
   - A. Vena cava
   - B. Duodenum
   - C. Kidney
   - D. Ureters
   - E. Aorta
   - F. Pancreas
   - G. Kidney
   - H. Descending colon
3. Organs in the pelvis (page 1822, Figure 36-2C)
   - A. Iliac vessels
   - B. Uterus
   - C. Rectum
   - D. Sigmoid colon
   - E. Bladder

Fill in the Blank

1. evisceration; abdominal (page 1832)
2. Grey Turner sign (page 1831)
3. Cullen sign (page 1831)
4. diaphragm; compromise (page 1833)
5. pancreas; retroperitoneum (page 1834)
6. hollow (page 1822)
7. penetrating; blunt (page 1834)
8. peritonitis (page 1824)

Identify

1. a. Chief complaint: Patient denies any complaint. Emergency medical services (EMS) was called by police for a possible stab wound.
   b. Vital signs: Pulse is 120 beats/min and regular; skin is ashen, cool, and diaphoretic; oxygen saturation is 90%; BP is 86/60 mm Hg; and sinus tachycardia appears on the ECG.
   c. Pertinent negatives: Patient denies chest pain or other injuries.
2. a. Chief complaint: Evisceration, abdominal trauma
   b. Vital signs: Pulse is 100 beats/min and irregular; skin is pale, warm, and dry; oxygen saturation is 97% on room air; BP is 160/90 mm Hg.
   c. Pertinent negatives: Patient currently denies chest pain.

Ambulance Calls

1. The evaluation of a patient who has abdominal trauma must be systematic, keeping the entire patient in mind and prioritizing injuries accordingly. (pages 1828–1831)
   a. The MOI, including damage to the vehicle and type of seat belt worn (if any) if the patient is the victim of a motor vehicle crash
   b. The patient's complaints referable to the abdomen—specifically, complaints of nausea, vomiting, hematemesis, or abdominal pain
   c. External signs of abdominal injury, such as abrasions, contusion, seat belt marks, lacerations, or evisceration
   d. Tenderness or rigidity to palpation
2. The case of evisceration described in this question is based on an actual case.

   Injuries:
   a. Bruise over the right lower ribs
   b. Small bowel evisceration
   c. Avulsion in the right side of the abdomen
   d. Fractured right elbow

   The published case report does not record which care was given at the scene, but the care that should have been given at the scene is based on the fact that this patient is in shock.

   Priorities:
   a. Administer 100% oxygen.
   b. Anticipate vomiting, and have suction at hand.
   c. Assist ventilations with a bag-valve mask.
   d. Cover the eviscerated bowel with sterile dressings; use an occlusive dressing over the wet sterile dressings, or use sterile universal dressings that have been soaked in sterile saline. Cover the dressings, in turn, with a towel, to minimize heat loss across the wound.
   e. Immobilize the spine, taking care not to place any straps across the eviscerated bowel. Include the right arm within the straps, to hold the fractured elbow immobile.
   f. Start transport.
   g. Start two large-bore IV lines en route, and run in lactated Ringer's solution as rapidly as possible.
3. The principles of managing an impaled object in the abdomen are fundamentally the same as those for an impaled object anywhere else: Leave the impaled object in place. (page 1832)
   a. Administer oxygen.
   b. Stabilize the impaled object in place. Buttress it on all sides with universal dressings or with triangular bandages formed into "doughnut" rings. Then, tape the buttress material securely so that the knife cannot move in any direction.
   c. Start transport.
   d. Start an IV line en route.
   e. Discuss analgesia with medical control.

True/False

1. F (page 1824)
2. T (page 1837)
3. T (page 1831)
4. F (page 1832)
5. T (page 1829)
6. T (page 1829)
7. T (page 1831)
8. T (page 1836)
9. T (page 1836)
10. F (page 1837)

Fill in the Table

1. Organs of the abdomen and their location (page 1822)

Organ	Location
1. Liver	1. **Peritoneal cavity**
2. Spleen	2. **Peritoneal cavity**
3. Stomach	3. **Peritoneal cavity**
4. Duodenum	4. **Retroperitoneal space**
5. Kidney	5. **Retroperitoneal space**
6. Aorta	6. **Retroperitoneal space**
7. Uterus	7. **Pelvis**
8. Rectum	8. **Pelvis**
9. Bladder	9. **Pelvis**

Short Answer

1. a. kidneys (page 1825)
b. liver (page 1833)
c. bladder (page 1836)
d. liver (page 1833)

Chapter 37: Orthopaedic Trauma

Matching

Part I

1. U (page 1879)
2. T (page 1864)
3. S (page 1851)
4. R (page 1849)
5. Q (page 1864)
6. E (page 1847)
7. D (page 1878)
8. C (page 1845)
9. B (page 1848)
10. A (page 1854)
11. Z (page 1851)
12. Y (page 1851)
13. X (page 1863)
14. W (page 1850)
15. V (page 1865)
16. J (page 1849)
17. I (page 1867)
18. H (page 1845)
19. G (page 1850)
20. F (page 1867)
21. P (page 1849)
22. O (page 1848)
23. N (pagc 1879)
24. M (page 1850)
25. L (page 1879)
26. K (page 1863)

Part II

1. T (page 1849)
2. S (page 1868)
3. R (page 1871)
4. Q (page 1846)
5. P (page 1849)
6. J (page 1878)
7. I (page 1865)
8. H (page 1866)
9. G (page 1847)
10. F (page 1872)
11. E (page 1847)
12. D (page 1864)
13. C (page 1856)
14. B (page 1850)
15. A (page 1850)
16. Z (page 1875)
17. Y (page 1850)
18. X (page 1851)
19. W (page 1879)
20. V (page 1867)
21. O (page 1849)
22. N (page 1878)
23. M (page 1865)
24. L (page 1865)
25. K (page 1849)
26. U (page 1851)

Part III

1. R (page 1867)
2. Q (page 1878)
3. P (page 1864)
4. O (page 1851)
5. N (page 1865)
6. M (page 1879)
7. L (page 1854)
8. K (page 1845)
9. Z (page 1852)
10. Y (page 1869)
11. X (page 1851)
12. W (page 1849)
13. D (page 1848)
14. C (page 1869)
15. B (page 1875)
16. A (page 1849)
17. V (page 1868)
18. U (page 1867)
19. T (page 1878)
20. S (page 1849)
21. J (page 1845)
22. I (page 1849)
23. H (page 1854)
24. G (page 1850)
25. F (page 1846)
26. E (page 1878)

Part IV

1. H (page 1869)
2. A (page 1847)
3. B (page 1867)
4. F (page 1874)
5. D (page 1867)
6. E (page 1876)
7. G (page 1848)
8. C (page 1847)

Multiple Choice

1. B (page 1844)
2. D (page 1845)
3. B (page 1847)
4. A (page 1847)
5. D (page 1851)
6. D (page 1877)
7. B (pages 1852–1855)
8. D (page 1858)
9. A (page 1864)
10. B (page 1868)

Labeling

1. Types of fractures (page 1848, Figure 37-2)
   - **A.** Transverse fracture of the tibia
   - **B.** Oblique fracture of the humerus
   - **C.** Spiral fracture of the femur
   - **D.** Comminuted fracture of the tibia
   - **E.** Greenstick fracture of the fibula
   - **F.** Compression fracture of a vertebral body

Fill in the Blank

1. **a.** fascia (page 1864)
   - **b.** arthritis (page 1878)
   - **c.** glomerular filtration (page 1865)
   - **d.** scaphoid (page 1867)
   - **e.** boxer's (page 1867)

f. mallet (page 1867)
g. patella (page 1872)
h. Thompson (page 1877)
i. pectoral girdle (page 1884)

2. The signs and symptoms of a fracture are usually not terribly subtle:
   a. Unnatural shape: DEFORMITY (page 1848)
   b. Reduced length: SHORTENING (page 1850)
   c. Fracture of the small finger: BOXER'S FRACTURE (page 1867)
   d. Numbness and tingling: PARESTHESIAS (page 1854)
   e. Grating: CREPITUS (page 1851)
   f. Devastating consequence of musculoskeletal injuries: DISABILITY (page 1863)
   g. Protecting from movement: GUARDING (pages 1850–1851)
   h. Hurts to touch it: POINT TENDERNESS (page 1854)
   i. Patient with a fracture may report this: Heard a SNAP (page 1871)
   j. Seen in open fracture: EXPOSED BONE ENDS (page 1851)

Identify

1. a. Chief complaint: Right ankle pain; severe wrist pain. The patient denies loss of consciousness or head or neck pain. The patient denies any respiratory distress and any current chest discomfort. He denies any medical condition that may have caused him to fall. He adamantly states that he simply slipped on ice and fell.
   b. Vital signs: His baseline vital signs reveal a pulse of 116 beats/min and irregular, respirations of 16 breaths/min nonlabored, oxygen saturation on room air at 98%, and blood pressure (BP) of 150/90 mm Hg. ECG is rapid atrial fibrillation. PERRLA. Normal capillary refill of < 2 seconds. Skin color is normal, and skin is warm and dry.
   c. Pertinent negatives: By questioning the patient, you discover that he has a previous medical history of angina, atrial fibrillation, and hypertension. He also takes one 81-mg aspirin tablet per day and an antihypertensive medication.
2. a. Chief complaint: The patient tripped on a curb in the parking lot. She complains of bilateral wrist injuries and is found in extreme pain. You notice that both her wrists appear bruised and deformed.
   b. Vital signs: The patient's initial vital signs indicate she is conscious and alert. Her skin is slightly ashen and diaphoretic, and she has positive distal motor and neurologic sensations in both hands. She denies other injuries. Her capillary refill is > 2 seconds, and she has bilateral radial pulses that appear to be equal. Her BP is obtainable only by palpation at 86 mm Hg. Her oxygen saturation is 96% on ambient air. She denies taking any medications or having any allergies.
   c. Pertinent negatives: The patient denies loss of consciousness or head or neck pain. She denies any respiratory distress and any current chest discomfort. She denies any medical condition that may have caused her to fall.
3. a. Chief complaint: A farm mishap where a tractor rolled on top of and is pinning a 64-year-old man. The patient is unresponsive, with airway compromise.
   b. Vital signs: Patient is unresponsive, with a GCS < 8. He has delayed capillary refill and sinus tachycardia of 128 beats/min. His BP is 64 mm Hg by palpation.
   c. Pertinent negatives: There are no pertinent negatives indicated.

Complete the Patient Care Report (PCR)

Show the completed PCR to your instructor to obtain feedback on your completion of the form.

Ambulance Calls

1. The presence of some injuries may also give clues to the possible presence of other injuries that share the same mechanism of injury.
   a. The young man's calcaneal fracture mandates that you check for fracture of the other calcaneus as well as fracture of the lumbar vertebrae, especially around L1–L2. (page 1847)
   b. The 50-year-old woman in the head-on collision has the classic dashboard injury. The same forces that smashed up the knee may well have acted anywhere along the femur to cause a femoral fracture or to ram the femur backward, producing a fracture or dislocation of the hip. (page 1847)
   c. The 60-year-old man who fell sideways onto his outstretched hand probably has a scaphoid fracture, in which the forces are transmitted from the hand, along the radius and ulna, through the elbow, and up the humerus into the shoulder. Look for injuries anywhere along that axis—specifically, fracture of the distal radius/ulna, fracture/dislocation of the elbow, fracture of the shaft of the humerus, fracture/dislocation of the shoulder, or fracture of the clavicle. (page 1847)

d. The obvious fracture in the construction worker is the fracture of the scapula, which is a tip-off to the powerful forces involved in the injury. Thus, you need to start looking for rib fractures, vertebral fractures, and damage to underlying soft tissues (eg, pulmonary contusion, renal injury). (page 1847)

2. It's all well and good to memorize the signs and symptoms of musculoskeletal injuries, but what counts is whether you can recognize the injuries when you see them and whether you then take the appropriate action.

a. For the boy who fell off his skateboard: (page 1867)

(1) The most likely field diagnosis is a fractured elbow. If you want to be more exact, you could specify that it's a supracondylar fracture of the humerus, but probably it won't be possible (or necessary) in the field to know exactly what is broken and what isn't. The fact that the elbow is involved in a fracture is reason enough to feel a sense of urgency.

(2) Yes, there is a special danger in this case—the danger of the patient developing Volkmann ischemic contracture as a result of the blood supply to his forearm being jeopardized. He's already showing signs of a compromised blood supply (his hand is cool and pale), and the broken end of the humerus is probably pinching his radial nerve as well (he has a sensory loss in the distribution of the radial nerve). Those are danger signals!

(3) If this boy is to retain the use of his right hand, urgent measures must be taken to restore the blood supply to the area. Those measures are best taken by an expert—an orthopaedic surgeon—in the hospital. If you are close to the hospital, splint the elbow as you found it, and hit the road. Notify the hospital personnel of your ETA so that they can summon an "orthopod" (ie, orthopaedic surgeon) to be standing by in the emergency department (ED). If you are any distance from the hospital, however, contact medical command for orders; you may be instructed to apply traction along the axis of the humerus and straighten the elbow slightly, until the patient's hand "pinks up."

b. The boy's mother tripped over his skateboard in her haste to assist him (there's a lesson in that!). She's done something to her wrist. (pages 1867–1868)

(1) The most likely field diagnosis is a Colles fracture—that is, a fracture of the distal radius and ulna. The "dinner-fork deformity" is a classic sign of Colles fracture, as is the way the woman walked over to you, holding the injured wrist in her other hand and using her body as a splint.

(2) There is not ordinarily any special danger in a Colles fracture, although you must, as always, check the circulation and neurologic function distal to the injury, just to be certain.

(3) A padded aluminum ladder splint, bent into a right angle at the elbow and supported in a sling, is probably the most comfortable splint for this woman. Alternatively, you may use an air splint (provided it comes up over the elbow) or a padded board splint. In either of those two cases, transport the woman supine, with her splinted arm supported on a pillow, to elevate the injured part.

c. This case is another classic dashboard injury. (page 1876)

(1) The most likely diagnosis is posterior dislocation of the hip. That outcome is what one would expect given the mechanisms of injury (deceleration forces, femur driven backward), and the patient has characteristic signs: The affected hip is flexed, adducted, and internally rotated, and the leg appears shorter than the leg on the uninjured side.

(2) Yes, there is a particular danger associated with posterior hip dislocation—two dangers, in fact. The most feared complication is avascular necrosis of the head of the femur, which leads to total destruction of the hip joint. There is also the danger of damage to the sciatic nerve and consequent foot drop.

(3) The most important treatment for a dislocated hip is early reduction of the dislocation. If you are within 20 minutes or so of the hospital, the best thing to do is to immobilize the patient on a long backboard, generously padded with pillows, and transport immediately. If you are at a considerable distance from the hospital, contact medical control. If you are given instructions to do so, try once to reduce the dislocation.

d. The other patient from the same crash was the driver, found unresponsive. (pages 1868–1871)

(1) The most likely orthopaedic field diagnosis in this case is a fractured pelvis. In addition, this patient has some other very serious, even life-threatening injuries. Loss of consciousness in a patient with trauma means head injury until proven otherwise, and head injury in multitrauma means spinal cord injury until proven otherwise.

(2) Yes, indeed, there is a particular danger in this case—several, in fact. First, the patient is unresponsive, so his airway is in jeopardy. Second, he seems to be in shock, perhaps from blood loss related to his pelvic fracture but perhaps from blood loss elsewhere as well.

(3) After the scene size-up, conduct a primary survey on this patient. The steps in the primary survey involve obtaining a general impression and implementing the "MS-ABC Priority Plan" of searching for and managing life threats.

General impression: unresponsive male trauma patient.

MS: U—unresponsive to pain

A—Open the patient's airway (chin lift or jaw thrust); insert an oropharyngeal airway to help keep it open.

B—Determine whether the patient is breathing adequately; if not, assist his breathing with a bag-mask device. In any event, give supplementary oxygen.

C—Assess the circulation (pulse, capillary refill in children), and control external bleeding.

Priority: High

Given the patient's condition, you won't have time to do a lot more in the field than the following:

(a) Manage the ABCs.

(b) Secure the patient to the backboard or scoop.

(c) Start transport.

(d) En route, get a set of vital signs if you haven't done so already.

(e) Start at least one and preferably two large-bore IV lines, and run a 500-mL fluid challenge.

(f) Complete the secondary assessment and physical exam as best you can.

(g) Keep the patient warm.

e. Only when you get back to base does your partner mention how much his ankle is hurting. (page 1851)

(1) The most likely diagnosis is a sprained ankle, although you can't be 100% sure without an x-ray.

(2) There is no particular danger associated with a sprained ankle.

(3) The treatment is to immobilize the ankle (eg, air splint, pillow splint), apply a cold pack, elevate the ankle, and transport your partner to the ED to be checked over.

f. The high school quarterback who ended up under a pile of 225-pound linemen was subject to significant crushing forces. (pages 1874–1875)

(1) The most likely diagnosis is a posterior sternoclavicular dislocation.

(2) Yes, there is a particular danger in this case—namely, damage to critical underlying structures. In fact, there is already evidence that such damage has occurred: The boy says he is "choking," which is an indication of possible tracheal damage.

(3) The most important aspect of this boy's treatment will be expeditious transport to the hospital. Administer supplementary oxygen en route. If he is comfortable lying down, keep him supine, with his left arm abducted and a pillow or rolled towel under his left shoulder; that position may take the pressure off the trachea or whatever structures are being compressed by the proximal end of the clavicle.

g. The pedestrian received a direct blow to the shin. (page 1873)

(1) The most likely diagnosis is an open fracture of the tibia, probably a transverse fracture.

(2) Yes, there is a particular danger associated with tibial fracture—the development of compartment syndrome. Indeed, the patient's paresthesias suggest that there may already be pressure on the sensory nerves supplying the foot.

(3) To treat the patient in the field, apply manual traction to straighten out the angulation, and splint the limb (padded board splint, long-leg air splint). Keep the patient supine so that you can elevate the injured leg. Apply cold packs. Transport the patient without delay, and notify the receiving hospital to have an orthopaedic surgeon standing by.

h. In today's less-than-tranquil society, gunshot wounds are frequent sources of musculoskeletal trauma. (page 1872)

(1) The most likely diagnosis in this case is a fractured femur. The location of the wound and the shortening of the injured leg are the tip-offs.

(2) Yes, there is a particular danger in this case. Aside from the danger of shock that attends every femoral fracture, this patient apparently has some compromise to the distal circulation (the dorsalis pedis pulse is weak). There may also be a danger to you if the person who did the shooting is still wandering around with a loaded gun. Did you bother to check that possibility before you ran over to attend the patient?

(3) This case requires setting priorities:

(a) Administer supplemental oxygen.

(b) Cover the open wound(s) with sterile dressings.

(c) Immobilize the injured leg in a traction splint.

(d) Start transport.

(e) Start a large-bore IV line en route to the hospital.

(f) Keep rechecking the dorsalis pedis pulse. Document all your findings.

(4) The purposes of splinting in general are as follows:

(a) To relieve pain

(b) To prevent further injury

(c) To help control bleeding (page 1858)

i. The skier who ended up at the bottom of a pileup doubtless experienced a hyperextension injury of the leg. (pages 1876–1877)
   (1) The most likely diagnosis is dislocation of the knee (it may also be fractured).
   (2) Yes, there is a particular danger associated with that diagnosis—the danger of damage to the popliteal artery and consequent ischemic damage to the lower leg.
   (3) The treatment under these circumstances—where you are on the ski slopes, at some distance from a hospital—is to try once to reduce the dislocation, before muscle spasm makes it impossible to do so. Use a traction splint if you have one available. Otherwise, apply manual traction to the long axis of the leg. Then, get the patient to the hospital as quickly as possible, and notify the hospital in advance of your impending arrival.

3. a. When dealing with a severely injured patient, knowing what to do is not enough. You have to know what to do first, and what to do next, and what to do after that. If you remember the alphabet, you'll be in good shape.
   Step 15. Start an IV line.
   Step 9. Take the vital signs.
   Step 6. Cut away the trouser leg. (You will want to control the bleeding in the leg if it is excessive, which is part of step C, Circulation.)
   Step 3. Determine whether the patient is breathing (he is) (step B, Breathing).
   Step 13. Secure the patient to a backboard or scoop.
   Step 7. Put manual pressure on the bleeding site (part of step C, Circulation).
   Step 2. Open the airway (chin lift) (step A, Airway).
   Step 14. Start transport.
   Step 10. Move the patient to a backboard or scoop.
   Step 5. Check for a carotid pulse (pulse is present) (first part of step C, Circulation).
   Steps 11 and 12. Check for a dorsalis pedis pulse on the right. (You need to do this both before and after you have applied the splint.)
   Step 1. Do the AVPU "mental status" check (the "mental status" in the MS-ABC Priority Plan).
   Step 4. Check for an open or tension pneumothorax (part of checking the adequacy of breathing, step B).
   Step 8. Put a pressure dressing over the open wound on the leg. (In practice, you'll do this whenever the dressing material becomes available.)

   In actual practice, you will be carrying out some of the preceding steps very nearly simultaneously. While holding the airway open and observing the movements of the chest, for instance, you will also have a finger on the carotid pulse. But it is useful to consider the actions separately to review priorities.

b. At least one step has been omitted: The patient was not given supplemental oxygen!

4. An open fracture of the tibia is a serious injury with serious potential complications (such as compartment syndrome), but it does not pose an immediate threat to life, nor are there any signs so far of other injuries that do jeopardize the patient's life. (pages 1872–1873)

a. Steps to be taken in the field:
   (1) Conduct a rapid trauma assessment.
   (2) Cover the wound on the leg with a sterile dressing.
   (3) Straighten and splint the fractured leg.
   (4) Start a large-bore IV line (or could be done en route).

b. Steps to be taken en route:
   (1) Communicate with medical control or the receiving hospital.
   (2) Recheck the pulse and sensation distal to the fracture every 5 minutes.
   (3) Start a large-bore IV line (if not done yet).

True/False

1. T (page 1859)
2. T (page 1861)
3. T (page 1859)
4. T (page 1872)
5. T (page 1859)
6. T (page 1853)
7. T (page 1861)

Fill in the Table

1. (Table 37-4, page 1858)

Potential Blood Loss From Fracture Sites	
Fracture Site	**Potential Blood Loss (mL)**
Pelvis	**1,500-3,000**
Femur	**1,000-1,500**
Humerus	**250-500**
Tibia or fibula	**250-500**
Ankle	**250-500**
Elbow	**250-500**
Radius or ulna	**150-250**

Short Answer

1. Compartment syndrome may be heralded by any or several of the six Ps, which are symptoms and signs of an ischemic limb (page 1864):
   a. Pain—the earliest and most reliable sign
   b. Pallor
   c. Pulselessness
   d. Paresthesias
   e. Paresis or paralysis
   f. Pressure

2. In examining the patient injured on the ski slope, it's a good idea to start by eliciting his chief complaint. Although his deformed right knee may be the most obvious injury, there may be other injuries that are bothering the patient more. If you don't ask, you may not find out. In conducting the physical assessment, pay particular attention to the following issues (pages 1852–1855):
   a. The position in which the extremities are found; as always, compare the injured limb to the uninjured limb.
   b. The circulatory status of the injured limb—check the following:
      (1) Skin condition
      (2) Capillary refill
      (3) Distal pulses (anterior tibial and dorsalis pedis)
   c. The neurologic status of the injured limb—check the following:
      (1) Sensation to pinprick over the heel and dorsum of the foot
      (2) Motor function: ability to plantar flex and dorsiflex the foot

3. Equipment to grab and take with you when you rush to the side of a severely injured patient should include the following:
   a. Long backboard with at least three straps
   b. Cervical collar and head immobilizer (eg, blanket roll)
   c. Portable oxygen and suction
   d. Oropharyngeal and nasopharyngeal airways
   e. Pocket mask or bag-mask device
   f. Wound kit
   g. Stethoscope, BP cuff, and flashlight

Chapter 38: Environmental Emergencies

Matching

Part I

1. Z (page 1895)
2. Y (page 1891)
3. X (page 1889)
4. W (page 1923)
5. P (page 1891)
6. O (page 1891)
7. N (page 1904)
8. M (page 1896)
9. I (page 1890)
10. H (page 1913)
11. G (page 1912)
12. F (page 1904)
13. A (page 1908)
14. B (page 1920)
15. C (page 1906)
16. D (page 1919)
17. U (page 1900)
18. T (pages 1916–1917)
19. S (page 1913)
20. R (page 1912)
21. E (page 1915)
22. L (page 1902)
23. K (page 1911)
24. J (page 1912)
25. Q (page 1890)
26. V (page 1907)

Part II

1. V (page 1898)
2. U (page 1928)
3. T (pages 1907–1908)
4. S (page 1908)
5. R (page 1890)
6. K (page 1912)
7. J (page 1895)
8. I (page 1896)
9. H (page 1892)
10. G (page 1895)
11. F (page 1893)
12. E (page 1901)
13. D (page 1900)
14. C (page 1900)
15. B (page 1912)
16. A (page 1897)
17. Z (page 1896)
18. Y (page 1916)
19. X (page 1912)
20. W (page 1898)
21. Q (page 1889)
22. P (page 1890)
23. O (page 1908)
24. N (page 1889)
25. M (page 1920)
26. L (page 1920)

Part III

(Table 38-2, page 1893)

1. HL
2. HP
3. HL
4. HL
5. HP
6. HP
7. HL
8. HP
9. HL
10. HP

Multiple Choice

1. D (page 1895)
2. C (page 1890)
3. B (page 1891)
4. A (pages 1893–1894)
5. D (pages 1896–1898)
6. A (page 1902)
7. B (page 1904)
8. B (page 1913)
9. C (page 1918)
10. D (page 1900)

Labeling

1. Dangerous snakes
   (page 1925, Figure 38-24)
   A. Rattlesnake
   B. Copperhead
   C. Cottonmouth
   D. Coral snake

Fill in the Blank

1. **a.** For the human body to maintain a nearly constant core temperature, it must balance heat loss with heat production.

Sources of Body Heat	Ways of Shedding Heat
1. Basal metabolism	1. Radiation
2. Exercise	2. Convection
3. Absorption of heat	3. Conduction
4. Evaporation of sweat	

b. The body's mechanisms for dissipating excess heat have certain limitations. First, all of the mechanisms depend on **peripheral vasodilation** to shunt blood from the core to the body surface. Furthermore, to be effective, three of the body's cooling mechanisms require a temperature gradient between the body and the outside. None of these three mechanisms—**radiation**, **convection**, or **conduction**—can work if the outside is not at least a few degrees cooler than the body core. Finally, one of the body's cooling mechanisms is dependent on the ambient humidity. When the humidity is high, that mechanism—namely, **evaporation of sweat**—is ineffective in lowering the core temperature.

c. A hatless hiker standing still on a mountaintop on a windless day loses heat from his head by **radiation**. A breeze picks up. Now the hiker loses heat by **convection** as well.

d. A white-water enthusiast who capsizes his canoe in a swift-running stream loses body heat by **conduction**.

e. A soldier on maneuvers in the desert in ambient temperatures of more than 37.7°C (100°F) can shed heat only by **evaporation of sweat**. (pages 1891–1892)

Identify

1. **a.** Chief complaint: Fell through ice
   b. Vital signs: Patient is shivering. ECG rhythm is regular with Osborn waves.
   c. Pertinent negatives: None
   d. *Students should provide three of the following:*
      (1) Time in water
      (2) Patient temperature
      (3) Neurologic assessment
      (4) Amount of alcohol ingested and when
      (5) Any drugs taken
      (6) Blood glucose (pages 1902–1904)
   e. B. (Conduction) This is the transfer of heat from a hotter object to a cooler object by direct physical contact. (page 1891)
   f. A fluid bolus (unless otherwise contraindicated) (page 1906)

Complete the Patient Care Report (PCR)

Show the completed PCR to your instructor to obtain feedback on your completion of the form.

Ambulance Calls

1. **a.** The patient probably had a heat syncope episode, which occurs in people who are under heat stress and then experience peripheral vasodilation, which possibly may be exacerbated by dehydration. One group in which this seems prevalent is those attending mass outdoor gatherings. An additional contributing factor may be alcohol intake (beer). Some other factors that should be considered but that might not yet be identified are medical conditions, such as diabetes, drug intake, and amount of physical exertion done by the patient. (page 1895)
   b. Maintain the airway and provide oxygen, place the patient in a cool environment in the supine position, and provide fluid replacement either orally or by IV administration. (page 1895)
   c. If the patient does not quickly respond in the supine position, suspect heat exhaustion or heatstroke. (page 1895)
2. **a.** The fullback who is acting "crazy" after practicing on a hot, humid afternoon is most probably experiencing exertional heatstroke. You were fortunate to be able to record a temperature and obtain conclusive evidence. In many cases, the patient is too combative to allow you to measure the temperature, and you can only suspect the diagnosis on the basis of the patient's symptoms and signs alone. (page 1897)
   b. The steps in managing exertional heatstroke in this patient are as follows:
      (1) Move him to a cooler environment, preferably your air-conditioned ambulance with the fans blowing.
      (2) Strip off his clothing and football gear.
      (3) Apply ice packs to his flanks while massaging his neck and torso. Spray the patient with tepid water, and keep a fan blowing in his direction.
      (4) Start an IV line, and administer a bolus of fluid (unless otherwise contraindicated).
      (5) Monitor temperature and cardiac rhythm.
      (6) Be prepared for seizures.
      (7) Transport without delay. (pages 1898–1899)
3. **a.** The running back writhing in pain most likely has heat cramps. (pages 1893–1894)
   b. The steps in treating him are as follows:
      (1) Tell the coach to stop massaging the player's legs!
      (2) Move the patient to a cooler environment.
      (3) If he is not nauseated, give him salt-containing fluids to drink (at least a quart). If the patient is too nauseated to take the fluids by mouth, start an IV line and infuse normal saline rapidly (consult medical control for the IV rate).
      (4) Do not allow the patient to return to practice that day. He should go home and rest in a cool place. Instruct him to seek medical attention if he develops headaches, dizziness, nausea, or severe fatigue. (pages 1894–1895)

4. a. The quarterback may indeed be coming down with mononucleosis, but it could be fatal to miss a case of heat exhaustion. (pages 1895–1896)

b. You should treat him in the field as follows:

(1) Move the patient to a cooler environment.
(2) Remove most of his clothing, down to his undershorts, and sponge him with cool water.
(3) Start an IV line and run it wide open.
(4) Monitor cardiac rhythm and vital signs.
(5) Transport to the hospital. (page 1896)

c. By now, one would think the coach would have reached the conclusion that football practice in the searing heat is not healthy for a teenager. You should suggest to him that if he must conduct practice during the "dog days" of August, he should schedule the heavy-exertion activities during the hours of early morning and late afternoon.

5. a. The baby at the supermarket is suffering from classic heatstroke. The inside of an automobile that is parked in the sun in a 37.7°C (100°F) external temperature can very quickly reach a temperature of around 82°C (180°F)—not high enough to bake a cake, perhaps, but certainly high enough to bake a baby. This infant is in severe danger and may die. (pages 1896–1897)

b. Treatment is extremely urgent:

(1) Open the airway. Intubate as soon as you have a chance.
(2) Administer supplemental oxygen.
(3) Strip off all the baby's clothing.
(4) Spray and fan the baby continuously until you reach the hospital.
(5) If you are able to do so, start an IV line en route to the hospital with 5% dextrose in half normal saline. Consult medical control for local orders on flow rate and/or boluses of fluid.
(6) Monitor rectal temperature.
(7) Transport without delay. (pages 1897–1899)

6. This scenario only happens to paramedics—a ski vacation turns into a search-and-rescue mission.

a. The first skier has deep frostbite. You do not really have the means to rewarm his leg in the field, nor can you ensure that it will not freeze again during transport to the ski lodge. (pages 1900–1901)

b. The management is as follows:

(1) Move the patient to a sheltered place, such as that cabin behind the trees, until the snowmobile comes.
(2) Give him some calories, preferably a candy bar or some other carbohydrate source. Give him a hot, sweet drink if you are carrying a thermos.
(3) Leave the frostbitten extremity frozen. Do not attempt any rewarming in the field.
(4) Pad the frostbitten leg to prevent it from being bruised during transport.
(5) Protect the rest of the patient's body from the cold with insulating blankets. (page 1901)

c. The second skier has a more superficial frostbite. (page 1900)

d. The management is as follows:

(1) Move the patient to a sheltered place, such as that cabin behind the trees, until the snowmobile comes.
(2) Give him some calories, preferably a candy bar or some other carbohydrate source. Give him a hot, sweet drink if you are carrying a thermos.
(3) Try to warm the frostbitten foot with your hands (or by putting it in your armpit!).
(4) Splint the frostbitten leg to prevent it from being bruised during transport.
(5) Protect the rest of the patient's body from the cold with insulating blankets. (page 1901)

e. The third lost skier has developed severe hypothermia. Only his very occasional breathing tips you off that he is not (yet) in cardiac arrest. (pages 1902–1904)

f. The management is as follows:

(1) As long as his airway is not obstructed, it is best not to touch the patient at all until the ambulance arrives. Send someone down to the road to intercept the ambulance, help carry equipment, and guide the paramedics to the patient.
(2) Move the patient very gently onto the stretcher, and carry the stretcher very gently to the ambulance.
(3) Maintain the airway manually until the patient has been well ventilated with 100% oxygen by bag-mask device for at least 3 minutes. Then, intubate the trachea rapidly and smoothly.
(4) Apply monitoring electrodes, and check the cardiac rhythm. If asystole should occur, start cardiopulmonary resuscitation (CPR), but give basic life support (BLS) only. If you see ventricular fibrillation (VF) on the monitor, give one shock, resume CPR immediately for a 2-minute cycle, and then attempt to deliver another shock. Continue until three shocks have been given. If VF persists, put the defibrillator away and just continue BLS all the way to the hospital. It is important that CPR be uninterrupted, with quality compressions at a rate

of at least 100 per minute. Medical control can be contacted to determine whether additional shocks from the defibrillator should be provided.
   (5) If the patient's clothing is wet, gently cut away wet clothing and replace it with dry blankets.
   (6) Notify the receiving hospital of the nature of the case and your estimated time of arrival (ETA).
   (7) Keep the ambulance interior at a temperature of approximately 15.5°C (60°F).
   (8) Instruct the driver to make it a smooth ride to the hospital. (pages 1904–1907)

7. The speedboat driver who plunged into cold lake water is a likely candidate for hypothermia by the process of conduction. Heat loss is 25% faster in water than in air and can occur after relatively short exposure because of the rapidity with which water conducts heat away from the body. In managing such a case, you should observe these guidelines:
   a. Try to prevent the victim from exerting himself. Toss him a rope and pull him to shore, or send one of the other boats over to haul him aboard and bring him ashore. In any case, discourage him from thrashing about in the water.
   b. As soon as you have the victim ashore, carry him to a sheltered place, preferably the inside of your ambulance, and cut away his wet clothes. Be sure to keep him absolutely still.
   c. Monitor his cardiac rhythm.
   d. Cover him with insulating materials, and cover those with blankets.
   e. Wrap chemical hot packs in towels, and place them in his armpits and near the groin.
   f. Give him a hot, caffeine-free, sugary drink.
   g. Keep him recumbent.
   h. Transport him to the hospital. (pages 1904–1906)

8. The "vagrant" in the bus station represents a classic example of the kind of case that is too often misdiagnosed.
   a. Any patient found in the circumstances described must be suspected to have one of the following conditions:
      (1) Hypothermia
      (2) Hypoglycemia
      (3) Stroke
      ... or all of the above until proved otherwise.
   b. In view of those possibilities, the steps in management are as follows:
      (1) Administer warmed, humidified oxygen (if available).
      (2) Complete the rapid medical assessment. Obtain vital signs, and check for injuries, paying particular attention to the head.
      (3) Start an IV line (using warmed IV fluid).
      (4) Give 50% dextrose, 50 mL IV (or equivalent).
      (5) Monitor the patient's cardiac rhythm.
      (6) Cover the patient with warm blankets.
      (7) Transport to the hospital.

9. a. Ask if the headache is throbbing and worse over the temporal or occipital areas and if it is exacerbated by a Valsalva maneuver. If the answer to any of these questions is yes, there is a likelihood the patient has acute mountain sickness. (pages 1918–1920)
   b. *Students should list four of the following:*
      (1) Dyspnea at rest
      (2) Cough
      (3) Weakness or decreased exercise performance
      (4) Chest tightness or congestion
      (5) Central cyanosis
      (6) Audible crackles or wheezing in at least one lung field
      (7) Tachypnea
      (8) Tachycardia (page 1920)
   c. (1) Give supplemental oxygen until the condition improves.
      (2) Descend as soon as possible, with minimal exertion.
      (3) A portable ventilator can be used, if available, if descent is not possible or no oxygen is accessible. If you cannot descend, give your friend nifedipine, and add dexamethasone if neurologic deterioration occurs. (pages 1920–1921)

10. a. The diver ascended from his dive without exhaling constantly to vent air from the lungs, or he held his breath during the ascent. The result is that he probably has sustained pulmonary overpressurized syndrome (POPS), also known as "burnt lungs," which has likely led to the development of an arterial gas embolism (AGE). (pages 1915–1916)

b. (1) Ensure an adequate airway, intubate if a BLS airway is not effective (fill the cuff with saline if the patient is to be placed in a hyperbaric chamber).
(2) Administer 100% supplemental oxygen.
(3) Transport the patient in the supine position (use ground transport if cabin pressure is an issue).
(4) Establish an IV line en route.
(5) Place on an ECG monitor.
(6) Have medication ready for seizures and dopamine for hypotension, and follow your local protocol for direct referral to a hyperbaric chamber facility. (pages 1915–1916)

c. Decompression sickness (pages 1916–1917)

True/False

1. F (page 1901)
2. T (page 1900)
3. T (page 1901)
4. T (page 1924)
5. F (page 1901)
6. T (pages 1899–1900)
7. T (page 1895)
8. F (pages 1896–1897)
9. F (page 1897)
10. T (page 1891)

Short Answer

1. Heat is a form of cardiovascular stress because the body responds to heat by vasodilation. Increasing the diameter of the blood vessels increases their volume; in turn, the heart must increase its output to prevent a fall in BP. The heart increases output by increasing both its rate and stroke volume, which inevitably means an increase in cardiac work. (page 1891)

2. A person's risk of developing significant heat illness in response to heat stress can be increased by the following factors (*students should provide five of the following*):
a. High ambient temperature
b. High humidity
c. Obesity
d. Diabetes
e. Alcoholism
f. Impaired vasodilation
g. Impaired ability to sweat
h. Heavy or tight clothing
i. Drugs such as diuretics and some tranquilizers (page 1893)

3. a. The dog days of summer also put you at risk of heat illness, especially if you have to carry heat-stricken, 300-pound patients down four flights of stairs. So, take some precautions to protect yourself on very hot days (*students should provide five of the following*):
(1) Acclimatize whenever possible. Maintain personal fitness.
(2) Limit time spent in heavy activity in personal protective equipment (PPE; eg, wildland duties in bunker gear), especially during the hottest parts of the day or season. Paramedics working in hot climates should have appropriate summer uniforms.
(3) Maintain hydration, eat appropriately, and rest. Avoid beverages with a high sugar and caffeine content. Some ambulances are equipped with an on-board refrigerator for hot weather. Otherwise, carry a portable cooler, fill it about half full with crushed ice, and stock it with sports drinks or other salt-containing drinks for patients and the crew.
(4) Develop or research standards on activities in hot weather from professional organizations (eg, National Fire Protection Association, Occupational Safety and Health Administration, American College of Sports Medicine, Wilderness Medical Society).
(5) Improve your own physical fitness, both in terms of cardiovascular endurance and muscular strength.
(6) Seek medical attention at the first symptom of heat illness. (page 1899)

b. Of course, to seek attention at the first symptom of heat illness, you have to know what the symptoms are! *Students should provide four of the following:*
(1) Headache
(2) Fatigue or lack of energy
(3) Dizziness
(4) Nausea or vomiting
(5) Weakness
(6) Abdominal cramping (page 1896)

4. Let's hear it for all the mothers out there! They've been right all along.
  a. "Don't go out without a hat and scarf; it's freezing out there."
  Most heat loss from the body occurs from the head and neck. By trapping some of that heat within insulating layers, a hat and scarf can reduce convective heat loss from above the shoulders. (page 1891)
  b. "Stop rolling around in the snow. You'll get a death of a chill."
  Snow conducts heat away from the body faster than air does. And when the snow melts and your clothes get wet, cooling by conduction is even faster. (page 1891)
  c. "Get out of those wet clothes this minute."
  Wearing wet clothing promotes heat loss by conduction while the clothes remain wet and by evaporation as the clothes dry. (page 1891)
  d. "Those skates are much too tight. Your toes will fall off."
  Anything that interferes with the circulation to the extremities predisposes them to frostbite. (page 1900)
  e. "Make sure you wear your windbreaker. It's blowing a gale out there."
  Exposure to the wind increases heat loss by convection. (page 1891)
  f. "Eat. Eat. You have to have something to keep you going in this weather."
  Metabolic heat production requires fuel, so you need to maintain your caloric intake, especially in the form of carbohydrates, before anticipated exposure to cold temperatures. (page 1890)

5. It's important to follow your mother's advice because, by itself, the body does not have a lot of ways to defend itself against the cold. The three ways it can do so are as follows:
  a. By peripheral vasoconstriction, to shunt blood away from the body shell to the body core
  b. By shivering, to increase heat production by skeletal muscle
  c. By increasing the basal metabolic rate, to increase overall metabolic heat production (page 1892)

6. Some people are more likely to develop cold injury than others are.
  a. Factors that predispose a person to frostbite include the following:
    (1) Inadequate or tight clothing, especially tight shoes or gloves
    (2) Smoking
    (3) Hunger, fatigue, or dehydration
    (4) Hypothermia (generalized cooling)
    (5) Coming in direct contact with cold objects (page 1900)
  b. Many factors predispose a person to experiencee hypothermia. *Students should provide four of the following:*
    (1) Old age
    (2) Infancy
    (3) Alcoholism
    (4) Chronic illness
    (5) Poor planning for outdoor activity; unpreparedness
    (6) Trauma (pages 1902–1903; see Table 38-5 for a full list)

7. Even our nursery rhyme companions were in danger of cold exposure:
  a. When the three little kittens lost their mittens, they became most vulnerable to frostbite of the paws.
  b. While sitting on an ice-cold tuffet, Miss Muffet was losing heat by conduction from her bottom to the tuffet and by radiation, mostly from her head and neck, to the surrounding atmosphere. If there was any breeze, she was losing heat by convection as well.
  c. Jack Sprat has a greater risk of hypothermia than his wife does because he has less natural insulation.
  d. Little Jack Horner had the right idea eating his Christmas pie before going out into the cold because he knew that one needs calories to increase internal heat production in cold weather.
  e. When the wind blows, the cradle rocks, and Baby loses heat by convection.

Fill in the Table

1. The slang expression "Cool it!" means to take it easy, to simmer down. That is precisely what happens to the major systems of the body when cooled: They all slow down. These are the factors that predispose to cold illness. (Table 38-5, page 1902)

Increase Heat Loss	Impair Thermoregulatory Mechanism	Decrease Heat Production
Cold water submersion	Dehydration	**Hypothyroidism**
Wet clothes	Parkinson disease or dementia	Age (very young or very old)
Wind-chill temperature	**Multiple sclerosis**	**Hypoglycemia**
Impaired judgment from drugs/alcohol	Anorexia nervosa	**Malnutrition**
Vasodilation	Central nervous system (CNS) bleeding or ischemia, spinal cord injury with neurogenic shock	Inability to shiver and immobility
Diabetic peripheral neuropathies	**Multisystem trauma**	
	Drugs interfering with vasoconstriction	

Section 8: Shock and Resuscitation

Chapter 39: Responding to the Field Code

Matching

1. B (page 1953)
2. C (page 1944)
3. E (page 1945)
4. F (page 1945)
5. H (page 1957)
6. I (page 1959)
7. J (page 1944)
8. K (page 1945)
9. G (page 1973)
10. D (page 1947)
11. L (page 1945)
12. A (page 1948)

Multiple Choice

1. C (page 1945)
2. B (page 1946)
3. D (page 1947)
4. B (page 1947)
5. D (page 1950)
6. B (page 1953)
7. C (page 1956)
8. D (page 1958)
9. A (page 1950)
10. C (page 1969)

Labeling

1. CPR devices (pages 1967–1968, Figures 39-10, 39-11, and 39-12)
   A. AutoPulse load-distributing band device
   B. Thumper CPR system
   C. Lucas 2 mechanical piston device
2. Resuscitation pyramid (page 1947, Figure 39-2)
   A. Drugs
   B. Endotracheal (ET) tube, laryngeal mask airway (LMA), Combitube
   C. Ventilations (proper rate and visible chest rise)
   D. Single shock for VF/VT
   E. High-quality compressions (fast, deep, full recoil)

Fill in the Blank

1. Thumper (page 1967)
2. advanced airway (page 1967)
3. impedance threshold device (page 1968)
4. asynchronous; 6 (page 1966)
5. asystole; PEA (page 1959)
6. vasopressor (page 1964)

Identify

1. a. Chief complaint: Sudden cardiac arrest
   b. Vital signs: Initially none, then after ROSC; with a BP of 108/p and pulse of 96 regular
   c. Pertinent negatives: No prior heart attack, no allergies
   d. Epinephrine 1:10,000 and amiodarone
   e. Links in the chain of survival
      (1) Recognition and activation of the emergency response system
      (2) Immediate high-quality CPR
      (3) Rapid defibrillation
      (4) Basic and advanced emergency medical services (EMS) care
      (5) Advanced life support (ALS) and postarrest care (page 1945)

Complete the Patient Care Report (PCR)

Show the completed PCR to your instructor to obtain feedback on your completion of the form.

Ambulance Calls

1. a. High-quality compressions are the priority. A successful resuscitation is built around compressions with little to no interruptions. Change out the compressor every 2 minutes to assure a fresh compressor. (page 1972)

b. The roles of the code team leader may include all of the following:
   (1) Obtaining the patient's history and performing the physical examination
   (2) Interpreting the ECG
   (3) Keeping track of the time
   (4) Making a medication decision following the algorithm
   (5) Clearly delegating tasks to code team members
   (6) Completing documentation after the resuscitation attempt
   (7) Talking with medical control
   (8) Controlling the resuscitation scene
   (9) Fostering the concepts of crew resource management (CRM) (page 1972)
c. The code team member may be called on to perform all of the following roles (and more):
   (1) Ventilator
   (2) Active compressor
   (3) On-deck compressor
   (4) Other support personnel (pages 1972–1973)

2. a. As a paramedic, it is your responsibility to start CPR in all patients who are in cardiac arrest, with only two general exceptions:
- You should not start CPR if the patient has obvious signs of death, such as absence of a pulse and breathing, along with any one of the following findings: rigor mortis, dependent lividity, putrefaction, or evidence of nonsurvivable injury such as decapitation, dismemberment, or burned beyond recognition.
- You should not start CPR if the patient has obvious signs of death, such as absence of a pulse and breathing, along with any one of the following findings: rigor mortis, dependent lividity, putrefaction, or evidence of nonsurvivable injury. You should also not start CPR if the patient and his or her physician have previously agreed not to resuscitate. If CPR has been started and a valid DNR or a medical order for life-sustaining treatment (MOLST) form is presented to you by family, then resuscitative efforts may be withheld. (page 1969)

b. The significance of bystander CPR, even if only chest compressions, is that if applied properly, it can double, if not triple, the chance of survival. (page 1947)

3. a. For situations where advanced life support (ALS) personnel are present to provide care for an adult in out-of-hospital cardiac arrest, the ALS termination of resuscitation rule was established to consider terminating resuscitative efforts before ambulance transport if all of the following criteria are met:
   (1) The arrest was not witnessed by anyone.
   (2) Bystander CPR was not provided.
   (3) There is no ROSC after complete ALS care in the field.
   (4) No AED shocks were delivered. (page 1971)

b. The details that might lead you to ask if the patient has a DNR order or was in hospice care could best be expressed by the following quotes from the narrative:
   (1) "only 100 pounds"—Often terminal patients have lost a lot of weight and are very frail.
   (2) "hospital bed in the living room"—Those beds are large and often do not fit on the upper floors of the home. If set up on the first floor, the patient can be easily cared for while accessible to the entire family.
   (3) "been suffering for a long time"—This is an indication of a potential terminal illness.
   (4) "Dad wouldn't have wanted all this"—Hopefully, he had discussed his wishes with his physician previously and has a DNR or MOLST in place!

True/False

1. T (page 1966)
2. T (page 1966)
3. T (page 1966)
4. F (page 1969)
5. T (page 1964)
6. F (page 1970)
7. T (page 1968)
8. F (pages 1968–1969)
9. F (pages 1956–1957)
10. T (page 1963)

Short Answer

1. *Students should list five of the following recommendations:*
   a. Establish a national cardiac arrest registry.
   b. Foster a culture of action through public awareness and training.
   c. Enhance the capabilities and performances of EMS systems.
   d. Set national accreditation standards related to cardiac arrest for hospitals and health care systems.
   e. Adopt continuous quality improvement programs for cardiac arrest response in EMS.

f. Accelerate research on pathophysiology, new therapies, and translation of science for cardiac arrest.
g. Accelerate research on the evaluation and adoption of cardiac arrest therapies.
h. Create a national cardiac arrest collaborative to raise the visibility of cardiac arrest for policy makers and members of the public. (page 1959)

2. A five-person team can be organized as follows:
a. Compressor 1—Responsible for performing high-quality chest compressions, stays in position and compresses for 2 minutes and then rests for 2 minutes (for the duration of the time the patient is pulseless), may assist with application of the mechanical chest compression device or other adjunct to circulation, provided Compressor 2 is continuing uninterrupted compressions.
b. Compressor 2—Responsible for performing high-quality chest compressions, stays in position and compresses for 2 minutes and then rests for 2 minutes (for the duration of the time the patient is pulseless), may assist with application of the mechanical chest compression device or other adjunct to circulation, provided Compressor 1 is continuing uninterrupted compressions.
c. Ventilator—Responsible for providing ventilations at a ratio of 30:2, ensuring visible chest rise with each ventilation (1 second in duration). May need to briefly suction the patient as necessary, and then as appropriate will switch over to the ATV. Will assist with the transition from BLS airway to advanced airway (not a high priority). Once an advanced airway is placed, ventilates once every 6 seconds to achieve visible chest rise over a 1-second duration for each ventilation.
d. Code team leader—Responsible for initial ECG analysis and defibrillation with a single shock (200 J). Responsible for overall timing of the code and reassessment after 2 minutes of cycles of CPR with the interruption not to exceed 10 seconds. After the initial shock (or ascertaining "no shock" rhythm), proceeds to establish IV or IO access, then begins administration of a vasopressor every 3 to 5 minutes, helps to transition the airway from BLS to an advanced airway, and continues with single shocks every 2 minutes if the patient is still in VF or pVT. Makes the decision with input from the code team and medical control that the resuscitation should be terminated if there is no ROSC in the first 15 to 30 minutes. If there is ROSC, administers the appropriate antidysrhythmic, ensures appropriate ventilations, and assists the team in preparing for transport.
e. EMS field supervisor—Brings in the Thumper or other adjunct to circulation and works with one of the compressors to transition the patient to mechanical CPR compressions with minimal interruption. Assists the medic with IV or IO, advanced airway placement, and preparation of medications and contacts medical control, per local protocols. (pages 1972–1973)

Fill in the Table

Paramedics should know the key elements of CPR for adults, children, and infants from the 2015 Guidelines. (Table 39-4, pages 1962–1963)

Key Elements of CPR for Adults, Children, and Infants			
Procedure	**Age 9 to Adult**	**Age 1-8 Years**	**Younger Than 1 Year[a]**
Circulation			
Recognition	Unresponsive with no breathing or only agonal (gasping) respirations		
Pulse check	**Carotid artery**	**Carotid artery**	Brachial artery
Compression location	In the center of the chest (lower half of the sternum)	In the center of the chest (lower half of the sternum)	**Just below the nipple lin**e
Hand placement	Heel of both hands	**Heel of one or both hands**	Two-fingers or two-thumb encircling-hands technique
Compression depth	At least 2 in. (5 cm); not to exceed 2.4 in. (6 cm)	At least one-third of anterior-posterior diameter of chest; approximately 2 in. (5 cm)	**At least one-third of anterior-posterior diameter of chest; approximately 1.5 in. (4 cm)**
Compression rate	**100-120/min**		
Chest wall recoil	Allow full chest recoil in between compressions. No **leaning**! Rotate rescuers delivering compressions every 2 min		
Interruptions	Limit interruptions in delivery of chest compressions to less than 10 s		

Key Elements of CPR for Adults, Children, and Infants			
Procedure	**Age 9 to Adult**	**Age 1-8 Years**	**Younger Than 1 Year[a]**
Compression-to-ventilation ratio (until an advanced airway is inserted)	**30:2 (one or two rescuers)**	**30:2** (one rescuer); **15:2** (two professional rescuers)	
Airway			
Airway positioning	Head tilt-chin lift maneuver; jaw-thrust maneuver if **spinal injury** is strongly suspected		
Breathing			
Untrained rescuer	Compressions only		
Ventilations without advanced airway	2 breaths with a duration of **1 s** each, with enough volume to produce **chest rise[b]**		
Ventilations with advanced airway	1 breath every 6 seconds (10/min) **Asynchronous** with chest compressions; duration of 1 s each with enough volume to produce chest rise	*Age 1 month to the onset of puberty:* 1 breath every 6-8 s (8-10 breaths/min); chest compressions delivered continuously at a rate of at least 100/min with no pauses for ventilations; duration of 1 s each, with enough volume to produce visible chest rise	
Rescue breathing	1 breath every **5-6 s** (10-12 breaths/min)	1 breath every **3-5 s** (12-20 breaths/min)	1 breath every **3-5 s** (12-20 breaths/min)
Defibrillation			
Device	Adult AED	Use **pediatric dose-attenuator** unit if available; if unavailable, then use adult unit	Use **manual defibrillator** if available; if unavailable, use unit with pediatric dose attenuator; if neither is available, then use adult unit
Procedure	Attach AED as soon as it is available. If two rescuers are available, then one should immediately begin CPR while the second retrieves and applies the AED. Minimize CPR interruptions. Resume CPR immediately after shock, beginning with **chest compressions.**		
Airway Obstruction			
Foreign body obstruction	Responsive: **abdominal thrusts** Unresponsive: **CPR[c]**	Responsive: **abdominal thrusts**	Responsive: **back slaps and chest thrusts**

Abbreviations: AED, automated external defibrillator; CPR, cardiopulmonary resuscitation.

[a] Excluding newborns, in whom arrest is usually the result of asphyxiation and requires the rescue ventilations.

[b] Pause compressions to deliver ventilations.

[c] Look in the mouth for objects before delivering breaths in a patient with a known airway obstruction.

Data from: Kleinman ME, Brennan EE, Goldberger ZD, et al. Part 5: Adult basic life support and cardiopulmonary resuscitation quality: 2015 American Heart Association Guidelines Update for Cardiopulmonary Resuscitation and Emergency Cardiovascular Care. *Circulation.* 2015;132(suppl 2):S414-S435; Atkins DL, Berger S, Duff JP, et al. Part 11: Pediatric basic life support and cardiopulmonary resuscitation quality: 2015 American Heart Association Guidelines Update for Cardiopulmonary Resuscitation and Emergency Cardiovascular Care. *Circulation.* 2015;132(suppl 2):S519-S525.

Chapter 40: Management and Resuscitation of the Critical Patient

Matching

Part I

1. M (page 1993)
2. L (page 2006)
3. K (page 1997)
4. J (page 2007)
5. I (page 1988)
6. Z (page 1989)
7. Y (page 1999)
8. X (page 1985)
9. W (page 2013)
10. V (page 1988)
11. P (page 1983)
12. O (page 1985)
13. N (page 1999)
14. H (page 2009)
15. G (page 1993)
16. F (page 2011)
17. E (page 1985)
18. U (page 1990)
19. T (page 2009)
20. S (page 1991)
21. R (page 1982)
22. Q (page 1999)
23. D (page 2011)
24. C (page 1993)
25. B (page 1988)
26. A (page 1993)

Part II

1. J (page 1988)
2. I (page 2006)
3. H (page 1983)
4. G (page 1988)
5. F (page 1999)
6. W (page 1983)
7. V (page 1996)
8. U (page 1988)
9. T (page 1988)
10. S (page 2010)
11. E (page 2009)
12. D (page 2013)
13. C (page 2010)
14. B (page 1988)
15. R (page 1991)
16. A (page 1996)
17. Q (page 1988)
18. P (page 2009)
19. O (page 2011)
20. N (page 2009)
21. M (page 1989)
22. L (page 2011)
23. K (page 1983)

Multiple Choice

1. C (page 1982)
2. B (page 1983)
3. B (page 1984)
4. D (page 1985)
5. B (page 1985)
6. D (page 1988)
7. B (page 1988)
8. C (page 1989)
9. A (page 1990)
10. C (page 1990)
11. B (page 1990)
12. C (page 1992)
13. D (page 1996)
14. B (page 1999)
15. C (page 1999)

Labeling

1. Relationship between the organism and the cells (page 1992, Figure 40-6)
   - **A.** Organism (human in this case)
   - **B.** Organ systems (organs with similar functions)
   - **C.** Organs (tissues with similar functions)
   - **D.** Tissues (cells with similar functions)
   - **E.** Cells (smallest unit of the organism)

Fill in the Blank

1. anchoring (page 1985)
2. compensate; shunting (page 1991)
3. sphincters (page 1991)
4. chemoreceptors (page 1993)
5. aerobic; anaerobic (page 1993)
6. alpha 1; alpha 2; increasing (page 1993)
7. renal; necrosis; oliguria (page 1997)
8. irreversible (page 1999)
9. cardiac tamponade (page 2004)
10. Cardiogenic (page 2007)

Identify

1. Chief complaint: Chest pain
2. Vital signs: Sinus bradycardia rate of 52 beats/min, crackles in the base of the lungs. Respirations are 24 breaths/min, blood pressure (BP) is 80/56 mm Hg, skin is diaphoretic and clammy. Patient is alert with oxygen administration and is PERRLA.
3. Pertinent negatives: No pulse at wrist, no ectopy on 12-lead ECG

Complete the Patient Care Report (PCR)

Show the completed PCR to your instructor to obtain feedback on your completion of the form.

Ambulance Calls

1. In assessing the state of perfusion:
   a. You can judge *peripheral* perfusion by checking distal pulses in an adult, and/or capillary refill in a child.
   b. The best indicator in the field of *perfusion of vital organs* is the patient's state of consciousness (mental status).
2. You are called to a concert to attend a bleeding, unresponsive man. The band is still playing so it is very noisy and there are a number of potentially intoxicated concertgoers surrounding the patient. The police are attempting to provide you a pathway to the patient. *Remember the priorities of the primary survey:* A-B-C or C-A-B.

   Before you even enter the concert, make certain that the police have the situation under control. Always look first to your own safety!
   a. Open the patient's airway.
   b. Check whether he is breathing. If not, start artificial ventilation.
   c. Check whether he has a pulse. If he does not have a pulse, start external chest compressions.
   d. Cut away the patient's trouser leg, and find the source of his bleeding. When you've found it, control the bleeding by applying direct pressure on the wound, preferably over a sterile dressing. Check quickly for other lower extremity injuries.
   e. Transfer the patient to the vehicle (he should be on a backboard by now).
   f. Begin transport to the hospital, and start an IV infusion en route. Complete your rapid secondary assessment as time permits.
3. This patient earns his "load-and-go" status by virtue of uncontrollable bleeding from the femoral artery and developing shock.
   a. Steps to be taken at the scene:
      (1) Seal the open wound of the neck.
      (2) Administer supplemental oxygen.
      (3) Try at least to slow the bleeding from the groin by using pressure dressings and a hemostatic dressing if one is available.
      (4) Communicate with medical control or the receiving hospital.
   b. Steps to be taken en route:
      (1) Start two large-bore IV lines with rapid infusion of fluids.
      (2) Complete a physical exam (as time permits).
      (3) Recheck vital and neurologic signs every 5 minutes.
4. Abdominal evisceration is certainly an attention-getter, but it does not pose an immediate threat to life, whereas shock can.
   a. Steps to be taken at the scene:
      (1) Administer supplemental oxygen.
      (2) Complete the physical exam.
      (3) Cover the eviscerated organs with sterile dressings soaked in sterile saline and an occlusive dressing.
   b. Steps to be taken en route:
      (1) Communicate with medical control or the receiving hospital.
      (2) Start a large-bore IV line with normal saline.
      (3) Recheck vital and neurologic signs every 5 minutes.
5. An open chest wound is considered a critical injury because it prevents adequate ventilation of the lungs.
   a. Steps to be taken at the scene:
      (1) Seal off the sucking chest wound with an occlusive dressing taped on three sides.
      (2) Administer supplemental oxygen; assist ventilations as needed.
      (3) Communicate with medical control or the receiving hospital.
   b. Steps to be taken en route:
      (1) Complete a physical exam.
      (2) Start an IV with fluids.
      (3) Recheck vital and neurologic signs every 5 minutes.

6. Your primary survey has not given you much information regarding *where* precisely this woman has been injured, but the primary *has* given you unmistakable evidence that the patient is in shock (restlessness, profuse sweating). Don't be fooled by the slow pulse—bradycardia occurs sometimes with intra-abdominal bleeding. *And don't wait for the BP to fall before you decide that the patient is in shock!*
   a. Steps to be taken at the scene:
      (1) Manually stabilize the head/neck, and apply a cervical collar.
      (2) Administer supplemental oxygen.
      (3) Conduct the rapid secondary assessment.
      (4) Immobilize the patient on a scoop stretcher.
      (5) Prepare for rapid transport to the appropriate facility.
   b. Steps to be taken en route:
      (1) Complete a physical exam.
      (2) Start two large-bore IV lines and run a fluid challenge.
      (3) Communicate with medical control or the receiving hospital.
      (4) Conduct a reassessment, rechecking vital and neurologic signs every 5 minutes.

True/False

1. T (page 2006)
2. F (page 2006)
3. T (page 2007)
4. T (page 2007)
5. F (page 2009)
6. T (page 2010)
7. T (page 2007)
8. T (page 2011)
9. T (page 2011)
10. T (page 1998)

Short Answer

1. M: Medication overdose/noncompliance
   T: Tumor, trauma, toxins
   S: Seizures or stroke
   H: Hypoxia, hyperthermia/hypothermia, hyperglycemia/hypoglycemia, hypertensive crisis, hypovolemia, hyperkalemia/hypokalemia
   I: Infection and uremia
   P: Psychiatric or behavioral disorders (page 1984)
2. Karl Weick's "five-step process" for communicating intuitive decisions and obtaining feedback from team members includes:
   a. Here is what I think we are dealing with.
   b. Here is what I think we should do.
   c. Here is why.
   d. Here is what we should keep our eyes on.
   e. Now talk to me. Are there any other concerns? (page 1985)

Fill in the Table

1. The "H and T" questions of cardiac arrest (Table 40-2, page 1987)

Reversible Causes of Cardiac Arrest	Questions to Ask Your Team
Hypovolemia	Does this patient have any evidence of internal or external bleeding or fluid loss?
Hypoxia	How well is the patient oxygenating? Could there have been a respiratory event that led to this cardiac arrest?
Hydrogen ion (acidosis)	Is there any reason for metabolic or respiratory acidosis in this patient?
Hypokalemia/hyperkalemia	Does this patient undergo renal dialysis? Might the electrolytes be altered (ie, is the patient on a liquid diet)?
Hypothermia	Does the patient feel cold to touch? If so, obtain the core body temperature.
Hypoglycemic/hyperglycemic	Does the patient have diabetes? What is the blood glucose level?
Tension pneumothorax	Does the patient have bilateral breath sounds? Is the patient becoming difficult to ventilate? Consider the need for chest decompression.

Reversible Causes of Cardiac Arrest	Questions to Ask Your Team
Tamponade (cardiac)	Is there penetrating trauma to the patient's heart? Consider the need for pericardiocentesis or ultrasound (in the emergency department).
Toxins	Consider substance abuse (ie, narcotics or opiates). Consider naloxone (Narcan) intravenously/intramuscularly/intranasally.
Thrombosis (pulmonary)	Does the patient have a history of blood clots? Does the patient smoke and/or take birth control? Has the patient had a recent long-bone immobilization?
Thrombosis (coronary)	Does the patient have a large acute myocardial infarction developing? Is this patient a candidate for percutaneous coronary intervention (PCI)?
Trauma	Is there a mechanism of injury for life-threatening trauma?

2. Compensated versus decompensated shock (Table 40-4, page 1999)

Compensated Shock	Decompensated Shock
• Agitation, anxiety, restlessness • **Sense of impending doom** • Weak, rapid (thready) pulse • Clammy (cool, moist) skin • **Pallor with cyanotic lips** • **Shortness of breath** • Nausea, vomiting • Delayed capillary refill in infants and children • **Thirst** • **Normal blood pressure**	• Altered mental status (verbal to unresponsive)[a] • **Hypotension** • **Labored or irregular breathing** • Thready or absent peripheral pulses • Ashen, mottled, or cyanotic skin • **Dilated pupils** • Diminished urine output (oliguria) • **Impending cardiac arrest**

[a]Mental status changes are late indicators.

3. Types of shock (Table 40-7, page 2006)

Type of Shock	Examples of Potential Causes	Signs and Symptoms	Assessment and Treatment
Cardiogenic	Inadequate heart function Disease of muscle tissue Impaired electrical system Disease or injury	Chest pain Irregular pulse Weak pulse Low BP Cyanosis (lips, under nails) Cool, clammy, mottled, or flushed skin Anxiety Rales Pulmonary edema Hepatomegaly	**If lungs are clear and protocols allow, then administer a fluid challenge of 200 mL (to increase preload)** **Consider CPAP/BPAP**
Obstructive	Mechanical obstruction of the cardiac muscle causing a decrease in cardiac output 1. Tension pneumothorax 2. Cardiac tamponade	Dependent on cause: • Dyspnea • Rapid, weak pulse • Rapid, shallow breaths • Decreased lung compliance • Unilateral, decreased, or absent breath sounds • Decreased BP • JVD • Subcutaneous emphysema • Cyanosis • Tracheal deviation toward affected side • Beck triad (cardiac tamponade): – JVD – Narrowing pulse pressure – Muffled heart tones	**Dependent on cause:** • **Administer fluid at a KVO rate** • **Consider chest decompression (injured side for suspected tension pneumothorax)** • **Consider immediate transport for pericardiocentesis for cardiac tamponade (a procedure that is NOT done in the field)**
Septic	Severe bacterial infection	Warm, unstable skin temperatures Tachycardia Low BP	**Administer fluid boluses to maintain radial pulses** **Consider sepsis alert program if protocol exists in your region** **Consider medications depending on the existence of warm versus cold shock**
Neurogenic	Cervical or thoracic spinal cord injury, which causes widespread blood vessel dilation	Bradycardia (slow pulse) or normal pulse Low BP Signs of neck injury	**Administer warmed IV fluids to maintain radial pulses** **Consider vasopressors, steroids, or vagal blocker per local protocols**
Anaphylactic	Extreme life-threatening allergic reaction	Develop within seconds Mild itching or rash Burning skin Vascular dilation Generalized edema Coma Rapid death	**Determine cause of anaphylaxis** **Administer epinephrine IM or a vasopressor** **Administer fluid at a KVO rate** **Consider bronchodilator or antihistamine**

Type of Shock	Examples of Potential Causes	Signs and Symptoms	Assessment and Treatment
Psychogenic (fainting)	Temporary, generalized vascular dilation Anxiety, bad news, sight of injury or blood, prospect of medical treatment, severe pain, illness, tiredness	Rapid pulse Normal or low BP	**Determine duration of unresponsiveness** **Suspect head injury if patient is confused or slow to respond**
Hypovolemic	Blood or fluid loss	Rapid, weak pulse Low BP Change in mental status Cyanosis (lips, nail beds) Cool, clammy skin Increased respiratory rate	**Control external bleeding** **Provide fluid resuscitation en route** **After initial fluid resuscitation, consider use of vasopressors to maintain the BP**
Respiratory insufficiency	Severe chest injury, airway obstruction	Rapid, weak pulse Low BP Change in mental status Cyanosis (lips, nail beds) Cool, clammy skin Increased respiratory rate	**Seal hole in chest** **Stabilize impaled objects** **Assure adequate ventilation; consider positive pressure ventilation** **Administer fluid at a KVO rate**

Abbreviations: BP, blood pressure; CPAP/BPAP, continuous positive airway pressure/bilevel positive airway pressure; IM, intramuscularly; JVD, jugular venous distention; KVO, keep vein open.

Section 9: Special Patient Populations

Chapter 41: Obstetrics

Matching

Part I

1. X (page 2027)
2. W (page 2052)
3. V (page 2028)
4. U (page 2040)
5. T (page 2043)
6. L (page 2039)
7. K (page 2027)
8. J (page 2053)
9. I (page 2054)
10. H (page 2043)
11. E (page 2029)
12. D (page 2053)
13. C (page 2029)
14. B (page 20432)
15. A (page 2040)
16. F (page 2048)
17. G (page 2028)
18. Z (page 2027)
19. Y (page 2043)
20. S (page 2042)
21. R (page 2037)
22. Q (page 2039)
23. P (page 2034)
24. O (page 2027)
25. N (page 2041)
26. M (page 2037)

Part II

1. N (page 2052)
2. M (page 2049)
3. L (page 2043)
4. K (page 2043)
5. J (page 2027)
6. T (page 2027)
7. S (page 2030)
8. R (page 2027)
9. Q (page 2055)
10. P (page 2027)
11. Z (page 2055)
12. Y (page 2030)
13. X (page 2037)
14. W (page 2031)
15. V (page 2042)
16. O (page 2041)
17. U (page 2027)
18. I (page 2041)
19. H (page 2041)
20. G (page 2038)
21. F (page 2053)
22. B (page 2029)
23. C (page 2030)
24. D (page 2040)
25. E (page 2039)
26. A (page 2037)

Part III

1. N (page 2056)
2. M (page 2027)
3. L (page 2028)
4. K (page 2054)
5. E (page 2040)
6. D (page 2054)
7. C (page 2041)
8. B (page 2043–2044)
9. H (page 2040)
10. G (page 2044)
11. F (page 2036)
12. A (page 2038)
13. J (page 2039)
14. I (page 2039)

Multiple Choice

1. A (page 2040)
2. D (page 2042)
3. A (page 2032)
4. C (pages 2043–2044)
5. B (page 2048)
6. D (page 2049)
7. A (page 2050)
8. B (page 2039)
9. C (page 2029)
10. A (page 2031)

Labeling

1. Structures of the pregnant uterus (page 2029, Figure 41-2)
   - **A.** Placenta
   - **B.** Umbilical cord
   - **C.** Amniotic cavity
   - **D.** Uterus
   - **E.** Lumen of uterus

Fill in the Blank

1. amniotic sac (page 2029)
2. increases (page 2031)
3. increases (page 2031)
4. Gestational hypertension (page 2037)
5. habitual abortions (page 2040)
6. Placenta previa (page 2042)
7. abruptio placenta (page 2042)
8. first stage (page 2043)
9. transverse (page 2054)
10. Magnesium sulfate (page 2049)

Identify

1. Chief complaint: "I am bleeding from my vagina."
2. Vital signs: Pulse is 110 beats/min and thready, respirations are 24 breaths/min, blood pressure (BP) is 100/70 mm Hg, and the patient is pale and diaphoretic.
3. Pertinent findings: Patient is 35 years old, in her third trimester, multiparity with previous cesarean sections. The blood is bright red; she is painless and thirsty and says she is weak. The vital signs and physical examination reveal signs of shock.

Complete the Patient Care Report (PCR)

Show the completed PCR to your instructor to obtain feedback on your completion of the form.

Ambulance Calls

1. a. The 22-year-old who has passed blood and tissue through the vagina and is showing signs of hemorrhagic shock is most likely having an **incomplete** abortion (answer C). The passage of tissue indicates some sort of abortion, and the fact that she is continuing to bleed suggests there is still tissue in the uterus. (page 2040)
   b. She should be treated for shock because her vital signs indicate that she is already in shock:
      (1) Keep the woman recumbent, lying on her left side.
      (2) Administer 100% supplemental oxygen via nonrebreathing mask at 15 L/min.
      (3) Provide rapid transport to a definitive care facility, notifying the facility of the patient's condition en route.
      (4) Start an IV lifeline of normal saline with a large-bore IV catheter. Infuse at a rate necessary to maintain BP. An additional IV lifeline may be indicated.
      (5) Establish an electrocardiogram (ECG) and obtain baseline vital signs. Do not attempt to examine the woman internally or pack the vagina with trauma pads.
      (6) Use loosely placed trauma pads over the vagina in an effort to staunch bleeding.
      (7) Collect all products of conception that need to be collected and presented to the ED. (page 2041)
2. a. The 32-year-old woman has good reason to be "feeling poorly": She is carrying a dead fetus in her uterus; that is, she has a **missed** abortion (answer D). Her history is typical: a threatened abortion earlier in the pregnancy that seemed to get better, but failure of the pregnancy to develop normally. By 6 months, her uterine fundus should be palpable above the umbilicus, just barely above the pelvic brim. (page 2041)
   b. The prehospital management of missed abortion is simply to transport the patient to the hospital while providing emotional support. At the hospital, surgical evacuation of the uterus will be required. (page 2041)
3. a. The primigravida with painless vaginal bleeding is experiencing a **threatened** abortion (answer A). The absence of contractions indicates that the abortion is not yet inevitable. (page 2040)
   b. The prehospital treatment of threatened abortion is simply to transport while providing emotional support to the patient. (page 2041)
4. a. The 16-year-old who went to the backstreet abortionist has suffered one of the most common results: **septic** abortion (answer E). This patient already has signs of septic shock, and she may die. (page 2041)
   b. The prehospital management is to treat for shock:
      (1) Keep the woman recumbent, lying on her left side.
      (2) Administer 100% supplemental oxygen via nonrebreathing mask at 15 L/min.
      (3) Provide rapid transport to a definitive care facility, notifying the facility of the patient's condition en route.
      (4) Start an IV lifeline of normal saline with a large-bore IV catheter. Infuse at a rate necessary to maintain BP. An additional IV lifeline may be indicated.
      (5) Establish an ECG and obtain baseline vital signs. Do not attempt to examine the woman internally or pack the vagina with trauma pads.
      (6) Use loosely placed trauma pads over the vagina in an effort to staunch bleeding. (page 2041)
5. a. The 26-year-old veteran of three previous miscarriages is probably correct; she seems to be having yet another miscarriage—that is, an **imminent** abortion (answer B). The severe cramping and uterine contractions that accompany her vaginal bleeding bode ill for the continuation of the pregnancy. (page 2041)
   b. The prehospital treatment of imminent abortion is expectant treatment for shock:
      (1) Keep the woman recumbent, lying on her left side.
      (2) Administer 100% supplemental oxygen via nonrebreathing mask at 15 L/min.
      (3) Provide rapid transport to a definitive care facility, notifying the facility of the patient's condition en route.

(4) Start an IV lifeline of normal saline with a large-bore IV catheter. Infuse at a rate necessary to maintain BP. An additional IV lifeline may be indicated.
(5) Establish an ECG and obtain baseline vital signs. Do not attempt to examine the woman internally or pack the vagina with trauma pads. (page 2041)

6. This case concerns a 36-year-old grand multipara with third-trimester bleeding.
a. Three possible causes of third-trimester bleeding are:
(1) Abruptio placenta
(2) Placenta previa
(3) Uterine rupture (pages 2042–2043)
b. In this particular case, the most likely diagnosis is **placenta previa**. (page 2042)
c. Among the characteristic features of placenta previa manifested by this patient are the following:
(1) *Painless* vaginal bleeding. (There is severe pain with placental abruption or uterine rupture.)
(2) *Bright red* blood. (In abruption, bleeding is dark.)
(3) The *fetus remains viable.*
(4) The *abdomen* is *soft and nontender.* (page 2043)
d. The steps in prehospital management are (page 2043):
(1) Keep the woman recumbent, lying on her left side.
(2) Administer 100% supplemental oxygen via nonrebreathing mask at 15 L/min.
(3) Provide rapid transport to a definitive care facility, notifying the facility of the patient's condition en route.
(4) Start an IV lifeline of normal saline with a large-bore IV catheter. Infuse at a rate necessary to maintain BP. An additional IV lifeline may be indicated.
(5) Establish an ECG and obtain baseline vital signs. Do not attempt to examine the woman internally or pack the vagina with trauma pads.
(6) Use loosely placed trauma pads over the vagina in an effort to staunch bleeding. (page 2043)

7. a. The woman with the fainting spells is most probably suffering from **supine hypotensive syndrome** (answer E) because her pulse and BP improved very quickly after she turned to her side and took the weight of her uterus off her inferior vena cava. Nonetheless, you cannot take the chance of missing a concealed hemorrhage. Women whose volume status is already marginal are most vulnerable to supine hypotensive syndrome, so you will have to treat this patient as someone who might develop hemorrhagic shock. (page 2036)
b. The prehospital management is as follows:
(1) Administer supplemental oxygen.
(2) Keep the patient in the recumbent position, with the bulk of her uterus to the side to avoid vena cava syndrome.
(3) Start an IV with saline.
(4) Transport to the hospital as soon as possible.
(5) Obtain an ECG. (page 2036)

8. a. The woman who fell in a downtown department store has a chief complaint unrelated to her pregnancy—a twisted ankle. The careful examination reveals a very serious problem that is related to her pregnancy—**preeclampsia** (answer B), as manifested by edema and hypertension. (page 2037)
b. The initial prehospital treatment is as follows:
(1) Splint the injured ankle.
(2) Transport the woman in semi-Fowler position (as long as this does not cause any dizziness).
(3) Start an IV line en route so that it will be there if you need it. Pain medications should be discussed with medical control before being administered.
c. You did need that IV line—when the woman proceeded to have a grand mal seizure and develop full-blown eclampsia. The steps to take at that point are:
(1) Protect the patient from injury during the tonic–clonic phase of the seizure.
(2) Ensure an adequate airway.
(3) Administer supplemental oxygen.
(4) Contact medical control for orders. You may be asked to give magnesium sulfate 10%, 2–4 g IV.
(5) Notify the receiving hospital. If the woman's seizures cannot be controlled, it may be necessary to take her straight to the operating room for an emergency cesarean section. (page 2037)

9. When *two* pregnant women are involved in a motor vehicle crash, the responders face quadruple trouble!

a. Some of the changes during pregnancy that make a woman more vulnerable to injury or that affect her response to injury include the following *(students should list five)*:

(1) Elevation of the diaphragm effectively pushes the abdominal contents into the chest so that abdominal organs are more apt to be injured after a blow to the chest.

(2) Forward, upward displacement of the bladder renders it more vulnerable to injury.

(3) The uterus becomes more susceptible to injury as it enlarges and occupies more space in the abdomen.

(4) Vascular volume may increase by as much as 50%, so the pregnant woman can lose a lot of blood (and the fetus can be in big trouble) before she shows signs of shock.

(5) Relative tachycardia and hypotension make it difficult to interpret the pregnant woman's vital signs after injury.

(6) Redistribution of blood flow to the pelvic area means that a pregnant woman will bleed much more profusely from injuries such as pelvic fracture.

(7) Delayed gastric emptying during pregnancy makes a pregnant woman more likely to vomit and aspirate after injury. (pages 2058–2059)

b. You find the *driver* of the car conscious but with evidence of steering wheel trauma to the abdomen and indications of impending shock (thirst, tachycardia, slight hypotension). She must be treated for shock and regarded as a load-and-go emergency:

(1) Ensure an adequate airway.

(2) Administer oxygen by nonrebreathing mask if the patient is responsive.

(3) Assist ventilations as needed, and provide a higher minute volume than usual.

(4) Control external bleeding promptly. Splint any fractures.

(5) Start one or two IV lines of normal saline. Use large-bore catheters and microdrip sets. Administer a bolus if signs and symptoms of hemodynamic compromise are present, with the goal of maintaining BP. Remember that a larger volume of fluid is necessary for the pregnant patient.

(6) Notify the receiving hospital of the patient's status. Also indicate your estimated time of arrival (ETA).

(7) Transport the woman in the lateral recumbent position. If she is on a backboard, tilt the backboard 30 degrees to the left by wedging pillows beneath it. This will cause the uterus to shift, taking the weight off the inferior vena cava and improving venous return to the heart. (pages 2058–2059)

c. The pregnant *passenger* does not seem to be seriously injured, although her complaints of neck pain ("whiplash") should prompt appropriate measures to stabilize the cervical spine. In any case, you cannot conclude that there is no injury to the fetus. Only careful evaluation in the hospital, and observation over several hours, can establish that fact. (page 2059)

10. Deciding whether you have time to transport a woman in active labor to the hospital is a judgment call, and there is room for debate in some of these situations. As a general rule, you will have a lot more time with nulliparas. Multiparas can progress very rapidly through labor, so the margin for error is smaller. (page 2044)

a. D. The urge to move the bowels indicates that the fetal head is already in the birth canal and delivery is imminent. The delivery may be complicated by fetal infection because the amniotic sac ruptured several hours ago.

b. D. As a general rule, when a woman who has had eight babies tells you that the baby is coming, she knows what she is talking about! Complications seen more commonly in grand multiparas include uterine rupture and postpartum hemorrhage.

c. T. In this case, you should have plenty of time. The woman is a beginner, and her contractions are still quite widely spaced. Make sure to obtain a full set of vital signs, as there is always a potential for complications.

d. D. No doubts here: The woman is crowning! If she has had two previous cesarean sections, she could be at increased risk for uterine rupture during labor. Also, you have to inquire why she needed the cesarean sections in the first place (eg, fetus in the wrong position, very large fetus, late delivery date).

e. T. This woman may not even be in labor. Her contractions sound suspiciously like Braxton-Hicks contractions. If you sit around waiting for her to deliver, you might spend several weeks at the scene! Although this is not a complication, it is a consideration in this case.

f. D. With the contractions coming at only 2-minute intervals in a multipara, you cannot afford to take a chance. The potential complications more likely in a twin birth include cord prolapse, breech presentation, and postpartum hemorrhage. The babies are also likely to be small and to require the kind of special care given to premature babies.

11. Science has not yet established the precise mechanism that stimulates a woman to go into labor, but any experienced emergency medical technician (EMT) or paramedic can attest to the fact that one thing that can stimulate labor is shopping! That is why paramedics frequently find themselves delivering babies in department stores.

- **a.** When the baby's face is found to be covered by the intact amniotic sac, you should tear open the amniotic sac, either with your fingers or a forceps, and carefully peel it away from the baby's face. Then, suction the baby's nostrils and mouth with a bulb aspirator. (page 2047)
- **b.** When the umbilical cord is found *tightly* wound around the baby's neck, the only thing you can do is put two clamps on the cord, 2 inches apart, and cut the cord between the clamps. (page 2055)
- **c.** The steps to take from that point on are as follows:
  - (1) Guide the baby's head downward to allow delivery of the upper shoulder.
  - (2) Guide the baby's head upward to allow delivery of the lower shoulder.
  - (3) Wipe the baby's mouth and nose free of blood and mucus, and suction out the mouth and nostrils again.
  - (4) Tell the mother and all the salespersons in the lingerie department if the newborn is a boy or a girl.
  - (5) Dry the baby, cover it with a blanket, and put it on the mother's abdomen.
  - (6) Record the time of birth and the Apgar score while you await the delivery of the placenta.
  - (7) When the placenta separates, instruct the mother to bear down.
  - (8) *After the placenta has delivered*, massage the uterus, and put the baby to the mother's breast.
  - (9) Clean up, put a sanitary pad between the mother's legs, bid farewell to the women in the lingerie department, and transport the patient. (page 2047)

12.
- **a.** You are dealing with a breech presentation. That smooth presenting part with a crack down the middle is the buttocks, not a head! (page 2054)
- **b.** Management is as follows:
  - (1) Position the mother with her buttocks at the edge of the bed or stretcher and her legs flexed.
  - (2) Allow the buttocks and trunk of the baby to deliver spontaneously. *Do not pull on the baby.*
  - (3) Once the baby's legs are clear, support the baby's body on the palm of your hand and volar surface of your arm.
  - (4) Lower the baby slightly so that it very nearly hangs by its own weight downward; that will help the head pass through the pelvic outlet. You can tell when the head is in the vaginal canal because you will be able to see the baby's hairline at the nape of its neck just below the mother's symphysis pubis.
  - (5) When you can see the baby's hairline, grasp the baby by the ankles and lift it upward in the direction of the mother's abdomen. The head should then deliver without difficulty.
  - (6) If the baby's head does not deliver in 3 minutes, the baby is in danger of suffocation, and immediate action is indicated. Suffocation may occur when the baby's umbilical cord is compressed by its head against the birth canal, which cuts off the baby's supply of oxygenated blood from the placenta, and the baby's face is pressed against the vaginal wall, which prevents it from breathing on its own. Place your gloved hand in the vagina, with your palm toward the baby's face. Form a V with your fingers on either side of the baby's nose, and push the vaginal wall away from the baby's face until the head is delivered.
  - (7) Do not attempt to pull the baby out forcibly or allow an explosive delivery. If the head does not deliver within 3 minutes of establishing the airway, provide rapid transport to the hospital, with the mother's buttocks elevated on pillows. If at all possible, try to maintain the baby's airway throughout transport in the manner described. En route, alert the hospital so that it can have the appropriate personnel on hand when the mother arrives. (page 2054)

13. Prolapsed umbilical cord occurs in only about 1 of every 300 deliveries, but it is more likely with a premature birth. You must do the following:

- **a.** Position the woman supine with her hips elevated as much as possible on pillows.
- **b.** Administer 100% supplemental oxygen via a nonrebreathing mask.
- **c.** Instruct the woman to pant with each contraction, which will prevent her from bearing down.
- **d.** With two fingers of a gloved hand, gently *push the presenting part* (not the cord) back up into the vagina until it no longer presses on the cord.
- **e.** While you maintain pressure on the presenting part, have your partner cover the exposed portion of the cord with dressings moistened in warmed normal saline.
- **f.** Try to maintain that position, with a gloved hand pushing the presenting part away from the cord, throughout urgent transport to the hospital. (page 2055)

14.
- **a.** The special measures required in delivering twins, as opposed to a single birth, are:
  - (1) Wait for the second birth after the first is complete. Meanwhile, keep the first baby warm on the mother's abdomen, covered with a blanket.
  - (2) Treat both babies as you would premature newborns, paying scrupulous attention to their warmth, prevention of bleeding, and protection from contamination. (page 2052)

b. The mother's risk factor for postpartum hemorrhage is the very fact of her twin pregnancy. The placenta covers a larger area in a twin pregnancy, and the uterine muscles become overstretched, so they contract less efficiently. (page 2052)

c. Other risk factors for postpartum hemorrhage include *(students should list three of the following)*:
   (1) Prolonged labor
   (2) Retained products of conception
   (3) Grand multiparity
   (4) Multiple pregnancy
   (5) Placenta previa
   (6) A full bladder
   (7) Lacerations
   (8) Uterine atony (page 2056)

d. The steps that should be taken to manage postpartum hemorrhage in the field are as follows:
   (1) Continue uterine massage.
   (2) Put either or both babies to the breast to start nursing.
   (3) Contact medical control to consider administration of oxytocin.
   (4) Begin transport, and notify the receiving hospital.
   (5) Start another IV with a large-bore catheter to infuse crystalloid rapidly.
   (6) Manage external bleeding from perinatal tears with a sanitary napkin and direct pressure. (page 2056)

True/False

1. F (page 2044)
2. T (page 2036)
3. F (page 2045)
4. T (page 2046)
5. F (page 2048)
6. F (page 2048)
7. T (page 2054)

Short Answer

1. Fetal alcohol syndrome classically requires the following three abnormalities:
   a. Poor growth
   b. Facial abnormalities
   c. Central nervous system abnormalities (page 2029)

Fill in the Table

1. (page 2044, Table 41-2)

The Stages of Labor: Nullipara Versus Multipara		
Stages of Labor	**Nullipara**	**Multipara**
First stage	**8 to 12 h**	**6 to 8 h**
Second stage	**1 to 2 h**	**30 min**
Third stage	**5 to 60 min**	**5 to 60 min**

2. (page 2034, Table 41-1)

False Labor Versus True Labor		
Parameter	**True Labor**	**False Labor**
Contractions	**Regularly spaced**	Irregularly spaced
Interval between contractions	Gradually shortens	**Remains long**
Intensity of contractions	**Gradually increases**	Stays the same
Effects of analgesics	Do not abolish the pain	**Often abolish the pain**
Cervical changes	**Progressive effacement and dilation**	No changes

Chapter 42: Neonatal Care

Matching

Part I

1. H (page 2080)
2. G (page 2080)
3. F (pages 2078–2079)
4. E (page 2076)
5. X (page 2099)
6. W (page 2095)
7. V (page 2095)
8. U (page 2095)
9. T (pages 2094–2095)
10. D (page 2100)
11. C (page 2072)
12. B (page 2075)
13. O (page 2076)
14. A (page 2076)
15. I (page 2101)
16. N (page 2071)
17. M (page 2071)
18. L (pages 2098–2099)
19. K (page 2081)
20. J (page 2099)
21. S (page 2092)
22. R (page 2094)
23. Q (page 2102)
24. P (page 2071)

Part II

1. G (page 2101)
2. F (page 2109)
3. E (page 2070)
4. A (page 2095)
5. N (page 2076)
6. M (page 2071)
7. L (page 2109)
8. K (page 2074)
9. J (page 2109)
10. C (page 2092)
11. D (page 2070)
12. Z (page 2102)
13. Y (page 2071)
14. X (page 2094)
15. W (page 2087)
16. V (page 2091)
17. P (page 2071)
18. O (page 2070)
19. H (page 2079)
20. I (page 2079)
21. B (page 2071)
22. U (page 2101)
23. T (page 2098)
24. S (page 2071)
25. R (page 2098)
26. Q (page 2087)

Multiple Choice

1. D (page 2071)
2. A (page 2071)
3. C (page 2075)
4. C (page 2077)
5. D (page 2088)
6. A (page 2102)
7. D (page 2094)
8. C (page 2089)
9. A (page 2087)
10. D (page 2080)

Fill in the Blank

1. shunts; foramen ovale (page 2071)
2. acrocyanosis (page 2076)
3. term (page 2076)
4. Pierre Robin (page 2079)
5. 40; 60; hypocapnia; pneumothorax (page 2080)
6. obstruction; choanal atresia (page 2078)
7. decompression; orogastric; diaphragmatic (page 2081)
8. seizure; newborn (pages 2091–2092)
9. Malrotation (page 2095)
10. resuscitation; fontanelle (page 2094)
11. clavicle (page 2099)
12. viral infection (page 2095)

Identify

1. a. The five types of seizures:
   (1) Subtle seizure
   (2) Clonic seizure
   (3) Tonic seizure
   (4) Spasms
   (5) Myoclonic seizure (page 2092)

   b. From the mother's description, this was most likely a multifocal clonic seizure.
2. a. If the baby is apneic (ie, has a 20-second or longer respiratory pause) or has a pulse rate less than 100 beats/min after 30 seconds of drying and stimulation and supplemental free-flow (blow-by) oxygen:
   (1) Begin PPV by bag-mask device, being sure to use a newborn-sized bag mask.
   (2) Use caution when squeezing the bag to avoid inadvertently delivering too much volume, potentially resulting in a pneumothorax. (page 2076)

b. Chest compressions are indicated if the pulse rate remains less than 60 beats/min despite positioning, clearing the airway, drying and stimulation, and 30 seconds of effective PPV:

(1) With the thumb (two-rescuer) technique, two thumbs are placed side by side over the sternum between the nipples, and the hands encircle the torso. With the two-finger (one-rescuer) technique, the tips of the index and middle fingers are placed over the sternum between the nipples and the sternum is compressed between the fingers and a hand behind the baby's back.

(2) The depth of compression is one-third of the anteroposterior diameter of the chest. Your fingers should remain in contact with the chest at all times but allow full chest recoil.

(3) In neonates, the chest compressions occur in synchrony with artificial ventilation, which you continue during chest compressions. (pages 2083–2084)

Ambulance Calls

1. If you were expecting problems in delivering this 38-year-old multipara, you were right. So be prepared! (page 2073)

a. Equipment categories to be prepared for newborn resuscitation would include:

(1) Suction equipment
(2) Ventilation equipment
(3) Intubation equipment
(4) Medications
(5) Umbilical vessel catheterization equipment
(6) Miscellaneous

b. When the baby's head delivers and is found to be covered with meconium:

(1) Clean the mouth and nostrils with sterile gauze.
(2) Use a bulb aspirator to suction the mouth and nostrils only if needed. (page 2088)

c. The initial Apgar score would be:

(A) = 0
(P) = 1
(G) = 0
(A) = 0
(R) = 1
Total = 3 (page 2075)

d. Steps in the neonatal resuscitation pyramid, from top to bottom, include:

(1) Warm, dry, position, suction, stimulate
(2) Oxygen
(3) Establish effective ventilation: bag mask or endotracheal (ET) tube.
(4) Chest compressions
(5) Medications (page 2077)

2. *Return of the Spider Monster* is not recommended viewing for an impressionable woman in the third trimester of pregnancy. Look what can happen!

a. When you find yourself holding a premature newborn infant who had the temerity to be born before you could even open your OB kit, take the following steps:

(1) Suction the mouth and nostrils with a bulb syringe.
(2) Quickly dry the baby with whatever you have available.
(3) As soon as possible, wrap the baby in something warm.
(4) When your partner brings the OB kit, clamp and cut the cord. (page 2074)

b. Hypothermia represents an increased risk for morbidity and mortality. However, if the newborn appears otherwise healthy, it is appropriate to clamp and cut the cord. It may also be necessary to cut and clamp the cord to resuscitate in the prehospital setting. (page 2074)

c. To prevent the baby from becoming hypothermic, take the following steps:

(1) Dry the baby thoroughly.
(2) Place a cap on the baby's head.
(3) Cover the baby with a warm blanket.
(4) Keep the baby on the mother's body.
(5) In the ambulance, turn on the heaters full blast until the ambient temperature increases to approximately 35°C (95°F), even if it's summer. (pages 2074–2075)

3. Do you suspect this case is exaggerated—that teenage girls don't give birth on the toilet? In fact, this scenario is based on an actual case managed by real paramedics.
   a. Immediately upon rescuing the infant from the toilet, you must do the following:
      (1) Dry off the baby, preferably with warm towels, and cover with a warm blanket.
      (2) Suction the mouth and nostrils.
      (3) Stimulate the baby to breathe.
      (4) Clamp and cut the umbilical cord.
      (5) Administer supplemental oxygen. (pages 2071–2075)
   b. The indications for starting artificial ventilation are as follows:
      (1) Apnea
      (2) Heart rate less than 100 beats/min
      (3) Persistent central cyanosis despite 100% supplemental oxygen (page 2076)
   c. After a minute of artificial ventilation, you find the heart rate to be 84 beats/min. You should continue artificial ventilation only. (page 2076)
   d. When you check again, the pulse rate has dropped below 60 beats/min. At that point, you should start external chest compressions at 120 per minute. (page 2076)
   e. The indications for epinephrine are a heart rate persistently less than 60 beats/min despite adequate artificial ventilation with 100% supplemental oxygen and high-quality external chest compressions. (page 2076)

True/False

1. T (page 2074)
2. F (page 2080)
3. F (page 2090)
4. T (page 2084)
5. T (page 2097)
6. F (page 2077)
7. F (page 2084)
8. T (page 2090)
9. T (page 2095)
10. F (page 2088)

Short Answer

1. Catheterization of the umbilical vein (pages 2084–2085)
   a. Clean the cord with alcohol or another antiseptic. Place a sterile tie firmly, but not too tightly, around the base of the cord to control bleeding. Place a sterile drape over the site. Maintain sterile technique as much as possible.
   b. Prefill a sterile 3.5F to 5F umbilical vein line catheter (a comparable-size sterile feeding tube can be used in an emergency) with normal saline using a 3-mL syringe.
   c. Cut the cord with a scalpel below the clamp placed on the cord at birth about 1 to 2 cm from the skin (between the clamp and the cord tie).
   d. The umbilical vein is a large, thin-walled vessel usually found at the 12 o'clock position, as compared to the two thick-walled umbilical arteries usually found at 4 and 8 o'clock. Insert the catheter into this vein for a distance of 2 to 4 cm (less in preterm infants) until blood can be aspirated. If the catheter is advanced into the liver, the infusion of hypertonic solutions may lead to irreversible damage. If the catheter is advanced into the heart, dysrhythmias may develop.
   e. Flush the catheter with 0.5 mL of normal saline and tape it in place.
2. Intubate a neonate (page 2082)
   a. Be sure the newborn is preoxygenated by bag-mask ventilation with 100% supplemental oxygen prior to making an intubation attempt.
   b. Suction the oropharynx to remove any secretions.
   c. Place the laryngoscope blade in the oropharynx, and then visualize the vocal cords. Place the ET tube between the vocal cords until the black line on the tube is at the level of the cords.
   d. Confirm ET tube placement.
   e. Tape the ET tube in place.

Fill in the Table

1. (page 2092, Table 42-9)

Causes of Neonatal Seizures
• Hypoxic-ischemic encephalopathy
• **Intracranial infections (meningitis)**
• **Hypoglycemia**
• **Other metabolic disturbances**
• **Epileptic syndromes**
• **Intracranial hemorrhage**
• Development defects
• Hypocalcemia
• **Meningitis**
• **Encephalopathy**
• **Drug withdrawal**

Problem Solving

1. The Apgar score is 4.
2. The Apgar score is 13. (page 2075)

Chapter 43: Pediatric Emergencies

Matching

Part I

1. E (pages 2118–2120)
2. A
3. D
4. B
5. A, B
6. D, E
7. A
8. A, B, C, D, E
9. E
10. A, B, C, D, E
11. D
12. B
13. A
14. E
15. D

Part II

1. G (page 2143)
2. F (page 2187)
3. E (page 2147)
4. Z (page 2176)
5. Y (page 2176)
6. X (page 2166)
7. U (page 2127)
8. T (page 2168)
9. S (page 2194)
10. D (page 2141)
11. C (page 2129)
12. B (page 2168)
13. W (page 2170)
14. V (page 2178)
15. R (page 2141)
16. Q (page 2166)
17. P (page 2144)
18. A (page 2183)
19. J (page 2183)
20. K (page 2184)
21. L (page 2168)
22. H (page 2144)
23. I (page 2194)
24. O (page 2140)
25. N (page 2176)
26. M (page 2168)

Part III

1. J (page 2176)
2. I (page 2124)
3. H (page 2169)
4. G (page 2183)
5. Z (page 2168)
6. Y (page 2168)
7. X (page 2178)
8. W (page 2170)
9. R (page 2137)
10. Q (page 2173)
11. P (page 2170)
12. O (page 2144)
13. F (pages 2165–2166)
14. E (page 2128)
15. D (page 2169)
16. C (page 2173)
17. V (page 2128)
18. U (page 2143)
19. T (page 2137)
20. S (page 2137)
21. B (page 2173)
22. A (page 2173)
23. N (page 2170)
24. M (page 2144)
25. L (page 2126)
26. K (page 2168)

Multiple Choice

1. C (page 2184)
2. C (page 2187)
3. D (page 2124)
4. D (page 2126)
5. B (page 2127)
6. D (page 2128)
7. A (page 2133)
8. D (pages 2193–2195)
9. C (page 2195)
10. C (pages 2145–2147)
11. C (page 2183)
12. D (page 2184)
13. A (page 2184)
14. D (pages 2184–2185)
15. D (pages 2184–2185)

Labeling

(page 2154, Figure 43–16)

A. Earlobe
B. Xiphoid process
C. Costal margin

Fill in the Blank

1. tolerated; oropharyngeal (page 2146)
2. blow-by technique (page 2147)
3. ventilation; airway management (page 2148)
4. teeth; aspiration (page 2150)
5. bradycardia; pulse oximeter (page 2151)
6. hypovolemic; distributive; cardiogenic (page 2156)
7. hypovolemic; tachypnea; mottled (page 2156)
8. mucous membranes; turgor; delayed (page 2156)
9. compartment syndrome; injury; infection (page 2158)
10. congenital; rhythm (page 2160)
11. cardiopulmonary; monitor (page 2164)
12. SIDS (page 2186)

Identify

1. **a.** Chief complaint: Respiratory distress (probably the croup).
   b. Vital signs: Normal capillary refill, oxygen saturation of 95%, conscious and alert, audible stridor.
   c. Pertinent negatives: Age-appropriate behavior, recognizes her mother.
2. **a.** Chief complaint: Infant unrestrained and ejected during fatal motor vehicle crash.
   b. Vital signs: Age-appropriate level of consciousness (LOC), skin color normal, skin is warm and dry. Normal capillary refill, oxygen saturation of 96%, pulse rate of 150 beats/min.
   c. Pertinent negatives: No obvious external bleeding; assessment is unremarkable.
3. **a.** Chief complaint: Seizure, probably a febrile seizure.
   b. Vital signs: Skin ashen, warm, and dry. A rectal temperature of 100.3°F. Patient responds to pain. Her oxygen saturation is 98%. Pupils are sluggish but equal. Patient has equal bilateral breath sounds. The remainder of the exam is unremarkable.
   c. Pertinent negatives: The patient's mother denies any other medications, history, or allergies to medications. She further denies any recent injury or trauma to the child.

Complete the Patient Care Report (PCR)

Show the completed PCR to your instructor to obtain feedback on your completion of the form.

Ambulance Calls

1. The scene of a collision where a child has been injured is probably the most stressful environment that a paramedic will enter.
   a. (1) Fracture of the left femur
   (2) Ruptured spleen
   (3) Injury to the right side of the head
   b. Perhaps the most challenging element to deal with at a collision scene like the one described is the feelings and behaviors of the child's parents.
   (1) Obviously, there is no "correct" answer to the question of how you feel when assaulted by an angry parent. The average paramedic, however, will probably feel angry.
   (2) What you do with your feelings is another matter, and there is a correct way to handle the situation and an incorrect way. The correct way is as follows:
   (a) Mentally count to 10 before you reply to the angry father.
   (b) Stay calm.
   (c) Don't raise your voice.
   (d) Try to enlist the father's help in caring for the child; give him something constructive to do, such as fetching the backboard from the ambulance or folding triangular bandages into cravats.
   c. The child's vital signs are normal for his age (answer 3). The slight tachycardia is easily explained by the pain and excitement of the situation.
2. When 2-year-old Tammy starts barking in the middle of the night, it's a great attention-getter.
   a. The vital signs are abnormal for her age. There is tachycardia and tachypnea.
   b. The most likely diagnosis is croup. (pages 2140–2141)
   c. The steps of prehospital management are as follows:
   (1) Give humidified supplemental oxygen while you set up a nebulizer.
   (2) Nebulized epinephrine is available in two formulations: racemic epinephrine and L-epinephrine. The dose for racemic epinephrine (2.25%) is 0.5 mL mixed in 3 mL of normal saline. The dose for L-epinephrine is 0.25 to 0.5 mg/kg of the 1 mg/mL (1:1,000) solution (maximum, 5 mg/dose); this form can be diluted with normal saline to bring the volume to 3 mL. (page 2141)
   (3) Place the child in a position of comfort.
   (4) Notify the receiving hospital of the case.
   (5) Transport without delay.
3. Diffuse wheezing and respiratory distress in a child under 1 year of age are the tip-offs in this case.
   a. The vital signs are abnormal. The baby has tachycardia, tachypnea, and a slight elevation in BP. (page 2135)
   b. The most likely diagnosis is bronchiolitis. (pages 2143–2144)

c. The steps of prehospital management are as follows:
   (1) Give humidified oxygen.
   (2) Assist ventilations gently with a bag-mask ventilator.
   (3) Consult medical command as to whether to give a trial of bronchodilators.
   (4) Keep the intubation kit handy in case of apnea.
   (5) Monitor cardiac rhythm.
   (6) Transport without delay. (pages 2143–2144)

4. a. When little Bobby develops severe respiratory distress and signs of airway obstruction over a very short time, and he does not have a high fever, the most likely diagnosis is foreign body obstruction of the airway—that is, choking.

b. The steps of managing a choking child are as follows:
   (1) Kneel on one knee behind the child, and circle his or her body by placing both arms around the child's chest. Prepare to give abdominal thrusts by placing your fist just above the patient's umbilicus and well below the xiphoid process. Place your other hand over that fist.
   (2) Give the child rapid, distinct abdominal thrusts in an upward direction. Be careful to avoid applying force to the lower rib cage or sternum.
   (3) Repeat this standing technique until the child expels the foreign body or becomes unresponsive.
   (4) If the child becomes unresponsive, place him or her supine on a firm, flat surface and inspect the airway using the head tilt–chin lift maneuver. If you can see the foreign body, try to remove it. Do not perform blind finger sweeps.
   (5) Attempt rescue breathing. If the first attempt fails, reposition the head and try again.
   (6) If the airway remains obstructed, begin CPR with chest compressions at a 30:2 compression/ventilation ratio and prepare for immediate transport. If you manage to clear the airway obstruction in an unresponsive child (older than 1 year), but he or she remains apneic and pulseless, begin CPR and attach the automated external defibrillator (AED) as soon as possible, using appropriately sized AED pads. If you are unable to relieve the obstruction after several attempts, transport the patient immediately.
   (7) If the child loses consciousness, start CPR. Initiate transportation. Consider direct laryngoscopy to remove the foreign body under direct vision. (pages 2139–2140)

5. A sudden, severe sore throat along with a high fever should start some warning lights blinking in your brain.

a. The vital signs are abnormal. The child has both tachycardia and tachypnea, not to mention his very high fever.

b. The most likely diagnosis is epiglottitis. (page 2141)

c. The steps in prehospital management are as follows:
   (1) Approach the child very gently so as not to disturb him.
   (2) Give humidified supplemental oxygen.
   (3) Place the child in a position of comfort.
   (4) Notify the receiving hospital to have the appropriate specialists standing by.
   (5) Transport without delay. (page 2141)

d. The special danger threatening this child is complete airway obstruction from epiglottal swelling, which may occur within minutes. (page 2141)

6. The little boy having an asthmatic attack during nature study is already in bad shape by the time you arrive on the scene.

a. Five signs that suggest he is in bad shape:
   (1) Drowsiness (a sign of carbon dioxide retention)
   (2) Pulsus paradoxus of 40 mm Hg
   (3) Cyanosis, indicating hypoxemia
   (4) Hyperinflated chest, indicating obstruction to exhalation
   (5) Silent chest, indicating that practically no air is moving in and out (page 2142)

b. The steps in managing this case are as follows:
   (1) Give humidified supplemental oxygen by mask while preparing the nebulizer.
   (2) Start an IV.
   (3) Give a nebulized bronchodilator, such as 0.5 mL of albuterol in 3 mL of normal saline, with oxygen as the carrier gas.
   (4) Monitor cardiac rhythm.
   (5) Ask your dispatcher to notify the child's parents and request that they meet you in the ED.
   (6) Transport the child in a position of comfort. (pages 2142–2143)

7. Most calls you receive for asthmatic attacks will be for patients already known to have asthma. Such patients will not call for help unless there is something different about this particular attack.

a. Questions to ask in taking the history of a child having an acute asthmatic attack include the following:

(1) How long has the attack been going on?
(2) Which medications has the child already taken? When? At which dosage?
(3) How much fluid has the child managed to take?
(4) Does the child have any allergies?
(5) Has the child had any hospitalizations for asthma? If so, when? (pages 2142–2143)

b. It is easier to remember the medications to give in an acute asthmatic attack if you know what you are giving them for. When giving albuterol, you need to know:

(1) The contraindication in children: diabetes
(2) The possible adverse side effects: palpitations, tremors, nervousness, dizziness, nausea
(3) Administration and dosage: Metered-dose inhaler (MDI) with a spacer-mask device. Unit doses of 2.5 mg of albuterol premixed with 3 mL of normal saline are often used for nebulization and represent an acceptable starting dose for most young children. (pages 2142–2143)

8. There is no easy answer to the question of how to respond in a case of SIDS. Each case will be a little different, and your response should be guided by local protocols and personal judgment. You need to make a quick appraisal to decide whether the mother already realizes that the baby is dead. If not, it might be worth starting CPR, so that she can feel, afterward, that everything possible was done. If you do start CPR, do it right; go through all the steps as you would for a baby you expected to survive. Conversely, if you feel that the mother already knows that her baby is dead, it may be better to take the more difficult option, and that is to confirm her worst fears. Should you do so, you must be prepared to spend time with the mother and to deal with her grief.

As this case illustrates, when you do confront a case of "crib death," you will have to make an instant decision on the spot regarding how to proceed. If you have not prepared yourself ahead of time for such decisions, it could be one of the longest instants of your experience. (pages 2186–2187)

9. Seizures in children are a lot like seizures in adults, but they tend to be considerably more upsetting to all concerned.

a. Seizures in children may result from the following causes (*students should provide five of the following*):

(1) Head trauma
(2) Meningitis
(3) Fever
(4) Hypoglycemia
(5) Hypoxia
(6) Failure of a patient with known epilepsy to take prescribed medications
(7) Abuse of drugs (yes, in children) (page 2168)

b. There are specific questions to ask in taking the history of a child who has experienced a seizure (*students should provide five of the following*):

(1) Is this the child's first seizure?
(2) How many seizures has the child had today?
(3) Has the child had a fever? Stiff neck? Headache?
(4) Might the child have ingested a toxic product?
(5) Is there a family history of seizures?
(6) If the child is known to have seizures, did the child take his or her medication today?
(7) What did the seizure look like? (page 2169)

c. In performing the physical assessment of a child who has had a seizure, look in particular for the following signs (*students should provide five of the following*):

(1) Changes in the state of consciousness
(2) Skin temperature and moisture (febrile seizure?)
(3) Evidence of head trauma
(4) Equality and reactivity of the pupils
(5) Stiff neck
(6) Signs of injury sustained during the seizure (eg, dislocation of the shoulder) (page 2169)

d. From all of the information you obtain about this child, you conclude that he probably had a febrile seizure. The prehospital treatment is as follows:

(1) Maintain the airway.
(2) Transport him to the hospital. (page 2169)

10. This 14-year-old child is in status epilepticus.

a. The steps in treatment are as follows:

(1) Treatment at the scene will be limited to supportive care if the seizure has stopped by the time of your arrival.

(2) Status epilepticus requires more extensive intervention. For a child with ongoing seizure activity, open the airway using the head tilt-chin lift maneuver or the jaw-thrust maneuver. Very proximal airway obstruction is common during a seizure or postictal state because the tongue and jaw fall backward as a result of the decreased muscle tone associated with altered mental status.

(3) If the airway is not maintainable with positioning, consider inserting a nasopharyngeal airway.

(4) Suction for secretions or vomitus, and consider the lateral decubitus position in case of ongoing vomiting. Do not attempt to intubate during an active seizure because ET intubation in this setting is associated with serious complications and is rarely successful. You are better off using BLS airway management, stopping the seizure, and then considering the child's need for ALS airway support.

(5) Provide 100% supplemental oxygen to the patient, and start bag-mask ventilation as indicated for hypoventilation. Consider placing an NG tube to decompress the stomach if the patient requires assisted ventilation.

(6) Assess the child for IV-line sites. Measure the serum glucose level, and treat any documented hypoglycemia.

(7) Consider your options for anticonvulsant administration. (page 2169)

b. Diazepam is used to treat repeated seizures. The contraindications to giving diazepam are pregnancy, respiratory depression, hypotension, and previous ingestion of alcohol or sedative drugs.

11. Whenever you are called to deal with injury in an infant or very young child, you must always keep the possibility of child abuse in the back of your mind.

a. This particular story is suspicious because of the claim that the 10-month-old "stepped on a cigarette." At the age of 10 months, most babies are just beginning to stand up (while holding on) and are not yet walking, so it is difficult to imagine how a 10-month-old would manage to step on a cigarette.

b. Clues to child abuse include the following:

(1) Parental behavior: vague, evasive, hostile

(2) Discrepancies in the history

(3) Delay in seeking care

(4) A child who looks generally neglected (dirty, unkempt)

(5) A child who does not turn to his or her parents for comfort

(6) A child who does not cry

(7) The presence of multiple bruises in different stages of healing

(8) Injuries in and around the mouth

(9) Suspicious burns (as in the present case; or scald burns without splash marks)

(10) Fractures in an infant less than a year old (page 2184)

c. The steps in caring for this particular child are as follows:

(1) Put a sterile dressing on the burn.

(2) Transport the child to the hospital.

(3) Notify the physician in private of your suspicions.

(4) Fill out whatever legal forms are required.

(5) Document everything on your PCR. (pages 2184–2185)

d. If the parent refuses to permit you to transport the child, your service should have a policy established in advance to deal with such situations. Here are some suggestions:

(1) Try to persuade the parent to change his or her mind. Do so in a calm, professional manner.

(2) Call for law enforcement.

(3) Document the entire call, including a list of whom you notified, on your PCR.

Remember, the abused child may be in life-threatening danger. If you fail to report a suspected case of child abuse, the next call to the same address may be for a dead child. (pages 2184–2185)

12. The baby who fell from the balcony has sustained a serious head injury. (Did you notice the signs of increasing intracranial pressure?) The prehospital treatment is as follows:

a. Maintain an open airway (use an oropharyngeal airway if the baby becomes unconscious). Anticipate vomiting, and have suction at hand.

b. Administer supplemental oxygen.

c. Immobilize the spine with a baby backboard or a pediatric backboard with folded towels to elevate the baby's back slightly.

d. Start transport.

e. Ventilate the baby with a bag-mask device.

f. Notify the receiving hospital. (pages 2188–2189)

13. a. The infant removed from the smoky house fire should be intubated because he was unconscious in a smoky environment and, therefore, is at high risk for respiratory complications.

b. Other factors that put a pediatric fire victim at high risk for airway obstruction and that are therefore indications for early intubation include the following (*students should provide five of the following*):

(1) Stridor
(2) Wheezing
(3) Signs of respiratory distress
(4) Facial burns
(5) Singed eyebrows
(6) Red, edematous mouth
(7) Carbonaceous sputum (pages 2192–2193)

14. a. Abdominal thrusts (Heimlich maneuver) are recommended to relieve a severe airway obstruction in a conscious child. Have Johnny's mother call 9-1-1. Ideally, you will be able to successfully dislodge the peanuts and uneventfully return to the football game. But what if you can't?

b. Follow these steps to remove a foreign body obstruction from a conscious child who is in a standing position:

(1) Kneel on one knee behind the child, and circle his or her body by placing both arms around the child's chest. Prepare to give abdominal thrusts by placing your fist just above the patient's umbilicus and well below the xiphoid process. Place your other hand over that fist.
(2) Give the child rapid, distinct abdominal thrusts in an upward direction. Be careful to avoid applying force to the lower rib cage or sternum.
(3) Repeat this standing technique until the child expels the foreign body or becomes unresponsive.
(4) If the child becomes unresponsive, place him or her supine on a firm, flat surface and inspect the airway using the head tilt–chin lift maneuver. If you can see the foreign body, try to remove it. Do not perform blind finger sweeps.
(5) Attempt rescue breathing. If the first attempt fails, reposition the head and try again.
(6) If the airway remains obstructed, begin CPR with chest compressions at a 30:2 compression-to-ventilation ratio and prepare for immediate transport. If you manage to clear the airway obstruction in an unresponsive child (older than 1 year), but he or she remains apneic and pulseless, begin CPR. (pages 2139–2140)

True/False

1. F (page 2118)
2. F (page 2121)
3. F (page 2118)
4. T (page 2127)
5. T (page 2121)
6. T (page 2143)
7. F (page 2146)
8. F (page 2191)
9. F (page 2152)
10. T (page 2150)
11. T (page 2160)
12. F (page 2151)
13. T (page 2192)
14. F (page 2189)
15. T (page 2162)

Short Answer

1. Signs of hypovolemia and shock in infants and children include the following (*students should list six of the following*):

a. Listlessness or lethargy
b. Pale, mottled, or cyanotic skin
c. Delayed capillary refill (longer than 2 seconds)
d. Collapsed veins
e. Poor skin turgor
f. Compensatory tachypnea
g. Cool extremities
h. Sunken eyes
i. Dry mucous membranes (page 2156)

2. Load-and-go situations in children include the following:

a. Ominous MOI regardless of how the child looks on scene
b. Unstable or compromised airway
c. Child in shock
d. Difficulty breathing
e. Severe neurologic disability (page 2189)

Fill in the Table

1. (page 2134)

Pediatric Physical Examination	
Body Area	**What I Am Looking for in Particular**
Head	**Look for bruising, swelling, and hematomas. Significant blood can be lost between the skull and the scalp of a small infant. Assess the anterior fontanel in patients younger than 2 years. Temporary bulging of the anterior fontanel may be seen during periods of crying, coughing, or vomiting. The presence of a bulging fontanel in a quiet infant suggests elevated intracranial pressure (ICP) caused by meningitis, encephalitis, or intracranial bleeding. A sunken fontanel suggests dehydration.**
Neck	**Examine the trachea for swelling or bruising. Note the use of accessory muscles and the presence of a stoma. Suspect bacterial or viral meningitis if the child cannot move his or her neck and has a high fever.**
Chest	**Examine the chest for penetrating injuries, lacerations, bruises, or rashes. Note the presence of vascular access devices. If the pediatric patient is injured, feel the clavicles and every rib for tenderness or deformity. An infant with rib fractures will often display paradoxical crying; that is, he or she may cry when held and be calm when not touched.**
Abdomen	**Inspect the abdomen for distension. Gently palpate the abdomen and watch closely for guarding or tensing of the abdominal muscles, which may suggest infection, obstruction, or intra-abdominal injury. Note any tenderness or masses. Look for any seat-belt abrasions or bruising. Be suspicious of bruising on the abdomen of a nonambulatory child; this finding is highly suspicious for nonaccidental trauma. In an infant, a common finding is a range of active, tinkling bowel sounds when the stethoscope is placed on the belly. Because patients react to cold stimuli, warming the diaphragm of your stethoscope before placing it on the skin might yield a more accurate result. You can percuss an infant's abdomen as you would an adult's; however, you might note a more tympanic sound.**
Extremities	**Assess for symmetry. Compare both sides for color, warmth, size of joints, swelling, and tenderness. Put each joint through full range of motion while watching the eyes of the pediatric patient for signs of pain, unless there is obvious deformity of the extremity, suggesting a fracture.**

2. (page 2122, Table 43-3)

Pediatric Respiratory Rates	
Age	**Respiratory Rate (breaths/min)**
Infant	**30 to 53**
Toddler	**22 to 37**
Preschool-aged child	**20 to 28**
School-aged child	**18 to 25**
Adolescent	**12 to 20**

Data from: American Heart Association (AHA). Vital signs in children. In: AHA. *Pediatric Advanced Life Support*. Dallas, TX: AHA; 2015.

3. (page 2122, Table 43-4)

Pediatric Pulse Rates	
Age	**Pulse Rate (beats/min) [Awake]**
Infant	**100 to 180**
Toddler	**98 to 140**
Preschool-aged child	**80 to 120**
School-aged child	**75 to 118**
Adolescent	**60 to 100**

Data from: American Heart Association (AHA). Vital signs in children. In: AHA. *Pediatric Advanced Life Support*. Dallas, TX: AHA; 2015.

4. (page 2135, Table 43-11)

Normal Blood Pressure for Age	
Age	**Minimal Systolic Blood Pressure (mm Hg)**
Infant	**72 to 104**
Toddler	**86 to 106**
Preschool-age child	**89 to 112**
School-age child	**97 to 120**
Adolescent	**110 to 131**

Data from: American Heart Association (AHA). Vital signs in children. In: AHA. *Pediatric Advanced Life Support*. Dallas, TX: AHA; 2015.

5. (page 2184, Table 43-25)

CHILD ABUSE Mnemonic	
Mnemonic	**What the Letter Represents**
C	**Consistency of the injury with the child's developmental age**
H	History consistent with injuries
I	**Inappropriate parental concerns**
L	Lack of supervision
D	**Delay in seeking care**
A	Affect
B	**Bruises of varying stages**
U	Unusual injury patterns
S	**Suspicious circumstances**
E	Environmental clues

Problem Solving

1. Minimal systolic blood pressure = 70 + (2 × age in years)
   - **a.** 82 mm Hg
   - **b.** 89 to 112 mm Hg
   - **c.** 89 to 112 mm Hg (page 2135)
2. **a.** 5.5 mm
   - **b.** 6.25 mm (page 2151)
3. **a.** The initial energy setting is 2 J/kg or 36 joules. (page 2165)
   - **b.** Subsequent defibrillations should occur at 4 J/kg or 72 joules. (page 2165)
4. **a.** Epinephrine should be given by the intramuscular (IM) route at a dose of 0.01 mg/kg of the 1 mg/mL (1:1,000) solution, to a maximum dose of 0.3 mg. This patient should be given 0.01 mg/kg or the maximum dose of 0.3 mg of 1 mg/mL (1:1,000) solution. (page 2140)
   - **b.** Diphenhydramine dose: 1 to 2 mg/kg IV to a maximum of 50 mg, or 27 to 50 mg IV. (see the Volume 1 Appendix, *Emergency Medications*)
   - **c.** Bronchodilators may be delivered by nebulizer or metered-dose inhaler (MDI) with a spacer-mask device. Unit doses of 2.5 mg of albuterol premixed with 3 mL of normal saline are often used for nebulization and represent an acceptable starting dose for most young children. (page 2142)

Chapter 44: Geriatric Emergencies

Matching

1. C (page 2209)
2. H (page 2207)
3. G (page 2225)
4. B (page 2225)
5. R (page 2235)
6. T (page 2236)
7. W (page 2238)
8. U (page 2222)
9. V (page 2232)
10. F (page 2223)
11. D (page 2208)
12. N (page 2236)
13. E (page 2235)
14. A (page 2240)
15. I (page 2235)
16. J (page 2213)
17. K (page 2241)
18. S (page 2211)
19. L (page 2207)
20. M (page 2236)
21. O (page 2226)
22. P (page 2232)
23. Q (page 2210)

Multiple Choice

1. B (page 2207)
2. A (page 2208)
3. C (page 2209)
4. A (page 2209)
5. D (page 2229)
6. C (page 2211)
7. D (page 2213)
8. D (page 2220)
9. A (page 2236)
10. D (page 2218)

Labeling

1. Upper GI system (page 2228, Figure 44-5)
   - **A.** Liver
   - **B.** Gallbladder
   - **C.** Duodenum*
   - **D.** Pancreas
   - **E.** Jejunum
   - **F.** Colon
   - **G.** Esophagus*
   - **H.** Stomach*
   - **I.** Ileum
   - **J.** Rectum
2. Lower GI system (page 2228, Figure 44-6)
   - **A.** Liver
   - **B.** Gallbladder
   - **C.** Duodenum
   - **D.** Pancreas
   - **E.** Jejunum
   - **F.** Colon*
   - **G.** Esophagus
   - **H.** Stomach
   - **I.** Ileum
   - **J.** Rectum*

Fill in the Blank

1. Older; emergency (page 2207)
2. just getting old (page 2208)
3. cardiovascular; aging; deconditioning (page 2209)
4. respiratory; reductions (page 2208)
5. nephron units; filtering (page 2212)
6. appetite; saliva; dryness (page 2211)
7. intervertebral; compression fractures; height (page 2213)
8. Ménière disease; cycles; months (page 2211)
9. Wrinkling; resiliency; drier; fragile (page 2212)
10. morbidity; mortality; 70 (page 2221)

Identify

1. a. Chief complaint: Right-sided midthigh pain
   b. Vital signs: Her pulse is 84 beats/min and very irregular. Her oxygen saturation is 88% on room air. BP is 106/86 mm Hg. The patient's skin turgor is poor. Pupils are PERRLA. An ECG shows a sinus rhythm with frequent PVCs and short runs of VT (with a pulse).
   c. Pertinent negatives: She denies chest pain, shortness of breath, dizziness, nausea, or vomiting. She also denies a trip and fall. The area appears to be clear of obstacles, rugs, or other obvious trip hazards.
2. a. Chief complaint: Patient is conscious but not alert to person, place, or day, so his mental status is "V."
   b. Vital signs: Blood glucose of 66 mg/dL. His pulse rate is 92 beats/min and regular, BP is 160/72 mm Hg. His skin is warm and moist, and his oxygen saturation is 96% on room air.
   c. Pertinent negatives: There is minimally detectable damage to the vehicle as well as the vehicles that were struck.

Complete the Patient Care Report (PCR)

Show the completed PCR to your instructor to obtain feedback on your completion of the form.

Ambulance Calls

1. As noted, one way to try to make sure you don't miss any important symptoms is to conduct a review of systems, which should include questions such as the following (*students should list 10 of the following*): (page 2218)
   a. Have you had any pain or discomfort in your chest (cardiovascular system)?
   b. Have you had any fluttering in your chest or fast heartbeats (cardiovascular system)?
   c. Have you been short of breath (respiratory systems)?
   d. Have you been coughing (respiratory system)?
   e. Have you had any dizzy spells (neurologic system)?
   f. Have you fainted (neurologic system)?
   g. Can you explain the reason for calling 9-1-1 (neurologic system)?
   h. Have you had any difficulty speaking (neurologic system)?
   i. Have you had any severe headaches recently (neurologic system)?
   j. Have you noticed any unusual weakness or odd sensations in your arms or legs (neurologic system)?
   k. Have you had any changes in your appetite (gastrointestinal system)?
   l. Have you gained or lost any weight (gastrointestinal system)?
   m. Has there been any change in your bowel movements (gastrointestinal system)?
   n. Have you had any nausea or vomiting (gastrointestinal system)?
   o. Have you had any pain or difficulty in urinating (genitourinary system)?
   p. Have you noticed any change in the color of your urine (genitourinary system)?
   q. Have you noticed any changes in the frequency of urination (genitourinary system)?
2. One of the most frequent geriatric calls is for a patient who has fallen.
   a. Questions to ask in taking the history might include the following: (page 2239)
      (1) If the patient fell, from what height?
      (2) Did the patient have any symptoms beforehand, such as dizziness?
      (3) If the patient was struck by a car, how fast was the car moving?
      (4) If the patient was the driver of a car involved in a crash, did he or she feel dizzy or black out before the crash?
      (5) Did the patient have any chest pain?
      (6) Did witnesses notice the car moving erratically before it crashed?
   b. The past medical history of an elderly patient may be quite extensive, and there isn't enough time in the field to elicit all the details. The things you need to know to render appropriate emergency care are: (pages 2218, 2239)
      (1) major underlying illnesses (eg, diabetes, angina)
      (2) recent hospitalizations (Where? What doctor?)
      (3) allergies
      (4) obtain a complete list of all medications the patient takes regularly. (Collect them all in a bag and take them with the patient to the hospital.)

c. In performing the GEMS environmental assessment, one should look in particular for the following *(students should provide six from the list)*: (page 2216)
   (1) Check the physical condition of the patient's home: Is the exterior of the home in need of repair? Is the home secure?
   (2) Check for hazardous conditions that may be present (eg, poor wiring, rotted floors, unventilated gas heaters, clutter that prevents adequate egress).
   (3) Are smoke detectors present and working?
   (4) Is the home too hot or too cold?
   (5) Is there an odor of feces or urine in the home?
   (6) Is bedding soiled or urine soaked?
   (7) Are pets well cared for?
   (8) Is food present in the home? Is it adequate and unspoiled?
   (9) Are liquor bottles present? If so, are they empty?
   (10) Are there burn patterns on the walls, cabinets, or floors?
   (11) Are there unsecured throw rugs that could result in falls?
   (12) If the patient has a disability, are appropriate assistive devices (eg, a wheelchair or walker) present and in adequate condition?
   (13) Does the patient have access to a telephone?
   (14) Are medications prescribed to someone else, expired, unmarked, or from many physicians?
   (15) If living with others, is the patient confined to one part of the home?
   (16) If the patient is residing in a nursing facility, does the care appear to be adequate to meet the patient's needs?

d. Older adults are more susceptible than younger people to *(students should provide three of the following)*:
   (1) subdural hematoma (page 2238)
   (2) compression of the cervical spinal cord (page 2238)
   (3) rib fracture (page 2238)
   (4) hip fracture (page 2238)

3. Factors related to GEMS social assessment:
   a. Assess activities of daily living (eating, dressing, bathing, toileting).
   b. Are these activities being provided for the patient? If so, by whom?
   c. Are there delays in obtaining food, medication, or toileting? The patient may complain of such a delay, or the environment may suggest a problem.
   d. Does the patient have regular visits from family members, live with family members, or live with a spouse?
   e. If in an institutional setting, is the patient able to feed himself or herself? If not, is food still sitting on the food tray? Has the patient been lying in his or her own urine or feces for prolonged periods?
   f. Does the patient have a social network? Does the patient have a mechanism to interact socially with others on a daily basis? (page 2216)

True/False

1. T (page 2208)
2. F (page 2210)
3. F (page 2214)
4. T (page 2210)
5. T (page 2210)
6. F (page 2213)
7. T (page 2219)
8. T (page 2209)
9. F (page 2225)
10. T (page 2240)

Short Answer

1. Among the attributes that make caring for the older adults particularly challenging are the following *(students should provide five of the following)*: (pages 2214–2215)
   a. Health care providers must know what is and what is not a part of the aging process.
   b. Signs and symptoms of disease may present differently in this population than in younger patients.
   c. A variety of acute illnesses from heart failure to an acute abdomen may present simply as delirium.
   d. In the older patient, there will likely be multiple problems—medical, psychological, and social.
   e. The symptoms of one disease or disability may alter or hide the symptoms of another condition.
   f. The presence of multiple underlying illnesses also makes it much more difficult for you to sort out which problem is causing which symptom.
2. Among the psychosocial stresses that accompany advancing age are the following:
   a. Retirement from work, with the attendant loss of community status, sense of usefulness, and the structure that a job gives to one's daily life (pages 2207–2208)
   b. Bereavement, as more and more friends (and often a spouse) die (page 2208)

3. A number of changes in the body occur as part of the normal aging process *(students should provide two changes per organ system).*
- **a.** Cardiovascular (page 2209)
  - (1) Left ventricle wall thickens.
  - (2) Arteriosclerosis contributes to systolic hypertension.
  - (3) Widening pulse pressure, decreased coronary artery perfusion, and changes in cardiac ejection efficiency
  - (4) Electric conduction system: SA node, AV node, and bundle of His become fibrotic, and the number of pacemaker cells in the SA node decreases, leading to bradycardia.
- **b.** Respiratory (pages 2208–2209)
  - (1) Decreased vital capacity
  - (2) Increased residual volume
  - (3) Decreased airflow
  - (4) Decreased arterial PaO_2
  - (5) Decreased cough, gag, and ciliary clearance
- **c.** Renal (page 2212)
  - (1) Decline in kidney size (weight) results from a loss of functioning nephron units and smaller filtering surface area.
  - (2) Aging kidneys respond sluggishly to sodium deficiency.
  - (3) Decreased thirst mechanism
  - (4) At risk for rapid dehydration as well as overhydration if exposed to large sodium loads
- **d.** Digestive (pages 2211–2212)
  - (1) Decreased sense of taste
  - (2) Decreased secretion of saliva and gastric juice
  - (3) Less efficient hepatic detoxification
- **e.** Musculoskeletal (pages 2213–2214)
  - (1) Decreased bone mass
  - (2) Decreased muscle mass
- **f.** Nervous (pages 2210–2211)
  - (1) Decreased visual acuity
  - (2) Loss of high-tone hearing
  - (3) Impaired proprioception
- **g.** Homeostatic (page 2213)
  - (1) Impaired temperature regulation
  - (2) Blunted febrile response to infection
  - (3) Impaired blood glucose control

4. Responses to illness common among the elderly and similar to ACS would include *(students should provide four of the following)*: (page 2221)
- **a.** Acute confusion or other change in mental status
- **b.** Weakness
- **c.** Dizziness
- **d.** Dyspnea
- **e.** Fatigue

5. A number of problems can be involved in taking a history from an older adult patient, but most of those obstacles can be overcome with a little patience, tact, and ingenuity.
- **a.** Obstacle: The patient has trouble hearing you.
  What you can do about it: Sit facing the patient, in good light, and speak slowly and clearly.
- **b.** Obstacle: Patient may not report important symptoms.
  What you can do about it: Conduct a review of systems to screen the major organ systems for serious abnormality.
- **c.** Obstacle: The patient has several chief complaints.
  What you can do about it: Ask, "What happened *today*?" or "What is bothering you the most?" and "How is it different from the way it was yesterday?"
- **d.** Obstacle: The patient is too confused to give a history.
  What you can do about it: Try to obtain information from the family or other caregivers.

6. AMI and heart failure occur commonly in older adults but are as likely as not to present with atypical signs and symptoms: (pages 2221–2222)

Condition	Possible Signs and Symptoms in Older Adults
Acute myocardial infarction	**Confusion, weakness, dyspnea, stroke, syncope, incontinence**
Heart failure	**Fatigue**

7. Conditions that may present as delirium in the older adult include the following: (page 2224)

D: Drugs or toxins (including intoxication or withdrawal)

E: Emotional (psychiatric)

L: Low PaO_2 (carbon monoxide poisoning, COPD, heart failure, acute coronary syndrome [ACS], pneumonia)

I: Infection (pneumonia, urinary tract infection [UTI], sepsis)

R: Retention of stool or urine

I: Ictal state (seizures)

U: Undernutrition (including vitamin deficiencies) or underhydration

M: Metabolism (thyroid or endocrine, electrolytes, kidneys)

S: Subdural hematoma

Fill in the Table

1. (page 2237, Table 44-4)

Causes of Falls in the Older Adults	
Cause	**Clues to Suggest This Cause**
Extrinsic (accidental)	Obvious environmental hazard at the scene, such as poor lighting, scatter rugs, uneven sidewalk, ice or other slippery surface
Intrinsic drop attacks	Sudden fall; patient found on the ground somewhat confused, often temporarily paralyzed and unable to get up; no premonitory symptoms
Postural hypotension	Fall when getting up from a recumbent or sitting position (Check medications the patient is taking, and ask about occult blood loss, such as presence of black stools. Measure BP in recumbent and sitting positions.)
Dizziness or syncope	Marked bradycardia or tachydysrhythmias
Stroke	Other characteristic signs of stroke, such as hemiparesis, hemiplegia, or aphasia
Fracture	Patient felt something snap before falling

2. (page 2231, Table 44-3)

Signs of Dehydration in Older Adults
Dry tongue
Longitudinal furrows in the tongue
Dry mucous membranes
Weak upper body musculature
Confusion
Difficulty in speech
Sunken eyes

Chapter 45: Patients With Special Challenges

Matching

Part I

1. N (page 2280)
2. M (page 2258)
3. L (page 2269)
4. K (page 2269)
5. J (page 2274)
6. Z (page 2262)
7. Y (page 2273)
8. X (page 2262)
9. W (page 2262)
10. V (page 2254)
11. I (page 2286)
12. H (page 2280)
13. G (page 2258)
14. F (page 2259)
15. E (page 2279)
16. U (page 2283)
17. T (page 2278)
18. S (page 2251)
19. R (page 2278)
20. Q (page 2287)
21. D (page 2251)
22. C (page 2280)
23. B (page 2283)
24. A (page 2283)
25. P (page 2258)
26. O (page 2280)

Part II

1. R (page 2283)
2. Q (page 2289)
3. P (page 2262)
4. O (page 2259)
5. N (page 2289)
6. J (page 2257)
7. I (page 2283)
8. H (page 2276)
9. D (page 2274)
10. C (page 2251)
11. B (page 2275)
12. A (page 2274)
13. Z (page 2284)
14. Y (page 2290)
15. X (page 2290)
16. W (page 2253)
17. V (page 2283)
18. M (page 2289)
19. L (page 2289)
20. K (page 2288)
21. G (page 2251)
22. F (page 2262)
23. E (page 2287)
24. U (page 2284)
25. T (page 2258)
26. S (page 2262)

Part III

1. I (page 2259)
2. H (page 2289)
3. G (page 2286)
4. F (page 2284)
5. M (page 2270)
6. L (page 2275)
7. K (page 2261)
8. J (page 2258)
9. E (page 2254)
10. D (page 2253)
11. C (page 2280)
12. B (page 2283)
13. A (page 2282)

Multiple Choice

1. D (page 2283)
2. B (page 2282)
3. D (page 2255)
4. C (page 2284)
5. C (page 2267)
6. C (page 2258)
7. D (page 2286)
8. B (page 2286)
9. B (page 2261)
10. D (pages 2266–2267)

Labeling

1. American Sign Language signs for common terms related to illness or injury (page 2281, Figure 45-23)
   - **A.** Sick
   - **B.** Hurt
   - **C.** Help
   - **D.** Ache/pain
   - **E.** Allergy (motion E1 followed by motion E2)
   - **F.** Breathe
   - **G.** Chest
   - **H.** Dizziness
   - **I.** Where
   - **J.** Write
2. Parts of the tracheostomy tube (page 2262, Figure 45-6)
   - **A.** Tubing to ventilator
   - **B.** Cuff inflation valve
   - **C.** Inflatable cuff
   - **D.** Flange
   - **E.** Outer cannula

Fill in the Blank

1. conductive; sensorineural (page 2280)
2. impairment; congenital (page 2280)
3. language; production; articulation (page 2283)
4. semantic; pragmatic (page 2283)

5. colostomy; intestinal (page 2269)
6. bariatrics; obesity (page 2259)
7. spina bifida; fetal neural (page 2289)
8. cystic fibrosis (CF); defective recessive (page 2287)
9. altered skeletal; contraction (page 2286)
10. myelomeningocele; development; spinal (page 2289)

Identify

1. a. Chief complaint: Terminally ill patient
   b. History of the present illness: Irregular breathing, apnea, unconscious
   c. Other medical history: DNR order
2. a. Chief complaint: Seizures
   b. History of the present illness: Seizures that haven't responded to rectal diazepam
   c. Other medical history: Down syndrome, multiple medications, seizures
3. a. Chief complaint: Fever
   b. History of the present illness: Cloudy urine, has a Foley catheter
   c. Other medical history: Quadriplegic, tracheotomy, colostomy, feeding tube, can't verbalize his complaints and concerns, uses a writing board, taking a steroid and antibiotic

Complete the Patient Care Report (PCR)

Show the completed PCR to your instructor to obtain feedback on your completion of the form.

Ambulance Calls

1. a. It's best to ask the patient how to move her in the safest and most comfortable manner. She may have a special lift or assist devices that will make the transfer easier for both the crew and herself. It is important to try to protect her dignity and privacy. Calling EMS can sometimes be embarrassing for a patient, especially when his or her deformity is revealed. It is often better to work as a team. If more assistance is required, it should be requested. The goal is to provide movement that is safe for the patient and the crew.
   b. The patient may have some level of paralysis, especially in her lower trunk and extremities (if present). The patient may have bowel control issues and may have a Foley catheter. Some patients have shunts placed in the brain to relieve excess cerebrospinal fluid. If the patient has suffered other injuries, she might not even know. (pages 2289–2290)
2. a. As with any patient who has had a seizure, your concern is to maintain adequate ABCs. Based on the primary survey, it is obvious that this patient probably needs aggressive airway and breathing support. This should be accomplished by opening the airway with a head tilt–chin lift maneuver. Suctioning is also important, as is high-flow oxygen. If the patient needs ventilatory assistance, a bag-mask device would be indicated. It would also be appropriate to transport the patient away from the crowd and concert to avoid an embarrassing episode when she regains consciousness. The patient's mom is probably well versed in her medical history and care. It is important to include the mother in any treatment decisions and have her assist as appropriate. If the patient doesn't recover in a reasonable period of time, transport to an appropriate hospital is required. (page 2279)
   b. The patient may present with a round head with a flat occiput; an enlarged, protruding tongue; wide-set eyes; and folded skin on either side of the nose. (page 2279)

True/False

1. T (page 2251)
2. F (page 2273)
3. T (page 2283)
4. T (page 2283)
5. F (page 2285)
6. F (page 2285)
7. F (page 2287)
8. F (pages 2288–2289)
9. T (page 2289)
10. T (page 2260)
11. T (page 2261)

Short Answer

1. Many of the patients a paramedic encounters have a hearing impairment. Sometimes this impairment is readily noticeable. (pages 2280–2282)
   a. The following clues would indicate to you that your patient may have a hearing impairment:
      (1) Presence of hearing aids
      (2) Poor word pronunciation
      (3) Failure to respond to your questions

b. How would you go about communicating with someone who has a hearing impairment? *Student should list five of the following eight.*
  (1) Face the patient; position yourself directly in front of the patient.
  (2) Ask the patient how he or she would like to communicate with you, such as by using American Sign Language.
  (3) Use written communication.
  (4) Speak slowly.
  (5) Use a normal tone of voice.
  (6) Try placing the earpieces of your stethoscope into the patient's ears while you speak into the bell ("reverse stethoscope" technique).
  (7) Have only one person interview the patient to avoid confusion.
  (8) Make sure the patient is using his or her hearing aid and that it is turned on. (pages 2280–2281)

2. *Student should list five of the following seven strategies.*
a. Request and plan for extra help.
b. Plan the safest and easiest exit route.
c. Avoid lifting the patient by one limb.
d. Use a team approach to coordinate and preplan each move.
e. Use specialized equipment if available.
f. Notify the receiving hospital.
g. Be respectful of the patient's dignity. (page 2260)

3. a. What are some of the main causes of visual impairments?
  (1) Congenital defects
  (2) Genetic factors
  (3) Acquired causes (eg, trauma, CVA, macular degeneration, glaucoma) (pages 2282–2283)

b. What can paramedics do to alleviate some of the fears felt by patients with visual impairments?
  (1) Make yourself known when entering the room and introduce yourself and others.
  (2) Tell the patient what is happening.
  (3) Identify noises.
  (4) Describe the situation and surroundings. (page 2283)

Fill in the Table

1. (page 2278, Table 45-3)

Known Causes of Development Disabilities
Genetic abnormality
Hypoxia, malnutrition, or toxic exposure during fetal development
Maternal trauma, hemorrhage, or infection during fetal development
Premature birth, low birth weight
Malnutrition
Abuse or neglect; improper treatment of common childhood illnesses
Neurologic insult, injury, or infection
Severe metabolic abnormality
Toxic exposure
Inadequate stimulation during childhood
Near drowning
Hyperthermia
Trauma or hypoxia during delivery
Traumatic injuries

Data from: Facts about developmental disabilities. Centers for Disease Control and Prevention website. https://www.cdc.gov/ncbddd/developmentaldisabilities/facts.html. Updated July 9, 2015. Accessed May 4, 2017; Pivalizza P, Lalani SR. Intellectual disability in children: evaluation for a cause. UpToDate website. http://www.uptodate.com/contents/intellectual-disability-in-children-evaluation-for-a-cause. Updated May 26, 2016. Accessed May 4, 2017; and Pivalizza P, Lalani SR. Intellectual disability in children: definition, diagnosis, and assessment of needs. UpToDate website. http://www.uptodate.com/contents/intellectual-disability-in-children-definition-diagnosis-and-assessment-of-needs?source=see_link. Updated August 15, 2016. Accessed May 4, 2017.

2. (page 2259, Table 45-2)

Causes of and Contributing Factors to Obesity
Poor dietary choices
Excessive food intake
Lack of exercise
Hormonal changes
Inadequate sleep
Low basal metabolic rate
Environmental toxins
Genetic predisposition
Cessation/reduction of cigarette smoking
Widespread dependence on air conditioning

Data from: Dare S, Mackay DF, Pell JP. Relationship between smoking and obesity: a cross-sectional study of 499,504 middle-aged adults in the UK general population. *PLoS One*. 2015;10(4):e0123579. https://www.ncbi.nlm.nih.gov/pmc/articles/PMC4401671/. Accessed May 4, 2017.

Section 10: Operations

Chapter 46: Transport Operations

Matching

Part I

1. G (page 2322)
2. G (page 2322)
3. A (page 2322)
4. A (page 2322)
5. G (page 2322)
6. G (page 2322)
7. A (page 2322)
8. A (page 2322)
9. G (page 2322)
10. G (page 2322)

Part II

1. E (page 2308)
2. T (page 2315)
3. U (page 2308)
4. G (page 2314)
5. J (page 2304)
6. K (page 2308)
7. F (page 2311)
8. L (page 2318)
9. M (page 2305)
10. Z (page 2305)
11. AA (page 2305)
12. N (page 2311)
13. Q (page 2321)
14. A (page 2320)
15. B (page 2306)
16. H (page 2311)
17. I (page 2311)
18. C (page 2314)
19. D (page 2307)
20. R (page 2309)
21. S (page 2309)
22. V (page 2308)
23. W (page 2311)
24. X (page 2309)
25. Y (page 2305)
26. BB (page 2308)
27. O (page 2318)
28. P (page 2322)
29. CC (page 2308)

Multiple Choice

1. B (page 2304)
2. B (page 2306)
3. C (page 2319)
4. B (page 2316)
5. C (page 2315)
6. C (pages 2320–2321)
7. C (page 2322)
8. A (page 2323)
9. C (page 2323)
10. D (page 2308)
11. D (page 2313)
12. B (page 2314)

Labeling

1. Landing zone (LZ) (page 2324, Figure 46-11)
   - **A.** The pilot's normal area of vision is the front of the aircraft, as the pilot faces forward, at 12 o'clock.
   - **B.** The pilot's blind area is the rear of the aircraft, as the pilot faces forward, between 6 o'clock and 3 o'clock.
   - **C.** Post a guard to the rear of the aircraft, 30 feet behind tail rotor, as the pilot faces forward, between 6 o'clock and 9 o'clock.
2. Helicopter hand signals

   (page 2325, Figure 46-13)
   - **A.** Move right
   - **B.** Move forward
   - **C.** Move rearward
   - **D.** Move upward
   - **E.** Move downward
   - **F.** Move left

Fill in the Blank

1. There's room for some discussion regarding what things are absolutely essential during the first few minutes with a patient who has been critically injured in a road collision. With experience, you may want to modify your list. In general, you will have to make a trade-off between all the equipment you would like to have immediately at hand and what you can carry comfortably during your first, hurried dash—often over difficult terrain—to the patient.

   ______ Long-leg air splint
   ______ Drug box
   __X__ Portable suction unit
   __X__ Oxygen cylinder
   ______ OB kit
   __X__ Pocket mask
   __X__ Oropharyngeal airways
   ______ Intravenous fluid bags
   __X__ Dressing materials

__X__ Large-bore IV cannulas
__X__ Head immobilizer
__X__ Self-adhering roller bandage
_____ Selection of board splints
_____ Wheeled cot stretcher
_____ ECG monitor
_____ Contact lens remover
__X__ Stethoscope
__X__ Flashlight
__X__ Triangular bandages
_____ Chemical cold packs
__X__ Cervical collar
_____ Traction splint
__X__ Nonrebreathing mask
__X__ Long backboard/straps
_____ Oral thermometer
__X__ Fire extinguisher
_____ Bed pan
__X__ Heavy-duty scissors
_____ Emesis basin
__X__ Handheld radio
_____ Adhesive bandages

Other equipment that might be needed: Depending on the circumstances, you might require some light rescue and extrication equipment. And you may prefer a bag-mask device to a pocket mask. Finally, emergency medical technicians (EMTs) and paramedics should, in this era of bloodborne diseases, don nonlatex or rubber gloves when they have to come in contact with a patient's blood or secretions.

Identify

a. Chief complaint: Deformity to left collarbone, possible internal trauma

b. Vital signs: Alert; respirations are 22 breaths/min, shallow; decreased left lung sounds, and Spo_2 94%. Pulse is 114 beats/min, heart monitor shows sinus tachycardia with PVCs, BP is 132/84 mm Hg. Pain is 9/10, PERRLA, skin is warm.

c. Pertinent negatives: No loss of consciousness, right lung sounds clear.
Walt and Dave did a great job in thinking on their feet. Because of the collarbone, a rigid cervical collar will not work. The use of the towels and tape is the next best thing. They also went to the regional trauma center. The patient has a few PVCs and decreased lung sounds on the left, which is consistent with the seat belt injuries. They should be watching the left chest for a possible pneumothorax and pericardial tamponade.

Complete the Patient Care Report (PCR)

Show the completed PCR to your instructor to obtain feedback on your completion of the form.

Ambulance Calls

1. a. Cory and Bill should have worked out their differences before arriving on the scene. They should know who is going to act as lead, and both of them should know what equipment to grab before leaving the squad. It is not a good idea to have a layperson digging through your squad looking for your equipment. Their actions on scene were very unprofessional and detrimental to the patient's outcome. (pages 2309–2310)

b. There were a few "unprofessional" moves they made while on the scene. List them here:
(1) Not listening to the bystander (coworker)
(2) Late cervical spine immobilization
(3) Wasting 15 minutes before getting the stretcher, cervical collar, and scoop stretcher
(4) The couple of IV lines and the method of deciding who does what
(5) The "high five" after a procedure
(6) Thirty-four minutes on the scene

c. What kind of transport decision would you make right away? This patient needs to be at a trauma center. Most likely he has a head injury, and because he is unconscious as a result of a fall from a second-story roof, he is a definite regional trauma center candidate. If air medical is available and able to get the patient to the trauma center more quickly than by ambulance, they should be called within the first minute of arriving on the scene. Cory and Bill should be thinking of the "Golden Hour (Golden Period)" when treating this patient. (page 2320)

2. a. Jeff and Larry should know better than to skip checking the emergency vehicle. You should always recheck after every change in crews. Tires can leak during downtime; people forget to refuel. A turn signal may be working in the morning but may quit sometime during the day. Checking the emergency vehicle also mentally prepares you for the coming shift. It gives you confidence in your equipment because *you* know that it is ready to go, instead of relying on someone else. Everything should be checked once a day. (pages 2306–2308)

b. A visual check should include a quick walk around to ensure that there are no flat tires or fluids dripping from the engine. Many services have a checklist beside the emergency vehicle so that you can see when the last check was made on the unit and the equipment. The responding crew could have someone in the back check other equipment on the way to the scene. Every department is different, so make sure you understand the checks that are designed for your unit, and make sure when your call is over that all supplies are stocked and ready for the next call. (pages 2306–2308)

True/False

1. F (page 2304)
2. T (page 2304)
3. T (page 2305)
4. F (page 2306)
5. F (page 2307)
6. T (page 2308)
7. F (page 2309)
8. T (page 2312)
9. F (page 2318)
10. T (page 2322)

Short Answer

1. Make sure you have a detailed street and area map in the driver's compartment.
2. Even if you routinely use global positioning system (GPS), there should be a backup map.
3. Be familiar with the roads and traffic patterns in your district.
4. Be aware of construction and school zones and avoid them if you can. (page 2313)

Fill in the Table

(Tables 46-3 and 46-4, pages 2320–2321)

Advantages and Disadvantages of Using Helicopter Transport	
Advantages	**Disadvantages**
• Reduced transport time • **Ability to access patients in remote areas** • **Availability of medical crew with advanced skills and equipment**	• **Weather- or environment-related challenges** • Altitude limitations • **Airspeed limitations** • Aircraft cabin size limitations • Terrain that poses landing challenges • **Cost** • Patient condition that is not suited to helicopter transport • Restrictions on the number of responders • **Potential for crash**

Chapter 47: Incident Management and Mass-Casualty Incidents

Matching

Part I

1. V (page 2334)
2. U (page 2344)
3. T (page 2333)
4. S (page 2344)
5. R (page 2341)
6. Z (page 2345)
7. Y (page 2338)
8. X (page 2337)
9. W (page 2344)
10. A (page 2344)
11. B (page 2336)
12. C (page 2351)
13. D (page 2337)
14. E (page 2333)
15. F (page 2343)
16. Q (page 2333)
17. P (page 2337)
18. O (page 2339)
19. N (page 2349)
20. M (page 2339)
21. G (page 2337)
22. H (page 2335)
23. I (page 2351)
24. L (page 2334)
25. K (page 2336)
26. J (page 2338)

Part II

1. I (page 2348)
2. H (page 2343)
3. G (page 2335)
4. F (page 2336)
5. A (page 2339)
6. B (page 2343)
7. P (page 2336)
8. O (page 2342)
9. N (page 2345)
10. M (page 2342)
11. L (page 2343)
12. E (page 2346)
13. D (page 2339)
14. C (page 2343)
15. K (page 2337)
16. J (page 2337)

Multiple Choice

1. C (page 2235)
2. B (page 2236)
3. C (page 2340)
4. C (page 2342)
5. D (page 2343)
6. A (page 2346)
7. C (pages 2350–2351)
8. D (page 2348)
9. A (page 2349)
10. B (page 2340)

Labeling

1. Diagram of an MCI (page 2345, Figure 47-8)
   A. Incident
   B. Extrication area
   C. Triage area
   D. Treatment area
2. The JumpSTART pediatric MCI triage algorithm (page 2350, Figure 47-13)
   A. Immediate (red)
   B. Deceased (black)
   C. Deceased (black)
   D. Immediate (red)
   E. Immediate (red)
   F. Immediate (red)
   G. Immediate (red)
   H. Delayed (yellow)

Fill in the Blank

1. multiple-casualty incident (page 2333)
2. ICS; span of control (page 2335)
3. finance (page 2337)
4. safety; PIO; liaison (page 2339)
5. Preparedness; planning (page 2340)
6. transportation (page 2343)
7. primary; secondary (pages 2345–2346)
8. rapid (page 2348)
9. Jump (page 2349)
10. staging (page 2343)

Identify

1. Chief complaint: Impaled object in left buttock
2. Vital signs: Respirations are 20 breaths/min, oxygen saturation is 97%, lungs are clear, pulse is 98 beats/min, sinus rhythm is normal, BP is 136/88 mm Hg, patient is 7/10 on scale for pain, skin is warm and dry.
3. Pertinent negatives: Remained alert the whole time, not a lot of bleeding, which indicates a tamponade effect inside where the wood is pressing against the veins and arteries.

Your patient provides a small challenge because of the need to stabilize him to a backboard or scoop stretcher as a result of the blast knocking him down. However, the impaled object is not letting you lay him flat. This is where you do the best job possible and move him as little as possible. A scoop stretcher may be a better tool to use to "pick up" the patient.

Ambulance Calls

1. This call may be the most stressful event you ever respond to. Remember to take care of yourself as soon as possible, and debrief. Don't be a hero; take your turn in the rehab section. Don't become a victim! Stay on top of scene safety, and don't get lulled into a false sense of security. Stay on your toes!
   a. Everyone's answers may be different because there are no right or wrong answers here. Work as a group to develop a list of the best items to carry.
      (1) Communication radio
      (2) Multi tool
      (3) Gloves
      (4) Pen and paper
      (5) Flashlight
      (6) AM/FM radio
      (7) Trauma bandages
      (8) Pocket face mask
      (9) Leather gloves
      (10) Orange vest (page 2338)
   b. Once again, there will be a lot of different answers. Two heads are always better than one. Tell them help will be coming soon, to stay away from downed power lines, and not to move patients unless they are in extreme danger. Try to account for everyone in the area. Stay in a group. Do not go back into a destroyed building.
   c. Remember, anything can become a hazard during a disaster, including people, animals, burst water and gas mains, downed electrical lines, fires, falling debris, sewage, and the weather. Can you think of any others?
2. a. If you have emergency management people that are trained for this, they should take command. If the fire station is unharmed, it would make a great central command post. The nursing home should also have a command post that reports back to central command because of the large volume of people in that area. The fire station can also serve as a rehab center or staging area because a lot of supplies are already there. The fire station will be a logical gathering area for incoming help.
   b. Because the high school has not been touched, it would be a logical place to go. It has large open spaces and a large kitchen that could be used to feed people. Churches, community buildings, libraries, and senior citizen centers are all good places to use. Check to see if the local grocery store is able to start bringing food and water to your chosen site.
3. a. Your emergency response team should have a list of these agencies and phone numbers to call for help right away. If your dispatch center is still operating, it may have already alerted these agencies. Red Cross Disaster Services will probably be the first to arrive. You may have church agencies and state and local governmental agencies that will also respond.

True/False

1. F (page 2343)
2. T (page 2338)
3. T (page 2351)
4. F (page 2344)
5. F (page 2336)
6. T (page 2339)
7. T (page 2338)
8. T (page 2341)
9. F (page 2346)
10. T (page 2349)

Short Answer

1. In the first stage of the START triage system, you will use a strong, commanding voice to shout out to the victims. You need to tell them that if they can walk or are uninjured, they should move to a specific landmark away from the disaster site. In this way, you have just effectively triaged all the walking wounded into one area without actually looking at each patient. (page 2349)
2. In the second stage of START, you begin with the first patient you reach. Assess the respiratory status by opening the airway. If the patient is not breathing, tag the person black, and move to the next patient. A patient breathing faster than 30 breaths/min should be tagged red. If the breathing rate is less than 30 breaths/min, move on to the assessment of the

circulatory system. If the person has no radial pulse, tag him or her red; if not, move again to the neurologic assessment. If the patient is unconscious or unable to follow a simple command, tag him or her red. If the person can follow the command, tag the person yellow, and move on to the next patient. (page 2349)

3. Children and infants may not be able to understand your commands. Children with special needs will be confused and need to be taken to the treatment center as soon as possible. Remember that children go into cardiac arrest because of respiratory arrest; therefore, the assessment process is a little different for children. (page 2349)
4. Always take advantage of a debriefing after a large incident. It can really help to manage stress after the initial event. Encourage participation, but do not force people to attend. The quicker you can return to active work after an incident, the better off you will be in the long run. (page 2351)

Fill in the Table

(page 2338, Table 47-2)

MCI Equipment and Supplies*	
Airway control	PPE (gloves, face shield, HEPA or N95 mask) **Oral airways, nasal airways** **Suction units (manual units)** Rigid-tip Yankauer and flexible suction catheters Laryngeal mask airway, i-gel or King LT airway, ET tubes[a] **Laryngoscope and blades**[a] Commercial tube holder, tape, syringes, stylet[a] $ETCO_2$ device
Breathing	**Pocket mask and one-way valve** Bag-mask devices (adult and child), spare masks Oxygen delivery devices (nonrebreathing mask, cannula, extension tubing) **Oxygen tank, regulator** **Occlusive dressings** Large-bore IV catheter for thoracic decompression[a]
Circulation	**Dressings, bandages, tape** Sphygmomanometer, stethoscope Burn dressings, burn sheets, sterile water for irrigation **One-handed commercial tourniquets** Hemolytic dressings 1,000-mL bags of normal saline, IV start kits, catheters[a]
Disability	**Rigid collars (universal size)** Head beds, wide tape, backboard straps **Flashlights, spare batteries**
Exposure	Space blanket to cover patients Scissors
Logistic/Command	Sector vests (triage, treatment, transport, staging, command, rescue) Pads of paper, pencils, pens, markers **Triage tags or kits used by your regional system** Assessment cards Tarps: red, yellow, green, black

[a]These items could be packaged in an advanced life support (ALS) kit.

Chapter 48: Vehicle Extrication and Special Rescue

Matching

Part I

1. R (page 2382)
2. Q (page 2374)
3. P (page 2363)
4. O (page 2364)
5. N (page 2384)
6. Z (page 2380)
7. Y (page 2379)
8. X (page 2384)
9. W (page 2384)
10. V (page 2384)
11. D (page 2382)
12. C (page 2361)
13. B (page 2369)
14. A (page 2366)
15. U (page 2381)
16. T (page 2367)
17. S (page 2361)
18. M (page 2370)
19. L (page 2362)
20. K (page 2366)
21. E (page 2371)
22. F (page 2380)
23. G (page 2364)
24. H (page 2366)
25. I (page 2378)
26. J (page 2371)

Part II

1. L (page 2373)
2. K (page 2361)
3. J (page 2363)
4. P (page 2371)
5. O (page 2364)
6. N (page 2369)
7. M (page 2363)
8. I (page 2361)
9. H (page 2386)
10. G (page 2367)
11. A (page 2371)
12. B (page 2379)
13. C (page 2366)
14. D (page 2386)
15. F (page 2371)
16. E (page 2379)

Multiple Choice

1. B (page 2361)
2. D (page 2361)
3. A (page 2362)
4. C (page 2364)
5. A (page 2363)
6. B (page 2365)
7. B (page 2369)
8. C (page 2368)
9. D (page 2371)
10. D (page 2373)

Labeling

1. Posts of a vehicle (page 2368, Figure 48-4)
   - **A.** C post
   - **B.** B post
   - **C.** A post
2. Wood cribbing designs (page 2372, Figure 48-12)
   - **A.** Step chocks
   - **B.** Wedges
   - **C.** Box crib
   - **D.** Shims

Fill in the Blank

1. airbag; hazard (page 2376)
2. steering column (page 2376)
3. frontal; dash (page 2376)
4. confined space (page 2378)
5. Hydrogen sulfide (page 2378)
6. shoring (page 2379)
7. self-rescue position (page 2380)
8. reach out (page 2381)
9. swift; drive (page 2381)
10. low-angle (page 2382)

Identify

1. Chief complaint: Decreased level of consciousness, trauma to left side region
2. Vital signs: Verbally responsive, BP 102/68 mm Hg, pulse of 116 beats/min and thready at the wrist, sinus tachycardia. Skin is pale and cool. Oxygen saturation is 96%. Respirations are 24 breaths/min and shallow with diminished lung sounds in left side. Pupils are equal, round, and regular in size, but they are slow to react to light.
3. Pertinent negatives: Negative halo test

Complete the Patient Care Report (PCR)

Show the completed PCR to your instructor to obtain feedback on your completion of the form.

Ambulance Calls

1. To answer this question, you need to apply a lot of the information you have learned in the past chapters. How well did you do?
   a. The steps to take are as follows:
      (1) Assess the scene for:
         (a) Hazards
         (b) Missing patients (Could a front-seat passenger who was not wearing a seat belt have been thrown through that shattered front windshield?)
      (2) Call for help. At the least, you will need the police department, the fire department, and perhaps additional help in the extrication.
      (3) Once the hazards have been dealt with, gain access to the patient. Try all the doors first.
      (4) Enter the vehicle and start care. Specifically:
         (a) Open the airway by lifting the head into neutral position; if possible, have one of your crew take up a position in the back seat where he or she can apply a cervical collar and hold the patient's head in a neutral position.
         (b) Administer supplemental oxygen.
         (c) Quickly check the chest for signs of pneumothorax or sucking chest wound.
         (d) Control external hemorrhage by direct pressure.
         (e) Start a large-bore IV line with lactated Ringer's or normal saline.
         (f) Cover open wounds.
         (g) Splint fractures.
      (5) As soon as disentanglement is complete, remove the patient on a long backboard or scoop, and transfer the patient to the ambulance.
      (6) Notify the receiving hospital.
      (7) Transport. This is a "load-and-go" situation.
      (8) If possible, start another IV line en route.
   b. (1) Once the patient has been transferred to the hospital, you have to clean up the ambulance and equipment.
      (2) Restock all kits used.

True/False

A lot of extrication is common sense.

1. F (page 2366)
2. T (page 2366)
3. T (page 2366)
4. T (page 2365)
5. T (page 2364)
6. T (page 2365)
7. F (page 2374)
8. F (page 2374)
9. F (page 2366)
10. F (page 2373)

Short Answer

1. a. Awareness: You need to be trained in recognizing hazards at the scene and being able to call for the appropriate assistance, such as the power company, or calling for the correct rescue team.
   b. Operations: You will be working in the area directly outside of the rescue zone. This area helps to assist the people working on the rescue. An example would be a rehab zone for a diving team.
   c. Technician: This is where you are directly involved in the rescue operation. It could be high-angle rappelling or swift-water rescue. You will be the person saving the patient from the incident. (page 2361)
2. a. Be equipped, prepared, and ready to meet the expectations of your role.
   b. Maintain situational awareness.
   c. Work as a team.
   d. Follow the golden rule of public service. (page 2362)
3. Gear that is standard for a water rescue is a personal flotation device, thermal protection, a helmet appropriate for water rescue, a cutting device, a whistle, contamination protection (if necessary), and foot protection (ie, wetsuit-type booties). (page 2381)

4. Side glass versus windshield: Tempered glass is used in the side windows and the rear window. This glass will break in small pieces by using a spring-loaded punch in the corner. A windshield has laminated glass, which will not break and must be cut using an axe or a glass saw because of the plastic that is between the layers of the glass. Remember to cover your patient and to tell the patient before attempting to remove or break glass around him or her. (pages 2373–2374)

Fill in the Table

(page 2386)

The Hartford Consensus: THREAT	
T	**Threat suppression**
H	**Hemorrhage control**
R	**Rapid**
E	**Extrication to safety**
A	**Assessment by medical providers**
T	**Transport to definitive care**

Chapter 49: Hazardous Materials

Matching

Part I

1. G (page 2407)
2. F (page 2421)
3. E (page 2411)
4. M (page 2421)
5. L (page 2420)
6. K (page 2403)
7. D (page 2403)
8. C (page 2399)
9. B (page 2421)
10. A (page 2418)
11. H (page 2408)
12. I (page 2421)
13. J (page 2403)
14. N (page 2407)
15. Z (page 2498)
16. Y (page 2415)
17. X (page 2416)
18. W (page 2414)
19. V (page 2418)
20. U (page 2421)
21. O (page 2418)
22. P (page 2418)
23. Q (page 2418)
24. R (page 2415)
25. S (page 2407)
26. T (page 2410)

Part II

1. G (page 2417)
2. F (page 2417)
3. E (page 2403)
4. D (page 2406)
5. C (page 2417)
6. M (page 2415)
7. L (page 2414)
8. K (page 2414)
9. J (page 2414)
10. I (page 2414)
11. A (page 2398)
12. B (page 2416)
13. H (page 2417)
14. Z (page 2415)
15. Y (page 2402)
16. N (page 2416)
17. O (page 2418)
18. P (page 2408)
19. X (page 2416)
20. W (page 2406)
21. V (page 2418)
22. U (page 2422)
23. Q (page 2409)
24. R (page 2409)
25. S (page 2409)
26. T (page 2409)

Part III

1. S (page 2416)
2. R (page 2416)
3. Q (page 2415)
4. P (page 2415)
5. N (page 2410)
6. M (page 2421)
7. L (page 2417)
8. K (page 2417)
9. O (page 2416)
10. J (page 2417)
11. T (page 2403)
12. B (page 2404)
13. C (page 2415)
14. D (page 2414)
15. E (page 2420)
16. I (page 2416)
17. H (page 2419)
18. G (page 2415)
19. F (page 2416)
20. A (page 2403)

Multiple Choice

1. B (page 2407)
2. A (page 2409)
3. D (page 2416)
4. C (page 2418)
5. D (page 2422)
6. B (page 2399)
7. C (page 2405)
8. D (page 2411)
9. A (pages 2410–2412)
10. A (page 2420)

Fill in the Blank

1. awareness level (page 2399)
2. ensure your safety (page 2400)
3. authority having jurisdiction (page 2399)
4. information (page 2400)
5. agricultural; insecticides (page 2400)
6. bill of lading; waybill (page 2403)
7. primary; secondary (page 2415)
8. Primary contamination (page 2415)
9. Secondary contamination (page 2415)
10. local effect; systemic (page 2415)

Identify

1. a. Based on the information provided in the *ERG*, this product is highly toxic and may be fatal if inhaled or absorbed through the skin.
   b. Specialized protective clothing with SCBA is required. Structural fire fighter clothing will provide only a limited amount of protection. Most paramedics and ambulances don't carry the proper clothing unless it is a specialized unit with specially trained personnel.

c. Based on the information given, the ambulance and stopped nearby traffic are in immediate danger. It's important to relocate upwind and to set up a staging area at a safe distance, as determined by incident command and the parameters of the guidebook. It's also advisable to begin requesting the allocation of additional resources and personnel based on the life-threatening nature of the incident.

2. The photos show the four levels of protection in the following order: Level B, Level A, Level D, Level C.

   Level A provides the greatest protection from exposure to hazardous substances. These suits look like an astronaut's suit because they are fully encapsulating. These suits fully cover and protect the SCBA worn by hazardous materials technicians. The suits are rigorously tested by the manufacturers to determine resistance and permeability to many chemicals.

   Level B is called for when the technician needs protection from splashes and inhaled toxins. It is not fully encapsulating like Level A is, and it is worn with SCBA. Level B suits are often worn by the hazardous materials decontamination team.

   Level C is designed to protect against a known agent. The equipment provides splash protection and is worn with an air-purifying respirator that must have filters specifically chosen to provide protection against the known agent. Offering eye and hand protection and foot coverings, Level C protection could be used during transport of patients with the potential of secondary contamination.

   Level D is typically not worn in hazardous materials incidents but may be used by some personnel in the cold zone. (pages 2411–2414)

Ambulance Calls

1. a. (pages 2417–2419)
      (1) Your safety comes first.
      (2) The decision to do an emergency decontamination
      (3) The need to do a mass decontamination
2. a. Three potential sources of information regarding the nature of the train's cargo are the following:
      (1) The USDOT placard on the side of each car
      (2) The waybill or the consist carried by the conductor
      (3) The conductor (pages 2401–2403)
   b. Once you know that you are dealing with a hazardous cargo, you should take the following precautions:
      (1) Protect yourself first!
      (2) Isolate the incident as much as possible to avoid the risk of further harm to other people.
      (3) Notify your dispatcher and other EMS, fire, or law enforcement responders that a hazardous materials incident is in progress.
      (4) Inform incoming responders of what you observe about wind direction, terrain features, and a safe response route. (page 2410)

True/False

1. Transport accidents involving radioactive materials are likely to increase in frequency, so it is important to have a clear plan of action for such events and to know what you should and should not do at the scene.
   a. T (page 2400)
   b. F (page 2422)
   c. F (page 2401)
   d. T (page 2403)
   e. T (page 2403)
2. It is just as important to know what *not* to do at a hazardous materials incident as to know what *to* do.
   a. F (page 2421)
   b. T (page 2415)
   c. F (page 2419)
   d. F (page 2422)
   e. T (page 2422)

Short Answer

1. a. Name of the chemical
   b. Potential fire and explosion and/or health hazards of the chemical identified.
   c. The isolation distance and the protective actions required for the chemical identified (pages 2401–2402)

2. a. CHEMTREC
   b. Bill of lading
   c. Waybill
   d. Hazardous materials warning labels, placards, and markings
   e. Safety data sheet (pages 2401–2403)
3. The most important step in dealing with a hazardous materials incident is recognizing that a hazardous materials situation exists in the first place. If you have to wait until you start to feel sick from your own exposure to a poisonous material before you figure out that the situation might be dangerous, you've waited too long.
   a. Two-car collision downtown: If either of those cars is on fire, you may be dealing with toxic products of the combustion of automobile upholstery. (page 2421)
   b. Apartment-house fire: Not immediately likely, but the products of combustion do contain soot, carbon monoxide, carbon dioxide, water vapor, formaldehyde, cyanide compounds, and many oxides of nitrogen. (page 2421)
   c. Three municipal workers collapsed in a sewer: The sewer could be a low-oxygen environment, and there is a lot of potential for chemical inhalation. (page 2421)
   d. Two police officers injured in a riot: The presence of hazardous materials would depend on whether tear gas or pepper spray was used.
   e. Fire in a garden supply store warehouse: There are many dangerous chemicals stored and sold at a garden supply company. Was there any exposure to pesticides? (page 2421)
   f. Semitrailer overturned on the interstate. If the semitrailer is carrying hazardous materials, they could have leaked, and there may be an increased risk of fire.
   g. Two "men down" on the maintenance staff of the municipal swimming pool. This scene could include a chlorine leak.
   h. Freight train struck car on level crossing. Until you know what freight the train was carrying, you should suspect a possible hazardous materials situation.
   i. Fire in a furniture factory. A furniture factory not only carries a big fire load of wood but also stains and finishes that may be hazardous.

Chapter 50: Terrorism Response

Matching

Part I

1. U (page 2435)
2. T (page 2447)
3. S (page 2447)
4. R (page 2455)
5. Q (page 2455)
6. Z (page 2437)
7. Y (page 2455)
8. X (page 2443)
9. W (page 2437)
10. V (page 2445)
11. P (page 2446)
12. O (page 2439)
13. N (page 2437)
14. M (page 2447)
15. L (page 2442)
16. C (page 2450)
17. B (page 2457)
18. A (page 2455)
19. D (page 2436)
20. E (page 2449)
21. K (page 2447)
22. J (page 2443)
23. I (page 2451)
24. H (page 2451)
25. G (page 2452)
26. F (page 2455)

Part II

1. H (page 2451)
2. G (page 2442)
3. F (page 2443)
4. E (page 2455)
5. D (page 2434)
6. Z (page 2455)
7. Y (page 2455)
8. X (page 2453)
9. W (page 2451)
10. V (page 2442)
11. N (page 2451)
12. M (page 2443)
13. L (page 2437)
14. K (page 2445)
15. J (page 2445)
16. I (page 2451)
17. U (page 2443)
18. T (page 2442)
19. S (page 2441)
20. C (page 2447)
21. B (page 2457)
22. A (page 2437)
23. R (page 2441)
24. Q (page 2443)
25. P (page 2444)
26. O (page 2455)

Part III

1. K (page 2444)
2. J (page 2453)
3. I (page 2442)
4. H (page 2458)
5. G (page 2456)
6. U (page 2453)
7. T (page 2447)
8. S (page 2441)
9. R (page 2442)
10. Q (page 2448)
11. F (page 2444)
12. E (page 2448)
13. D (page 2441)
14. C (page 2443)
15. B (page 2442)
16. P (page 2449)
17. O (page 2442)
18. N (page 2442)
19. M (page 2444)
20. L (page 2433)
21. A (page 2452)

Multiple Choice

1. C (page 2447)
2. D (page 2437)
3. A (page 2442)
4. A (page 2442)
5. B (page 2443)
6. A (page 2445)
7. B (page 2448)
8. D (page 2451)
9. C (page 2451)
10. A (page 2455)

Labeling

1. Alpha, beta, and gamma radiation (page 2455, Figure 50-16)
   - **A.** Gamma
   - **B.** Beta
   - **C.** Alpha

Fill in the Blank

1. Weapon of mass destruction (page 2441)
2. covert (page 2437)
3. secondary (page 2440)
4. Route of exposure (page 2442)
5. Nerve agents (page 2443)
6. German (page 2443)
7. lymphatic (page 2451)
8. Anthrax (page 2450)
9. castor bean (page 2452)
10. Points of distribution (pages 2453-2454)

Identify

1. Chief complaint: Trauma, organophosphate poisoning
2. Vital signs: Alert to start but loses consciousness as the poisoning progresses. Heart rate is 50 beats/min, BP is 98/66 mm Hg, oxygen saturation is 88%, respirations are 9 breaths/min.
3. Pertinent negatives: There are no pertinent negatives.

   Always look around before running into the scene. You never know what people are carrying in the truck. It is no fun to become a patient yourself!

Complete the Patient Care Report (PCR)

Show the completed PCR to your instructor to obtain feedback on your completion of the form.

Ambulance Calls

1. **a.** This train derailment could be a terrorist attack. You need to be thinking about what kind of attack it was and be prepared for the type of scene you will be entering.
   (1) Chemical—Not very likely at this scene.
   (2) Biologic—Probably not this scene, but you never know what the train is carrying.
   (3) Radiologic—Not very likely at this scene.
   (4) Nuclear—No signs of radiation, so you should be okay here.
   (5) Explosives—This is the best bet here; either the tracks were blown up or something inside the train blew to cause the derailment. Be careful because there may be some secondary explosions. (page 2433)

   b. You can designate someone to walk toward the vehicles, but instruct the person to stay clear of the vehicles. Feel free to use the public address (PA) system on one of the ambulances to make an announcement. It is a good idea for the person to be wearing a bright color because people will be able to see him or her. Appoint that person, and tell the person he or she is the leader. Have the person remain standing so that the walking wounded have someone to walk toward. If you have enough responders, you can designate one of them. They can wave a white towel or some type of flag; whatever your solution, get the walking wounded cleared out of the wreckage as soon as possible! (page 2440, and Chapter 47, *Incident Management and Mass-Casualty Incidents*)
2. **a.** Chlorine, which is used a lot in swimming pools, is what is leaking and causing the green haze. It will have the smell of bleach. (page 2443)

   b. Before getting out, you'd better call for help. First, you need members of a hazardous materials team or at least firefighters to go into the pool area with their self-contained breathing apparatus (SCBA) gear and bring out any missing lifeguards. Leave all your windows up, and use your external public address (PA) system to direct the children standing around to walk upwind and away from the pool. Have them follow the ambulance until you are a safe distance away.

   c. With chlorine gas, complete airway obstruction can occur as a result of pulmonary edema. Provide oxygen as needed, and be prepared to intubate if necessary. (page 2443)

True/False

1. F (page 2456)	**3.** F (page 2449)	**5.** T (page 2447)	**7.** F (page 2443)	**9.** T (page 2435)
2. T (page 2455)	**4.** F (page 2448)	**6.** T (page 2449)	**8.** T (page 2458)	**10.** T (page 2439)

Short Answer

1. Five of the following seven should be listed: (page 2437)

   a. Major sporting events, concerts, ceremonies, and parades where large crowds are gathered.

   b. Locations where damage or destruction will create extreme fear, such as nuclear power plants and research facilities, chemical factories, biologic laboratories, and petroleum distillation and storage facilities.

   c. Locations where attacks will provoke extreme emotional reactions, such as day-care centers, schools, health care facilities, abortion clinics, and churches.

   d. Locations that are critical to transportation, such as airports, subway or train stations, tunnels, and bridges.

   e. Critical industry and infrastructure, such as power plants, water treatment plants, manufacturing facilities, shipping facilities, dams and reservoirs, power lines, and natural gas lines.

f. Locations of symbolic significance, such as local, state, and federal government buildings; financial buildings; corporate headquarters; military installations; monuments; and national parks.

g. Locations vital to emergency response, including police stations, fire stations, dispatch centers, command centers, emergency medical services (EMS) facilities, and hospitals.

2. Sources of radiologic material can be found in these locations: (page 2455)
   a. Hospitals
   b. Colleges and universities
   c. Chemical and industrial sites
   d. Power plants

Fill in the Table

1. Nerve agents
(Table 50-2, page 2446)

Name	Code Name	Odor	Special Features	Onset of Symptoms	Volatility	Route of Exposure
Tabun	**GA**	Fruity	Easy to manufacture	Immediate	Low	Both contact and vapor hazard
Sarin	**GB**	None (if pure) or strong	Will off-gas while on victim's clothing	Immediate	High	Primarily respiratory vapor hazard; extremely lethal if skin contact is made
Soman	**GD**	Fruity	Ages rapidly, making it difficult to treat	Immediate	Moderate	Contact with skin; minimal vapor hazard
VX agent	**VX**	None	Most lethal chemical agent; difficult to decontaminate	Immediate	Very low	Contact with skin; no vapor hazard (unless aerosolized)

2. Chemical agents
(Table 50-3, page 2448)

Class	Military Designation	Odor	Lethality	Onset of Symptoms	Volatility	Primary Route of Exposure
Vesicants	Mustard (H) Lewisite (L) Phosgene oxime (CX)	**Garlic (H)** **Geranium (L)**	Causes large blisters to form on victims; may severely damage upper airway if vapors are inhaled; severe, intense pain and gray skin discoloration (L, CX)	**Delayed (H)** **Immediate (L, CX)**	Very low (H, L) Moderate (CX)	Primarily contact; with some vapor hazard
Pulmonary agents	Chlorine (CL) Phosgene (CG)	**Bleach (CL)** **Cut grass (CG)**	Causes irritation; choking (CL); severe pulmonary edema (CG)	**Immediate (CL)** **Delayed (CG)**	Very high	Vapor hazard
Nerve agents	Tabun (GA) Sarin (GB) Soman (GD) VX agent (VX)	**Fruity or none**	Most lethal chemical agents can kill within minutes; effects are reversible with antidotes	**Immediate**	Moderate (GA, GD) Very high (GB) Low (VX)	Vapor hazard (GB) Both vapor and contact hazard (GA, GD) Contact hazard (VX)
Cyanide agents	Hydrogen cyanide (AC) Cyanogen chloride (CK)	**Almonds (AC)** **Irritating (CK)**	Highly lethal chemical gases; can kill within minutes; effects are reversible with antidotes	**Immediate**	Very high	Vapor hazard

3. Symptoms of persons exposed to nerve agents (Table 50-1, page 2445)

Mnemonic: SLUDGEM	
S	Salivation
L	**Lacrimation**
U	Urination
D	**Defecation**
G	Gastrointestinal distress
E	**Emesis**
M	Miosis
Mnemonic: Killer Bs	
B	Bradycardia
B	**Bronchorrhea**
B	Bronchospasm

Chapter 51: Disaster Response

Matching

1. V (page 2480)
2. U (page 2483)
3. T (page 2483)
4. S (page 2481)
5. R (page 2468)
6. Z (page 2468)
7. Y (page 2483)
8. X (page 2481)
9. W (page 2482)
10. Q (page 2482)
11. A (page 2483)
12. P (page 2468)
13. O (page 2479)
14. N (page 2483)
15. M (page 2474)
16. H (page 2466)
17. G (page 2483)
18. F (page 2482)
19. E (page 2476)
20. D (page 2480)
21. L (page 2478)
22. K (page 2466)
23. J (page 2466)
24. I (page 2476)
25. C (page 2466)
26. B (page 2474)

Multiple Choice

1. D (page 2466)
2. B (pages 2466–2470)
3. B (page 2468)
4. A (page 2469)
5. C (pages 2473–2474)
6. B (page 2475)
7. A (page 2478)
8. C (page 2481)
9. D (page 2482)
10. B (page 2483)

Fill in the Blank

1. preplanning; all-hazards (page 2466)
2. mutual aid agreement (page 2468)
3. transportation; log (page 2471)
4. hospitals; readjust (page 2472)
5. briefing; briefing; media (page 2473)
6. after-action report (page 2474)
7. casualty collection points (page 2476)
8. emergency operations center (page 2474)
9. heavy; vegetables (page 2482)
10. epidemic; pandemic (page 2483)

Identify

1. Chief complaint: Critical thermal burns and potential respiratory involvement
2. Vital signs: Respiration is 24 breaths/min and shallow; oxygen saturation is 96%; lungs are clear; pulse is 110 beats/min; heart monitor shows sinus tachycardia; BP is 108/68 mm Hg; PERRLA; patient is 10/10 on scale for pain; skin is pale, cool, and moist.
3. Pertinent negatives: He denies taking any drugs and has no allergies. He has no ectopy on his ECG.

   In addition to almost losing his life and spending a month in the burn unit, he is ultimately convicted of arson for destroying over a million dollars in property. Fortunately, no one else was injured in the blaze.

Ambulance Calls

1. This call may be one of the most stressful events you have responded to in your EMS career thus far. Remember to take care of yourself and your crew during the entire response so that you do not become a patient also. It is hot in there for the patients and will become exhausting for you, too. Keep drinking fluids! As for those patients "trapped" in the hot environment: remove their hot clothing, give them water, and undo the restraints as long as there is no potential for the patients to fall down.
   a. There are many correct responses to this question. Here are six *(students should list four)*:
      (1) Vigilance is the key. If possible, work in pairs, monitoring each other for heat-related problems.
      (2) Water must be consumed at all times. Small, constant sips of water throughout the day are best. You may also consider some electrolyte fluid replacement in addition to the water.
      (3) Small, more frequent meals are better than large ones. Eat foods that are heavy in fluids, such as vegetables and fruits.
      (4) Set up "water trains." As you empty water bottles, have them refilled. Your agency must ensure that it has a good, clean source of water. Use of water buffalo trailers, lister bags, and portable water backpacks is advisable if outdoors.

(5) If you have air conditioning in your buildings or vehicles, use it.
(6) Wet towels placed on the head or on the body can help reduce body temperature. (page 2482)

b. Many medical problems are exacerbated by extreme heat. The following list provides examples but is not exhaustive *(students should list five examples)*:
(1) Circulatory problems
(2) Diabetes
(3) Cardiovascular problems
(4) Chronic obstructive pulmonary disease (COPD)
(5) Asthma
(6) Cardiac dysrhythmias
(7) The "traditional" heat emergencies such as heat exhaustion and heatstroke

True/False

1. F (page 2483)
2. T (page 2472)
3. T (page 2482)
4. F (page 2476)
5. T (page 2478)
6. T (page 2478)
7. T (page 2480)
8. F (page 2473)
9. T (page 2469)
10. T (page 2472)

Short Answer

1. The three phases of any plan of response:
a. Before the event (preplanning)
b. During the event
c. After the event (page 2466)

2. Considerations during a disaster should include inventory, mobilization of personnel, command setup or response, unification of command, personal protective and safety equipment, equipment resupply, triage and classification, patient tracking, assignment of personnel, personnel mental needs, personnel physical needs, hospital updates, providing and accepting relief, surveillance, weather conditions, media, legal issues, and unit leadership reinforcement. (page 2470)

Fill in the Table

1. Examples of natural and man-made disasters
(Tables 51-4 and 51-5, pages 2475 and 2483)

Natural Disasters	Man-Made Disasters
Forest and brush fires	**Structural fires**
Snowstorms and ice storms	Construction failures and building collapse
Tornadoes	**Power failures or disruptions**
Hurricanes	Riots, civil disturbances, and stampedes
Tsunamis	**Strikes and labor disputes**
Earthquakes	Sniper, shooter, and hostage situations
Landslides, avalanches, mudslides	**Explosions (intentional and unintentional)**
Cave-ins	Information technology (cyber) disruptions
Volcanic eruptions	**Incidents involving weapons of mass destruction**
Flooding	Hazardous materials incidents
Sandstorms and dust storms	
Prolonged cold weather	
Drought	
Heat wave	
Meteors and space debris	
Epidemics and pandemics	

Chapter 52: Crime Scene Awareness

Matching

1. H (page 2499)
2. G (page 2499)
3. A (page 2503)
4. F (page 2509)
5. C (page 2504)
6. B (page 2500)
7. L (page 2496)
8. K (page 2509)
9. I (page 2503)
10. D (page 2500)
11. E (page 2504)
12. J (page 2505)

Multiple Choice

1. C (page 2496)
2. C (page 2497)
3. A (page 2499)
4. C (pages 2499–2500)
5. D (page 2504)
6. B (page 2499)
7. B (page 2500)
8. C (page 2506)
9. D (pages 2502–2503)
10. A (page 2509)

Fill in the Blank

1. tunnel vision (page 2496)
2. 21; 10 (page 2496)
3. incident commander (IC) (page 2497)
4. A (pages 2498–2499)
5. primary; secondary (page 2499)
6. contact; cover (page 2500)

Identify

1. Errors in handling scene safety: Paramedics did not announce themselves at the front door, stood in front of the door to knock, did not identify a secondary exit, did not look for visible weapons (drawers in tables can conceal weapons, and the poker in the fireplace stand is a potential weapon), and both approached the patient (should have considered using contact and cover technique). (pages 2499–2500)
2. Warning signs of danger: Loud conversation inside (possible domestic violence), the patient arguing with the other person, and the person getting between you and a means of egress.
3. Potential evidence: Ceramic object is possible evidence and should not be brushed away with shoe. Also, the patient's shirt is potential evidence that should not be cut or ripped unless absolutely necessary to provide care and no alternative is available to access injuries. (pages 2509–2510)

Ambulance Calls

1. Listen for loud or threatening voices, glance through available windows for signs of a struggle, and look for visible weapons. Once at the door, stand to the doorknob side before knocking and announce yourself. Once inside, ask the person who answers to lead you to the patient. (page 2499)
2. a. The ambulance should be positioned a minimum of 21 feet behind the car at a 10° angle to the driver's side facing the shoulder. (page 2496)
   b. Before leaving the ambulance, the license plate number of the car should be given to the dispatcher. Also, notify the dispatcher of this information along with any additional information that might be helpful, such as the precise location. (page 2497)
   c. The incident commander, the person in the right front seat of the ambulance, should approach the rear passenger side of the car from the trunk to see that it is properly closed. Use a belly-in toward the motor vehicle, and stop at the C column (post) to look in the rear and side windows. Notice the number of people, and pay close attention to their hands. Look for weapons. At any sign of a weapon or other danger, retreat immediately to a safe area. (pages 2497–2499)
3. a. *Contact and cover* means you make contact with the patient to assess and provide care while your partner obtains patient information, gauges the level of tension, and warns you at the first sign of trouble. (page 2500)
   b. If you suspect that the location is a clandestine drug laboratory, immediately leave the house with the patient. Do not touch anything! Once clear of the lab, leave the area, and notify the appropriate personnel (police) as soon as possible without placing yourself in harm's way. (page 2500)
   c. Safety is a major issue for everyone because of the toxic nature of the material used, the highly flammable agents used, and the possibility of booby traps that are sometimes used to safeguard the illegal operations. (pages 2500–2501)

4. Alter the scene as little as possible while providing care. Be mindful of physical evidence such as bullet casings, weapons, and blood. Do not move or pick up items that might be evidence. When you remove a patient's clothes to expose wounds, do not cut through bullet holes. Once you have removed the patient's clothes, do not shake the clothing because valuable evidence, including trace evidence, may fall off the clothing or from the pockets. (pages 2509–2510)

True/False

1. F (page 2509)
2. T (page 2500)
3. F (page 2499)
4. F (page 2499)
5. F (page 2497)
6. T (page 2496)
7. T (page 2498)
8. F (page 2496)
9. T (page 2502)
10. F (pages 2500–2501)

Short Answer

1. a. Number of aggressors involved
   b. Number and type of injuries
   c. Number and type of weapons involved
   d. Make, color, body style, and license number of any vehicle involved
   e. Direction of travel if vehicle leaves scene before law enforcement arrives (page 2499)
2. a. Highly flammable properties of materials
   b. Toxic nature of chemicals and materials used
   c. Booby traps (fragmentation and incendiary devices) (pages 2500–2501)
3. a. Glove box
   b. Under the front dash
   c. Armrest
   d. Under either side of the seat
   e. In the center console
   f. In side-door pockets
   g. Next to driver's right thigh (page 2498)
4. A secondary exit could be used if the primary exit is blocked or an alternate means of egress is needed because of a threat or danger. A rear door or, in an emergency, a window can be used as a secondary exit. (page 2500)
5. *Cover* includes objects that are usually impenetrable by bullets. *Concealment* includes objects that hide you until you can assess the situation and find cover. (page 2500)
6. a. Cover *(students should list three of the following)*
      (1) Trees
      (2) Mail collection boxes
      (3) Dumpsters
      (4) Utility poles
      (5) Curbs
      (6) Vehicles
      (7) Depressions in the ground
   b. Concealment
      (1) Tall grass
      (2) Shrubbery
      (3) Dark shadows (page 2504)
7. At this stage, you are in grave danger. You must assume that the person on the other end of the gun will use violence if you do not follow instructions.
8. a. Testimonial evidence is oral documentation by a witness of a criminal act.
   b. Physical evidence ties a suspect to a crime and includes body materials, objects, and impressions. (page 2509)

Chapter 53: Career Development

Matching

1. D (page 2523)
2. E (page 2524)
3. B (page 2523)
4. C (page 2521)
5. A (page 2522)

Multiple Choice

1. C (page 2519)
2. D (page 2521)
3. C (page 2521)
4. B (page 2522)
5. C (page 2523)
6. D (page 2523)
7. B (page 2524)
8. A (page 2525)
9. B (page 2526)
10. D (page 2520)

Fill in the Blank

1. self-care; buddy-care (page 2524)
2. clinically; definitive; physically (page 2524)
3. management coordinators; incident (page 2525)
4. strategize; dreams (page 2527)
5. wellness; medication; adherence (page 2522)
6. bicycle; good; maintain (page 2523)

Ambulance Calls

1. Notify the dispatcher of the situation, and request that the police be dispatched. Do not enter the building aside from encouraging patrons to safely exit. Tactical paramedic training would have been helpful in this situation. (page 2523)
2. a. The CCP specialty training (page 2522)
   b. Training in vasoactive IV medications and hemodynamic monitoring (page 2522)
3. a. MIHP/CP (page 2522)
   b. Obtain medication inventory, and determine adherence to recommended guidelines. Monitor and manage chronic disease in the home setting. (page 2522)

True/False

1. T (page 2520)
2. T (page 2520)
3. F (page 2523)
4. F (page 2526)
5. T (page 2526)
6. F (page 2522)
7. T (page 2522)
8. T (page 2524)

Short Answer

1. a. Growth in the middle-aged and older adult population and age-related health emergencies in these age groups
   b. The increased lifespan for patients with special health care needs, including patients with chronic or debilitating conditions who are living at home and who depend on technology
   c. The increased demonstrated success of advanced life support (ALS) providers in administering life-saving interventions in the prehospital environment
   d. The increase in the roles, responsibilities, and education levels of prehospital providers and the increase in the number of conditions in which they can effectively intervene, creating an increased need for providers with a higher level of education, preparation, and training
   e. The increasing number of specialized medical facilities and the need for transport and transfer of patients with specific conditions to these facilities for ongoing care
   f. The creation of nontraditional roles for paramedics. Some of these roles are within the larger health care system (eg, EDs, urgent care clinics), whereas others are in locations, such as cruise ships, Hollywood movie sets, oil rigs, and schools.
   g. The increase in the number of suicides, the increase in the availability of lethal drugs on the streets, and the rise in violent crime and terrorist activities (pages 2519–2520)

2. *Students should list five of the following:*
   a. NAEMT
   b. NASEMSO
   c. NAEMSE
   d. ACCT for Patients
   e. NAOTM
   f. IAFCCP
   g. WMS
   h. NEMSMA
   i. IPMBA
   j. NEMA
   k. HIRA (page 2520)
3. **a through e.** Student should list short-term goals and thoughts on action steps to achieve the goals.
   f through j. Student should list long-term goals and thoughts on action steps to achieve the goals.
   The student should have some feedback on the goals and plan from instructor and/or mentor. (pages 2520–2521)